DR. LINFORD   SPRING.

D1824005

DR. LINFORD   SPRING.

DR L. C. SPRING
Clerklands Surgery
Vicarage Lane
Horley, Surrey
Tel Horley 783802

GENERAL PATHOLOGY
Principles and Dynamics

GENERAL PATHOLOGY
Principles and Dynamics

DONALD WEST KING, M.D.
Richard T. Crane Professor in Pathology
Pritzker School of Medicine
The University of Chicago

Sometime:

Francis Delafield Professor of Pathology
College of Physicians & Surgeons
Columbia University in the City of New York

CECILIA M. FENOGLIO, M.D.
Professor of Pathology
College of Physicians & Surgeons
Columbia University in the City of New York

JAY H. LEFKOWITCH, M.D.
Assistant Professor of Pathology
College of Physicians & Surgeons
Columbia University in the City of New York

Illustrated by Jay H. Lefkowitch, M.D.

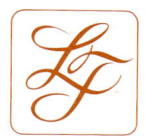

Lea & Febiger · 1983 · Philadelphia

Lea & Febiger
600 South Washington Square
Philadelphia, PA 19106
U.S.A.

Cover: Electron Micrograph. Contracted ventricular muscle from the apical septum (×24,500). Courtesy of Dr. John J. Fenoglio, Jr. and Ms. Arline Albala, Department of Pathology, College of Physicians and Surgeons, Columbia University, New York.

Library of Congress Cataloging in Publication Data

King, Donald West.
General pathology.

Bibliography: p.
Includes index.
I. Pathology. I. Fenoglio, Cecilia M.
II. Lefkowitch, Jay H. III. Title. [DNLM:
1. Pathology. QZ 4 K52g]
RB111.K56   1983   616.07   82-14883
ISBN 0-8121-0845-0

Line Illustrations Copyright © 1983 by Jay H. Lefkowitch, M.D.

Copyright © 1983 by Lea & Febiger. Copyright under the International Copyright Union. All Rights Reserved. This book is protected by copyright. No part of it may be reproduced in any manner or by any means without written permission of the Publisher.

PRINTED IN THE UNITED STATES OF AMERICA

Print Number: 5   4   3   2   1

This book is dedicated to those faithful faculty members we have known who have maintained a healthy perspective and a thoughtful appreciation for all aspects of their teaching, research, and diagnostic responsibilities.

———

I would rather discover one causal explanation than have rule over the Persians fall to me.

—DEMOCRITUS

Preface

This book was written for students of pathobiology. By "students" we mean not only medical students, but all faculty of the basic and clinical medical sciences. As the decade of the 1980's unfolds, we are at the crossroads of exciting developments in molecular biology, immunology, ultrastructural pathology, neurobiology, virology, clinical diagnosis, and therapeutics. It was in the spirit of integrating new concepts with classic cellular pathology as introduced by Rudolph Virchow that this text was written.

We have approached recent advances in the field of general pathology by considering five major areas: cellular injury, tissue injury (inflammation), agents of disease, neoplasia, and aging. A final chapter with six sections is included for those desiring a more extensive discussion of cellular injury and response. We have integrated the basic principles of immunology and hemostasis with the inflammatory process and have discussed agents of disease both generally and in relation to specific diseases. By evaluating clinical prototypes of injurious agents such as sickle cell disease (genetic), myocardial infarction (physical), celiac disease (nutritional), viral hepatitis (infectious), alcohol toxicity (drug), and myasthenia gravis (immune) from the molecular level through ultrastructure and histopathology to clinical presentation, we have aimed at presenting a unified approach to the multiple factors involved in the pathogenesis of disease.

The illustrations, figures, and tables are integral parts of the book. They are designed to clarify and supplement the text as well as to provide a unifying perspective of disease.

We would like this book to serve as a stimulus for intellectual curiosity and as a pleasurable introduction to an understanding of the basic mechanisms of disease.

DONALD WEST KING, M.D.
CECILIA M. FENOGLIO, M.D.
JAY H. LEFKOWITCH, M.D.

New York City

Acknowledgments

We are indebted to Ms. Jane Hundgen who persevered through years of our updating, reorganizing, and rewriting to produce the finished text. We must also commend Ms. Susan Coppock for her assistance not only in preparing the manuscript, but also in extensive reference work in the library. In addition, the typing of the manuscript could not have been accomplished without the help of Ms. Barbara John, Ms. Fausta Weir, and Ms. Hartley Humphries. Our colleagues in this and other institutions, here and abroad, have generously contributed illustrative material which we have acknowledged as it appears. We also thank the various authors and editors of medical journals and texts whose tables, charts and graphs we have reproduced. We were greatly helped by Drs. Susan Fox, Deborah Rund, and Peter Kelsey as well as Ms. Alison Moore, Ms. Ruth Ann Kava, and Ms. Mindi Steinhardt in the text preparation. The expert photographic talents of Ms. Ida Nathan and Mr. Ulises Martin were invaluable to the production of the book.

D.W.K.
C.M.F.
J.H.L.

Contents

Chapter 1

CELLULAR INJURY AND RESPONSE

If thou couldst, doctor, cast
The water of my land, find her disease,
And purge it to a sound and pristine health
I would applaud thee to the very echo.

—Macbeth V, iii

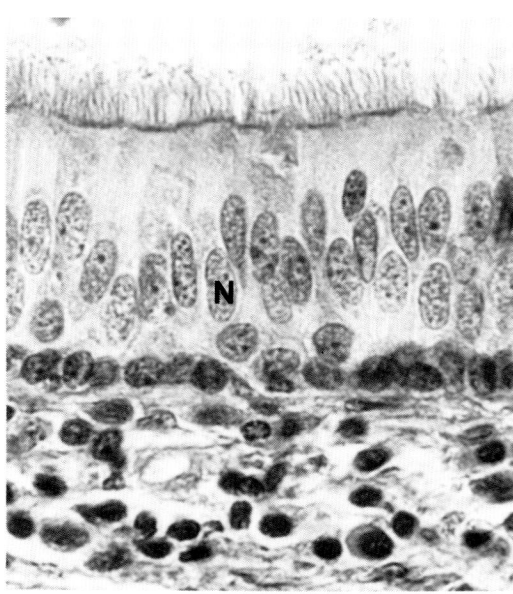

Figure 1–1. The cell is the unit of structure and function for the organism. Each cell contains a nucleus (N) with its genetic material. The cells exist within an architectural framework dictated by cellular structures.

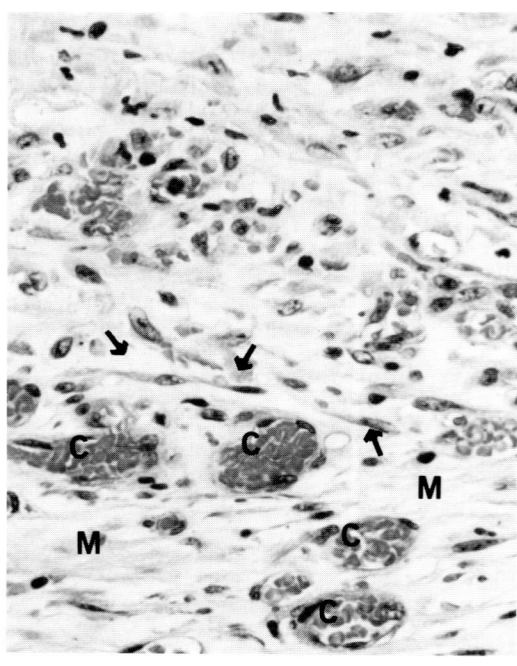

Figure 1–2. The connective tissue with capillaries (C) illustrated here demonstrates two cellular resources: the extracellular space and the vascular space. Fibroblasts (arrows) exist in a matrix (M) of collagen, hyaluronic acid, and other substances and receive nutrients and oxygen from the vascular spaces (C).

DISEASE AND THE CELL

Pathobiology may be thought of as a continuum of normal biology.[1] The cell is the unit of structure and function for the organism (Fig. 1–1). All intra- and extracellular products must originate in a cell. During disease processes, there are no new intermediary pathways involving metabolites, substrates, enzymes, or products that have not been seen previously in normal cells. Abnormal gene products resulting from mutations, usually lethal, and only occasionally heritable, are exceptions to this principle.

During the life of an organism, somatic mutations may produce alterations in the genome that can result in abnormal cell products. Usually, these are recognized and rejected as "nonsense" products and are then degraded by the cell's normal metabolic machinery. Minor errors generally do not interfere with cellular function. Germ-cell mutations that are not repaired may be lethal or may appear in offspring as inborn errors of metabolism. Many of these are subclinical; some have probably not been described and may never even be recognized in a patient. In similar fashion, incorporation of viral genetic material into the host genome may change the nature of the host cell's nucleic acid content or its synthetic products.

Over a period of millions of years, the cell has been exposed to multiple environmental influences and has dealt with them to one degree or another. This has been possible by the development of a body of information in the cell's genome that enables it to recognize and react to these extrinsic stimuli. The cell's compensatory capacity may, in turn, depend on its resistance to environmental insults.

An individual cell is the point of attack for environmental insults. In addition to its innate defenses, the cell reacts within the framework of three other resources: *the extracellular space*, the *vascular space*, and an ability to *differentiate* cells to perform specialized tasks (Fig. 1–2).

Role of the Extravascular Space

The extra- and intravascular spaces contain substances produced by cells that may initially protect the cell from environmental influences. Keratin, collagen, elastin, hyaluronic acid, and proteoglycans, which are present in an orderly tissue architecture, are examples.[2] They provide a framework on which new cells regenerate and new tissue is formed following injury. The extracellular space also provides an area for the interaction of nutritive substances, hormones, antibodies, and other humoral substances.

Role of the Vascular Space

The vascular space consists of *blood vessels, sinusoids,* and *lymphatics.* It supplies oxygen and other nutrients to cells. Toxic metabolites such as excess CO_2 and lactic acid are

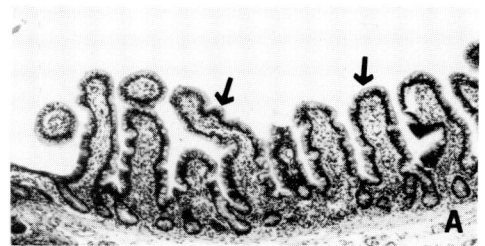

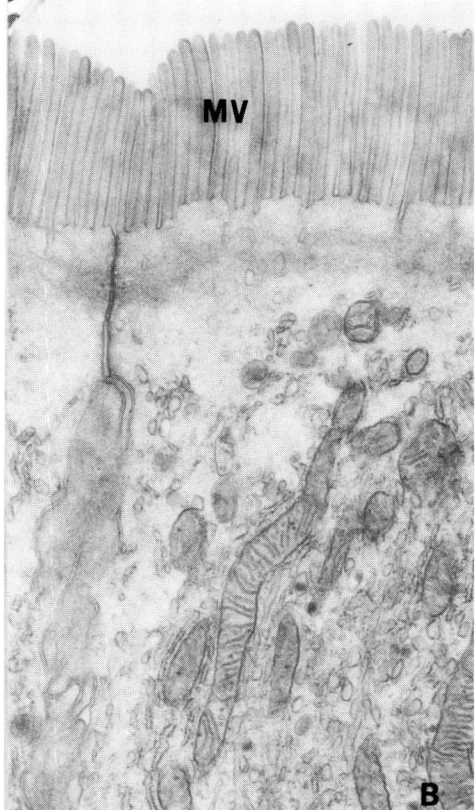

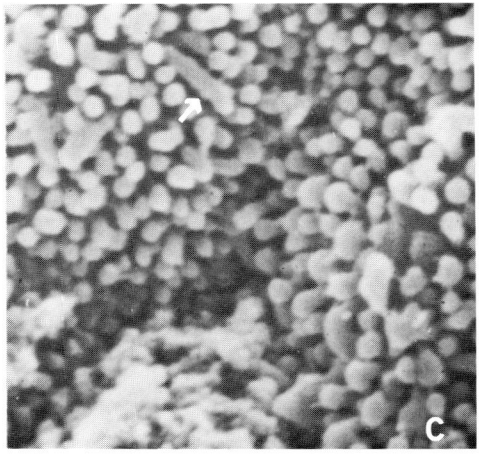

Figure 1–3. *A,* The absorptive surface area of the small intestine is increased by the presence of long, finger-like villi (arrows). *B,* It is also increased by long microvilli (MV) on the surfaces of the absorptive cells. *C,* These microvilli can also be seen in the scanning electron micrograph (arrow).

removed through the same channels. The vascular space contains proteins necessary for the clotting of blood as well as for hydrolyzing blood clots (fibrinolysis). These are of great importance in inflammation and repair. *Lymphatic channels* allow drainage of waste products, including fragmented cells and toxic metabolites, to local lymph nodes where the lymphoreticular cells participate in their hydrolysis and removal.[3]

Role of Differentiation

Another innate defense mechanism of the cell is its ability to differentiate into specialized forms (Fig. 1–3). Symbiotic supportive relationships among cells occur as a result of this differentiation. Cooperation between differentiated and undifferentiated cells in different organ systems permits survival of the organism. The intestinal tract is the principal site of nutritive substrate absorption. Waste products are secreted from the skin and the intestinal, respiratory, and urinary tracts. These sites are also responsible for maintaining water balance, ion control, and cellular and extracellular pH. The heart, partially dependent on regulation by the central nervous system (CNS), has the responsibility of ensuring that circulation continues. The liver synthesizes many of the plasma proteins, after metabolizing substrates derived from the intestinal tract. The endocrine neurotransmitter systems (for example, CNS, peripheral nervous system [PNS], hypothalamus, pituitary, thyroid, pancreas, adrenal, parathyroid, testis, ovary) exercise general and specific control over metabolism, reproduction, and homeostasis. The musculoskeletal system has both structural and metabolic roles.

Role of Cooperating Cells

In any inflammatory response, cells may have local or systemic effects. The latter are mediated by the synthesis and release of inflammatory substances such as prostaglandins, histamine, complement, and antibodies. All cells to some degree contribute to control, supportive, synthetic, or degradative functions, and the homeostasis of the entire organism depends upon cellular, tissue, and organ cooperation.[4]

Intrinsic Defense of the Cell

Despite a seemingly overwhelming complexity in the function of the mammalian organism, several simple principles of cell biology remain paramount. That all mammalian cells contain the same total amount of DNA implies that approximately the same gene content exists regardless of the number of chromosomes present. Although chromosome structure may differ among species in the amount and type of protein present, in chromosomal number and size, and even in number of DNA strands, the genetic code is identical for all.[5] In examining proteins such as the cytochromes that are common to several species, relatively few amino acid substitutions have been found.[6] The fidelity of the code is generally maintained after millions of years of evolution in all species.

Experiments by Gurdon with skin and intestinal nuclei from frogs[7] and by Mintz with cells of teratoma in mice[8] have shown that the nuclear DNA from a single differentiated or undifferentiated cell is capable of supplying and expressing all the genetic material necessary for reproduction of an intact animal (Fig. 1–4). Nevertheless, newer knowledge elucidating *jumping genes* and *splicing of RNA* indicates that the DNA sequence in different cells of the same individual may not be identical, as illustrated by the finding that only a single clone of immune cells can produce a specific antibody.

The ability, both theoretic and potential, of cells to overcome injurious agents remains inherent in the genetic information assembled over millions of years. In addition to protecting cells from injury, the genetic material also determines the ultimate life span of different species. Al-

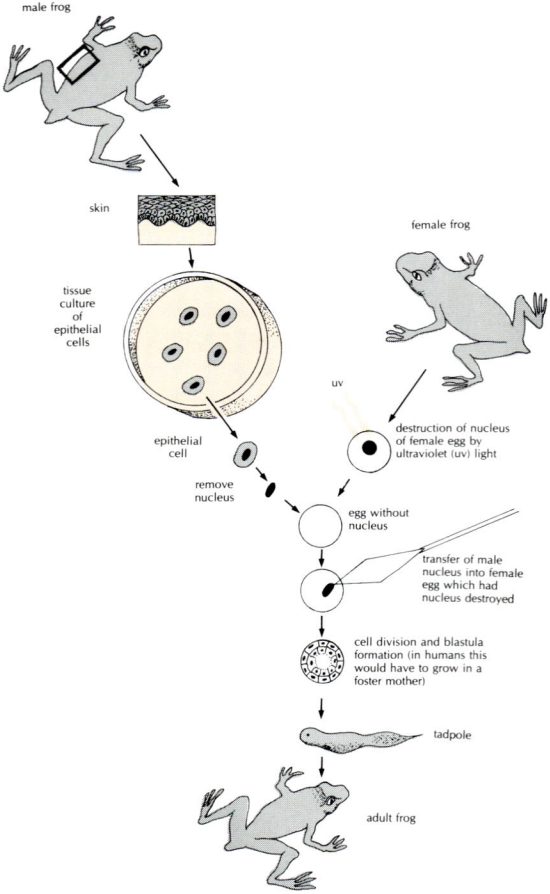

Figure 1–4. Experiments by Gurdon with nuclei from epithelial cells from frog skin demonstrated that nuclear DNA from differentiated cells can supply the necessary genetic material for reproduction of an intact amphibian.

though much can be done to prevent and alleviate disease before death, it is unlikely that the genetically determined life span of the human species can be extended.

ATTACK ON THE CELL

Agents of Injury

In a later chapter, we discuss the effect of various classes of injurious agents on the cell. For ease in dealing with these various agents, we have classified them into six major groups (Fig. 1–5): (1) *genetic* agents (congenital injuries acquired largely in somatic cells and those mutations transmitted through the germ cells); (2) *nutritional* defects in the cell resulting from extracellular deficits or metabolic failures within the cell itself; (3) *physical* agents, such as an imbalance of gases, ions, and other physical factors such as heat and ultraviolet (UV) radiation; (4) *infectious* agents, such as bacteria, viruses, and fungi; (5) *drugs, chemicals, or hormones* either from the environment or synthesized endogenously; and (6) *immune* agents (products and reactions of the immune system).

Research in the past 20 years has clarified the effects of injurious agents on specific intracellular organelles and intermediary metabolic pathways. Every injurious agent must, however, first interact with the cell membrane before entering or exerting an effect on the cell.

Absorption and Entrance into the Cell

Fluid Mosaic Membrane Model

The *fluid mosaic* model of cell membrane structure (Fig. 1–6) has drastically altered our concepts concerning the molecular pathogenesis of disease.[9] One of the principal advantages of the model is that it envisions the entire membrane in a state of flux and modulation, changeable in ways that are to the cell's advantage in protecting itself against injurious agents.

Bacteria, viruses, parasites, drugs, hormones, antigens, antibodies, complement, and many other substances have specific attachment *receptor sites* on the membrane. The number of receptor molecules may vary at any one time. In many instances, these molecules control the susceptibility of a cell to injurious external substances. By altering its membrane pattern, the cell is able to modulate the effects of the agents on the cell.[10]

Once information is received at the cell surface, it may be channeled to other parts of the cell by transmembrane proteins or by activating other cell surface systems such as adenyl cyclase-cyclic adenosine monophosphate (cAMP).[11]

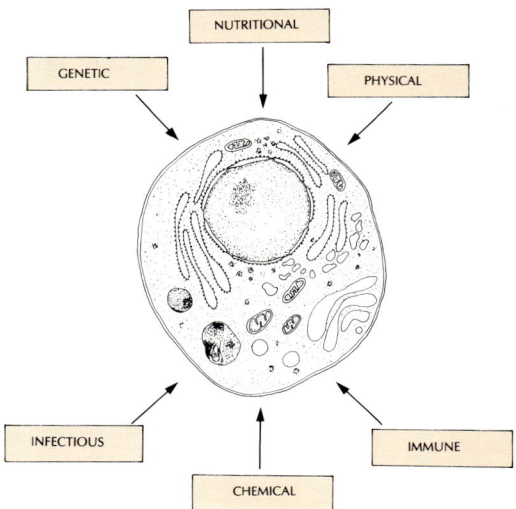

Figure 1–5. Six classes of cellular agents of injury.

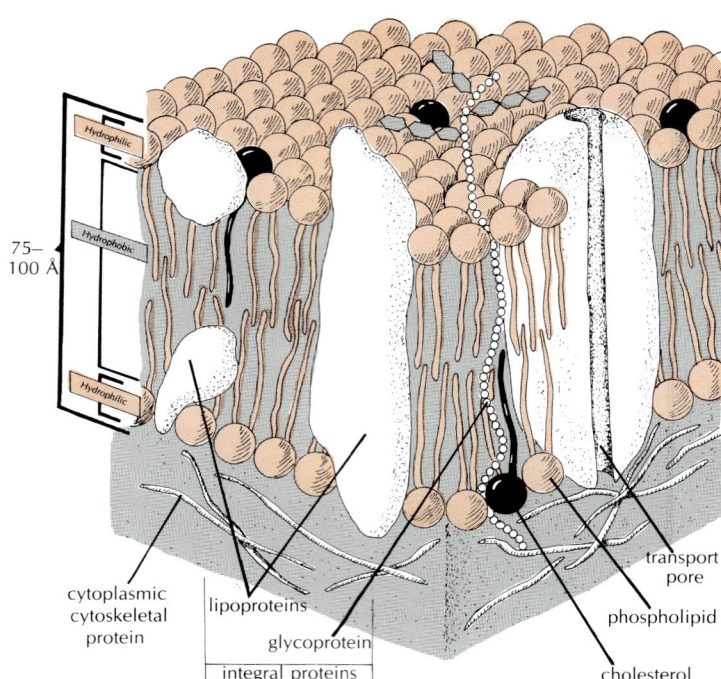

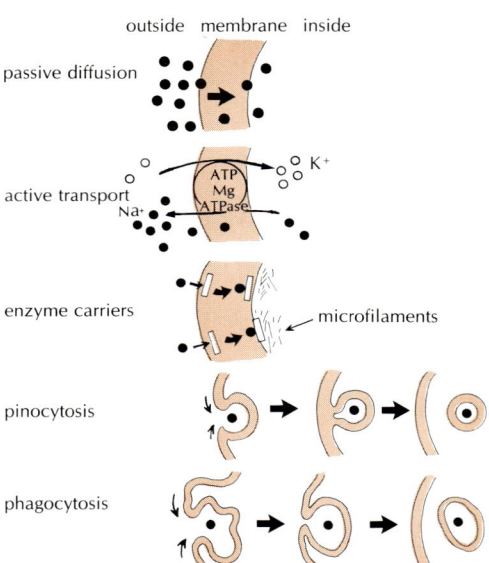

Figure 1–7. Modes of transport into the cell.

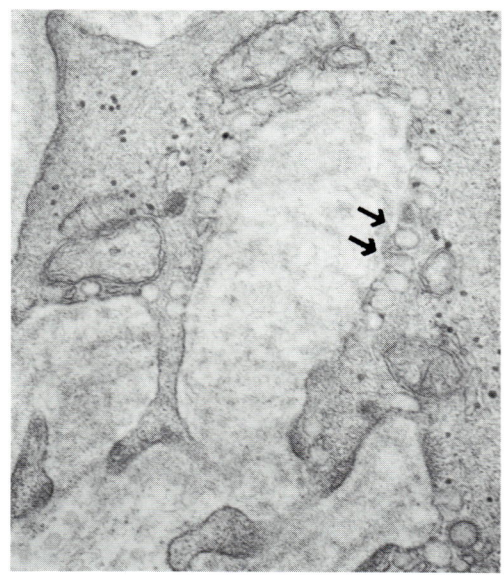

Figure 1–8. Pinocytotic vesicles (arrows) line the edge of this smooth muscle cell. They increase the absorptive surface of the cell.

Figure 1–6. In the fluid mosaic model of membrane structure, the trilaminar membrane consists of a bilayer of phospholipids and cholesterol through which pass various proteins, some of which contain transport pores. (Modified from Singer.)

Cell Membrane Transport

Substances usually pass into the cell by one of four mechanisms (Fig. 1–7): (1) *passive diffusion* (H_2O); (2) *active transport* (sodium and potassium via a calcium-magnesium-activated ATPase pump);[12] (3) by *enzyme carriers* requiring cooperation of microfilaments beneath the plasma membrane; and (4) *pinocytosis* or *phagocytosis*, requiring attachment sites, the cooperation of microfilaments, and an energy source.[13] Subsequent transfer of particles to the interior of the cell may involve microtubules.

Some injurious agents immediately block or disturb transport processes. For example, ouabain inhibits the sodium pump, cholera toxin causes a change in cAMP with increased fluid and electrolyte secretion, and antigen-antibody complexes with complement cause cell lysis. Other transport alterations appear later, during the final stages of cell injury.

General Response of Membranes to Injury

The cell may respond to injury by contraction or swelling, by formation of tenuous pseudopodal processes or blebs, or by altering movement and transport (Fig. 1–8). The cell may functionally increase or decrease the size of its membrane pores, change its internal, external, and underlying

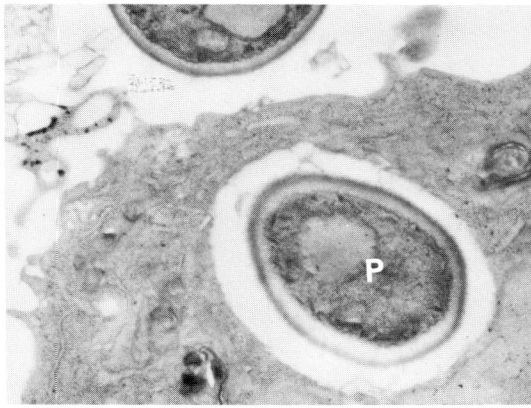

Figure 1–9. Transmission electron micrograph showing a phagolysosome (P) containing an undigested fungal spore.

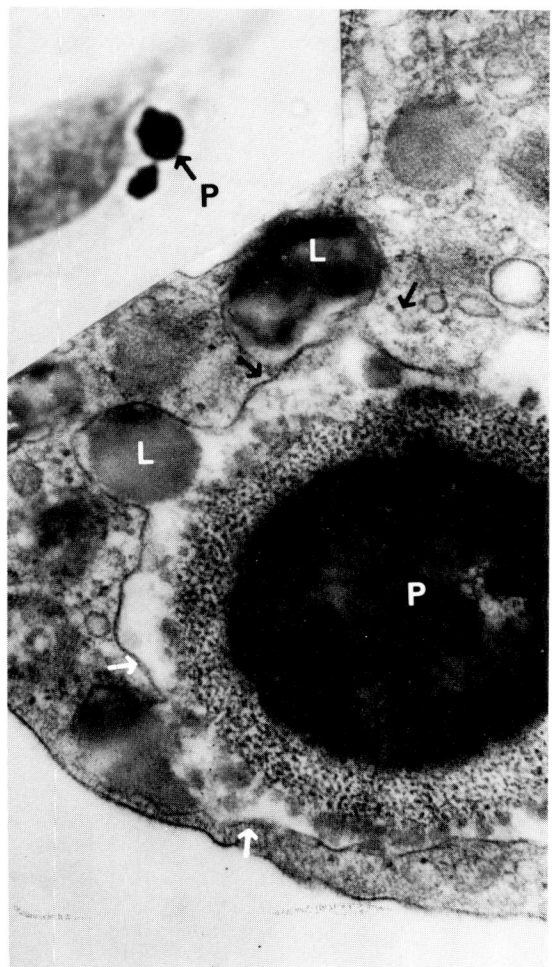

Figure 1–10. Phagolysosomes (P) in the cell may be visible histologically (inset) as well as ultrastructurally. Primary lysosomes (L) may be seen fusing (arrows) with the membranes of these particles.

membrane structure, and enhance or diminish admission or extrusion of molecular substances.

Cell membrane structure and function is under the local control of its immediate environment, including the effects of substrates, ions, pH, hormones, and temperature. Various unknown informational channels from other organelles such as the endoplasmic reticulum (ER), lysosomes, and mitochondria to the membrane also appear to be involved in the response to external stimuli.

Of all these factors, the central control of cell organelles by nuclear DNA is most important. It influences the cell's ability to modulate reactions, to repair damage by new synthesis, to retard transport processes, or to enhance membrane capabilities. At best, the cell responds to injury immediately, constantly, and vigorously. At worst, it dies.

Fate and Metabolism of Injurious Agents

Lysosomes, Autophagic Vacuoles, Hydrolysis

Pinocytosis and *phagocytosis* are two mechanisms of entry into the cell. Substances entering by these processes are usually rapidly enclosed by structures bounded by a single membrane (Fig. 1–9). These phagocytic particles are then escorted by microfilaments and microtubules to a region in the cytosol where they await fusion with lysosomal granules. The fusion of a lysosome with a phagosome results in a secondary lysosome *(phagolysosome)* (Fig. 1–10). The release and activation of hydrolytic lysosomal enzymes degrade foreign material into small metabolic products including amino acids, sugars, fatty acids, purines, and pyrimidines.[14] These molecules then pass back into the cytosol for reuse by the cell.

Cellular components, both molecules and organelles, undergo continual replacement. The factors that determine the normal half-life of specific macromolecules in the circulation and in cellular organelles are unknown, but each cell has a different synthetic capacity to respond to degradative reactions involving its constituents.

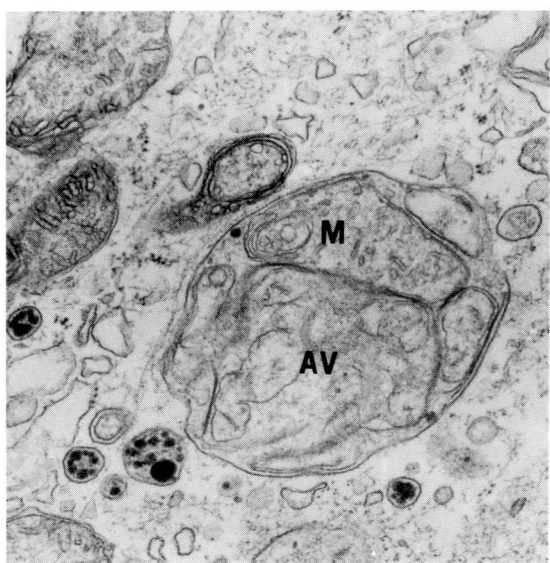

Figure 1–11. Autophagic vacuole (AV) containing portions of mitochondrion (M) and degenerating membranes.

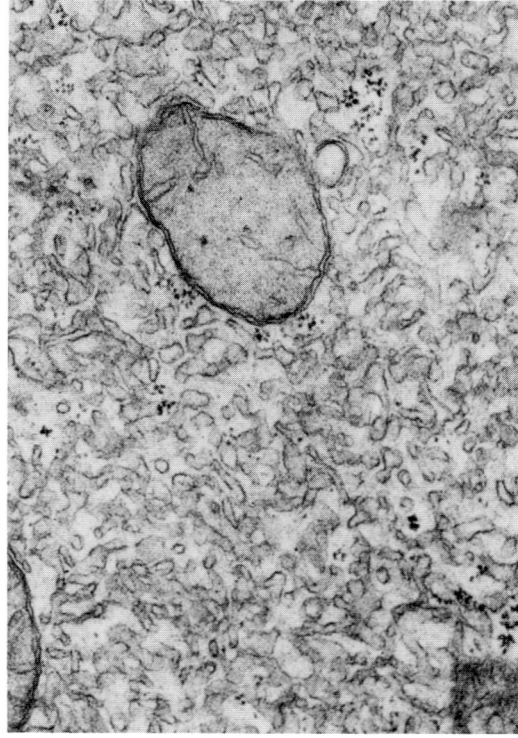

Figure 1–12. Proliferation of smooth endoplasmic reticulum surrounds a mitochondrion in barbiturate intoxication.

The major internal turnover and remodeling of cellular organelles take place in *autophagic vacuoles* (endogenous cytolysosomes)[15] (Fig. 1–11). Partially degraded substances in autophagosomes and undigested metabolites in *secondary phagolysosomes* may be either extruded by reverse phagocytosis or sequestered near the nucleus in enclosed vacuoles (*residual bodies* or *telolysosomes*). Some substances appear resistant to lysosomal degradation (ceroid and tubercle bacilli); in other situations, lysosomal enzymes are faced with too great a quantity of foreign material for degradation, for example in overwhelming infection. Lysosomes in some instances may also lack the proper hydrolytic enzymes to complete the degradative process (for example, as in glycogen storage disease).

Endoplasmic Reticulum

Substances that are not incorporated directly into a phagocytic lysosomal pathway may enter the cell by other transport processes and ultimately may be deposited in the cytosol. The cytosol contains enzymes for degradation of sugars (the glycolytic pathway) and free pools of small metabolites and substrates such as peptides, amino acids, sugars, fatty acids, and nucleic acid bases.

Harmful or foreign substances in the cell signal control mechanisms that are often located in the nucleus. Later, ribosomes activated by tRNA and mRNA initiate synthesis of hydrolytic and detoxifying enzymes and new membrane structural components. Following *barbiturate* intoxication, there is proliferation first of the smooth endoplasmic reticulum (SER) (Fig. 1–12) and then of the rough endoplasmic reticulum (RER) of the cell.[16] The former is responsible for synthesis of additional oxidative enzymes (*mixed oxidases*) required for drug detoxification. Bacteria stimulate the cells' ribosomes to increase synthesis of *lysosomal enzymes* necessary for digestion of their components.

Other cellular responses to various stimuli include increased glycogen production in the cytosol, as a result of excess glucose at the cell membrane, and synthesis of enzymes, coenzymes, and structural membrane proteins by the endoplasmic reticulum. An injurious stimulus sometimes results in the production of *abnormal macroglobulin* proteins or *excess proteins* such as light immunoglobulin chains.[17] These products are degraded, excreted, or sequestered and may result in disease.

Hyperplastic and *hypertrophic* compensatory organelle responses may be insufficient to offset the effects of injurious agents. If these responses fail, the cell's homeostatic control is impaired. Failure of ion pump transport mechanisms results in swelling of the cell. A manifestation of this phenomenon is the distended cisternae of the endoplasmic reticulum, known as *cloudy swelling*. These structures may rupture and coalesce to form large vacuoles, seen by light microscopy as *hydropic degeneration*.

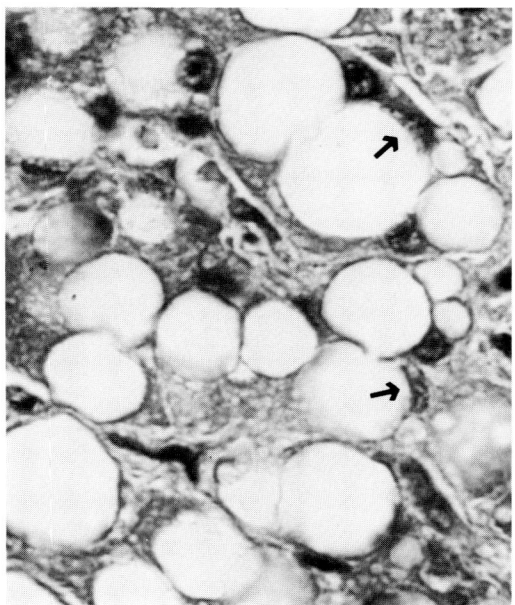

Figure 1–13. In steatosis of the liver, fat accumulations are so excessive that they distort the normal architecture of the cells and displace the nucleus to one side (arrows).

Certain substances such as *carbon tetrachloride* may produce injury so severe that complete *degranulation* and *disaggregation* of polysomes take place and protein synthesis ceases.[18] Early injury by a drug such as *puromycin*, however, may *inhibit protein synthesis* without producing marked structural alterations. The smooth endoplasmic reticulum may continue lipid synthesis, so that lipid molecules are assembled in the undamaged Golgi apparatus. When protein synthesis fails, essential components of lipoprotein molecules are not produced, and *fatty vacuoles* and inclusions may result[19] (Fig. 1–13). More severe injury ends in extensive damage to SER, RER, and Golgi membranes. Damaged ER may first be seen as areas of *focal cytoplasmic degeneration* (FCD) that later become incorporated into *autophagic vacuoles*.

Altered Energy Metabolism

Soluble Cytoplasm, Glycolysis

Resting cells maintain a minimum level of energy production for normal cellular function even when external requirements or demands are few. The *adenosine triphosphate (ATP)* obtained from the *glycolytic pathway* is sufficient for resting cells and for the performance of certain specialized functions. More complex cellular activity requires the production of additional energy by *mitochondria*. For example, the initial stage of phagocytosis occurs with energy obtained from the glycolytic pathway, but the energy needed for activation of lysosomes and myeloperoxidases requires aerobic metabolism.[20]

Mitochondria, Aerobic Respiration

Most metabolically active cells, especially heart, liver, kidney, endocrine, specialized muscle, and brain cells, must have an increased quantity of ATP production obtained through mitochondrial aerobic respiration and *oxidative phosphorylation* reactions. Mitochondria are particularly susceptible to injury by hypoxia, drugs, and nutritional agents.

Mitochondria are also particularly sensitive to injury by *drugs* that interfere with or *uncouple oxidative phosphorylation*. The comparatively minimal *protein synthesis* on mammalian mitochondrial ribosomes may be inhibited by drugs such as *chloramphenicol*, which also affects bacterial ribosomes, and *mitomycin*, which inhibits *DNA replication*.[21]

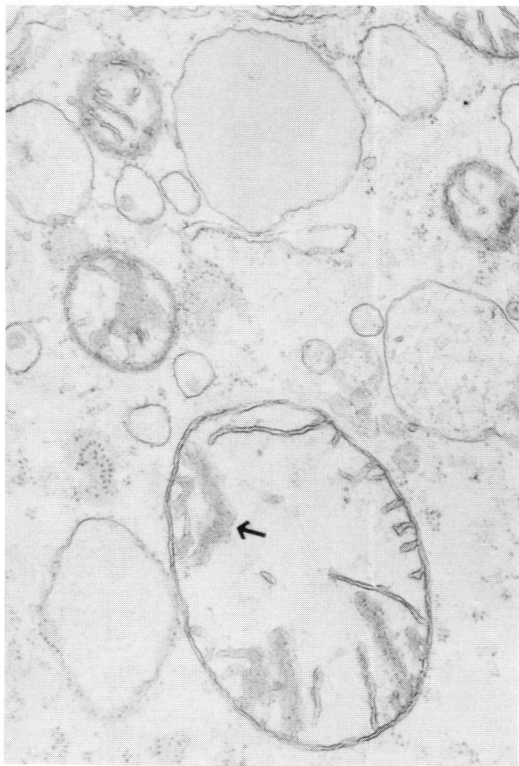

Figure 1–14. Irregularly swollen mitochondria in anoxia. Note the degenerating cristae (arrows).

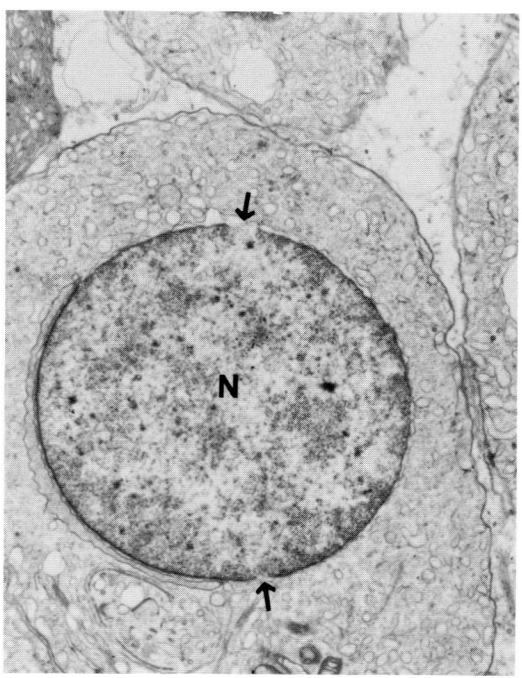

Figure 1–15. The nucleus (N) of the germ cell contains finely dispersed chromatin and is surrounded by the nuclear membrane. Nuclear pores are also visible (arrow).

Hypoxia or anoxia affects mitochondria initially by producing *condensation* and *contraction* of the matrix proteins and later by *swelling* and *unfolding* of the cristae, followed by *bursting* of the membranes[22] (Fig. 1–14). The diminished supply of ATP associated with severe hypoxic mitochondrial injury has far-reaching effects on protein synthesis and cell division. Its most profound initial effect is on *ion transport,* both at the inner mitochondrial membrane and at the cytoplasmic cell membrane.

Disturbance of Transcription, Control, Division

The nucleus (Fig. 1–15) is the key factor in all disease states, regardless of which cellular organelles are initially affected by the injurious agent. If the nuclear DNA is undamaged and the nuclear membrane remains relatively intact, with even a few ribosomes on the outside surface and mitochondria nearby, the nucleus is theoretically able to synthesize the RNA necessary to activate the protein-synthesizing machinery to initiate cellular repair. It can then, under the proper environmental conditions, replace all nuclear and cytoplasmic structures necessary for maintaining cell viability.

Transcription

Mechanisms by which chromosomes control cellular processes remain complex. Histone and acidic protein components of the chromosome are thought to have some regulatory roles.[23] It is possible that the cell is continually transcribing all its genes at a low level. Hormonal, environmental and cytoplasmic feedback mechanisms also regulate the production of gene products, which may be either increased or decreased to nondetectable amounts, if not completely repressed. In addition to the *transcriptional control* processes, substrate availability, ions, pH, metals (for example, magnesium, zinc, cobalt), as well as *feedback inhibition* and *allosteric inhibition* may also act at the translational level.

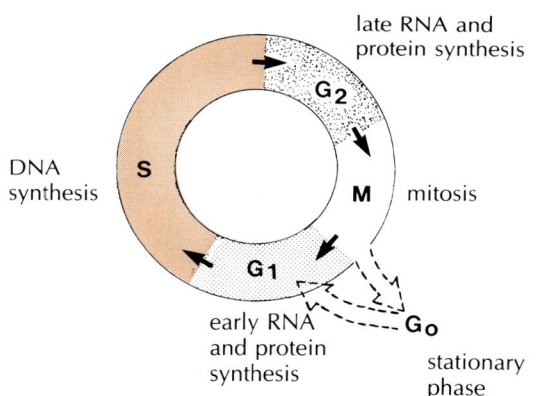

late RNA and protein synthesis

G_2

DNA synthesis

S

M mitosis

G_1

early RNA and protein synthesis

G_0

stationary phase

Control Mechanisms and Cell Cycle

The *nucleus* ultimately controls all facets of organelle response to injurious agents. It controls the initial absorption of an agent to the cell membrane through modulation of membrane receptors, by synthesis, recycling, assembly, and insertion. The nucleus controls synthesis of most structural and enzymatic proteins of the energy-generating systems of the mitochondria. It also regulates synthesis of the hydrolytic enzymes of the lysosomes, as well as enzyme carriers and microtubular networks for the general transport of small and large molecules throughout the cell. Finally, the nucleus directs the synthesis of enzymes necessary for the replicative process associated with cell division and codes directly for the structural and enzymatic proteins of the cell.

The cell's generation cycle consists of interphase and mitosis. Cells in *interphase* normally pass through 3 stages of the cell cycle, including G_1 (protein and RNA synthesis), S (DNA synthesis), and G_2 (continued RNA and protein synthesis).[24] The *mitotic* (M) period (*prophase, metaphase, anaphase,* and *telophase*) follows (Fig. 1–16). Interphase takes from 11 hours to many years, whereas mitosis is usually completed in less than an hour. Some cells (heart and brain) remain in a resting or stationary interphase period (G_0) forever while others (liver and kidney) stay at that point for varying periods of time.

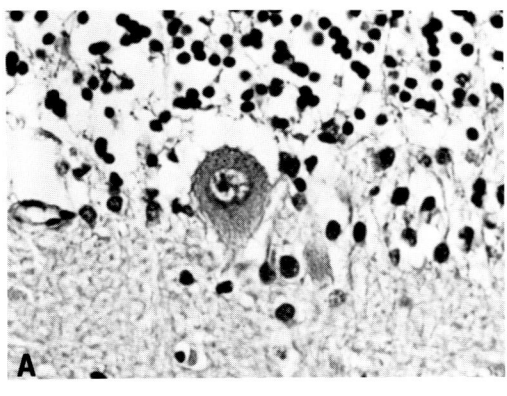

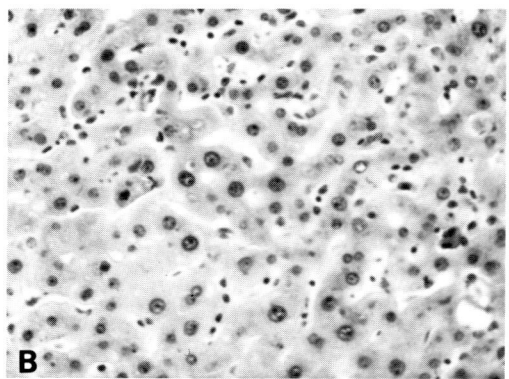

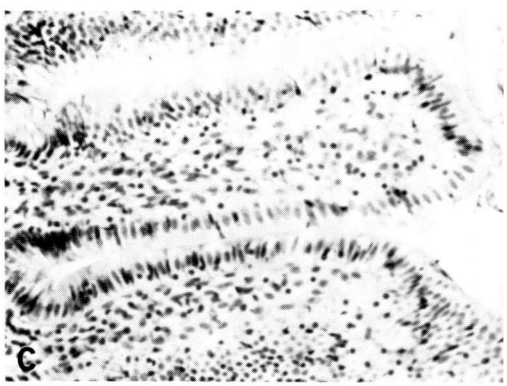

Figure 1–17. Postmitotic, reverting postmitotic, and intermitotic cells are shown. *A,* Neuron at center (Purkinje cell) from cerebellum is *postmitotic. B,* Hepatocytes of liver are *reverting postmitotic. C,* Gastrointestinal epithelium of small intestine villus is *intermitotic.*

Cells are generally classified as *postmitotic,* which are cells that never divide, such as heart and nerve cells, *reverting postmitotic,* or those that divide under the proper stimulation, such as endocrine, liver, kidney, and lung cells, and *intermitotic cells,* which are those in a constant state of division, such as gastrointestinal and genitourinary epithelium, bone marrow, and skin cells (Fig. 1–17).

Except for heart and nerve cells, which remain in the G_0 or stationary phase once they become mature, all other cells unwind portions of their DNA during replication, but this S period does not appear particularly vulnerable to injury. During transcription, some of the cell's genes are exposed in order to synthesize mRNA, tRNA, and rRNA. The genome is safer from injury during mitosis, when the DNA is in a contracted, condensed state, than during the G_1 and G_2 periods, when the DNA is partially uncoiled.

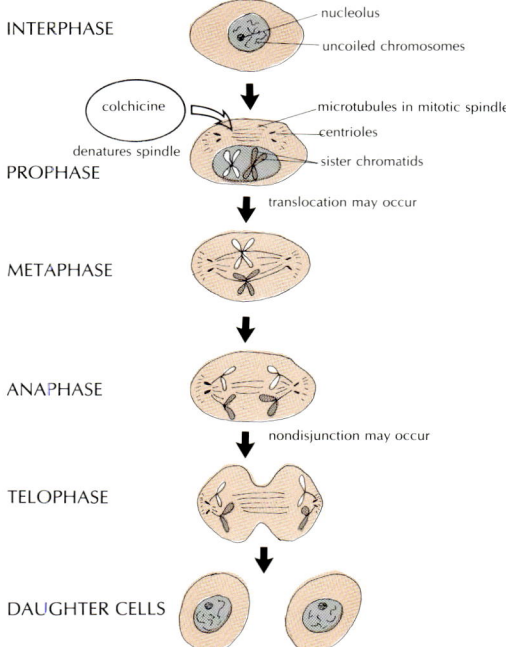

INTERPHASE — nucleolus — uncoiled chromosomes

colchicine — microtubules in mitotic spindle — centrioles

denatures spindle

PROPHASE — sister chromatids

translocation may occur

METAPHASE

ANAPHASE

nondisjunction may occur

TELOPHASE

DAUGHTER CELLS

Figure 1–18. Mitosis and sites of altered chromosome migration.

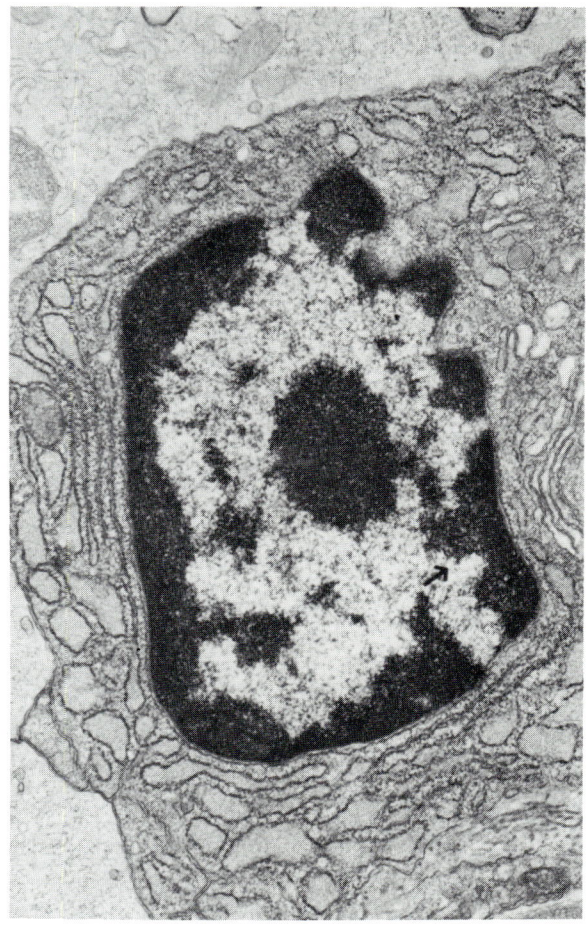

Figure 1–19. This electron micrograph of a mature plasma cell shows margination of the chromatin (arrow).

Effect of Injury on Chromosomes and DNA

Although the contracted chromosomal DNA is protected in the mitotic stage of division, the formation of the microtubular spindle, the attachment of the kinetochore or centromere to the spindle, and chromosomal migration provide opportunities for genetic abnormalities. Drugs such as *cytochalasin* and *colchicine*, which respectively affect the microfilaments and microtubules, are capable of interfering with and altering these processes.[25] *Translocation* may occur in prophase and *nondisjunctions* in anaphase (Fig. 1–18). Damage to DNA results either in cell death or in the production of somatic-cell or permanent germ-cell mutations.

The genome is protected from injury by a *reserve* of extra copies of certain *genes.* For instance, several hundred gene copies exist for rRNA and at least 60 separate genes for tRNA; however, most structural and enzymatic mRNA probably arises from a few copies of the gene (perhaps 2 to 4). Chromosomes cope with DNA injury by special *repair enzymes* known as exonucleases, endonucleases, polymerases, and ligases.[26] The opportunity for mistakes in gene repair is proportional to the extent of damage, the reserve capacity of the genome, and the effectiveness of the repair process.

Several drugs may interfere with DNA synthesis in the nucleus. This organelle is less affected than others by temperature, by hypoxic change, or by infectious agents, with the exception of viruses. Nutritional deficiencies only rarely cause nuclear injury, since the cell is able to synthesize many of its nuclear requirements and the nucleus may have first call on needed substrates.

Visible changes in nuclear morphology may indicate the cell's stage of activity or inactivity. *Margination* of chromatin on the nuclear membrane is accepted as representing condensation of DNA and an inactive (or single-purpose) genome (Fig. 1–19). This change occurs in multiple myeloma in which the cell is principally making immunoglobulins, following injury of all types, and in aged cells.

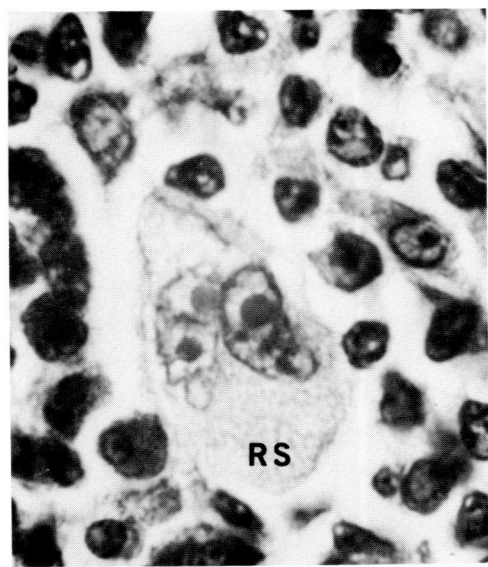

Figure 1–20. A binucleate Reed-Sternberg cell (RS) in Hodgkin's disease demonstrates multiple nucleoli.

Hyperplasia of chromosomes resulting in *hyperdiploidy* is seen in many growth processes, both in regenerating cells and in aneuploid cells of tumors.[27] An increase in nucleolar size and number is associated with growth and reflects amplification of ribosomes necessary for increased protein synthesis (Fig. 1–20). *Pleomorphism* of the nucleus and the presence of *nuclear vacuoles* containing water, sugar, protein, lipid, melanin, and iron are indications of nuclear injury, but are often reversible (Fig. 1–21).

Nuclear dysfunction is manifested by inhibition of division, and cessation of protein synthesis with resultant structural or functional deficiencies of cell organelles. Consequences of nuclear injury are slowed cellular movement, altered metabolic pathways, an increased number of telolysosomes, and eventually a failure of essential components as a result of inadequate synthesis or repair capability.

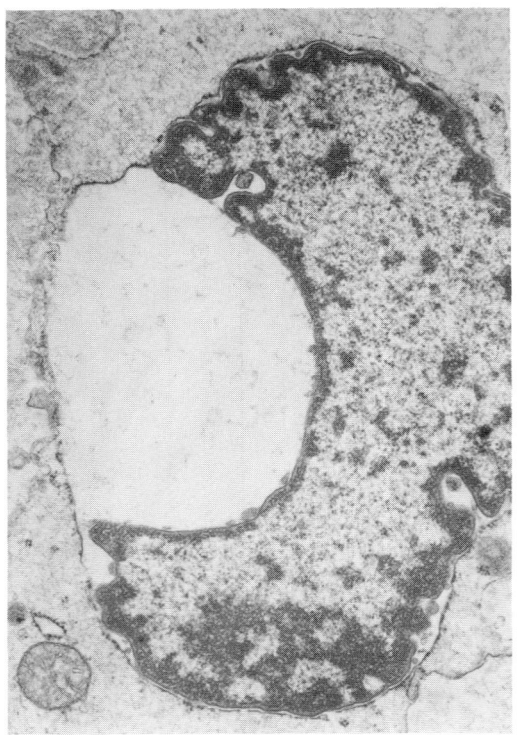

Figure 1–21. Intranuclear vacuole in a cell exposed to radiation.

RESPONSE OF THE CELL

Acute Injury and Recovery

Alterations in Organelles

Cells may be severely damaged by a variety of agents that cause many morphologic and biochemical changes.[28] For example, *vacuoles* containing water or lipid may be seen in the nucleus and cytoplasm (Fig. 1–22). As discussed, the cell may have *ribosomal disaggregation,* lack of formation of the mitotic apparatus, *swelling* of mitochondria, and membrane alterations associated with injury.

Postmitotic and reverting postmitotic cells often repair themselves and survive without apparent residual damage, particularly in younger individuals. Intermitotic cells with a shorter life span are often completely lost; they are replaced by division of stem cells.

Diversion of Metabolites, Regeneration

Another option of the injured cell is to cannibalize itself and other cells. By forming autophagic vacuoles, the cell self-digests less-needed organelles. It may degrade and use parts of other cells, for example in *erythrophagocytosis.* Homeostatic mechanisms operative at the tissue level may induce other cells in organs to provide needed metabolites. Fatty acids may be transported from cellular lipid stores, and amino acids may be diverted from the liver and skeletal muscles. A tissue such as muscle converts, for short periods of time, from *aerobic* to *anaerobic metabolism.* Intrinsic cell *regeneration,* including both *hyperplasia* and *hypertrophy* of organelles, and whole cell division contribute to tissue repair.

Chronic Injury

Cells are initially resistant to most forms of acute injury and usually recover completely. Because the cell may be exposed to injurious agents over continued periods of time, however, the outcome of cell injury may not only be either recovery or death, but also chronic disease. Persistent bacterial infection, constant autoimmune injury, poor nutrition, relative hypoxia, and chromosomal defects produced by drug or viral agents may adversely affect cells throughout a lifetime.

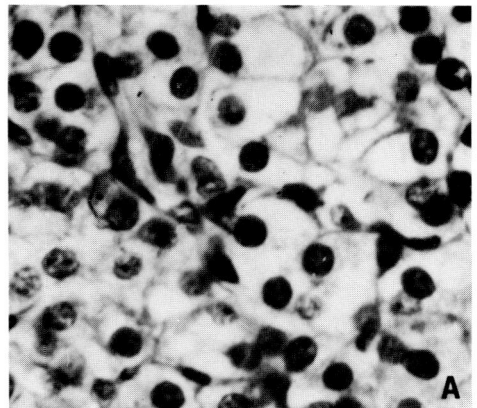
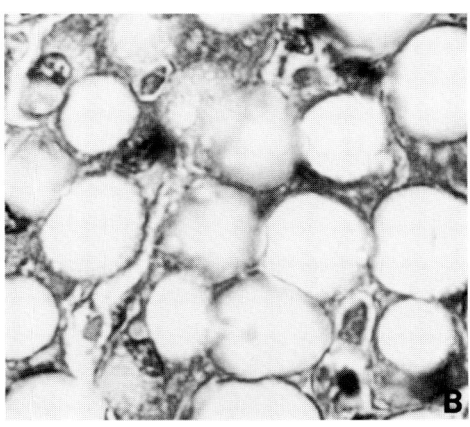

Figure 1–22. *A.* Water accumulation in cells produces cloudy swelling. Contrast this to the lipid inclusions that distort the cytologic architecture in *B.*

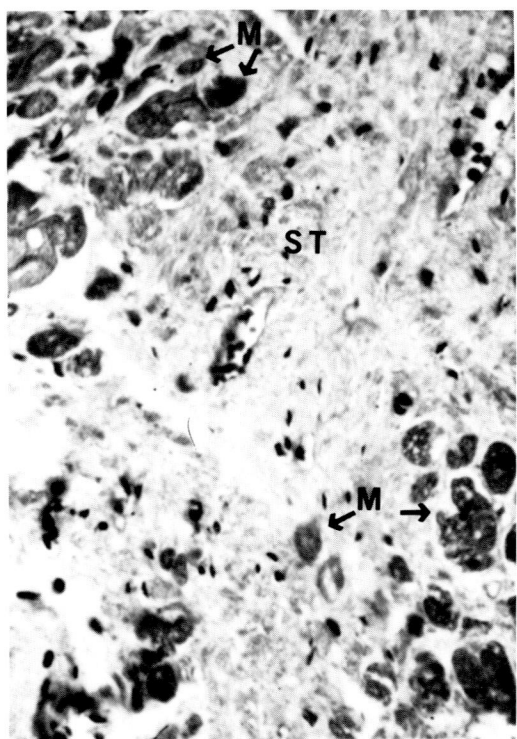

Figure 1–23. A healed myocardial infarct, with the formation of scar tissue (ST), has trapped some residual myocytes (M) (arrows).

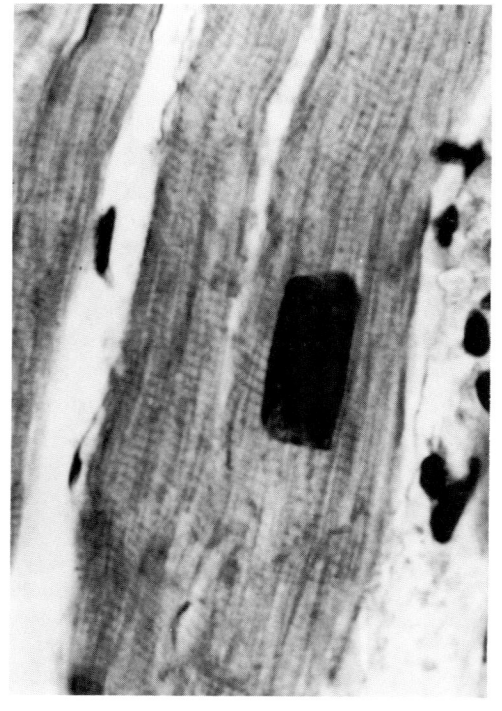

Figure 1–24. Hypertrophic cardiac myocyte in a patient with congestive heart failure.

Invalid Cells with Vacuoles and Inclusions

Chronically injured cells suffer alterations in intracellular organelles that may disappear, may persist during the life of the postmitotic cell, or in the intermitotic dividing cell may be transferred to daughter cells. Multiple nucleoli, altered chromosomal karyotypes, deficient or excess endoplasmic reticulum, megamitochondria, an increase in autophagic vacuoles, disruption and malfunction of the microtubular-microfilament system, and alterations in structure and function of the plasma membrane are all consequences of cell injury.[29]

In addition, the presence of *vacuoles* or *inclusions* containing water, carbohydrate, protein, lipid, nucleic acid, pigments, minerals, infectious agents, and hormones, as well as nonspecific structures such as crystals, particles, lamellar components, and fibrillary patterns,[30] are discussed in detail in Chapter 6.

Invalid cells may continue to serve structural roles despite ineffective functional states. We see this in the atrophic muscle following polio infection, in the trapped, hypoxic myocytes surrounded by collagen after a myocardial infarct (Fig. 1–23), in the few remaining thyroid follicle cells in Hashimoto's thyroiditis, and in the compensatory hyperplasia of bronchiolar cells in pulmonary fibrosis.

Hyperplasia, Hypertrophy, Metaplasia, Dysplasia, Neoplasia

If an injured cell does not die, atrophy, or recover completely, it may undergo other compensatory responses of *hyperplasia* (increase in number) or *hypertrophy* (increase in size). A cell stimulated by small doses of radiation undergoes hyperplasia. Heart cells, which are unable to divide, may undergo hypertrophy with nuclear enlargement and increased myofibrils (Fig. 1–24). Injured cells in the bronchus may undergo *metaplasia* (change in cell type from columnar to squamous) or *dysplasia* (alteration of normal cell and tissue morphology). Injured cells may also become transformed into *neoplastic* cells.

Cell Death

We describe *cell death* as an *irreversible alteration in cellular architecture.* Since many cells do not divide and cells can be frozen indefinitely, the criteria of division and metabolism are insufficient indices of permanent cell death. The most reliable test for a living cell in suspension is the exclusion of dye from the nucleus when cells are placed in a solution of trypan blue.[31] This test is, of course, a rough index and represents the culmination of a complex series of altered events.

Loss of cellular viability may occur with some injurious agents, although cell structure remains intact. For example, cells denatured by formaldehyde or red blood cells that have become dried retain normal morphologic characteristics, with none or few of the structural alterations associated with severe cell injury described by light or electron microscopic analysis.

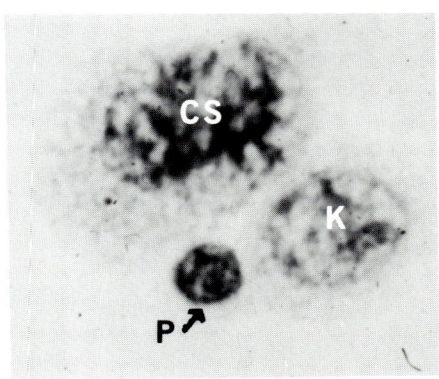

Figure 1–25. These three Ehrlich ascites cells show pyknosis (P), karyolysis (K), and cloudy swelling (CS).

Cell Organelle Destruction

Various morphologic and biochemical parameters of cell death are well described. Rupture of the plasma cell membrane, lysosomes, or mitochondria, swelling of the nucleus and nuclear membrane *(karyolysis)*, fragmentation of the chromatin *(karyorrhexis)*, and condensation of the chromatin *(pyknosis)* are morphologic signs of cell death (Fig. 1–25). Functional abnormalities include a decreased oxidative phosphorylation ratio, absence of amino acid incorporation, and altered cell membrane electrical activity.

Fate of the Cell

Pyknotic and *karyolytic* nuclei may be found in the cell for appreciable length of time, but eventually the majority of dead cells will be hydrolyzed by intra- or extracellular enzymes. Fragments of membranes, nuclei, mitochondria, and endoplasmic reticulum are phagocytized by wandering macrophages or are carried by the lymphatics and blood vessels to the lymph nodes, spleen, and liver, where phagocytosis and subsequent degradation also take place.

Tissue Necrosis

Following death of a cell, lysis often occurs rapidly. Cell proteins may clump together in denatured eosinophilic masses, usually seen in *coagulative necrosis,* often with a loss of nuclei. Some cells may be dissolved by hydrolytic enzymes, with intracellular rupture of lysosomes, as in *liquefaction necrosis.* A combination of liquefaction and denaturation also may be seen in coagulative necrosis.[33] Some organelles, such as the mitochondrion and the nucleus, may acquire calcium deposits *(calcific necrosis).* Cell membranes may degenerate into masses of membranous structures and fibrillary *myelin figures.* Under certain conditions, cells may persist intact for months in a mummified condition, especially if they contain large amounts of undegraded waxy material.

Death of the organism is associated with cessation of function of the heart and lungs (Fig. 1–26). With maintenance of cardiopulmonary activity through artificial mechanical devices, cessation of the brain's electrical activity becomes the legal criterion of death of the organism.[32]

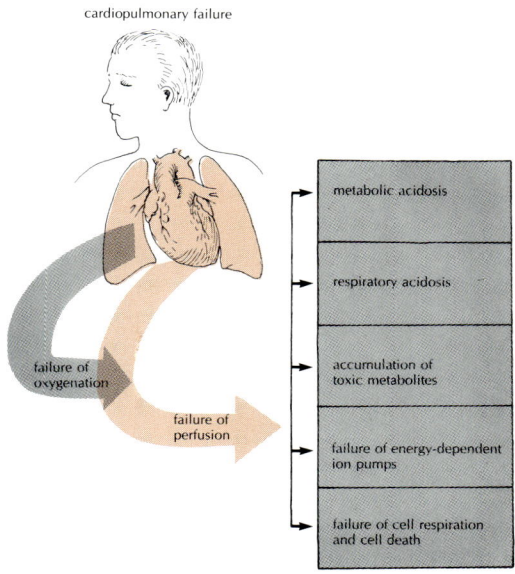

cardiopulmonary failure

failure of oxygenation

failure of perfusion

metabolic acidosis

respiratory acidosis

accumulation of toxic metabolites

failure of energy-dependent ion pumps

failure of cell respiration and cell death

Figure 1–26. Consequences of cardiopulmonary failure.

REFERENCES

1. King, D.W.: Symposium on effect of injury on the cell. Fed. Proc., *21*:1143, 1962.
2. Simon, G.T.: Ultrastructure of acute inflammation. Curr. Top. Pathol., *68*:11, 1979.
3. Hay, J.B.: Kinetics of the inflammatory response in regional lymph. Curr. Top. Pathol. *68*:33, 1979.
4. Cohen, S.: Cell mediated immunity and the inflammatory system. Hum. Pathol., 7:249, 1976.
5. Vendrely, R., and Vendrely, C.: La teneur du noyal cellulaire en acide désoxyribonucléique à travers les organes, les individus et les espèces animales. Experientia, 5:327, 1979.
6. Margoliash, E.: The molecular variations of cytochrome c as a function of the evolution of the species. Harvey Lect., *66*:177, 1972.
7. Gurdon, J.P.: The Control of Gene Expression in Animal Development. London, Oxford University Press, 1974.
8. Mintz, B.: Malignancy vs. normal differentiation of stem cells as analyzed in genetically mosaic animals. Adv. Pathobiol., *6*:153, 1977.
9. Singer, S.J., and Nicolson, G.L.: The fluid mosaic model of the structure of cell membranes. Science, *175*:720, 1972.
10. Catt, K.J., et al.: Hormonal regulation of peptide receptors and target cell responses. Nature, *280*:109, 1979.
11. Gallagher, J.P., and Shinnick-Gallagher, P.: Cyclic nucleotides injected intracellularly into rat superior cervical ganglion cells. Science, *198*:851, 1977.
12. Sweadner, K.J., and Goldin, S.M.: Active transport of sodium and potassium ions. Basic Sci. Clinicians, *302*:777, 1980.
13. Stossel, T.P.: Phagocytosis. N. Engl. J. Med., *290*:717, 1974.
14. deDuve, C., and Wattiaux, R.: Functions of lysosomes. Annu. Rev. Physiol., *28*:435, 1966.
15. Stossel, T.P.: Phagocytosis. N. Engl. J. Med., *290*:833, 1974.
16. Jones, A.L., and Fawcett, D.W.: Hypertrophy of the agranular endoplasmic reticulum in hamster liver induced by phenobarbital. J. Histochem. Cytochem., *14*:215, 1966.
17. Glenner, G.G.: Amyloid deposits and amyloidosis. The β-fibrilloses. N. Engl. J. Med., *302*:1283 and 1333, 1980.
18. Smuckler, E.A., Koplitz, M., and Striker, G.E.: Cellular adenosine triphosphate levels in liver and kidney during CCl_4 intoxication. Lab. Invest., *19*:218, 1968.
19. Lombardi, B.: Considerations on the pathogenesis of fatty liver. Lab. Invest., *15*:1, 1966.
20. Babior, B.M.: Oxygen-dependent microbial killing by phagocytes. N. Engl. J. Med., *298*:659, 1978.
21. King, M.E., Godman, G.C., and King, D.W.: Respiratory enzymes and mitochondrial morphology of the HeLa and L-cells treated with chloramphenicol and ethidium bromide. J. Cell Biol., *53*:127, 1972.
22. King, M.E., and King, D.W.: Respiratory enzyme activity and mitochondrial morphology of L-cells under prolonged oxygen deprivation. Lab. Invest., *25*:374, 1971.
23. Garel, A., and Axel, R.: Selective digestion of transcriptionally active ovalbumin genes from oviduct nuclei. Proc. Natl. Acad. Sci. U.S.A., *73*:3966, 1976.
24. Edmunds, L.N., Jr., and Adams, K.J.: Clocked cell cycle clocks. Science, *211*:1002, 1981.
25. Godman, G.C., and Miranda, A.F.: Cellular contractility and the visible effects of cytochalasin. Front. Biol., *46*:277, 1978.
26. Setlow, R.B.: Repair deficient human disorders and cancer. Nature, *271*:713, 1978.
27. German, J.: Studying human chromosomes today. Am. Sci., *58*:182, 1970.
28. King, D.W.: Introduction. *In* Ultrastructural Aspects of Disease. Edited by D.W. King. New York, Harper & Row, 1966.
29. Trump, B.F., McDowell, E.M., and Arstila, A.U.: Cellular reaction to injury. *In* Principles of Pathology. 3rd Ed. Edited by R.B. Hill and M.F. LaVia. New York, Oxford University Press, 1980.
30. Ghadially, F.N.: Ultrastructural Pathology of the Cell. Boston, Butterworth, 1975.
31. King, D.W., et al.: Cell death. IV. The effect of injury on the entrance of vital dye in Ehrlich tumor cells. Am. J. Pathol., *35*:1067, 1959.
32. Black, P.M.: Brain death. N. Engl. J. Med., *299*:393, 1978.
33. Farber, J.L.: Biology of disease. Membrane injury and calcium homeostasis in the pathogenesis of coagulative necrosis. Lab. Invest., *47*:114, 1982.

Chapter 2

INFLAMMATION AND REPAIR: MULTICELLULAR RESPONSE TO INJURY

And I'll repair the misery thou dost bear.

—King Lear, IV, i.

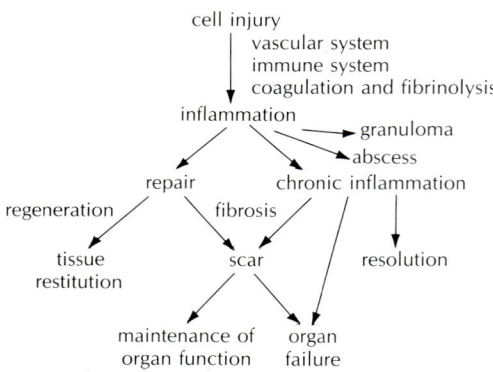

cell injury
vascular system
immune system
coagulation and fibrinolysis
inflammation → granuloma
→ abscess
repair   chronic inflammation
regeneration   fibrosis
tissue restitution   scar   resolution
maintenance of organ function   organ failure

Figure 2–1. Some of the possible pathways following cell and tissue injury.

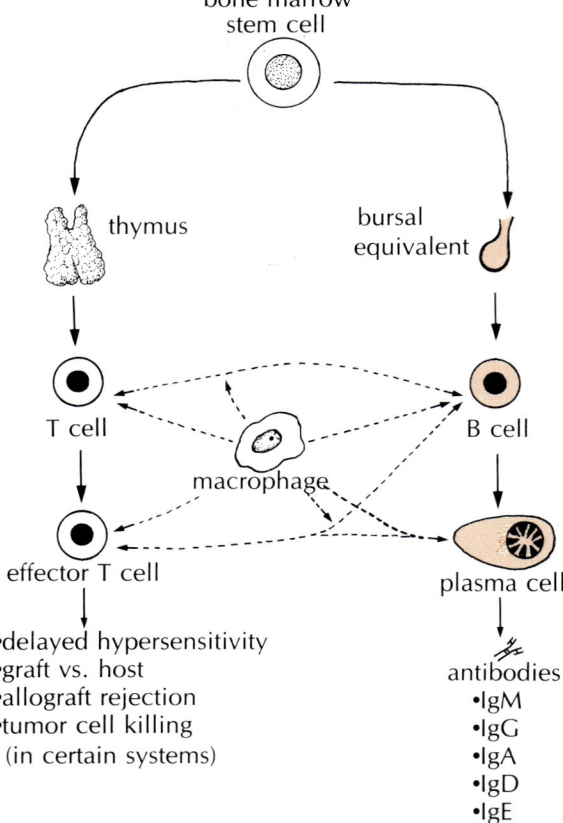

bone marrow stem cell

thymus   bursal equivalent

T cell   macrophage   B cell

effector T cell   plasma cell

•delayed hypersensitivity
•graft vs. host
•allograft rejection
•tumor cell killing
  (in certain systems)

antibodies
•IgM
•IgG
•IgA
•IgD
•IgE

Figure 2–2. Schematic diagram of lymphocyte maturation and functions. The processing of bone marrow stem cells by the thymus and bursal equivalent results in generation of effector T cells and plasma cells with respective roles in cell-mediated and humoral immunity. Interactions with macrophages are important at various stages in the generation of the immune response.

Injury, inflammation, and repair are the hallmarks of pathology. Knowledge of the basic phenomena, as well as the consequences, complications, and nuances of these processes, constitutes the basis for understanding many diseases (Fig. 2–1). *Inflammation is the host cell and tissue reaction to any injury.* An injurious agent or a damaged cell and normal inflammatory, hemostatic, and immune responses are the essential ingredients needed for inflammation to occur.

Inflammatory responses may be provoked by any of the agents previously discussed. Individual response to injury may vary widely for any given injurious agent, however, owing to the unique set of genetic, nutritional, physical, infectious, chemical, hormonal, and immune factors that make up that individual's internal and external milieu. Inflammatory and reparative processes are generally simultaneous, but one phase usually dominates when tissue is examined microscopically at any given time after injury. Although the inflammatory response varies depending upon the particular agent, the tissue, and the individual host characteristics, the final result is regeneration, the formation of scar tissue, or one of numerous complications.

For the purpose of discussion, we have divided this chapter into six sections: (1) the immune system; (2) acute inflammation, including the vascular and cellular responses; (3) coagulation and fibrinolytic phenomena associated with acute, subacute, and chronic inflammation; (4) repair, including healing by primary and secondary intention, regeneration, and scar tissue formation; (5) complications of repair, including abscess, chronic inflammation, and granulomata; and (6) factors affecting the inflammatory and repair processes.

IMMUNE SYSTEM

The immune system plays an important role in inflammation, in repair, and in the development and outcome of many disease processes. Indeed, in many diseases the multifaceted immune process is the primary mediator.[1,2]

The immune system (Fig. 2–2) arises from stem cells in the bone marrow that differentiate into two major classes of *lymphocytes (B and T)* and a larger mononuclear phagocytic cell known as a *monocyte.* Stimulation of these three cells by a foreign substance (an *"antigen"*), often a protein, provokes either a humoral response in the form of synthesis of an *antibody* or a cellular response that involves cell-cell interactions and production of additional synthetic products.

Other cells that participate in the immune response, particularly those producing chemical mediators, include *granulocytes* (neutrophils, eosinophils, and basophils), *mast cells,* and *platelets. Complement,* a multiprotein serum system, enhances the antigen-antibody interaction and contributes in

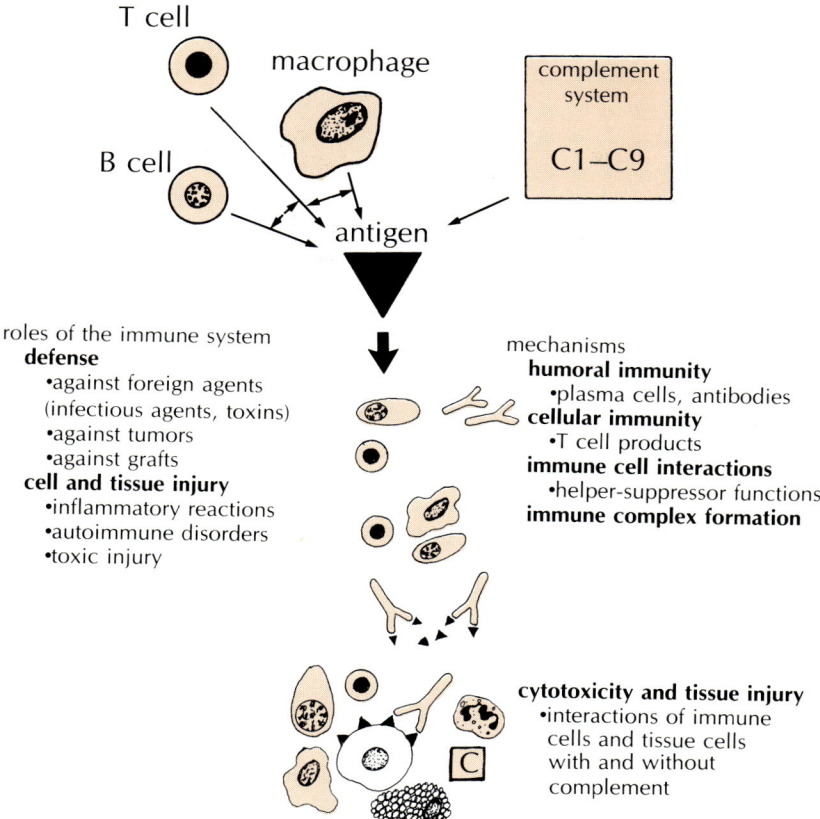

Figure 2–3. Functions of the immune system.

roles of the immune system
defense
- •against foreign agents (infectious agents, toxins)
- •against tumors
- •against grafts

cell and tissue injury
- •inflammatory reactions
- •autoimmune disorders
- •toxic injury

mechanisms
humoral immunity
- •plasma cells, antibodies

cellular immunity
- •T cell products

immune cell interactions
- •helper-suppressor functions

immune complex formation

cytotoxicity and tissue injury
- •interactions of immune cells and tissue cells with and without complement

many ways to the immune and inflammatory response (Fig. 2–3).

The immune response identified with antibody production was originally thought to be only a defense reaction. It is now known that it may be involved in both humoral and cellular reactions to exogenous and endogenous substances that are considered foreign to the host. Some of the reactions may produce serious injury in the host tissue, and these are discussed in Chapter 3.

Antigens

Definition and Structure

Antigens (Ag) may be proteins, carbohydrates, lipids, or nucleic acids. *Immunogens* are those antigens capable of eliciting a strong immune response. In general, these substances are large protein molecules or polysaccharides with molecular weights greater than 5000 daltons.[3] Antigenic determinants on proteins may represent only 5 to 7 amino acids. Smaller molecules, often carbohydrates, lipids, nucleic acids, or derivatives also act as antigenic determinants when attached to larger molecules and are called *haptens* (Fig. 2–4).[4]

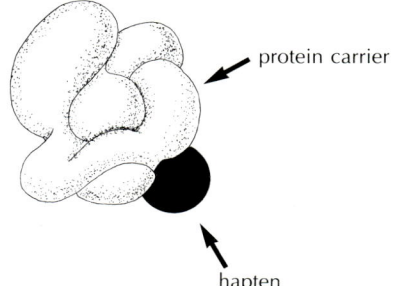

Figure 2–4. Small molecules (haptens) may function as immunogens when attached to larger protein carriers.

Extrinsic and Intrinsic Antigens

One classification of antigens uses specific terms to indicate whether an antigen originates in a foreign species or in the same species. This classification may be applied to grafts (Table 2–1). Antigens may also be classified as extrinsic, intrinsic, or occult. *Extrinsic antigens* are not a constituent of host cells, and include bacteria, viruses and their products, and transplanted foreign cells. Foreign substances, chiefly proteins, may be inhaled (ragweed), ingested (egg yolk), or absorbed through the skin (oil of poison ivy) and may provoke an immune response. *Intrinsic antigens* are derived from altered cell membranes or other organelles. *Occult antigens* are intra- or extracellular substances usually hidden from the immune system, but which may be unmasked by injury.

Antigenic molecules of cells are usually displayed on the outer sufaces of cell membranes, although they may leak from inside the cell under certain conditions. Oligosaccharide and carbohydrate groups attached to proteins in the form of glycoproteins in the bilayer cell membrane are often antigenic.

Membrane antigens expressed at any given moment reflect the state of cellular differentiation, the stage of the cell cycle, or the presence of other components of the immune system. Since the membrane is a fluid mosaic structure, it can be modulated or induced to move its antigenic molecules to different sites in the membrane, depending upon given requirements. Apparently, new or unmasked specific antigens may be seen as the result of neoplastic transformation of the cells, either by chemical carcinogens or by the integration of viral genetic material into the host cell genome.

Host cell products or components occasionally serve as antigens. This observation has led to the concept of autoimmunity, a violation of one of the original dogmas of immunology, that is, animals do not usually make antibodies to their own constituents.

The presence or development of immune complexes, immune deficiencies, hypersensitivity states, and autoimmune reactions are a few of the immune reactions associated with disease states. In some instances, both in fetal

Table 2–1. *Classification of Antigens*

| Origin of Antigen | Nomenclature | |
	Name of Antigen	Name of Graft
Foreign species	Heteroantigen	Heterograft or xenograft
Same species (genetically dissimilar)	Homoantigen	Homograft or allograft
Same species (genetically identical)	Isoantigen	Isograft
Same individual	Autoantigen	Autograft

and adult life, substances normally considered to be antigenic fail to stimulate an immune response. This state is known as *tolerance*.

Membrane Antigens

Histocompatibility (Transplantation) Antigens. The major histocompatibility complex (MHC) is found on chromosome 17 in the mouse as the H-2 complex and on chromosome 6 in man as the HLA complex.[5] Graft survival following transplantation, immune responsiveness, and disease susceptibility are the important functions in which the MHC plays a major role. Because of the wealth of investigative work on the murine system and because of its value as an experimental model, a discussion of the H-2 complex of the mouse is given in the following section.

Murine H-2 Complex. The H-2 complex, located on chromosome 17, is a series of genes controlling immunologic functions including graft rejection, immune responses to antigens, cell-cell interactions, resistance to certain infectious agents, and components of the complement (C) system (Fig. 2–5). The complex is characterized by regions bearing specific, linked marker genes localized to the right side of the centromere. K and D regions delineate the MHC, which spans a distance of 0.5 map units (0.5 centimorgan).[6]

The I region of the H-2 complex in the mouse contains: (1) the specific immune response (Ir) genes; (2) genes that regulate mixed lymphocyte culture (MLC) reactivity; and (3) genes that code for the Ia antigens on lymphocytes and macrophages.[7]

The Ia genes controlling cell surface antigens have been studied most extensively in mice and guinea pigs. That Ir genes strongly influence susceptibility to disease-causing agents is evidenced by their control over susceptibility to Gross murine leukemia virus and Friend leukemia virus. These genes also control the responses to T-dependent antigens.

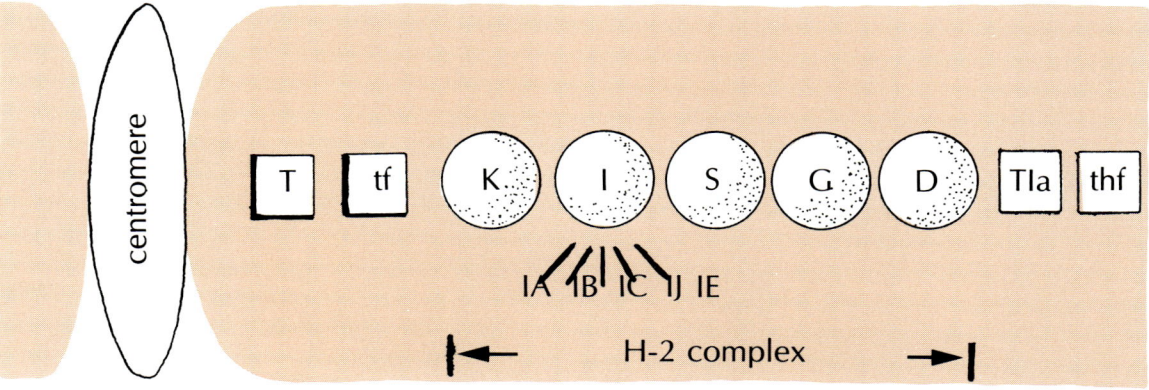

Figure 2–5. Schematic representation of the H2 histocompatibility complex of mice on chromosome 17 (K, I, S, G, D). Although IA, IB, IC, IJ, and IE antigens have been identified, the I gene locus does not appear to contain sufficient nucleotide bases to code for all these products. T, tf, Tla, and thf are nearby gene marker loci.

H-2K and H-2D genes code for serologically defined cell surface antigens on all cells. These cell surface glycoproteins contain galactose, glucosamine, mannose, fucose, and sialic acid. These antigens are consistently associated with tissue graft rejection between genetically different individuals. They are involved in the induction and effector stages of T-cell-mediated cytotoxicity (T-cell killer function).[8] Incompatibility of these loci is associated with rapid allograft rejection 10 to 14 days after the first graft and 5 to 6 days after the second.

Human HLA Complex. The human major histocompati-

Table 2–2. *HLA Specificities Recognized by the World Health Organization (Unofficial)*

HLA-A	HLA-B	HLA-C
A1	B5	CW1
A2	B7	CW2
A3	B8	CW3
A9	B12	CW4
A10	B13	CW5
A11	B14	CW6
AW19	B15	CW7
AW23	BW16	CW8
AW24	B17	
A25	B18	
A26	BW21	**HLA-D**
A28	BW22	
A29	B27	DW1
AW30	BW35	DW2
AW31	B37	DW3
AW32	BW38	DW4
AW33	BW39	DW5
AW34	B40	DW6
AW36	BW41	DW7
AW43	BW42	DW8
	BW44	DW9
	BW45	DW10
	BW46	DW11
	BW47	DW12
	BW48	
	BW49	
	BW50	**HLA-DR**
	BW51	
	BW52	DR1
	BW53	DR2
	BW54	DR3
	BW55	DR4
	BW56	DR5
	BW57	DRW6
	BW58	DR7
	BW59	DRW8
	BW60	DRW9
	BW61	
	BW62	DRW10
	BW63	
	BW4	
	BW6	

(Courtesy of Dr. Nicole Suciu-Foca, College of Physicians & Surgeons, Columbia University, New York.)

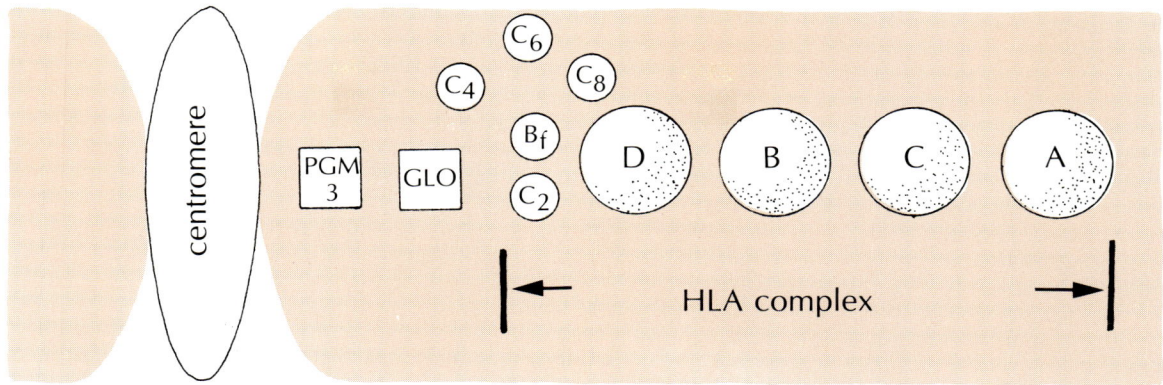

Figure 2–6. Schematic representation of the HLA complex of man (A, C, B, D) on the short arm of chromosome 6. Complement components (C2, C4, C6, C8, and Bf) are closely associated complement genes. Other nearby gene markers include phosphoglucomutase (PGM3) and glyoxalase (GLO).

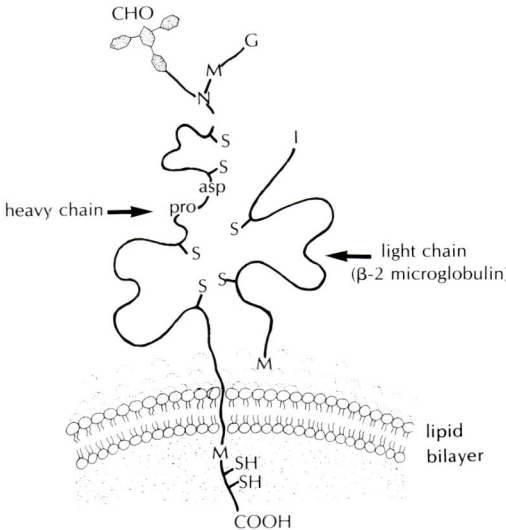

Figure 2–7. The structure of HLA-B7 antigen. (Modified from Orr, et al.: Structure studies of the membrane-associated products of the human major histocompatibility complex. *In* Aging, Cancer, and Cell Membranes. Edited by C. Borek, C.M. Fenoglio, and D.W. King. New York, Thieme-Stratton, 1980.)

bility complex (MHC or HLA complex) is an estimated series of 1000 genes found on chromosome 6, divided into 4 major loci (A, B, C, and D), which code for special cell surface glycoproteins known as HLA antigens (Table 2–2 and Fig. 2–6). Recent work indicates the presence of another specialized locus, the DR locus.[9]

Differences among the HLA glycoproteins in individuals provide the antigenic basis for tissue transplant rejection as well as for regulatory effects on immune responsiveness and disease susceptibility. The A, B, and C antigens are defined serologically, whereas D-locus markers can currently be recognized only by an in vitro lymphocyte culture test.

HLA-A, -B, and -C genes are closely linked, distinct gene loci that code for serologically detectable histocompatibility antigens. There are many antigen specificities at the A and B loci. Each locus also has certain alleles—two or more contrasting genes situated in the same locus in homologous chromosomes—with unofficial, unconfirmed designations ("W" or workshop) or blanks where the alleles have as yet to be defined.

HLA antigens are glycoproteins consisting of a "heavy" polypeptide chain (MW 45,000 daltons) noncovalently attached to a "light" chain (β-2 microglobulin) of 12,000 MW. That significant homology exists between β-2 microglobulin and immunoglobulin domains suggests an evolutionary or structural relationship between the HLA antigens and immunoglobulins[10] (Fig. 2–7).

The majority of the HLA antigen is outside the cell membrane, including the entire light chain and 75% of the heavy chain. The heavy chain is anchored in the cell membrane by a region of hydrophobic amino acids that passes through the membrane.[11]

These HLA antigens are integral proteins found in the plasma membrane of lymphocytes, platelets, and sperm.

These antigens are also found in cells of liver, intestine, lung, kidney, heart, as well as in saliva and serum.

The roles of the HLA antigens have been of primary interest with respect to their relationship to disease susceptibility.[12] Transplantation involves the interaction of serologically defined HLA antigens of the ABC gene loci, the ABO antigens, and the products of the D locus.

The HLA-D region contains 8 alleles controlling a strong mixed lymphocyte reaction (MLR) and coding for tissue matching antigens for transplantation. A second locus in the region of HLA-A may also stimulate low level MLR proliferative cell responses. HLA-DR antigens may be coded for by HLA-D or by a separate gene locus. In particular, antigens of MW 29,000 and 34,000 have been recovered from human lymphoblastoid B cells and are known as the HLA-DR antigens. They now have also been found in a variety of human tissues. These antigens appear to function analogously to murine Ia antigens as antigen receptors, in cell-cell interactions, or as self-recognition determinants.[13] The MB and MT antigens are a new group of B-cell alloantigens closely associated with HLA-DR antigens and may be a critical factor for survival of kidney transplants.[14]

HLA in Immune Disease. Certain authors have suggested theoretic mechanisms of the association of HLA with disease (Figs. 2–8 and 2–9). These include the following: (1) HLA antigens may function as cell surface receptors for viruses or toxins; (2) the similarity of configuration of viruses or toxins to HLA antigens (the molecular mimicry hypothesis) might render a host tolerant to specific injurious agents; (3) defective T-cell cytotoxicity may be induced by HLA-A or B; (4) immune response (Ir) and immune suppression (Is) genes in linkage disequilibrium with HLA-A, -B, or -D, may mediate production of a disease; and (5) disease susceptibility may be affected by abnormal structural genes for C components linked to the histocompatibility antigens. These genes affect cell-cell recognition and interactions and may modulate the pathogenesis of disease upon exposure to particular viruses, toxins, or environmental agents.[15]

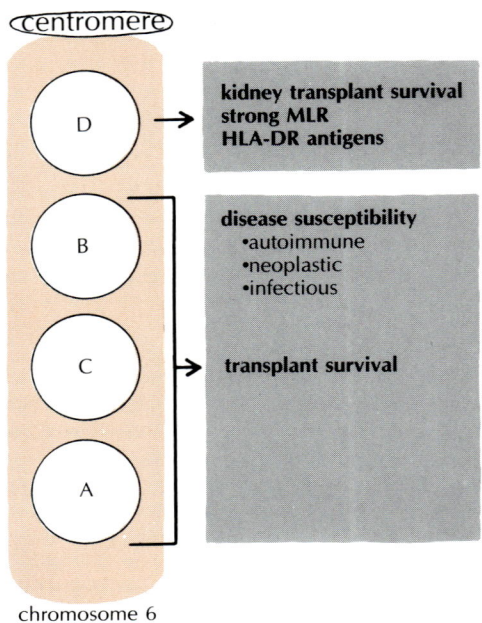

Figure 2–8. This figure depicts functions of cellular recognition and interaction controlled by the human HLA complex. (MLR, mixed lymphocyte reaction.)

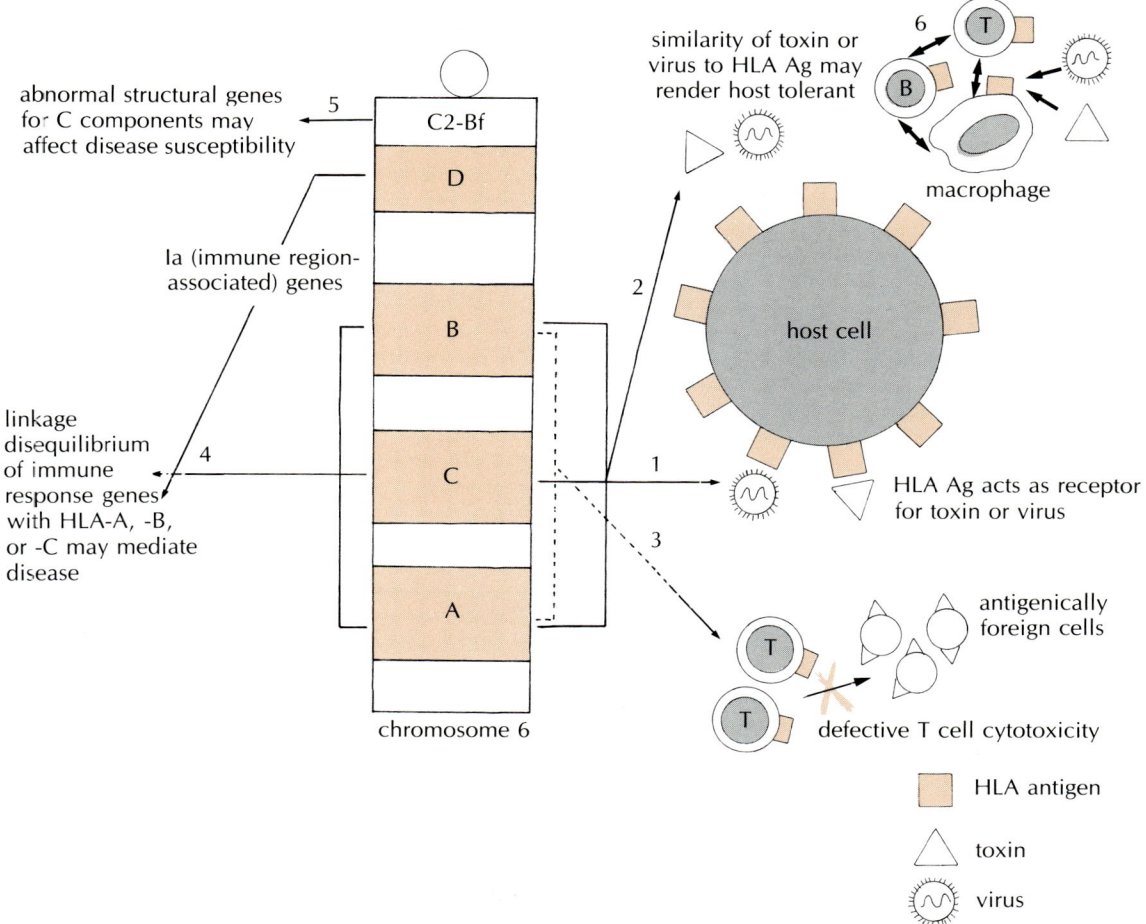

Figure 2-9. This schematic representation shows various roles of the HLA system in disease. (For details on numbers 1 to 6, see text.)

Although diseases of all organ systems have been associated with certain HLA antigens, clustering occurs in the skeletal, cutaneous, neuromuscular, endocrine, and gastrointestinal systems (Table 2-3). There is variation in strength and specificity of these associations. The strongest association, that between ankylosing spondylitis and HLA-B27, is so strong that it serves as a valuable aid to the diagnosis of this disorder even before characteristic x-ray changes develop. In comparison to those lacking antigen B27, persons with B27 have a hundredfold greater risk of developing ankylosing spondylitis, though only an eightfold greater risk of developing psoriatic arthritis.[16]

Specific HLA associations with diseases are especially well known, aside from that of ankylosing spondylitis and B27. Rheumatic heart disease as well as certain congenital cardiac malformations are associated with A2. Linkage disequilibrium is nonrandom association on the same chro-

Table 2–3. *Association of Disease with HLA*

Disease	HLA Antigen
Addison's disease	B8, DW3
Pernicious anemia	B7
Ankylosing spondylitis Reiter's disease, Uveitis, Reactive arthritis	B27
Arthritis	
Juvenile	DW4
Adult	B27
Rheumatoid	A2, CW3, DRW4, DR27
Celiac disease	A1, B8, BW35, DR23
Diabetes (Juvenile-onset, insulin-dependent only)	B8, BW15, DW3, DRW3, DRW4
Hemochromatosis	A3, B14
Hepatitis (chronic)	DRW3
Multiple sclerosis	A3, B7, DW2, DRW2
Myasthenia gravis	A1, B8, DRW8, DRW4
Psoriasis	CW6, B13
Retinoblastoma	B12, BW35
Sjögren's syndrome	B8
Thyrotoxicosis	
Caucasian	B8
Japanese	BW35

(Modified, with permission, from the Annual Review of Medicine, Volume 28. © by Annual Reviews, Inc.)

mosome of specific alleles at two closely linked loci. The extent to which an association exists between two alleles on a haplotype is measured by a value called Δ, which is equal to the difference between the observed frequency of the haplotype and the expected frequency. Linkage disequilibrium is displayed in the association of A2, CW3, DRW4, and DR27 with juvenile rheumatoid arthritis. In fact, a well-known triad in such linkage disequilibrium is the A1-B8-DW3 combination, which has associations with celiac disease, juvenile diabetes mellitus, myasthenia gravis, Addison's disease, Sjögren's syndrome, chronic active hepatitis, Graves' disease, and possibly systemic lupus erythematosus (SLE) (Table 2–3).

Although new implications of the HLA system in the mediation of hundreds of diseases exist, we are just realizing the complexity of HLA involvement with many other poorly identified genetic and environmental factors. HLA typing of donor and recipient in kidney and other tissue transplantation has received much clinical attention in the past. Recent advances in the treatment of bone marrow aplasias and other immunodeficiency states suggest the importance of HLA typing in successful bone marrow transplantation.[17]

Blood Group Antigens. The widely recognized need for blood donors with specific blood types to avoid transfusion reactions to foreign proteins illustrates the importance of identifying antigenic differences among cells. Red blood cells have specific glycoprotein molecules on their surfaces

Table 2–4. *Common Blood Groups*

Blood Group System	Antigens
ABO	(A, B, AB)
Rh	(Rh_1, R_1), (Rh_z, R_z), (Rh_2, R_2), (Rh_o, R_0)
	(rh, r) (rh', R'), (Rh_y, R_y)
MN	(M, N, Mn)
Ss	(S, s, Ss)
P	$(P_1, P_2,$ p)
Lutheran	(Lu^a, Lu^b)
Kell	(K^+, K^-)
Lewis	(Le^a, Le^b)
Kidd	(Jk^a, Jk^b)

(Modified from Davis, B., et al.: Microbiology. 3rd Ed. New York, Harper & Row, 1980.)

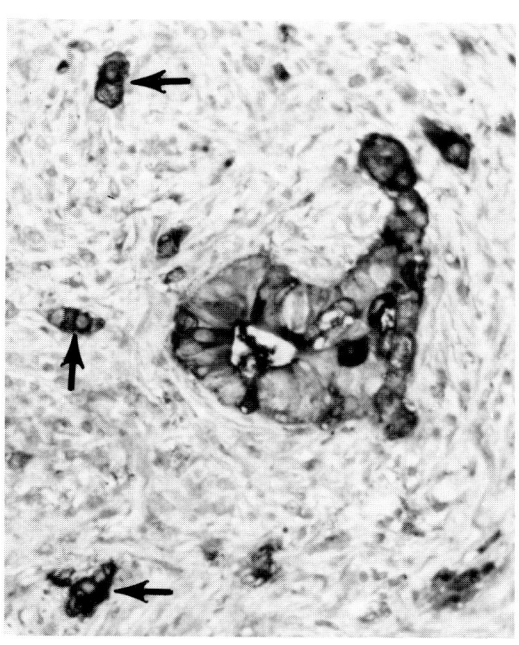

Figure 2–10. Immunoperoxidase demonstration of carcinoembryonic antigen in colon cancer cells. The glandular structure and isolated malignant cells (arrows) are positive.

that fall into several antigenic blood groups. The major groups making up the ABO system are A, AB, B, and O, although over 400 separate subgroups of blood types have been identified in several species and over 60 major blood groups are well known (Table 2–4).[18]

Tumor Antigens. These antigens may be of various types. Autochthonous tumors that arise spontaneously share antigens with other tumors of a similar histologic type. *Virally* induced tumors have cross-reacting antigenic determinants, and *chemically* induced neoplasms have unique or shared antigens.

Tumor-associated antigens *(TAA)* function as weak transplantation antigens and, therefore, are capable of eliciting immune responses. Differentiation or oncofetal antigens may be unmasked during neoplastic transformation; one is called *carcinoembryonic* antigen (CEA) (Fig. 2–10). These are poor immunogens because they were present in the host during embryonic life and failed to elicit an immune response.[19]

Antibodies

Structure

Antibodies are molecules that recognize antigens. They are members of the class of glycoproteins known as immunoglobulins (Ig) and are composed of 4 polypeptide chains: 2 identical *light chains*, each with about 214 amino acids, and 2 identical *heavy chains*, each containing about 440 amino acids (Fig. 2–11). The light chains contain 2 domains: a variable *V domain* and a constant *C domain*. The heavy chain has a variable domain and 3 constant domains. Immunoglobulins IgE and IgM each have 4 constant domains. The carboxyl-terminal (C-terminal) portions of the light and heavy chains are called the constant regions. These regions are nearly identical for antibodies in the same class.

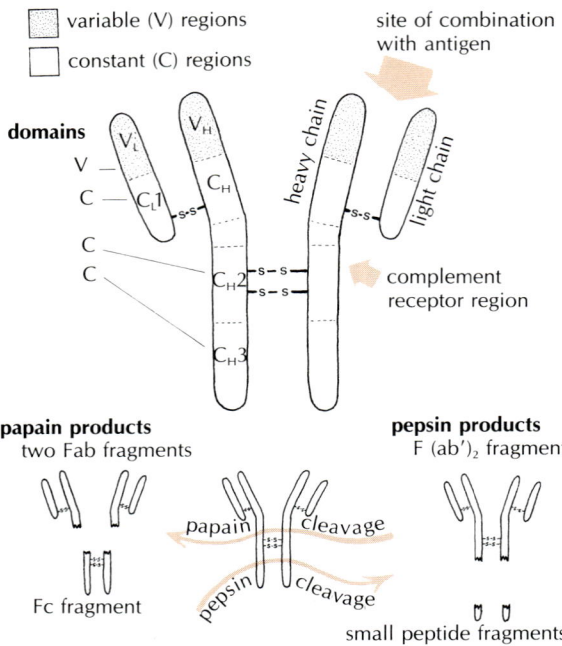

variable (V) regions

constant (C) regions

site of combination with antigen

domains

V

C

C

C

papain products
two Fab fragments

Fc fragment

pepsin products
F (ab')₂ fragment

papain cleavage

pepsin cleavage

small peptide fragments

Figure 2–11. The structure and components of the immunoglobulin (Ig) molecule. Cleavage of immunoglobulins by papain results in three fragments, two of which are univalent and can bind antigen (fragment antigen binding or Fab) to form soluble, non-precipitating, complexes. The third fragment (Fc) does not bind antigen. Pepsin cleavage produces a divalent fragment (F(ab')₂, which can precipitate with antigen. Amino acid sequences of various regions (domains) of the antibody molecule have been identified by enzymatic digestions.

The amino-terminal *(N-terminal)* portions of the light and heavy chains show significant differences in their amino acid sequences among individual species of antibodies. These are the variable regions of the light and heavy chains and combine to form the antibody combining site. The valence of the antibody is the number of titered antigen-binding sites per molecule. The affinity of the combining site is a measure of the strength of the antibody binding to the antigen.[20]

About 65% of the variable region of the heavy chain shows limited sequence variation, and 25 amino acid positions are absolutely *invariant*. There are also a number of *hypervariable regions*.[21] Broad areas of hypervariability comprise residues 24 to 25, 50 to 56, 89 to 97 in the light chain and 31 to 35, 50 to 65, and 95 to 102 in the heavy chain. These hypervariable regions are intimately associated with the antibody combining site.

The variable and constant regions of the heavy and light chains have the respective functions of antigen recognition and effector function. The *variable* regions of light and heavy chains fold and associate in such a way that the hypervariable regions are brought together to form large, antigen-binding surfaces. Different shapes of the antigen-binding surfaces have been found by x-ray crystallography. In addition, immunoglobulin folds have also been found to exist within the domains of the immunoglobulin chains.

Proteolytic digestion by trypsin, pepsin, or papain causes cleavage of the Ig molecules among globular domains. Cleavage of IgG by papain breaks the hinge region of the heavy chain into three fragments: two identical *Fab (antigen-binding fragments)* and one *Fc* portion. The latter contains the complement-binding site and the carbohydrate-binding site (Fig. 2–11).

Immunoglobulin Classes

The heterogeneous nature of serum immunoglobulins is appreciated when the serum of animals is studied by electrophoresis or by determination of the molecular weight of its components.

Five major classes of immunoglobulins are known: *IgG, IgM, IgA, IgD,* and *IgE*. The names of the classes are derived from the heavy chains: IgG (γ), IgM (μ), IgA (α), IgD (δ), and IgE (ε). The light chains are one of two types, κ or λ.

Table 2–5. *Characteristics of Immunoglobulins*

	IgG	IgA	IgM	IgD	IgE
Molecular weight	150,000	160,000	900,000	?150,000	190,000
Sedimentation coefficient	7S	7S	19S	7S	probably 7S
Number of antibody combining sites (valence)	2	2	5 or 10	probably 2	probably 2
Heavy chain type	γ	α	μ	δ	ε
Light chain type	κ,λ	κ,λ	κ,λ	κ,λ	κ,λ

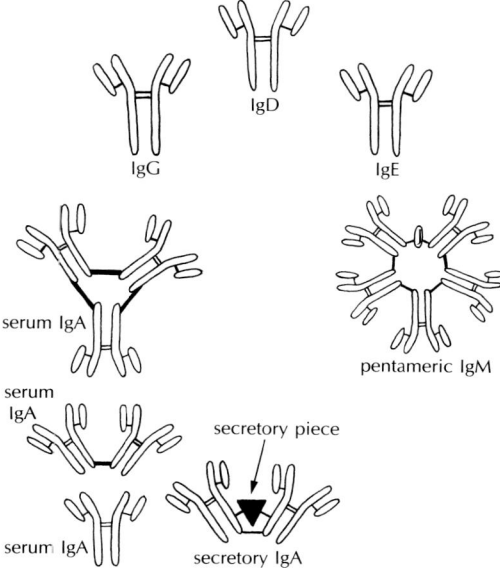

Figure 2–12. Comparative structures of the immunoglobulins.

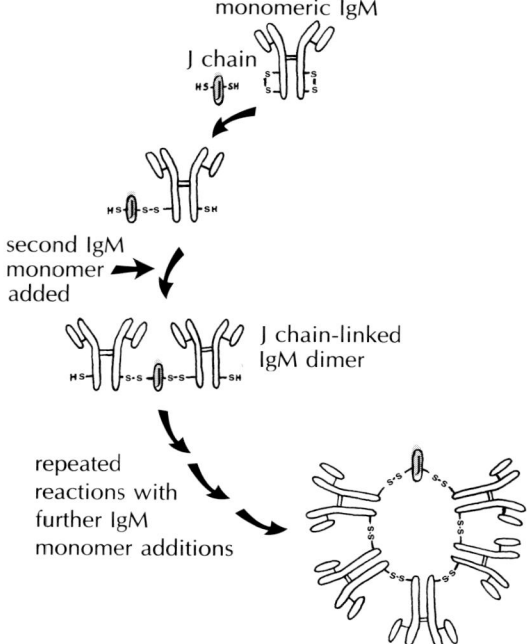

Figure 2–13. The mechanism of polymerization of pentameric IgM by disulfide linkage. (Modified from Chapius and Koshland, 1974.)

Each of these classes has specific molecular characteristics and functions (Table 2–5).

The immunoglobulin usually present in largest quantity is IgG, which is composed of two identical light chains (23,000 MW) and two identical heavy chains (53,000 MW). The dimer of light chain-heavy chain pairs (L-H)$_2$ is the basic structural unit of all other Ig molecules. The structures of the other classes and subclasses (IgG$_{1,2,3,4}$ and two subclasses of IgA) differ in the number and position of the disulfide bridges between the heavy chains.

Polymeric Immunoglobulins

Several of the immunoglobulins may exist in either monomeric or polymeric states (Fig. 2–12). IgA exists as a monomer on the cell and may be a dimer or a trimer in the serum. When found in tissue, IgA is often a dimer connected by a glycoprotein secretory piece. IgM exists as a monomer on the cell, but as a pentamer in the serum.

Pentameric IgM is the earliest antibody formed as a primary response to antigen. The presence of a linking component known as the J chain in the polymeric immunoglobulin (absent from the monomeric molecules), suggests that this J chain is important in the polymerization process (Fig. 2–13).

The *J chain* has a molecular weight of 25,000 and is folded within the polymeric structure so that few of its antigen determinants are exposed. J chains are biochemically identical among different Ig classes, but they are biochemically unique with respect to the rest of the Ig molecule. Interactions of SH groups of the J chain and monomeric (and later polymeric) Ig molecules allow the synthesis of the polymeric forms of immunoglobulin (IgA and IgM).[22]

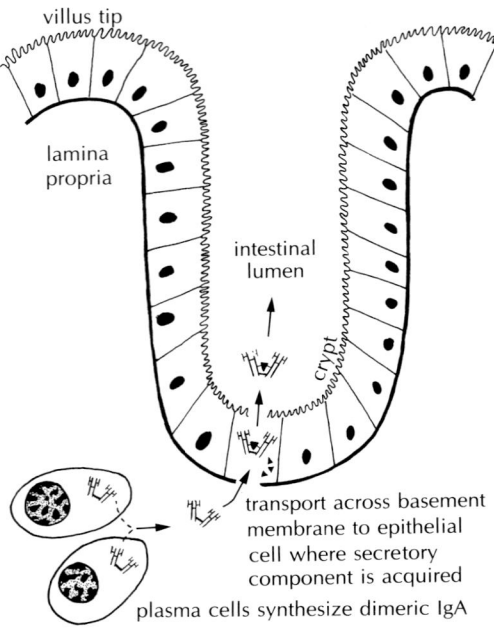

villus tip

lamina
propria

intestinal
lumen

crypt

transport across basement
membrane to epithelial
cell where secretory
component is acquired

plasma cells synthesize dimeric IgA

Figure 2–14. The mechanism of secretory IgA transport in the intestine.

Secretory Immunoglobulins

Subpopulations of immunoglobulin-secreting cells (immunocytes) exist in tissues. Within the submucosa of the gastrointestinal tract, respiratory tract, and salivary glands, immunocytes are present and produce dimeric IgA molecules connected by a J chain. These molecules later appear at the apices of columnar cells of the crypts of the gastrointestinal tract. The mucosal epithelial cells produce a glycoprotein called the *secretory component*, which has a specific affinity for two Ig molecules, the dimeric IgA and pentameric IgM[23] (Fig. 2–14).

The synthesis and transport of polymeric antibodies, IgA and IgM, into intestinal secretions have been carefully studied. IgA and IgM are synthesized in local plasma cells in the intestinal submucosa. Following release, IgA is assembled with J chains to form dimeric molecules in the crypt region. These molecules then diffuse through the basement membrane and are taken up into intestinal epithelium by a specific intracellular glycoprotein carrier system. Then they are linked to the secretory component and are released from the epithelial surface into secretions in the gut lumen by reverse pinocytosis.[24]

Complement

Complement makes up 10% of the serum globulins and consists of 9 major fractions that are important in antigen-antibody interaction. Complement is synthesized by various

Table 2–6. *Properties of the Complement Components*

Name	Molecular Weight
Classic pathway	
C1q	400,000
C1r	170,000
C1s	90,000
C2	117,000
C4	206,000
C3	180,000
C5	180,000
C6	95,000
C7	110,000
C8	163,000
C9	80,000
Alternate pathway	
Properdin	185,000
Factor B	95,000
C3 proactivator (C3PA)	
Factor D	25,000
C3 proactivator convertase (C3Pase)	
Complement regulators	
C1 inactivator	105,000
C3b inactivator	100,000
Anaphylatoxin inactivator	300,000

(Modified from Fudenberg, H.H., et al. (Eds.): Basic and Clinical Immunology. Los Altos, CA, Lange Medical Publications, 1976.)

Table 2–7. *Biologic Activities of Complement Components*

C1	Increase in association of Ag-Ab complexes
C3a	Chemotactic factor, anaphylatoxin
C3b	Adherence via receptor on lymphocytes and phagocytic cells—opsonin
	Activation of alternate pathway
	Stimulation of B lymphocytes to make mediators
	Stimulation of bone marrow leukocyte release
	Stimulation of release of Ag-Ab complexes from leukocyte surfaces
C5a	Chemotactic factor, anaphylatoxin
C5b67	Chemotactic factor, possible attack of unsensitized cells
C8	Slow membrane damage
C9	Rapid membrane damage

cells of the lymphoreticular system, particularly the liver, bone marrow, intestine, and spleen.[25] Some of the functional and biochemical properties of various complement components are indicated in Tables 2–6 and 2–7.

Gene Control of Complement

The major histocompatibility complex is important in the regulation of many immune reactions. We know that many of the complement genes appear to cluster on chromosome 6. The association of immune effector complement genes with the immune function MHC gene complex suggests a functional interaction between the two.[26]

Complement Activation: Classic Pathway

The complement system is triggered by the formation of antigen-antibody complexes, thereby initiating a cascade of proteolytic cleavage and protein-binding reactions. The distribution of antigens on cell surfaces has a major effect on complement activation and aggregation by IgG antibody. Certain components of complement interact with antigen and antibody to lyse cells. Complement is important in enhancing phagocytosis by opsonization (a process of adsorption of complement on leukocytes) and is also helpful in chemotaxis. It functions as an anaphylatoxin, triggering the kinin-mediated vasodilatation response, and acts as a parallel component of the coagulation system.[27]

Complement activation is a complex event that may be summarized as follows: (1) IgG or IgM binds to antigenic determinants on cells. (2) This binding exposes the complement-binding site of the Fc fragment of Ig. (3) C1q binds to the Ag-Ab complex. (4) This binding activates C1r, which cleaves C4. (5) The larger C4 fragment plus C1 cleaves C2 into C2a and C2b. (6) The C4b and C2a fragments (C3 convertase) combine to cleave C3 into C3a and C3b. C3a (MW 7000) is an anaphylatoxin, which dilates blood vessels

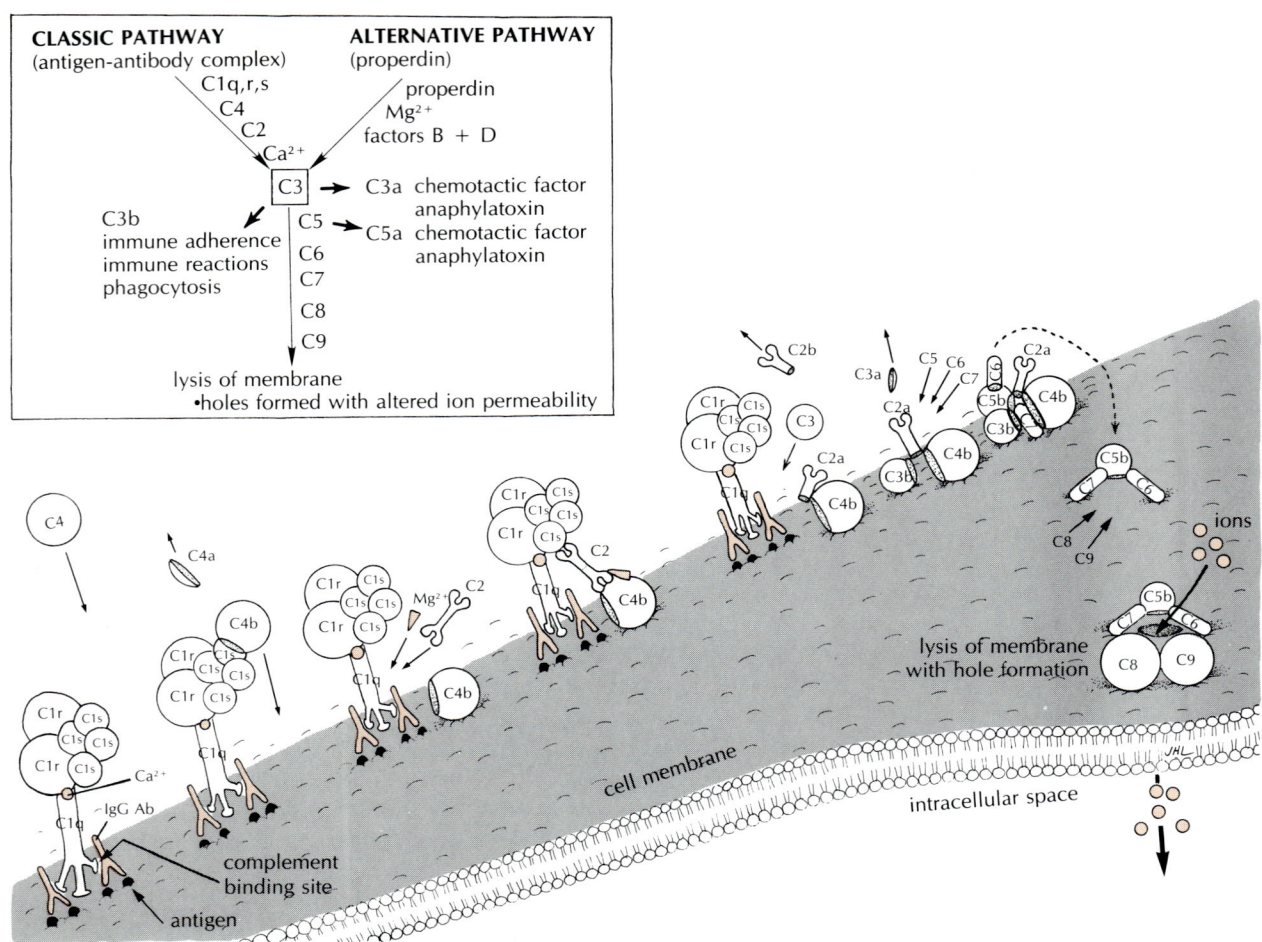

Figure 2–15. The complement (C) cascade.

and is also chemotactic for polymorphonuclear leukocytes. (7) C3b attaches to receptors over the entire cell membrane, promotes opsonization, and combines with the C4-C2 complex to cleave C5 into C5a and C5b. (8) C5b binds to the cell membrane and combines with C6 and C7 to form the C567 complex, which binds C8 and C9. The smaller C5a fragment acts like C3a. (9) C9 binding initiates lytic membrane damage by forming an ion-leakage pore[28] (Fig. 2–15).

The cell membrane is disrupted as the cell swells, and eventually osmotic lysis occurs. It has been suggested that complement acts as a detergent because the first event seen is the formation of a molecular grouping with a hydrophilic core in the cell membrane, surrounded by a hydrophobic rim. The hydrophobic rim interacts with lipid and thus interrupts the molecular bilayer. The disoriented lipid molecules allow free passage of water and soluble ions. The ultrastructural appearances of the membrane lesions resemble surface rings representing rearranged normal components of the membrane with formation of aggregates of

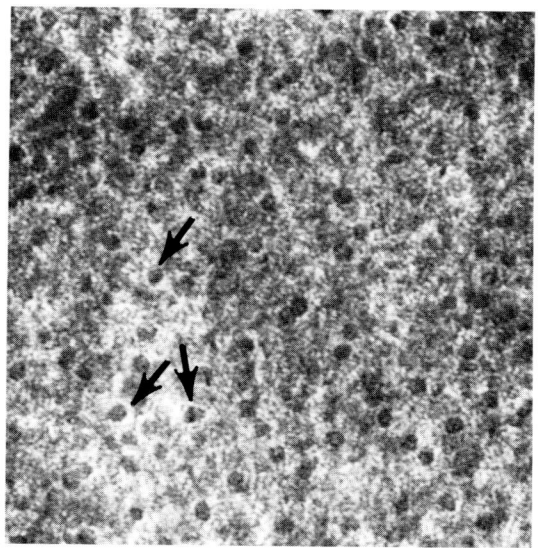

Figure 2–16. Negative staining demonstration of complement-mediated membrane lesions (holes) induced on a section of human red blood cell by the action of IgM antibody and human complement (arrows). (Courtesy of Charles H. Parkman and John P. Leddy, University of Rochester.)

globules and transient openings. These openings eventually permit osmotic lysis[29] (Fig. 2–16).

Complement Activation: Alternate Pathway

In 1954, Pillemer found an *alternate system* of complement activation, the *properdin system.*[30] This system is activated by aggregated IgG complexes, sugar moieties (for example, zymosan), and portions of bacterial membranes (that is, endotoxins). The alternate pathway of activation bypasses the need for antibody, C1, C4, or C2 and is important in the defense against gram-negative bacteria (Table 2–8 and Fig. 2–15).

Table 2–8. *Biologic Functions Following Alternate Pathway Activation*

Mediation of Arthus vasculitis

Leukotaxis

Platelet histamine release, lysis, and promotion of blood clotting in animals

Anaphylatoxin production

Immune adherence

Phagocytosis

Bactericidal activity

Erythrocyte lysis in paroxysmal nocturnal hemoglobinuria

Participation in renal damage of hypocomplementemic glomerulonephritis

The C3 convertase of the alternate pathway that cleaves C3 to C3a and C3b is formed at the cell membrane by interaction of the activating substance with factor D (an esterase analogous to C1s), factor B (analogous to C2a), C3, and Mg^{2+} ions and is stabilized by properdin. Once C3 cleavage occurs, C3b is then translocated to the cell surface with factors B and D. A second C3 convertase is bound to the cell surface and generates new polymolecular complexes containing two or more C3b molecules. C3b acts as a C5 convertase, which when stabilized by properdin itself, causes cleavage to C5a and C5b. The subsequent reactions, C5, C6, C7, C8, and C9, are identical to those in the classic pathway.[31]

Tissues of the Immune System

Thus far we have considered antigens, immunoglobulins, and complement, which function in immune responses. We have as yet to consider the cells concerned with interaction with antigen and antibody synthesis within the lymphoid organs, including the *central lymphoid tissues* (bone marrow and thymus) and the *peripheral lymphoid tissues* (spleen, ton-

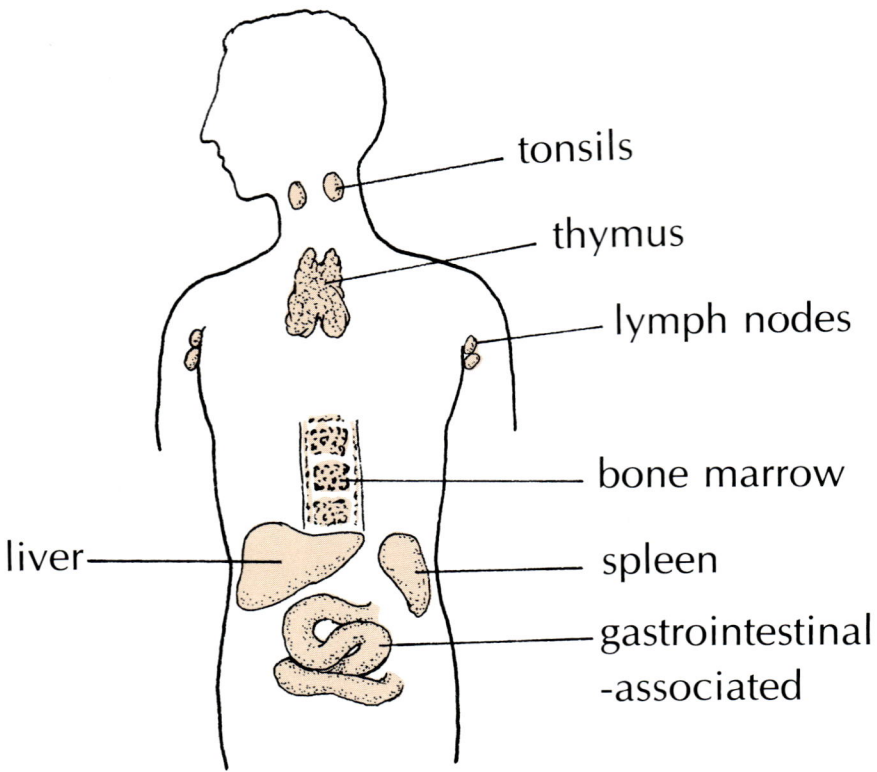

Figure 2–17. Tissues of the lymphoreticular system.

sils, lymph nodes, liver, and gastrointestinal tract)[32] (Fig. 2–17).

Bone Marrow

The bone marrow (Fig. 2–18) becomes populated with cells from the yolk sac early in fetal life. Immature stem cells proliferate there and give rise to leukocytic, erythrocytic, and megakaryocytic stem cells. During embryogenesis, the liver is the primary site of hematopoiesis.

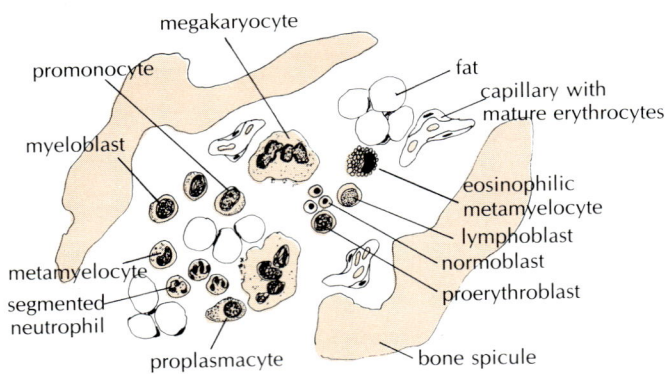

Figure 2–18. Cells of the bone marrow.

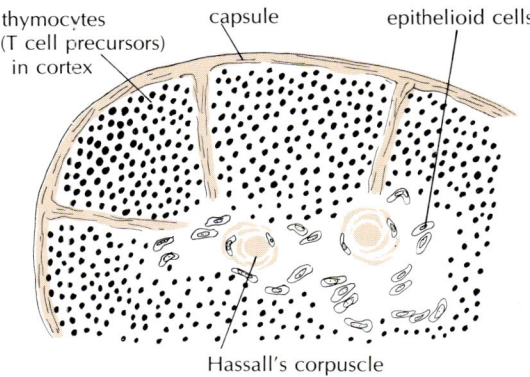

Figure 2–19. Thymus.

Thymus

The thymus (Fig. 2–19) arises from entoderm and mesoderm of the 3rd and 4th branchial pouches, which migrate into the mediastinum. Once the thymus is established, T-cell precursors from the bone marrow travel directly to it for further maturation by factors released by epithelial elements of the thymus. These cells rapidly acquire the surface markers and functional characteristics of mature thymocytes and later travel to predetermined T-cell domains in the peripheral lymphoid tissues.

The epithelium of the thymus presumably gives rise to some of the thymic hormones, including *thymopoietin* and *thymosin*. The latter substance was first identified by White and Goldstein, who noted its effect on T-cell maturation. One fraction of the thymic extract has been purified and contains a single active component. It is a polypeptide of 108 amino acids with a molecular weight of approximately 12,200 daltons. Eleven other active acidic polypeptides with molecular weights of 12,000 to 14,000 daltons have been identified.[33]

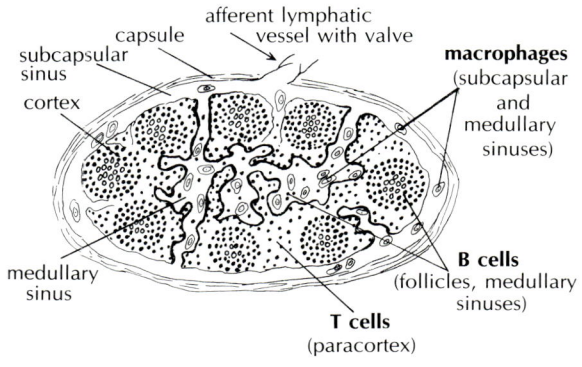

Figure 2–20. Lymph node.

Lymph Nodes

The resting lymph node (Fig. 2–20) is divided into *primary follicles* (B-cell regions) and an adjacent mantle of T-cells. The primary follicles are nodular aggregates of small lymphocytes within a network of dendritic macrophages. Lymphocytes enter the nodes through post-capillary venules and appear to recognize or be recognized by specific lymphocyte-endothelial cell-surface recognition units; then they return to their specific site in the nodes. The medulla also contains a reticular phagocytic network.

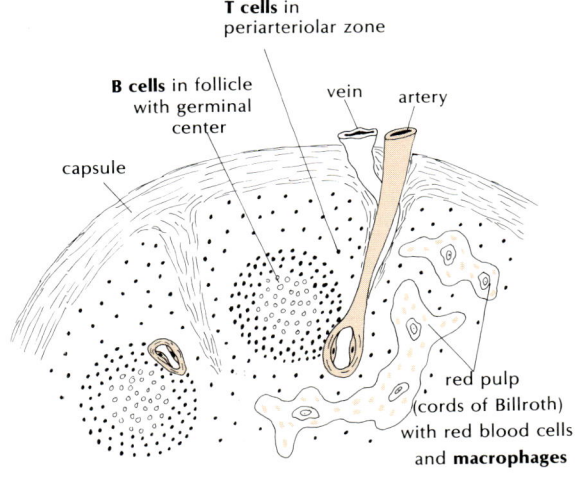

Figure 2–21. Spleen.

Spleen

The splenic architecture (Fig. 2–21) is analogous to that of the lymph nodes. The red pulp contains phagocytic macrophages, whereas the white pulp is the site of the lymphoid cells. The white pulp contains a central arteriole surrounded by a mantle of T lymphocytes and follicles of B cells. Lymphocytes enter the spleen from the circulation and travel to specific locales within it. B cells appear in the peripheral part of the periarteriolar sheath, the nearby splenic follicles, and the follicles and outer cortex of the lymph nodes. T cells lie in the central part of the periarteriolar sheath of the spleen and in the *paracortex* of lymph nodes (Fig. 2–20).[34]

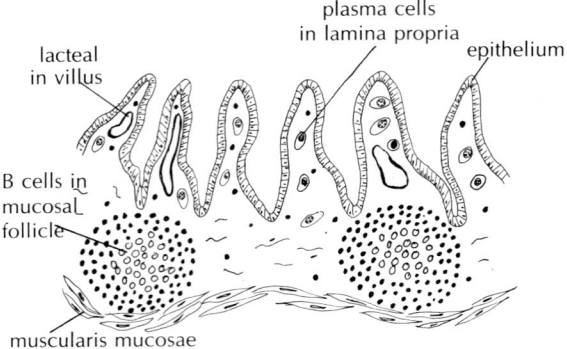

lacteal in villus — plasma cells in lamina propria — epithelium

B cells in mucosal follicle

muscularis mucosae

Figure 2–22. Peyer's patch (gastrointestinal-associated lymphoid tissue).

undifferentiated bone marrow stem cell

granuloblastic-monoblastic stem cell line — lymphoid stem cell line — erythroid stem cell line — megakaryocytic stem cell line

circulating monocytes and tissue histiocytes — granulocytes •neutrophilic •eosinophilic •basophilic — red blood cells — megakaryocyte with platelets

T cell   B cell

effector T cell   plasma cell

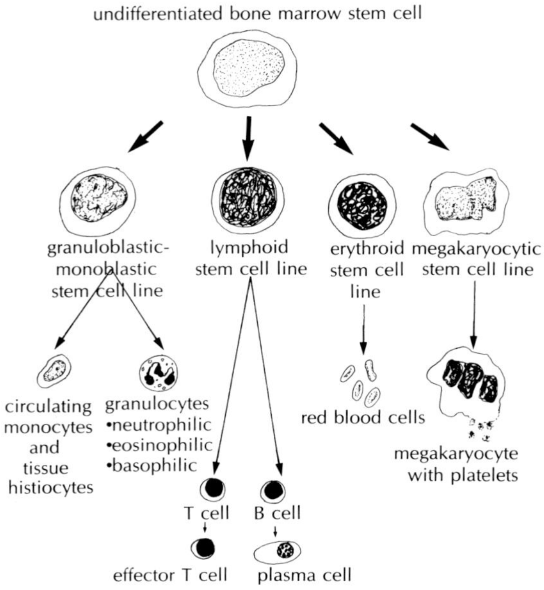

Figure 2–23. Stem cell lineage.

Gastrointestinal-Associated Lymphoid Tissue

The specialized lymphoid organs attached to the respiratory and gastrointestinal tracts include the adenoids, tonsils, *Peyer's patches* (Fig. 2–22), and appendix. These structures also have specialized postcapillary venules that serve as lymphocyte entry sites. The B cells and T cells migrate to their specific B and T domains within these tissues. We have already seen that these tissues have special roles with regard to the synthesis of the secretory immunoglobulins IgA and IgM (see Fig. 2–2).

Cells of the Immune System

The cells making up the immune system include stem cells, granulocytes, mast cells, lymphocytes, circulating monocytes, and tissue histiocytes.

Stem Cells

Undifferentiated stem cells are located in the bone marrow. Electron microscopic observations in the mouse have shown that these large basophilic cells have numerous mitochondria and free ribosomes, a well-defined Golgi apparatus, and a small amount of endoplasmic reticulum. These cells give rise to four major stem cell lines: *granuloblastic-monoblastic, lymphoid, erythroid,* and *megakaryocytic* stem cells (Fig. 2–23).

Granulocytes

Granulocytes normally comprise 60 to 70% of all white blood cells and consist of 3 classes: *polymorphonuclear leukocytes* (PMNs or neutrophils) whose principal function is phagocytosis and release of chemical mediators; *eosinophils,* which are also phagocytic and are involved especially in interactions with antigen-antibody complexes;[35] and *basophils,* with properties similar to those of mast cells.[36]

Mast Cells

Mast cells are found in the extravascular tissue and contain a host of chemical mediators for both immune and inflammatory responses, including histamine, serotonin, lysosomal enzymes, prostaglandin, and leukotrienes, alternately known as slow-reactive substance of anaphylaxis (SRS-A).[37]

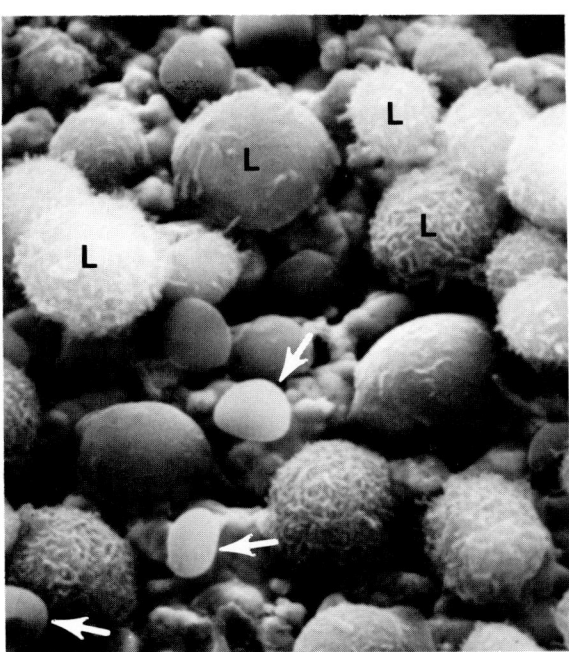

Figure 2–24. This scanning electron micrograph shows a mixed population of B and T lymphocytes (L) admixed with red blood cells (arrows).

Lymphocytes

All lymphocytes arise from a common lymphoid stem cell in the bone marrow. They then migrate to either the thymus or the bursal equivalent to mature and acquire specific surface markers and functional characteristics of T and B cells respectively (Fig. 2–24 and Tables 2–9 and 2–10). Cells without markers are called *null* cells.[38]

Table 2–9. *Distribution of Lymphocytes*

	B Cells (%)	T Cells (%)
Thymus	0	100
Thoracic duct lymph	15	85
Blood	10	90
Lymph nodes	30	70
Spleen	60	40
Bone marrow	40	? 60

Table 2–10. *Function of T and B Cells*

T Cells
  Help in antibody production by B cells
  Production of lymphokines
  Delayed hypersensitivity
    Reaction against intracellular bacteria, viruses, and parasites
  Killer T lymphocytes in cell-mediated immunity
    Allograft rejection
    Graft versus host reaction

B Cells
  Production of humoral antibodies IgM, IgG, IgA, IgD, and IgE

B Lymphocytes. B cells differentiate under the influence of the bursal equivalent, which may be the bone marrow. These cells then migrate to peripheral lymphoid organs, spleen (25 to 30%), tonsils, lymph nodes (10 to 20%), and gastrointestinal-associated lymphoid tissue. B cells are precursors to the major antibody secretory cells, i.e., differentiated plasma cells. They have Ia Ag, as do macrophages and activated T cells.[39]

T Lymphocytes. Other lymphoid stem cells pass to the thymus, where they are converted to thymocytes and, finally, to T cells. This process has been studied extensively in mice by Shortman and Jackson. They showed that most thymocytes (90%) are localized in the cortical region of the thymus. These cells displayed high levels of cortisone sensitivity and absence of immunologic activity. Another thymocyte subpopulation (10%) was present in the medullary area. These thymocytes were both cortisone-resistant and immunocompetent.[40] Although both the minor thymic subpopulation and the peripheral T lymphocytes in the mouse have similar properties (high level of *H-2 antigens*, low level of θ-*surface antigens*, and *cortisone resistance*), Asofsky found that they are functionally unique.[41]

The T lymphocytes that circulate in the blood are responsible for the major cell-mediated responses of the body. The classic example of these responses is the delayed hypersensitivity reaction in tuberculosis. These lymphocytes are also responsible for graft and tumor rejection, for the elaboration of soluble factors known as *lymphokines*, and for the initiation and suppression of antibody synthesis, in conjunction with B cells and macrophages.

Functional tests indicate that T cells may be divided into two major classes: *helper T cells* (T_H), which assist in B-cell activation, and *suppressor T cells* (T_s), which inhibit B-cell activation and regulate immune responses. T-cells secrete lymphokines and other factors. Suppressor-cytotoxic T cells (T_{killer} or $T_{cytotoxic}$ cells) may be stimulated to destroy tumors and allografts. These reactions are all antigen-dependent.[42]

Lymphokines. Activated *T lymphocytes* release a number of polypeptides called *lymphokines*. These substances activate other lymphocytes and macrophages, prevent their departure from the antigenic site, and stimulate the proliferation of other lymphocytes. Lymphocytes also produce *lymphotoxins*, which are nonspecifically cytolytic, arming factors, and agents such as *interferon* that interfere with viral replication (Table 2–11). Interferon may also have regulatory effects on T cells.[43]

Soluble mediators may also be produced by macrophages *(macrokines)* as well as B or T cells.[44] All are collectively known as *monokines*. Lymphocyte-activating factor pro-

Table 2–11. *Monokines and Their Properties*

Factor	Biologic Activity
Basophil chemotactin	Attraction of basophils
Eosinophil chemotactin	Attraction of eosinophils following interaction with immune complexes
Macrophage chemotactin	Attraction of macrophages
Neutrophil chemotactin	Attraction of neutrophils
Lymphocyte chemotactin	Attraction of other lymphocytes
Interferon	Antimicrobial activity
Macrophage activation factor (MAF)	Enhancing of macrophage motility and phagocytosis—arming of killer macrophages
Migration inhibition factor (MIF)	Prevention of macrophage migration in vitro
Mitogenic factor	Cause of blast transformation of lymphocytes
Interleukin I (produced by macrophages)	Lymphocyte-activating factor
Interleukin II (T-cell growth factor)	Stimulation of growth of T cell
Colony-stimulating factor (macrophage)	Stimulation of growth of lymphocytes

(Modified from Cohen, S.: The role of cell-mediated immunity in the induction of inflammatory responses. Am. J. Pathol., *88*:502, 1977.)

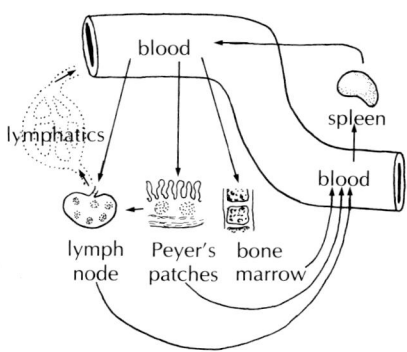

Figure 2–25. Recirculation of lymphocytes.

duced by macrophages stimulates synthesis of lymphokines in thymocytes.

Lymphocyte Recirculation. Small lymphocytes continually recirculate among the peripheral blood, the lymph nodes, and the thoracic duct (Fig. 2–25). The majority enter lymph nodes, bone marrow, spleen, and Peyer's patches. They then return to the blood and go to the spleen. These recirculation patterns occur within minutes. It is reasonable to assume that such rapid recirculation guarantees that these cells come into frequent contact with, and may synergistically interact with, other cell types.[45]

The various organs of the body have characteristic lymphocyte subpopulations, as we have described earlier. Discrepancies are found in the literature with regard to quantification, however, especially with regard to T cells, for which statistics obtained may reflect the specific assay methods used.

Identification of Lymphocyte Subpopulations. In mice, subpopulations of lymphocytes have been identified according to membrane antigen markers called $LyT_{1,2,3}$, TL, and Thy. They are found in specific parts of the lymph node and are associated with specific functions. The sites and their functions are noted in Tables 2–12 and 2–13.

Individual human B and T cells cannot be separated easily on a morphologic basis, although there appear to be some ultrastructural distinctions.[46] We know that there are several populations of helper T and suppressor T cells.

Table 2–12. *Sites of T-Cell Subclasses in Mice*

	Antigens		
	TL	Thy	Lyt
Bone marrow stem cells	–	–	LyT$^-$
Thymus	+	+	LyT1,2,3$^+$
Lymph node (cortex, paracortex)	–	+	LyT1$^+$
Lymph node (medulla)	–	+	LyT2,3$^+$

(From Cantor, H.: Personal communication. Cancer Biology I Seminar: Etiology, Diagnosis and Treatment. Aspen, Colorado, Institute of Pathobiology, July 23 to 27, 1979.)

Table 2–13. *Biologic Properties of T Cells in Mice*

Biologic Features	Ly1,2,3$^+$	Ly1$^+$	Ly2,3$^+$
Alloantigen recognition in MLC	+	+	+
Killer activity (in vivo) (T$_K$)	–	–	+
Helper amplifier potential with B cells (T$_H$)	(–)	+	–

(Modified from Cantor, H., and Boyse, E.A.: Functional subclasses of T lymphocytes bearing different Ly antigens. II. Cooperation between subclasses of Ly+ cells in the generation of killer activity. J. Exp. Med., *141*:1390, 1975.)

Lymphocytes have surface characteristics and functional properties that aid in their identification. The surface characteristics may relate to the presence of specific membrane markers or surface charges.[47]

Recently, basic biochemical differences have been described between the membranes of B cells and T cells, specifically the phospholipid and glycoprotein contents of the two cell types. T-cells have a preponderance of N-acetylgalactosamine and N-acetylglucosamine. B cells have a more even representation of fucose, mannose, glucose, galactosamine, N-acetylglucosamine, N-acetylgalactosamine, and N-acetylneuraminic acid.[48] These differences may allow the T cells and B cells to home selectively to differing sites and may also account for the differences in surface charges between the two populations of cells. Even these properties may not always be helpful in distinguishing B from T cells because these populations can be heterogeneous with respect to both function and surface markers.

Null Cells

Using surface markers, a third type of lymphocyte, a "null cell" or natural killer (N_K) cell, distinct from B and T cells, has been demonstrated. It is unclear whether null cells are a separate lineage of lymphocytes or merely immature T cells or B cells that have not yet acquired their full complement of cell surface markers. A second group of cytotoxic null cells (N_C) acts against leukemia, and a third type of null cell may destroy cells with the aid of antibody-dependent cellular cytotoxicity (ADCC). These cells lack B-cell membrane immunoglobulin, but have another B-cell marker, Ia antigen, and account for about 10% of circulating lymphocytes.[49]

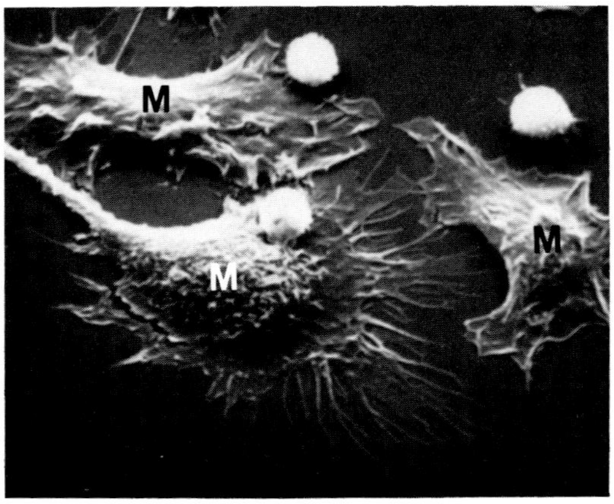

Monocytes and Histiocytes

The monoblastic stem cell differentiates from a monoblastic-granuloblastic stem cell and becomes either a *circulating monocyte* or a morphologically indistinguishable, fixed *tissue histiocyte*. Both are macrophages. The fixed tissue histiocyte is found lining the sinusoids of the spleen, lymph nodes, liver, and bone marrow.[50]

Mononuclear phagocytes *(macrophages)* (Fig. 2–26) have five properties (Fig. 2–27). Their functions[51] are aided by the immune receptors on their surfaces, which facilitate phagocytic processes. The first of these processes is phagocytosis of damaged cells and cellular debris. In this capacity, macrophages function in the normal debridement of wounds. Second, they are the first line of defense against facultative and obligate intracellular parasites. Third, macrophages interact with lymphocytes, particularly in presenting antigen to T and B cells in antibody synthesis, and fourth, in the cytolysis of foreign cells. Finally, macro-

Figure 2–26. This scanning electron micrograph shows peritoneal macrophages (M) attached to a coverslip. Three lymphocytes are also present.

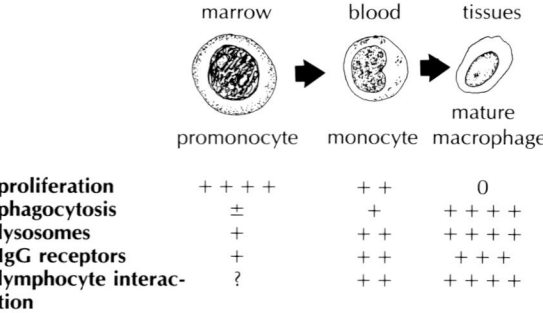

	marrow	blood	tissues
	promonocyte	monocyte	mature macrophage
proliferation	+ + + +	+ +	0
phagocytosis	±	+	+ + + +
lysosomes	+	+ +	+ + + +
IgG receptors	+	+ +	+ + +
lymphocyte interaction	?	+ +	+ + + +

Figure 2–27. Properties of the maturing monocyte. (Adapted from Cline and Golde.)

phages participate in the regulation and secretion of prostaglandins, other mediators, and enzymes.

Cell Surface Markers

The demonstration of surface markers has become a popular method of identifying lymphocytes because it allows their division into different subpopulations. These markers can be divided into two general categories: *surface receptors* and *surface antigens*. The former are recognized by their specific ability to bind certain labeled substances, whereas the latter are demonstrable by their reaction with specific antibodies directed at discrete membrane components.

Fc Receptors. These receptors are present on many mononuclear and nonmononuclear cells and are distributed along the cell membrane at 30-μm intervals.[52] Fc receptors may also be induced on cells that do not normally possess them by several of the DNA viruses, including herpes simplex virus (HSV), Epstein-Barr virus (EBV), and cytomegalovirus (CMV). The Fc receptor is important in cell-mediated cytotoxicity, a complement-dependent event with B-cell participation. Tumor cells coated with IgG subclasses confer a cytotoxic capacity on B cells in the presence of complement. This lysis is separate from complement-independent toxicity of T cells.

The presence of the Fc receptor on cells makes bacteria coated with specific antibody more readily phagocytized, especially in the presence of complement *(opsonization)* (see Fig. 2–38).

Under some circumstances, the binding of antibody to its target cell through the Fc receptor leads to release of specific cell products. For example, the binding of IgE to mast cells causes the release of histamine, SRS-A, and eosinophil chemotactic factor.[53]

Complement Receptors. These receptors are of two types and are structurally distinct. They have specificities for either *C3* or *C4* and are located on different molecules in the lymphocyte membrane.

Surface Immunoglobulin. The initial surface immunoglobulin (SIg) produced on B cells is either IgM, IgD, or both IgM and IgD and is recognized by heterologous antisera.[54] B cells may have both endogenous and exogenous immunoglobulins on their surfaces. The former are secreted by the individual cell; the latter are bound by Fc receptors.

These molecules are usually detected by the use of fluorescinated antibody techniques, labeling with ferritin, or lactoperoxidase iodination. Marchalonis also found an IgM-like molecule on the surface of T lymphocytes (IgT), but this evidence is controversial.[55] It has been shown that T cells may contain only a portion of the Ig molecule (that is, the variable region), which contains the antibody combining site.[56]

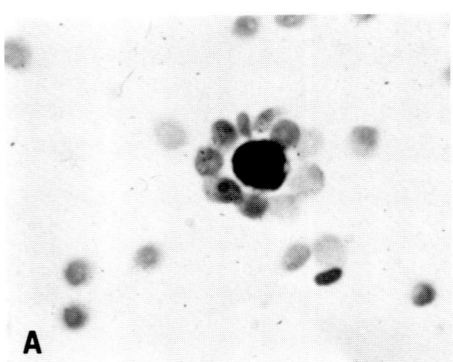

Figure 2–28. *A*, T lymphocyte rosette with sheep red blood cells.

Spontaneous Sheep Erythrocyte "E" Rosette. The most commonly used T-cell marker is the spontaneous sheep red blood cell *"E" rosette* (Fig. 2–28A). Not specific for T cells,[57] this marker is useful in classifying subpopulations of lymphocytes, especially in conjunction with other surface markers. Its formation is associated with OKT11 membrane receptor. In the presence of antibody (A) or complement (C) bound to B cells, sensitized red blood cells (erythrocytes or E) also form *"EA"* or *"EAC"* rosettes.

B-Cell Antigens. Recently, B-cell-specific antibodies have been identified in the sera of pregnant women. These sera recognize a set of antigens that used to be called SD-HLA antigens and are now referred to as DR antigens.

T-Cell Antigens. T cells have a number of specific surface antigens. The most common is the Thy antigen in the mouse; similar antigens are being investigated in humans. Recently, specific monoclonal human antibodies[58] to T-cell antigens have identified a specific function of T cells: OKT4 antibody binds helper T cells, whereas OKT8 antibody binds killer and suppressor T cells (Table 2–14).

Table 2–14. *Classification of OKT-Monoclonal Antibodies*

OKT1	T and B cells of chronic lymphocytic leukemia (CLL)
OKT3	T-cell antigen receptors
OKT4	Helper-inducer cells
OKT6	Cortical thymocytes
OKT8	Suppressor-killer cells
OKT9	Transferrin receptors
OKT10	Activated T cells, plasma cells
OKT11	E rosette receptor on T cells, NK cells

Other Receptors. Some mononuclear cells have receptors for the secretory component of IgA, the so called Sc-binding receptor.[59] Many mononuclear cells express receptors for a constellation of hormones. They may also express viral receptors. A receptor for EBV is characteristic of B cells.

Summary of Markers. Markers of *B lymphocytes* include surface membrane immunoglobulin *(SmIg), complement receptors, 7S IgG Fc receptors,* and receptors for *EBV. T cells* can be defined by their spontaneous *rosetting "E"* with sheep red blood cells (Fig. 2–28A) and by antisera specific for human T-*lymphocyte antigen* (Table 2–15). Receptors for the Fc portion of IgG and IgM may also be present on T cells. *Monocytes* have cytophilic IgG bound to their surfaces, bind aggregated IgG, form erythrocyte-antibody *(EA) rosettes* (indicating the presence of Fc receptor), and contain complement receptors. *Ia antigen* is a characteristic marker on B cells and macrophages, but is also seen on activated T cells (Fig. 2–28B).

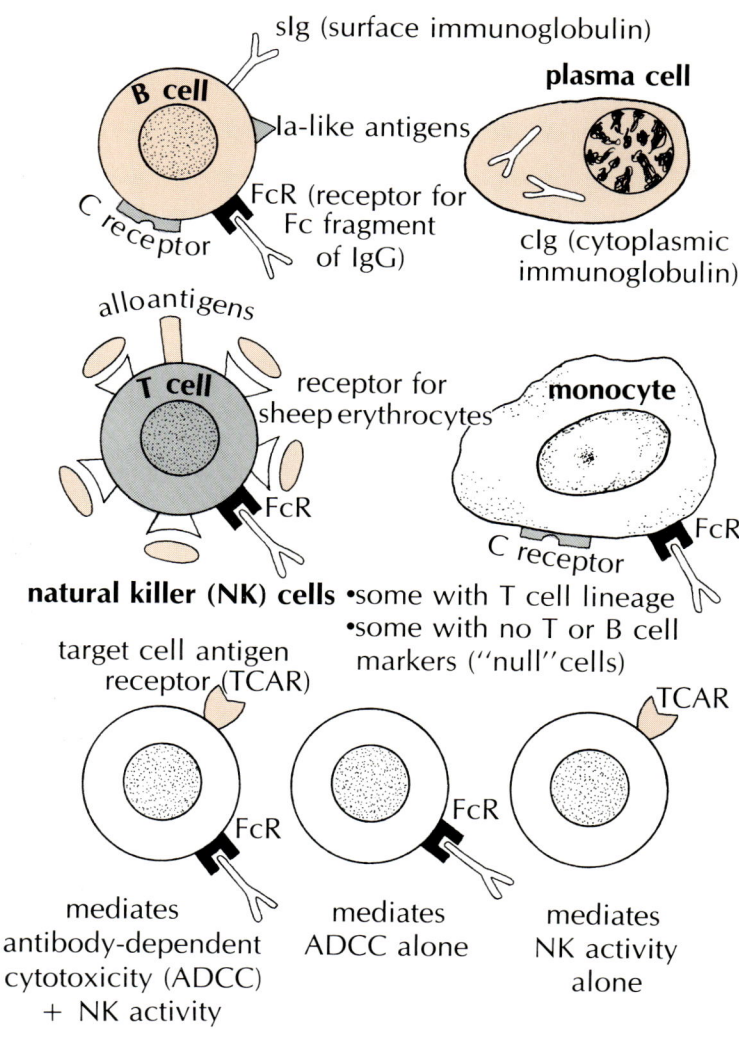

Figure 2–28 continued. B, Immune cells and their receptors.

Table 2–15. *Summary of Cell Surface Markers*

Markers	Null Cells	T Cells	B Cells	Monocytes
SmIg	−	−	+	±
Fc Receptor	−	±	+	+ +
C3 receptor	±	−	+	+
Rosette	−	E	EA(C)	EA(C)
Ia-like (DR) antigens	+	(activated T cells) +	+	(activated monocytes) +

SmIg, surface membrane immunoglobulin; Fc receptor, receptor of antibody of immunoglobulin; C3 receptor, third component of complement; E rosette, rosette with unsensitized (E) erythrocytes; EA(C) rosette, erythrocytes coated with antibody alone or with complement; Ia-like (DR) antigens, similar to murine Ia antigens, coded on HLA DR human locus.

Antibody Synthesis

Antigen Binding to Membranes

The mechanism of antigen binding to lymphocyte and macrophage cell membranes is unclear. Some believe that cross-linkage of the antigen with rearranged B-cell-surface antibody receptor molecules produces a signal that triggers the nuclear genome to transcribe appropriate antibodies.

Since antigen binding by B cells is easily demonstrated, we know a fair amount about antigenic activation of these cells. Much less is known about T cells, but antigen-specific receptors have been demonstrated on them as well. T cells apparently do not have an immunoglobulin receptor, and the nature of the idiotypic antigen-binding receptor is at present unknown.

Helper T cells are required to activate B-cell response to some antigens and are not required with others. Most antigens that require helper T-cell function for activation are known as *thymus-dependent antigens*, the activation response being controlled by the *Ir genes*. Certain thymus-independent antigens are represented largely by polymeric polysaccharide compounds.

Suppressor T cells are activated during normal antibody responses, and their inhibitory effects on B-cell antibody synthesis are antigen-specific in nature.[60]

Cellular Response to Antigens and Mitogens

At birth, most B cells bear monomeric IgM receptors. After the first two weeks of life, many cells contain IgD on their surface. It is believed that once B cells acquire IgD on their surface, they migrate to peripheral lymphoid tissues.

Binding of antigen to either B cells or T cells triggers a general cellular activation called blast transformation. Lymphoblastic cells proliferate and differentiate in the lymph nodes, often with concomitant release of specific and non-specific lymphokines.

Many substances *(mitogens)* that stimulate lymphocytes to undergo blast transformation have been identified[61] (Table 2–16). Mitogenic agents include lectins (plant proteins that bind to specific membrane carbohydrate groups), lipopolysaccharides (from the cell walls of gram-negative bacilli), chemical reagents, and antigens. Cells undergoing blast transformation show increased nuclear size, thymidine incorporation, and division.

Table 2–16. *Examples of Lymphocyte Mitogens*

Plant Extracts
  Phaseolus vulgaris (PHA)
  Canavalia ensiformis (ConA)
  Vicia fava (favin)

Bacterial Products
  Lipopolysaccharide (lipid A)
  Staphylococcal enterotoxin B
  Purified protein derivative (PPD)
  Streptolysin S

Antibody Reagents
  Anti-Ig sera
  Antilymphocyte sera
  Anti-$\alpha2$ macroglobulin
  Anti-$\alpha2$ microglobulin

Miscellaneous Chemicals
  Sodium metaperiodate
  Phorbol esters
  Ca^{++} ionophore (A23187)
  Metal ions (An, Hg N$_1$)
  Proteolytic enzymes (trypsin, papain)

(Modified from Cunningham, et al.: Structure and activities of lymphocytic mitogens. *In* Mitogens in Immunology. Edited by J.J. Oppenheim and D.L. Rosentereich. New York, Academic Press, 1976.)

Mitogenic stimulation requires that the mitogen bind to specific receptors on the cell membrane. This binding is followed by the transfer of a signal to the cell nucleus (probably involving the cyclic nucleotide system), which induces proliferation and differentiation. If B lymphocytes are incubated with mitogens in vitro, they will proliferate and produce antibodies. In vivo, they further differentiate into plasma cells with increased antibody production. In general, IgM is produced first, followed by IgG synthesis within a few hours.[62]

Examples of lectins include concanavalin A (ConA) and phytohemagglutinin (PHA).[63] Chemicals such as ionophore (A23187) and, to a lesser extent, periodate, are also mitogenic. These all increase cyclic adenosine monophosphate (cAMP), protein synthesis, and phosphorylation. Wheat germ agglutinin and latex, in contrast, increase cAMP but diminish phosphorylation. Activation by these latter agents thus inhibits a number of biochemical transport processes

Table 2–17. *Properties of Lectins*

Binding of sugars

Precipitation of polysaccharide and glycoprotein

Agglutination of erythrocytes, lymphocytes, tumor cells, microorganisms, viruses

Stimulation of lymphocytes

Inhibition of phagocytosis by granulocytes

Inhibition of fertilization of ovum by sperm

Insulin-like action on fat cells

Inhibition of fungal growth

(Modified from Sharon, N.: Lectins as mitogens. *In* Mitogens in Immunobiology. Edited by J.J. Oppenheim and D.L. Rosentereich. New York, Academic Press, 1976.)

that are stimulated by kidney bean and jack bean lectins. Further, prostaglandin E, theophylline, and isoproterenol increase cAMP, but do not effect phosphorylation. Other functions are summarized in Table 2–17.

Lectins may differentially stimulate cells of the B or T series.[64] T cells usually respond faster than B cells to kidney bean and jack bean mitogens. In general, pokeweed mitogen is more selective than the others in specifically activating B cells, but only polymerized polysaccharides (thymus-independent antigens) activate B cells directly. The lectin stimulus for B-cell division appears separate from the signal for antibody synthesis; the latter signal comes from a protein or group of proteins from activated T cells.

Antibody Synthesis in B Cells and Plasma Cells

During the first two days of antibody synthesis, antigen-specific lymphocyte clones are retained in the lymph nodes. T cells migrate into the T-cell-dependent regions of the lymph nodes, proliferate, and give rise to clones of memory and effector T cells. This process is accompanied by a proliferation of clones of memory and effector B cells. These cells in addition to activated macrophages form secondary follicles.

Macrophages first attach to antigens and apparently present the antigenic determinant in such a manner that an immunogenic signal is delivered to T cells. Binding is linked to the MHC and is an energy-dependent process. There is a need for the T lymphocyte to recognize both the antigenic determinant being presented by the macrophage and a product of the I gene (that is, the Ia antigen on the macrophage membrane). Later, the helper T lymphocyte must recognize the same Ia antigen on the B lymphocyte. For recognition to occur, direct physical interaction of the antigen-bearing macrophage and the T lymphocyte must take place (Fig. 2–29).

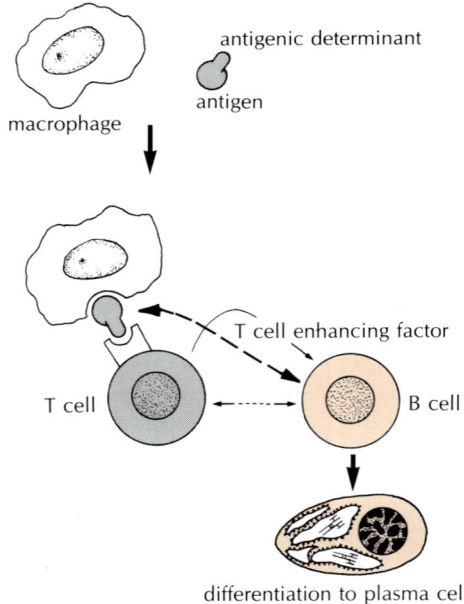

Figure 2–29. Antigen processing by immune cells.

The development of optimal antibody responses requires the active participation and interactions of antigen-specific helper T cells, antigen-specific macrophages that present soluble antigen determinants to both T and B cells. Sometimes, digestion and processing of particulate antigen are required before the soluble antigenic determinant is available. It appears that unless B cells are stimulated by two signals, antigen and helper T cells or a substance released from the T cell (enhancing factor), they will not synthesize antibody or differentiate into plasma cells. This helper function of the T cell depends on T and B cells' sharing certain products of the histocompatibility complex.

Once B cells have been stimulated by antigen and helper T cells, they may switch from IgD and IgM synthesis to IgE, IgG, or IgA synthesis.[65] These molecules (that is, *isotypes*) are the antigen-specific receptors on what now become *"memory B cells."* Following induction of the genome by antigen on the membrane, the Ig messenger RNA is transcribed in the nucleus and is transported to the cytoplasm where it becomes associated with ribosomes on the RER. The heavy and light polypeptide chains are translated from separate messengers. The peptides appear separately within the ER cisternae, are assembled into molecules covalently linked by disulfide bonds, and acquire carbohydrate components. The different Ig subclasses are the result of different genes and preferred pathways of assembly. In order to synthesize large amounts of antibody, further division and differentiation of the B cells are required. This process results in a population of plasma cells with a well-developed endoplasmic reticulum and Golgi complex.[66]

Capping is an in vitro antigen-binding phenomenon whose significance in vivo is unknown. Once an antigen is coupled to the receptor (IgM or IgG) molecule on the membrane with the help of macrophages and helper T cells, *aggregation* and then *patching* follows. Patching of labelled antigen-receptor complexes on the B lymphocyte's surface can occur at 4°C. Upon warming to 37°C, the label moves from patches over the surface of the cell and becomes concentrated over one pole. This process is known as capping[67] (Fig. 2–30).

Following antigen-antibody complexing, aggregation, patching, and capping, phagocytosis of the Ag-Ab complexes finally occurs.

The disappearance of the immunoglobulin receptor is not permanent. After incubation of cells in vitro and following new protein synthesis, receptors reappear on the cell surface in 6 to 12 hours.

Negative Controls on Antibody Synthesis. Following stimulation of the immune response by antigen, an antibody response, seen in six to seven days, increases during the next few weeks and then declines. The failure to sustain a maximum response suggests the presence of additional control mechanisms including *antigen catabolism, antigen masking* by *antibody, negative feedback*, the presence of inhib-

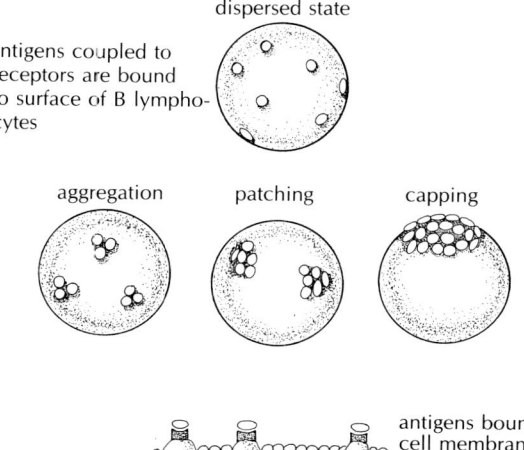

antigens coupled to receptors are bound to surface of B lymphocytes

dispersed state

aggregation   patching   capping

antigens bound to cell membrane Ig receptors are aggregated, patched, and capped by concerted actions of microfilaments and microtubules

Figure 2–30. Capping, an in vitro antigen binding phenomenon, relies on cell surface immunoglobulin (Ig) for antigen binding and movement of antigen through the fluid mosaic of the cell membrane.

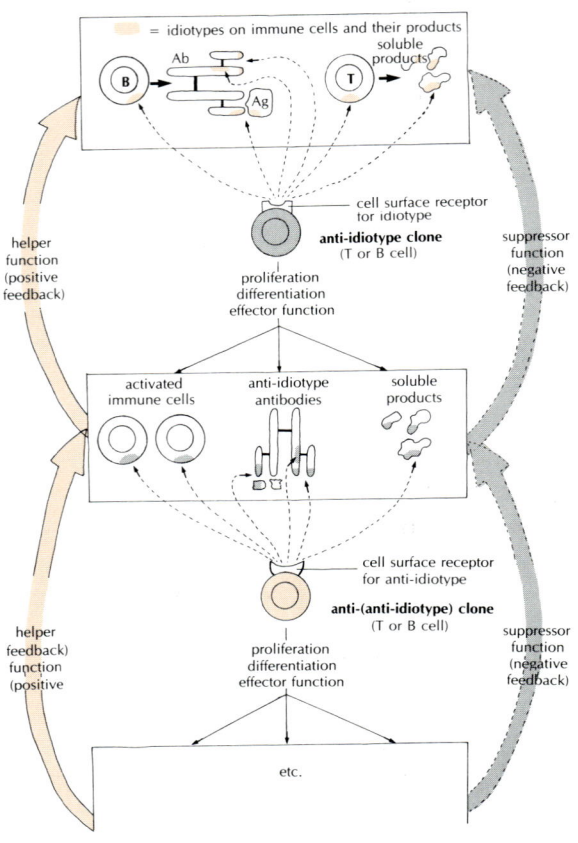

Figure 2–31. *A*, Interactions between idiotypes and anti-idiotypes provide homeostatic control over the immune system and may play pathogenic roles in autoimmune disease. At top, *idiotypes* (in color) are shown to be antigenic determinants on B and T cells and their soluble products, which are immunogenic. They elicit a response from *anti-idiotype clones* bearing surface receptors for idiotypes. The anti-idiotype clones may be B or T cells, and these cells, or their products, act on the immune system in helper or suppressor functions. Anti-idiotypes also reach the stage at which their antigenic determinants become immunogenic, thereby stimulating a response from *anti-(anti-idiotype) clones*. It appears likely that idiotype-anti-idiotype interactions comprise a circular, rather than unlimited, network for homeostatic control of immune reactions.

itory receptors on human lymphocyte cell surfaces, and the presence of suppressor T cells. The mechanisms that regulate immunity are as important as those that initiate it.

It is believed that one aspect of this control is regulated through a feedback system in which circulating antibody molecules specifically inhibit the differentiation of new antibody-synthesizing cells.[68] The Fc portion of the antibody molecule must be intact in order to suppress the immune response. Other postulated regulatory functions for Fc receptors include roles in the initial stages of antibody-mediated lymphocytotoxicity, in Ab synthesis, and in phagocytosis. The interaction of spleen cells with immobile antibody complexes leads to a 50% increase in cAMP. This increase may be the "off" signal to antibody synthesis by the cell by binding to receptors in a manner similar to the binding of insulin to cell receptors. Under conditions of lymphocyte activation, there is an increase in cGMP.[69]

The specific regulation of immune responses and specific suppressor activity is the direct result of antigenic stimulation. It is clear that both helper and suppressor cells appear to have important roles in immune regulation.[70] Abnormalities in negative control mechanisms probably play a role in tolerance and in autoimmune diseases.

Idiotypes and Anti-Idiotypes. Another mechanism for control of antibody synthesis and activity is the *idiotype-anti-idiotype network*.[68] This network exists because portions of immunoglobulin molecules or other antigen determinants (idiotypes) may themselves be immunogenic and generate synthesis of antibodies (anti-idiotypes). According to this scheme, classes of B or T cells possess surface receptors that recognize the following idiotypes on immunoglobulins: (1) idiotypes within the antibody's combining site; (2) idiotypes on the heavy chain, outside the combining site; and (3) idiotypes on the light chain in combination with the antigen bound to the combining site (Fig. 2–31A). The anti-idiotype clones (T or B cells) and their products, for example, lymphokines and antibodies, respond to idiotypes in either helper or suppressor functions, thereby enhancing or diminishing the immune response. Because of the great diversity of antibodies and therefore of potential idiotypes, a seemingly limitless network of idiotype-anti-idiotype interactions exists. These interactions function in the homeostasis of antibody responses by the host. In certain conditions, such as autoimmune diseases, abnormal idiotype-anti-idiotype interactions may play pathogenetic roles.[68]

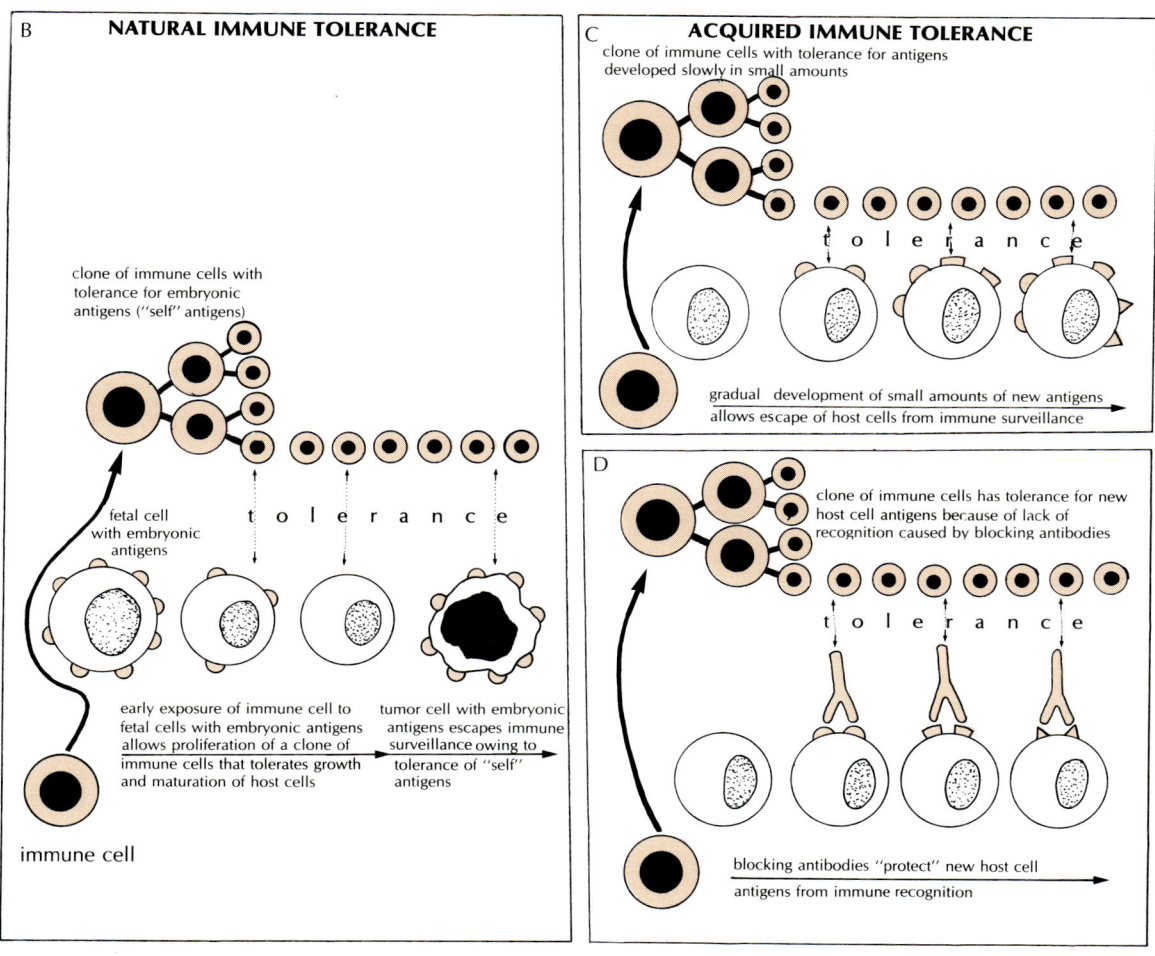

Figure 2–31 continued. *B*, Postulated mechanisms of the development of natural immune tolerance. *C* and *D*, Two postulated mechanisms mediating acquired immune tolerance.

Hormonal Modulation of Immune Response. We have previously discussed the action of antigens and mitogens on the membranes of lymphocytes and discussed some of their activating effects. *Hormones*, or other effector substances that act like hormones, also affect lymphocyte responsiveness[71] (Table 2–18).

Table 2–18. *Hormonal Modulation and Biochemical Alterations of Lymphocyte Membranes*

Hormone	Receptor Mechanism	Effect on Lymphocyte Metabolism
Insulin	+	↑ glucose and potassium transport
Norepinephrine Epinephrine	+ (α-adrenergic)	↑ glucose and potassium transport ↑ PHA-induced DNA synthesis
Isoproterenol Epinephrine	+ (β-adrenergic)	Inhibition of PHA-induced DNA synthesis (early) and stimulation (late)
Prostaglandin E₁	?	↓ PHA-induced DNA synthesis ↓ Lymphocytotoxicity
Acetylcholine	+ (muscarinic)	↑ RNA and protein synthesis ↑ Lymphocytotoxicity ↑ Lymphokine secretion
Adrenal corticosteroids	(cytoplasmic-nuclear receptors)	Inhibition of RNA and protein synthesis

(Adapted from Goodwin, J.S., Bankhurst, A.D., and Messner, R.P.: Suppression of human T-cell mitogenesis by prostaglandin. J. Exp. Med., *146*:1719, 1977.)

These substances usually do not dictate whether lymphocytes proliferate, but rather appear to function as a fine-tuning mechanism for maintaining homeostasis.

Gene Control of Antibody Synthesis and Diversity of Antibodies

Historically, the "instructive" theory of antibody synthesis stated that an antigen acted as a template for a standard unfolded γ globulin chain that could be molded to provide the appropriate complementary shape. Later, disulfide hydrogen bonding stabilized the shape of the molecule.

It is now believed that the information required for the synthesis of the different classes of antibodies is present in the genome. Once B cells are activated by antigen binding and a specific signal is sent to a structural gene in the nucleus, transcriptional and translational events result whereby immunoglobulin peptide chains, with the proper amino acid sequences, are synthesized. Depending on particular charged groups in the peptide chains, the peptides are folded spontaneously into tertiary configurations that present the specific antibody combining sites in the appropriate manner.

There is one family of genes specifying κ light chains, a second for λ light chains, and a third specifying various classes and subclasses of heavy chains. Genes within each family are linked, but the three families are not, and they are probably on separate chromosomes.

Variable and constant regions are coded for by separate genes. A small number of constant-region genes and a large array of variable genes exist. The V-region genes are encoded separately in the genome of both immunoglobulin-producing and uncommitted cells.

There are now known to be *J minigenes* and probably *D minigenes* in the heavy chain in addition to the *variable, constant,* and *intervening segments* of each gene coding for the *light* and *heavy chain.* Within the variable gene, Kabat et al. have classified four framework genes (FR4) and three complementary determining segments (CDR3), the latter representing the hypervariable regions.[72]

The problem of antibody diversity supplying millions of antibodies within a total genome estimated to range between 50,000 and 100,000 genes is now amenable to analysis[73,74]:

1. Approximately 300 to 500 germline cells have different κ light chains, and 200 to 300 germline cells are coded for different heavy chains.
2. Random somatic mutations during the life of stem cells capable of producing antibodies possibly account for additional thousands of antibodies.[75]
3. The properties of minigenes coding for different classes of light and heavy chains, variable, J, D, and intervening regions produce an almost infinite number of possible combinations when arranged in different sequences, especially when the germline and somatic mutation contributions to diversity are taken into consideration. They easily account for the 10^6 or 10^8 individual antibody molecules believed to be possible in the organism.[76,77]

Tolerance

Tolerance is an inability or failure of the immune mechanism to respond to antigenic stimulation with an appropriate response. Natural tolerance is present during fetal life. It is believed that presentation of the antigen before maturation of the immune stem cells precludes immune response at this time. Acquired immune tolerance occurs later, during adult life. It represents a lack of response to non-self-antigens with the assumption that organisms are normally tolerant to unaltered self-antigens.

Mechanisms

Tolerance is different from desensitization. The latter represents a temporary state of unresponsiveness induced by large dose of degraded antigen. Although current dogma states that the best toleragens are the poorest immunogens and the best immunogens are the poorest toleragens, some authors believe the opposite.[78]

Several suggestions have been advanced to explain the mechanism for tolerance (Fig. 2–31B to D), and these generally are divided into two categories: (1) direct *interaction* of toleragen and immunocyte is precluded as the appropriate clone may be deleted or may become exhausted, or there may be increased catabolism of the antigen; and (2) indirect effects include the presence of blocking antibodies to the antigen or to idiotypic receptors on the immune cell, both reactions preventing an appropriate immune response. Another indirect effect might be an increase in suppressor T cells, thus inhibiting antibody synthesis by B cells.

Tolerance to infectious agents and foreign tumor antigen is not advantageous to the patient, whereas tolerance to foreign graft antigens, poison ivy antigens, or toxins is of distinct benefit.

ACUTE INFLAMMATION

We have now discussed the basic immunology of the host including the role of cells, antibody, and complement, all of which contribute to the inflammatory response.

The immediate response to injury is *vascular*. After a fleeting moment of constriction of vessels, dilatation of arterioles and capillaries and, most prominently, postcapillary venules occurs. *Transudation*, the extravasation of fluid across the vessel wall, is followed by *exudation*, the transport of blood cells and plasma proteins. The increase in vascular permeability is mediated initially by *histamine* and later by *kinins* and *complement*.

Following vasodilatation with increased permeability, a cellular response in inflammation occurs. Concurrent with the dilatation of vessels and increased blood supply, products from the injured area stimulate the production of white blood cells, particularly polymorphonuclear leukocytes (*PMN*), in the marrow. Other factors attract cells to the site of injury (*chemotaxis*).

Initially, PMN *marginate* or *pavement* on the inner walls of the vessel and then pass through the widened pores between endothelial cells in a movement termed *emigration*. *Diapedesis* refers to the passing of red blood cells through the vessel wall. *Emperipolesis* denotes the movement of lymphocytes through the cytoplasm of endothelial cells rather than between the cells (Fig. 2–32).

Once the *polymorphonuclear leukocyte* reaches the site of injury it may phagocytose and digest injured cells, bacteria,

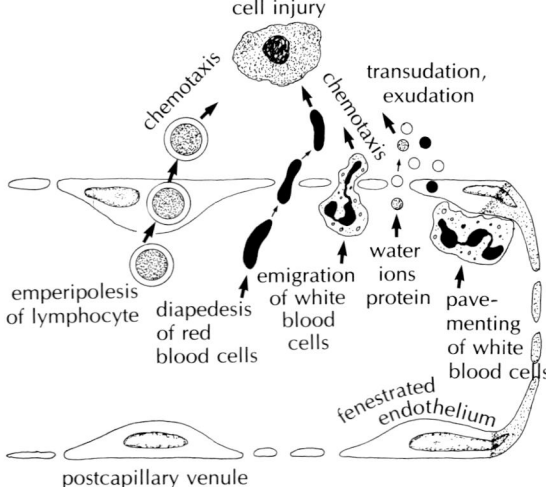

Figure 2–32. Cellular and fluid responses to inflammation.

or foreign protein. It may also rupture, releasing its lysosomal enzymes to destroy bacteria or to hydrolyze denatured protein. *Basophils,* which contain histamine granules, and *eosinophils,* whose lysosomal granules assist in digestion of antigen-antibody complexes, are much less common than neutrophils in most acute inflammatory reactions. Eosinophils are often seen in allergic states and in parasitic infections.

Later, chronic inflammatory cells arrive. *Monocytic macrophages* phagocytize fibrin, debris, dead PMN, and other foreign protein. *Lymphocytes* (B and T cells) are involved in a variety of immunologic defense reactions, and *plasma cells* (differentiated B cells) synthesize and secrete humoral antibody.

Local and Systemic Signs and Symptoms

Local signs and symptoms of inflammation include *rubor* (redness of the area associated with increased vascularity and increased blood flow to the area), *calor* (heat, also associated with increased blood flow and increased vascularity), *tumor* (swelling attributed to an increase in extra- and intracellular fluid), *dolor* (pain induced partially by chemical mediators and partially by edematous pressure on nerve endings), and *functio laesa* (partial or complete loss of tissue or organ function) (Fig. 2–33).

Malaise, anorexia, and fever are frequent systemic signs and symptoms of inflammation. Malaise and anorexia are often systemic symptoms of many diseases, and the mechanism is difficult to explain. Fever often results from pyrogens released by leukocytes, dead cells, infectious agents, and other substances that presumably affect the hypothalamus.[79] In addition to infectious agents, endotoxins, antigen-antibody complexes, lymphokines, and hormones (for example, etiocholanolone) may produce fever.

Classically, a *leukocytosis* follows cell injury; a granulocytic leukocytosis with a *shift to the left* (immature forms of PMN) is often present, especially with acute inflammatory processes associated with pathogenic bacteria in the blood (septicemia).

Initially, the leukocytosis results from a release of white blood cells, from tissue pools (that is, spleen and bone marrow). Leukocytosis is commonly seen in acute infection, for example, with streptococci and staphylococci, although it may occur under physiologically normal conditions, as following exercise. Immature cells in the bone marrow may be discharged as a result of *leukocyte releasing factor* (LRF) and a C3 fraction *(leukocyte mobilizing factor).* Other humoral blastogenic factors released from the inflammatory lesion stimulate division and maturation of stem cells.

Levels of neutrophils may be depressed in certain situations. Their proliferation may be inhibited by *chalones* produced by granulocytes. Autoimmune neutropenia, (presence of auto-antibodies to PMN) may involve increased

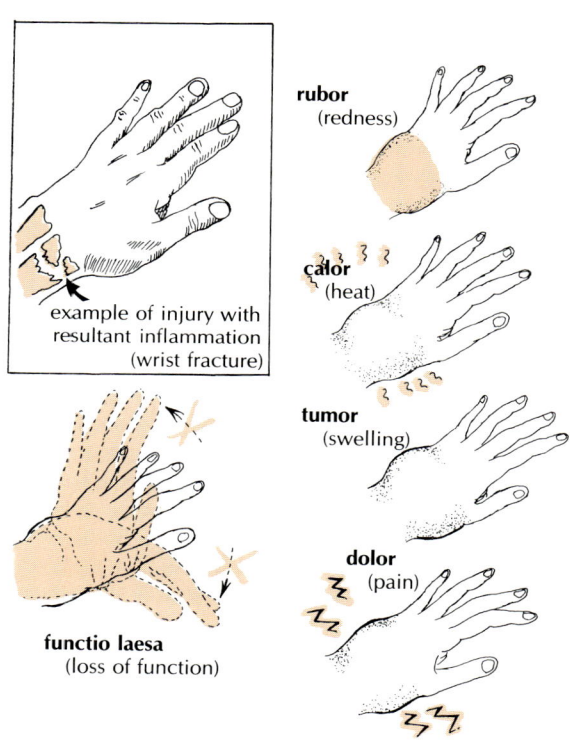

example of injury with resultant inflammation (wrist fracture)

rubor
(redness)

calor
(heat)

tumor
(swelling)

dolor
(pain)

functio laesa
(loss of function)

Figure 2–33. Five cardinal local signs of inflammation.

phagocytosis of neutrophils by mononuclear cells or heightened neutrophilic degradation through increased glucose oxidation rates.[80] *Neutropenia* commonly occurs following the use of cytotoxic chemotherapy, but may also be seen in various disorders such as typhoid fever and radiation exposure.

Monocytosis is seen in certain forms of leukemia and sometimes in chronic diseases, but is uncommon in infectious mononucleosis, which is a reaction of T cells to virus-infected B cells.

Lymphocytosis (increased circulating lymphocytes) is often seen with brucellosis, infectious mononucleosis, pertussis, and mumps. Lymphopenia is associated with typhoid fever, immune deficiency, and radiation therapy (Table 2–19). *Eosinophilia* is seen in allergic diseases (asthma, hay fever, dermatitis, angiitis) and in parasitic infections. *Basophilia* is seen only rarely and may be most prominent in basophilic leukemia.

Table 2–19. *Leukocytosis and Leukopenia*

Cells Affected	Leukocytosis	Leukopenia
Polymorphonuclear cells (neutrophils)	Bacterial infection	Autoimmune neutropenia Cytotoxic therapy
Monocytes	Viral and parasitic infection	Genetic disease

Lymphocytes	Infectious mononucleosis (T cells)
	Brucellosis
	Pertussis
	Mumps
		Typhoid fever
		Radiation therapy
		Immunosuppressive drugs
		Genetic diseases
		  Bruton's (B)
		  DiGeorge's (T)
		  Severe combined immune deficiency (SCID) (B and T)

Eosinophils	Allergy Dermatitis Parasites	Genetic disease (?)
Basophils	Leukemia	Genetic disease (?)

Vascular Response to Inflammation

The response to inflammation is by complex and often interrelated pathways, among which vascular, cellular, complement, coagulation, and kinin systems figure prominently. The vascular phase of inflammation involves increases in blood flow, vascular permeability, and lymphatic flow. Vascular permeability may be increased in inflammation as the result of a direct effect on the vessels, such as heat, or by chemically mediated action by other factors such as histamines released by mast cells or basophils or kinins activated in the serum or tissues.

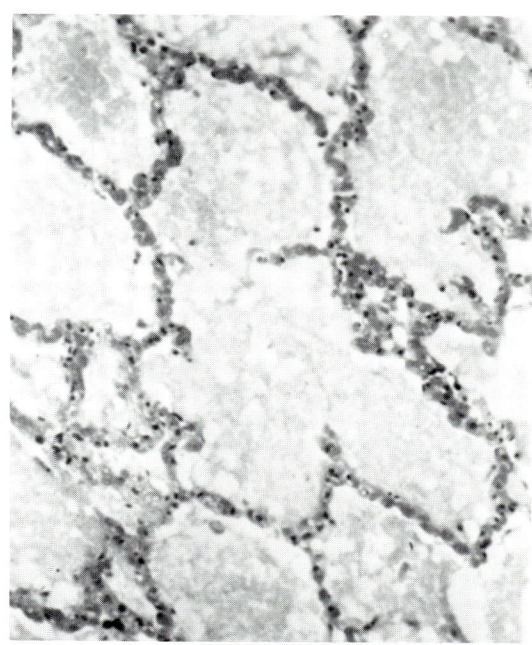

Figure 2–34. In this section of lung from a patient with pulmonary edema, the alveolar spaces contain large amounts of fluid.

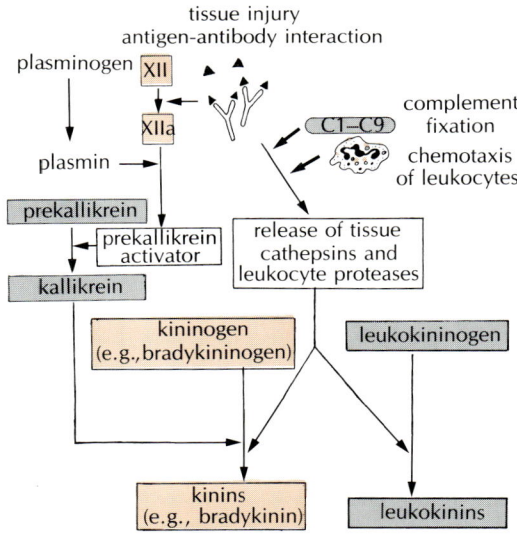

Figure 2–35. *A,* This figure shows the interaction of the kinin system with other components of inflammation. Injury causes activation of Hageman Factor XII as well as antigen-antibody interactions that fix complement. Plasmin and activated Hageman factor generate a prekallikrein activator that yields kallikrein. Kallikrein and tissue proteases (cathepsins) cleave kinins and leukokinins from kininogen and leukokininogen.

Transudate, Exudate, and Edema

The initial transitory vascular response to injury is an autonomic, neurogenic local constriction of the arterioles. The cause of the vasoconstriction is unknown. It is quickly followed by vasodilatation. Vasodilatation results in transudative and exudative fluid shifts involving movement of water, ions, and small amounts of serum proteins, including albumin, globulin, fibrinogen, complement, lipoproteins, and glycoproteins.

Three different types of fluid shift resulting in an increase in extracellular fluid (edema) are associated with inflammation: (1) *immediate-transient* edema, mediated particularly by histamine, which primarily affects postcapillary venules: (2) *immediate-prolonged* edema, as seen in burns; and (3) *delayed-prolonged* edema, which shows an initial transudation in the postcapillary venule followed several hours later by a more prolonged transudation from capillaries. This type of edema may result from bacterial toxins, radiation, and many exogenous and endogenous chemicals[81] (Fig. 2–34).

Vasodilatory Mediators

The transudation and extravasation of fluid through a postcapillary venule may occur in one of five ways: (1) actual destruction of the endothelial lining; (2) an increase in the intracellular gaps as a result of histamine and kinin-type mediators; (3) an increase in the transcellular leaking through caveolar channels seen in normal endothelium; (4) active pinocytotic transport, which is not well documented; and (5) actual secretion from the endothelial cell itself, as in cholera.

The principal soluble endogenous plasma mediators affecting vascular permeability (Fig. 2–35*A*) include kinins (bradykinin and lysylbradykinin) and the anaphylatoxin fractions (C3a and C5a) of complement. The latter act on mast cells to release histamine. Histamine causes contraction of actin in endothelial cells and in perivascular pericytes to widen intracellular gaps.

Other primary tissue vasodilators are amines such as histamine, 5-hydroxytryptamine (5-HT, serotonin), leukotrienes comprising slow-reacting substance of anaphylaxis (SRS-A), and perhaps prostaglandins, all found in mast cells (Table 2–20 and Fig. 2–35*B*). The group of compounds known either as slow reacting substance of anaphylaxis or slow reacting substance (SRS-A or SRS) consists of leukotrienes, which are oxidative metabolites of arachidonic acid derived from neutrophils, monocytes, and mast cells (Fig. 2–35*B*). Leukotrienes, particularly C4, D4, and E4, play active roles in inflammation and allergy by producing smooth muscle contraction, increased vascular permeability, neutrophil and eosinophil chemotaxis, and other changes.[82]

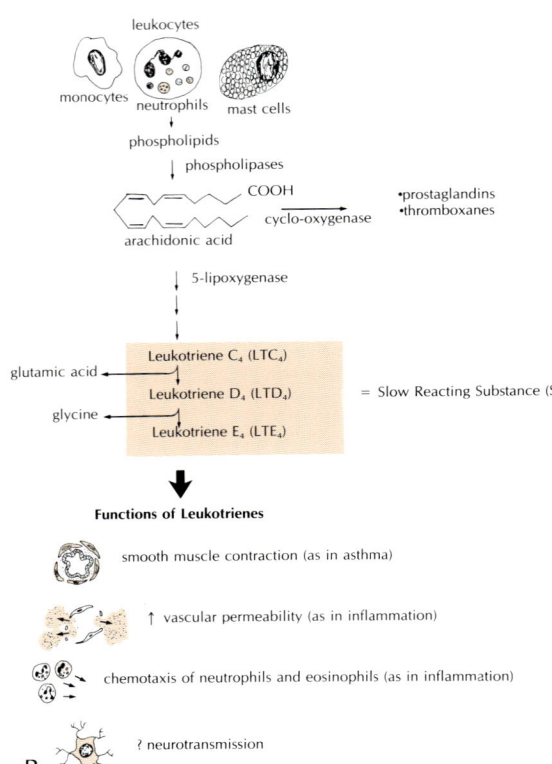

Origin	Mediators
Plasma	Kinins (bradykinin, C kinin, leukokinin)
	Anaphylatoxins (C3a, C5a)
Tissues	Vasoactive amines (histamine, 5-HT)
	Slow-reacting substance of anaphylaxis (SRS-A)
	Prostaglandins (PGE₁, PGE₂)
	Neutrophil lysosomal cationic proteins
	SH-dependent neutral proteases
	Lymphocyte-derived skin reactive factors
	Lymph node permeability factor (LNPF)
	Substance P (neurotransmitter)
	Neurotensin

(Modified from Ryan, G.B., and Majno, G.: Acute inflammation. A review.
Am. J. Pathol., 86:247, 1977.)

Figure 2–35 continued. B, Leukotrienes C4, D4, and E4 comprise slow reacting substance (SRS) and are derived by oxidation of arachidonic acid. The name "leukotriene" is used to indicate origin from leukocytes and the presence of three conjugated double bonds. Leukotrienes, as well as other metabolic products of arachidonic acid (prostaglandins, thromboxanes), are vasoactive substances involved in inflammation.

The *kinins* are especially important in vasodilatation during the immediate delayed phase of the vascular response. Their formation results from a sequence of events beginning with the splitting of Hageman factor (XII) with conversion of serum *prekallikrein* to kallikrein. *Kallikrein* can act on kininogens to form kinins including a nonapeptide called *bradykinin* (Fig. 2–35A). In addition to serum kallikrein, tissue kallikreins in the saliva, sweat, tears, urine, and feces may convert serum kininogens to *kallidin (lysylbradykinin)*, a decapeptide, which may then be converted to bradykinin. Kinins are ultimately degraded by kinases, another group of proteolytic enzymes.[83]

Secondary vasodilating substances active during the delayed phase of vasodilation include the globin permeability factor of Miles *(PF/dil)*, *lymph node permeability factors*, and *leukokines* generated by enzymes released from monocytes and other tissues acting on serum substrates.

Control of Mediators

Certain pharmacologic mediators (histamine, catecholamines, and prostaglandins of the E series) not only mediate vascular responses in inflammatory reactions, but also regulate the intensity of inflammation and immune reactions by inhibiting the release of lymphokines and lysosomal enzymes. Some evidence suggests that intracellular cAMP and cGMP are involved in release of mediators such as histamine and SRS-A.[84]

Cellular Response to Inflammation

Shortly after the vasodilatation phase, there is *migration* of white blood cells and infiltration of red blood cells into the area of injury (see Fig. 2–40). This migration principally occurs in the postcapillary venules, but may also be seen in capillaries and arterioles, depending on the extent of the inflammatory process.

The dilated capillary or venule in the inflammatory site contains a central core of sludged red blood cells, with *margination* or *pavementing* of white blood cells that adhere to the endothelial cells. This phenomenon may be due to increased "stickiness" of the white blood cells and increased absorption by the endothelial cells, either primarily or secondarily owing to the release of extracellular cement substances. The spaces may be widened by dilatation of the vessel, which pulls the endothelial gap junctions apart, by histamine-stimulated contraction of the endothelial cells, which contain actin fibrils, or possibly by retraction of the endothelial cells, which are connected to contracting *pericytes* that surround the capillary wall.[85]

Cell Types Involved

White blood cells, initially PMN, and later lymphocytes and macrophages, actively emigrate directly through the endothelial intercellular space and basement membrane to the site of injured cells.

Inflammation may be classified as *acute* or *chronic* depending on whether it lasts a few days or persists for months or longer. The histologic cellular response is also classified simplistically as acute or chronic inflammation. The presence of many PMN indicates an *acute* response (Fig. 2–36), whereas increased *lymphocytes* and *monocytes* indicate a *chronic* response. However, considerable overlap is always present. Acute inflammation is also seen superimposed on chronic inflammation.

In general, injury by most bacterial infections, chemicals, physical agents and some forms of immune injury produce an initial infiltration of PMN into injured tissue. Later, during the subacute and healing stages, monocytes, lymphocytes, and plasma cells enter the area. Viruses, rickettsiae, parasites, fungi, and mycobacteria classically and principally produce a monocytic and lymphocytic response. If damage to the cells is extensive or if the number and virulence of these organisms is overwhelming, a neutrophilic response is also seen, either initially or when widespread dissemination of the organisms takes place.

Chemotaxis and Chemotactic Factors

White blood cells are directly attracted to injurious agents or injured tissue by a process called *chemotaxis*. Adler[86] has identified chemoreceptors on E. coli that are influenced by different concentrations of galactose, glucose, ribose, aspartic acid, and serine. In Adler's system, chemotaxis is a result of both the temporal and spatial concentration of the substrate on the bacterial cell membrane.

Chemotaxis also occurs in mammalian tissues. Bessis has demonstrated that injured cells in serum-free medium have chemotactic influences.[87] Some investigators have suggested that this phenomenon results from release of cAMP,

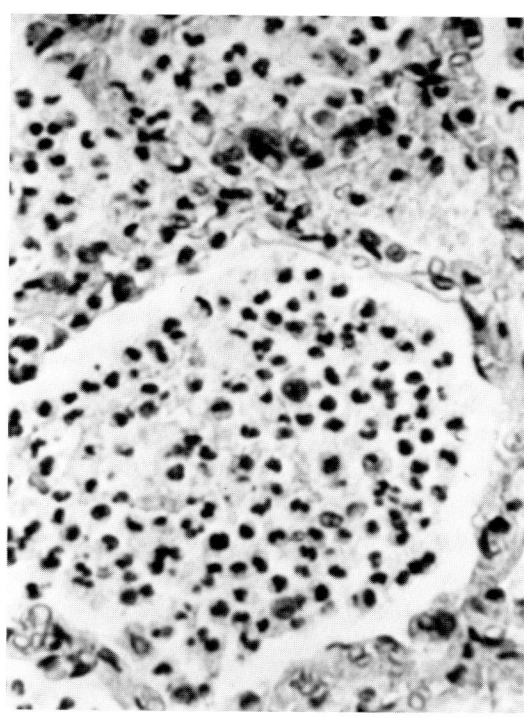

Figure 2–36. In this section of lung from a patient with pneumonia, note the intra-alveolar collection of inflammatory cells. Large numbers of polymorphonuclear leukocytes are present.

but others believe that it may be due to release of lysosomal products. Serum activated by minced tissue has a chemotactic component. Ryan has also shown that substances released from damaged tissue, after interacting with serum, attract PMN.[81]

Bacterial products, soluble split products of serum (but not serum protein), and degraded and denuded collagen are all chemotactic. Later in the inflammatory reaction, lysates of dead PMN, antigen-antibody complexes, and lymphokines are also chemotactic for other leukocytes. The most active chemotactic agents include bacterial and viral products, complement by-products, and kallikrein and other plasma proteins. The C5 component of complement, the most chemotactic complement fraction, attracts neutrophils, monocytes, and lymphocytes (Table 2–21).

Lysosomal cationic protein from PMN is chemotactic for monocytes. Histamine-release factor and neutral factors released from lysosomes from cells associated with tissue damage are also chemotactic for a variety of white blood cells. Various inactivators of chemotaxis have also been identified.[88,89]

Table 2–21. *Chemotactic Factors*

	Location and Derivation of Factors	
Cells Affected	*Cells*	*Serum*
Neutrophils	bacterial & viral products neutrophil-derived factor(s) leucoegresin lymphocyte-derived factor collagen fragments cyclic AMP	complement system by-products C5 fragments C3 fragments complex C567 kallikrein plasminogen activator fibrinopeptides fibrin degradation products prostaglandins (e.g., PGE_1)
Monocytes	bacterial products neutrophil lysosomal cationic protein lymphocyte-derived factor transfer factor	complement system by-products C5 fragments C3 fragments normal serum factor kallikrein plasminogen activator M. tuberculosis-treated serum
Eosinophils	bacterial products eosinophil chemotactic factors of anaphylaxis histamine lymphocyte-derived factor (in presence of immune complexes)	complement system by-products C5 fragments C3 fragments complex C567
Basophils	—	C5 fragments kallikrein lymphocyte-derived factor
Lymphocytes	lymphocyte product	—

(Modified from Ryan, G.B., and Majno, G.: Acute inflammation. A review. Am. J. Pathol., *86*:247, 1977.)

Cellular Action at the Site of Injury

Generally, the injured cell and the injurious agent are soon surrounded by a cellular infiltrate that consists initially of PMN and later of lymphocytes and monocytes. Some agents, characteristically viruses and mycobacteria, unless present in overwhelming concentration, bypass the neutrophilic phase or have only a transient initial PMN infiltrate.

Phagocytosis. Macrophages phagocytose and hydrolyze foreign proteins including bacteria, antigen-antibody complexes, and dead cell fragments and ingest soluble, injurious substances such as toxins by pinocytosis (Fig. 2–37).

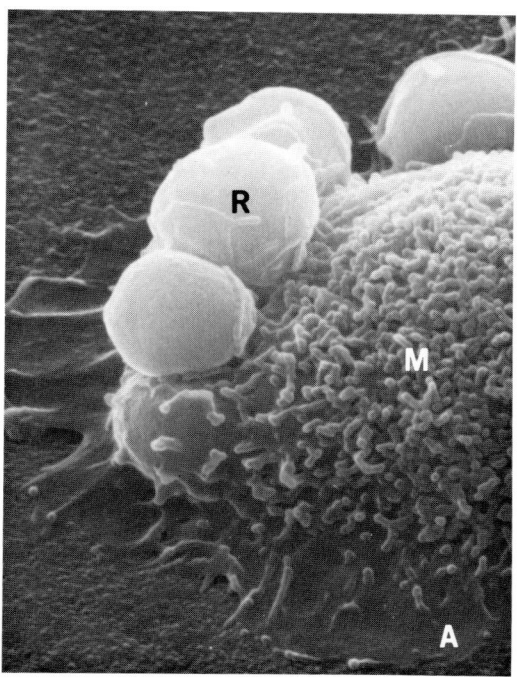

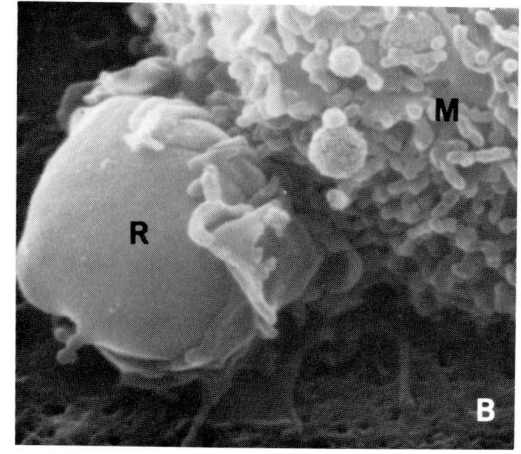

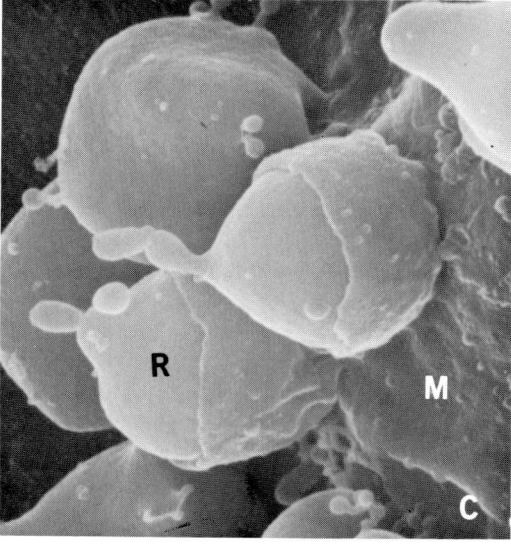

Figure 2–37. This scanning electron micrograph shows the progressive steps in phagocytosis. *A,* Red blood cells (R) attach to the surface of a macrophage (M). *B,* A veil of macrophage (M) membrane starts to enclose the red cell (R). *C,* The red blood cells (R) are almost totally engulfed by the macrophage (M). (Courtesy of Jan Orenstein, The George Washington University Center, Washington, D.C.)

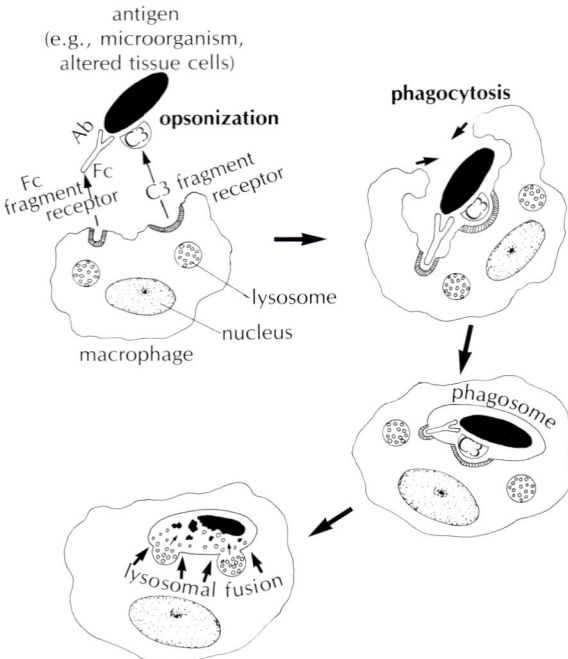

antigen
(e.g., microorganism,
altered tissue cells)

opsonization

phagocytosis

Fc fragment receptor

Fc

C3 fragment receptor

lysosome

nucleus

macrophage

phagosome

lysosomal fusion

Figure 2–38. Role of opsonization in phagocytosis. Host-derived immunoglobulins and complement fragments coat target substances and are recognized by membrane receptors on phagocytic cells.

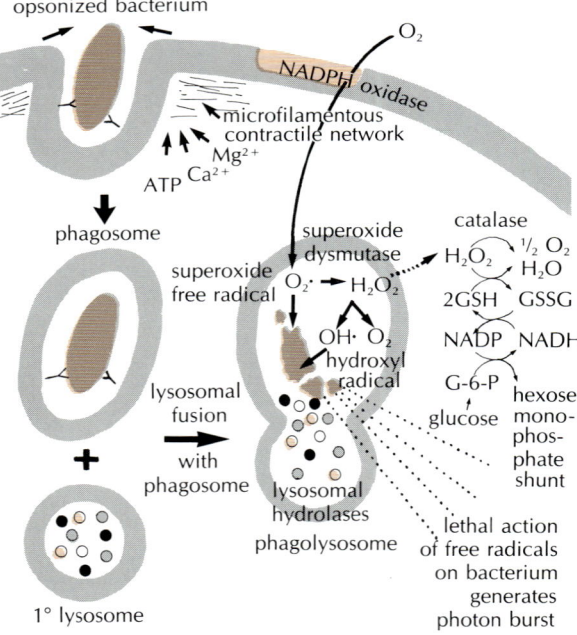

opsonized bacterium

O_2

NADPH oxidase

microfilamentous contractile network

Mg^{2+}

ATP Ca^{2+}

phagosome

superoxide dysmutase

catalase

H_2O_2

$\frac{1}{2} O_2$

H_2O

superoxide free radical

O_2^- → H_2O_2

2GSH GSSG

NADP NADH

OH· O_2
hydroxyl radical

G-6-P

glucose

hexose monophosphate shunt

lysosomal fusion

with phagosome

lysosomal hydrolases

phagolysosome

lethal action of free radicals on bacterium generates photon burst

1° lysosome

Figure 2–39. Uptake of oxygen, release of free radicals, and increased flow of glucose through the hexose monophosphate shunt, collectively known as the "respiratory burst," are major processes in phagocytosis. GSH, glutathione; G-6-P, glucose-6-phosphate.

Mobile phagocytes (neutrophils, eosinophils, and monocytes) are attracted to their targets by chemotaxis, and once they encounter the target substance, phagocytosis begins. Target substances are usually covered by a number of host-derived proteins belonging to the immunoglobulin and complement systems. These proteins function as *opsonins* and are recognized by specific receptors on the membranes of macrophages[90] (Fig. 2–38). Stossel divides phagocytosis into seven stages: (1) recognition of particle by membrane of phagocyte; (2) receipt by the cell of message for engulfment; (3) receipt of the message as signal for the cell to respond; (4) increased "stickiness" at area of contact with the particle and the membrane; (5) assembly of pseudopods; (6) movement of pseudopods; and (7) fusion of pseudopods.[91]

We have mentioned the role of opsonins in the first stage of this process. The second stage modulates activation of Fc receptors on the macrophage. Once bound to cells, the immune complexes are endocytosed and the surface receptors are regenerated. The adhesion of the particles in the fourth step may be nonspecific. As the targets come into contact with the phagocyte, evagination and invagination of the membrane ensues, with cytoplasmic processes extending over the surface of the particle.[92] The presence of intact microtubules is critical for these processes to occur. If PMN are overcome by the injurious agent, they may rupture, releasing lysosomal proteolytic enzymes to the extracellular fluid; this process produces liquefaction necrosis.

Following ingestion and formation of the phagosome, one of the two types of lysosomal granules of the PMN interacts with the engulfed particle to form a *phagolysosome*. The *primary lysosomal particle* is large and azurophilic and contains lysosomal enzymes including peroxidase, lysozyme, and cationic proteins. The smaller particle contains alkaline phosphatase, lysozyme, and peroxidase, in addition to other enzymes. Following formation of the phagolysosome, a burst of metabolic activity takes place, with a two- to threefold increase in oxygen consumption. Hydrogen peroxide, which is later degraded by catalase or oxidized by glutathione (GSH), is formed. It has been shown that the myeloperoxidase system, interacting with a halide (I^-, Cl^-, Br^-) (Fig. 2–39), enhances the effect of H_2O_2 against bacteria. A superoxide that is formed has also been found to be bactericidal.[93,94]

Eosinophils also contain lysosomal granules and are capable of phagocytosis. They are seen particularly in allergic reactions, in which they may phagocytize immune complexes. As previously mentioned, eosinophils are also prominent in parasitic infections and allergic dermatitides.

Monocytes and tissue histiocytes also phagocytose and hydrolyze foreign products. If unable to degrade injurious agents such as viruses, foreign bodies, resistant bacteria, or fungi, histiocytes may fuse with other monocytes, or their nuclei may divide without concomitant cellular division. These processes result in giant cell formation. Macrophages are also important in processing particulate antigens and in presenting antigenic determinants, in conjunction with T cells, to B cells for the production of specific humoral antibody. Macrophages have a significant immune cytolytic role in destroying foreign tissue cells such as tissue grafts and tumor cells.

Cellular Immune Reactions. B lymphocytes activated by antigen in tonsils, spleen, and lymph nodes may, after transformation into plasma cells, migrate and synthesize soluble antibodies directly at the site of inflammation. The differentiation, proliferation, and subsequent antibody synthesis occurs primarily in the spleen and lymph nodes, however. B cells are helped or suppressed in antibody synthesis by T lymphocytes derived from stem cells in the bone marrow and differentiated in the thymus. T cells are found in high concentration in the circulation as well as in specific sites in the lymph nodes.

Activated T cells in particular, but sometimes B cells and macrophages, produce a number of polypeptides called *lymphokines* or monokines, which activate other macrophages and lymphocytes, prevent their migration from the antigenic site, stimulate the proliferation of other lymphocytes, and modify immune responses.

The mechanism of interaction of these lymphokines with the cells of the immune system is unclear, but published evidence demonstrates a surface receptor for *migration inhibition factor* on B cells.[95] The binding of a lymphokine to a receptor may represent a prototype for these types of interactions.

Mast cells and basophils may release histamine-containing granules during inflammation and allergic responses. Other granules in these cells contain heparin, serotonin, and prostaglandin.

HEMOSTASIS, COAGULATION, AND FIBRINOLYSIS

Inflammation is a multifaceted phenomenon involving both the effects of injury to cells and tissue repair processes. Repair starts simultaneously with injury, but usually does not become the dominant pattern until the injurious agent is destroyed or inactivated and the necrotic tissue is being removed from the site of injury.

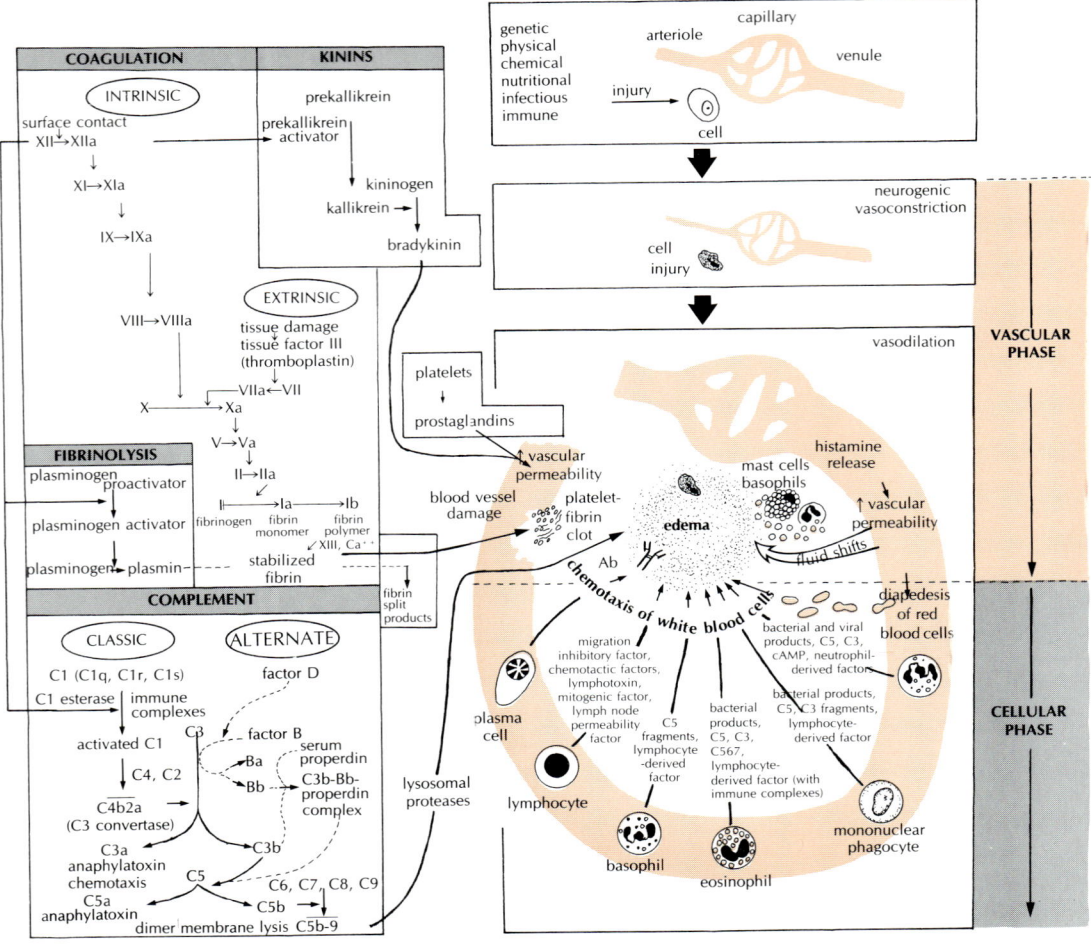

Figure 2–40. Components of the inflammatory response are shown. Cellular injury by various agents initiates the vascular and cellular phases of inflammation, which are closely interrelated to the coagulation, fibrinolyis, kinin, and complement systems.

As a result of a combined multicellular response, particularly of the white blood cells, the tissues produce vasodilatory, chemotactic, antimicrobial, and mitogenic factors, hormones (prostaglandins), and antibodies (Fig. 2–40). They attack and destroy injurious agents, remove injured cells and other products of the inflammatory process, and pave the way for the processes of repair. Because of the importance of the vascular response to inflammation, several hemostatic systems with local, as well as ramifying effects, are activated in injury and serve to preserve, as best as possible, architectural integrity and to facilitate repair.[96]

Blood coagulation, with the resultant formation of fibrin, plays an important role in inflammation, particularly in vessels, in which thrombosis may occur (Table 2–22). In tissue, the extracellular formation of fibrin in the area of inflammation, as well as in the lymphatics leading from it, may retard the spread of infectious agents and later may provide a framework for repair processes. In the acute inflammatory reaction, macrophages are able to engulf for-

Table 2–22. *Clotting Factor Nomenclature*

Factor	Definition
I	Fibrinogen
II	Prothrombin
III	Tissue thromboplastin
IV	Calcium
V	Labile factor (accelerator globulin)
VII	Stable factor (serum prothrombin conversion factor)
VIII	Antihemophilic globulin
IX	Plasma thromboplastin component (PTC) (Christmas factor)
X	Stuart-Prower factor
XI	Plasma thromboplastic antecedent (PTA)
XII	Hageman (contact) factor
XIII	Fibrin-stabilizing factor

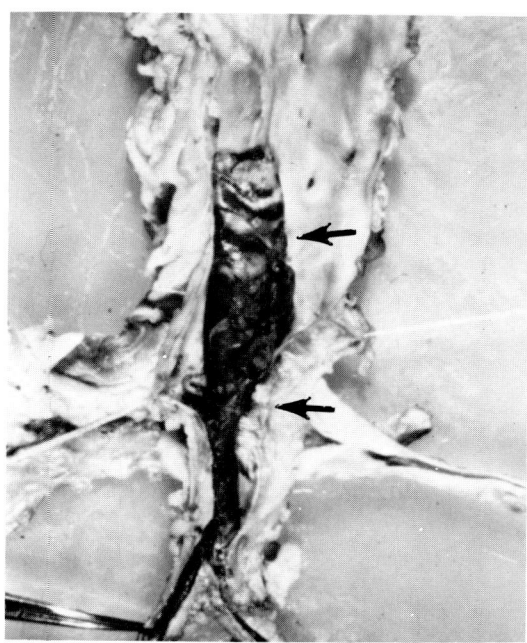

Figure 2–41. A thrombus (arrow) in the abdominal aorta extends into the iliac arteries.

eign material more easily when a surface such as that provided by fibrin is available. In granulation tissue and in chronic inflammation, fibrin serves as a scaffold on which fibroblasts lay down collagen. As noted previously, fibrin and ground substances form a barrier to invasion and spreading of infectious bacteria. Organisms (for example, streptococci) may release a fibrinolytic enzyme (such as streptokinase) to overcome this barrier.

Clotting is accentuated in the inflammatory reaction by ischemia, stasis, production of exo- and endotoxins, and various injurious agents causing cell damage.

Diseases classically associated with vessel clotting abnormalities include atherosclerosis (Fig. 2–41), diabetes, shock, gastrointestinal and liver disease, the Shwartzman reaction, disseminated intravascular coagulation (DIC), and carcinoma of the pancreas. Blood clots (thrombi) formed in vessels may break off and pass to other sites as emboli.

Hageman Factor

Coagulation is initiated by Hageman factor XII, which is also critical in activating kinins for vasodilatation, complement in the complement cascade,[97] and plasminogen proactivator for the activation of plasmin (fibrinolysin) (see Fig. 2–40).

This serum factor is synthesized by a variety of cells, including some tumor lines, and converts plasminogen to plasmin (fibrinolysin), which can split stabilized fibrin into fibrin-split products. Both plasmin and Hageman factor are presumably also capable of triggering, through an unknown intermediate, conversion of the C1 fraction of complement to C1 esterase, which in turn can activate the complement cascade.

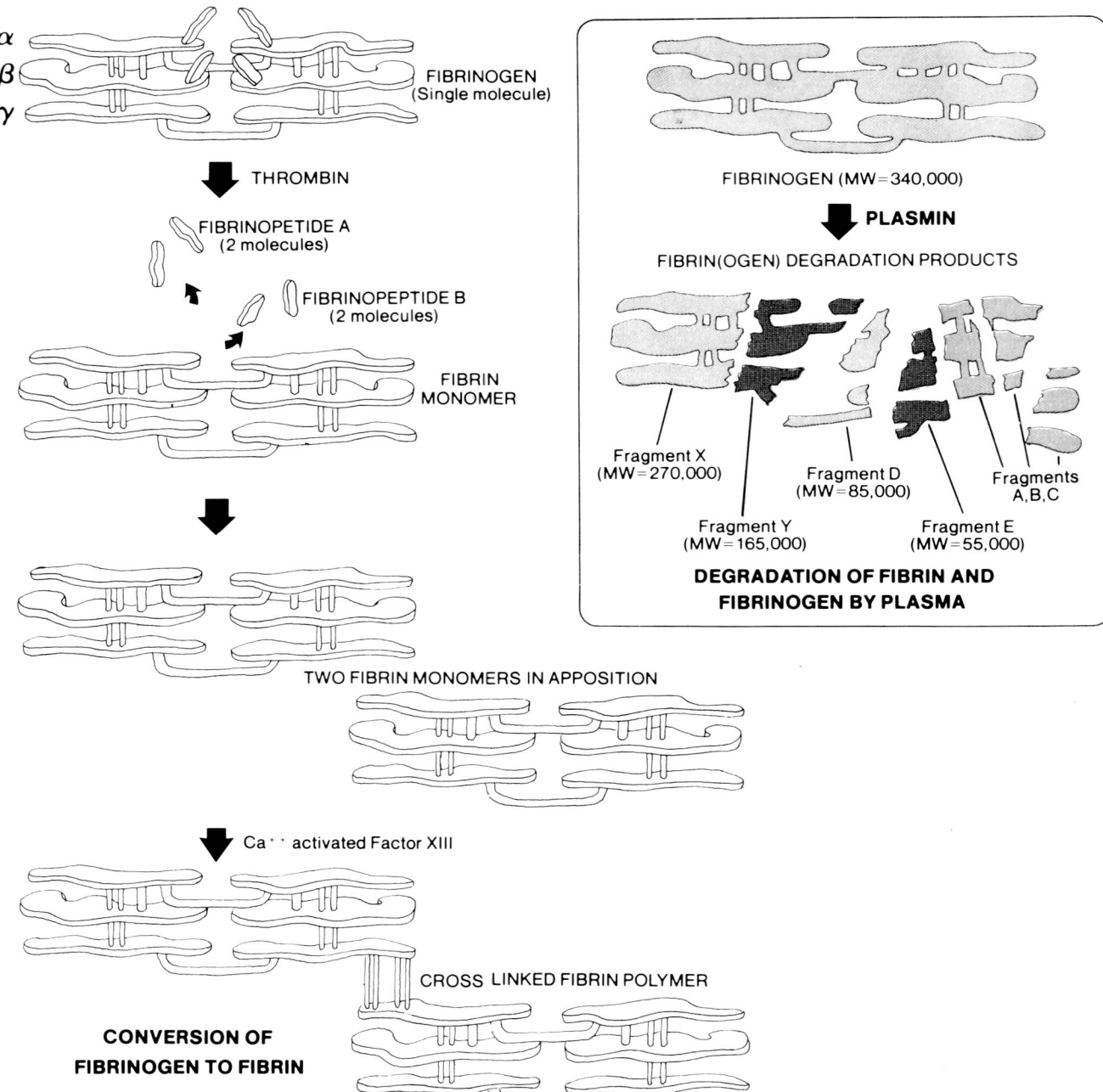

Figure 2-42. The formation of fibrin from fibrinogen is shown here. Fibrinogen normally exists as a dimer, each unit of which contains 3 individual polypeptide chains: A-alpha, B-beta, and gamma, with respective molecular weights of 67,000, 58,000, and 47,000 daltons.

Thrombin, a serine protease produced by proteolytic cleavage of prothrombin, acts at specific sites on the A-alpha and B-beta chains. This specific proteolytic action produces 2 molecules of fibrinopeptide A, 2 molecules of fibrinopeptide B, and leaves a large dimeric residue, known as fibrin monomer, composed of 2 alpha, 2 beta, and 2 gamma chains. The formation of fibrin monomer is the initiating event in the formation of a fibrin clot.

Fibrin monomer polymerizes spontaneously to form nonstabilized fibrin polymers that are crosslinked in the presence of calcium and activated factor XIII to form stabilized fibrin. Stabilized fibrin, as well as earlier forms of fibrin, and even fibrinogen itself, can undergo proteolytic fragmentation in the presence of plasmin.

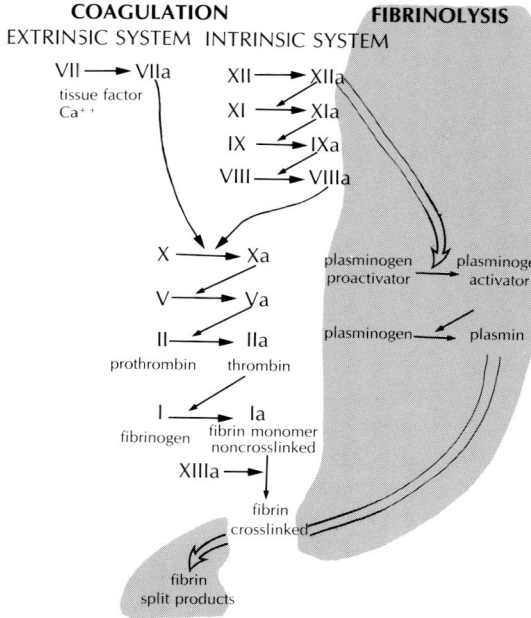

COAGULATION   FIBRINOLYSIS
EXTRINSIC SYSTEM INTRINSIC SYSTEM

Figure 2–43. Coagulation and fibrinolytic mechanisms.

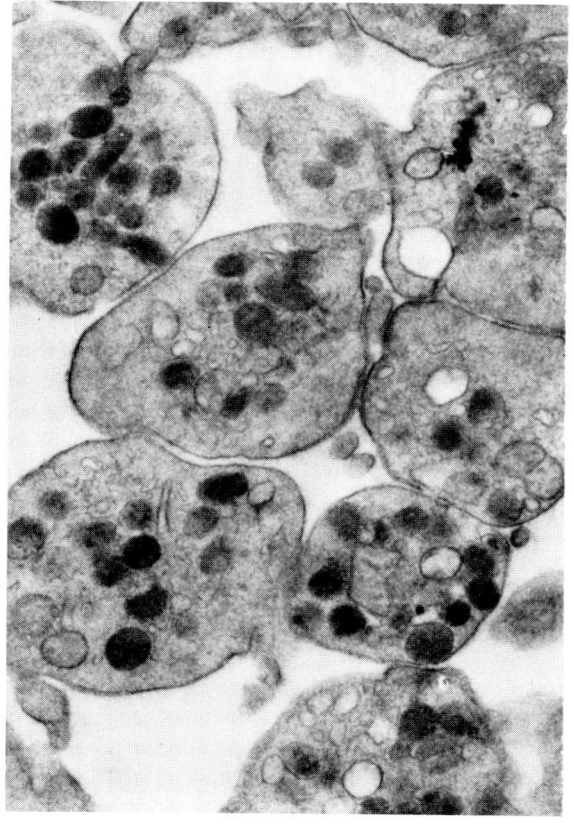

Figure 2–44. Electron micrograph showing platelets containing numerous electron dense granules.

Fibrinogen

Fibrinogen exists in the blood as a dimer, each unit of which consists of three polypeptide chains: α, β, and γ, with respective molecular weights of 67,000, 58,000, and 47,000 daltons. The release of fibrinopeptide A and fibrinopeptide B after thrombin action produces aggregation and end-to-end polymerization of fibrin monomer molecules[98] (Fig. 2–42).

Intrinsic and Extrinsic Fibrin Coagulation Pathways

The clotting mechanism proceeds by two pathways: *intrinsic* and *extrinsic* (Fig. 2–43). The intrinsic pathway is initiated by conversion of Hageman factor XII to factor XIIa. Factor XIIa acts on factor XI (plasma thromboplastic antecedent) which, when converted to factor XIa, converts factor IX (Christmas factor) to factor IXa. Factor IXa converts factor VIII (antihemophilic globulin) to factor VIIIa.

Antihemophilic globulin consists of three fractions: VIII-AHF, VIII-VWF (von Willebrand factor, necessary for normal platelet function), and factor VIII-AGN. Factor VIIIa converts factor X (Stuart-Prower factor) to factor Xa. This conversion also occurs following activation of factor VII (serum prothrombin conversion factor-SPCF or stable factor) to factor VIIa by tissue thromboplastin (factor III). Action of both factor VIIa and VIIIa on *factor X* is the point at which the intrinsic pathway joins the extrinsic pathway in a common integrated pathway leading to the formation of stabilized fibrin.

Factor Xa acts on factor V (an accelerator globulin) or labile factor which, when converted to factor Va, converts factor II (prothrombin) to Factor IIa (thrombin). Thrombin splits fibrinogen (factor I) to fibrin monomer (factor Ia), as shown in Figure 2–43. Fibrin monomer is then polymerized and, with the addition of calcium and factor XIII (fibrin-stabilizing factor), forms irreversibly polymerized stabilized fibrin. Plasmin (fibrinolysin) degrades stabilized fibrin to fibrin-split products.[99]

Platelets

Platelets (Fig. 2–44) are derived from *megakaryocytes* (large, multilobed, metachromatically staining cells, 35 to 40 microns in diameter) found in the bone marrow. Cytoplasmic fragments approximately 3 microns in diameter are continually broken off from the megakaryocytes. In the steady state, 4×10^{11} platelets leave the bone marrow and gain access to the peripheral blood. Platelets have an outer membrane 150-Å thick and contain a rough cytoskeleton and a poorly described network of microfilaments and microtubules.[100] An outermost fluffy mucopolysaccharide coat, with special adsorptive affinity for plasma factors I, V, VIII, XI, and XII, aids in the generation of thrombin when the intrinsic coagulation system is activated. Although a few mitochondria are present, the major energy source is glycolysis.

Platelets contain two major forms of granules: dense and light. Dense granules contain adenosine diphosphate (ADP) and vasoactive amines, including 5-hydroxytryptamine (serotonin) and heparin. Light granules contain a full complement of lysosomal enzymes. In addition, two other proteins are present: *thrombasthenin A*, which contains an actin-like protein, and *thrombasthenin B*, which contains a myosin protein. Rupture of the platelets will release either dense or light granules, or both. Platelets also secrete *prostaglandins, thromboxane A₂, mitogens, and permeability* factors[101] (Table 2–23).

Table 2–23. *Enzymatic Granules of Platelets*

Dense Granules
 ADP
 Vasoactive amines
 Serotonin
 Histamine
 Catecholamine

α *Granules (Light)*
 Lysosomal enzymes
 Cationic substances (vasopermeability)
 Thrombasthenin A (actin)
 Thrombasthenin B (myosin)
 Thrombospondin

Other
 Permeability factors
 Mitogens
 Thromboxane A₂
Gelsolin
Calmodulin

Clot Formation

Vascular clotting is often initiated by injury to the endothelial wall with exposure of the underlying collagenous basement membrane. A bleeding vessel initially constricts, and platelets quickly adhere at the disrupted edge.

Following formation of a temporary platelet clot, retraction takes place by means of thrombasthenin-induced contraction. Clotting follows an initial platelet aggregation within a vessel[102,103] (Fig. 2–45). The release of Hageman factor XII by denudation of collagen initiates the intrinsic pathway of fibrin formation in the vessel. Later, fibrin formation on the platelet surface attracts more platelets. White blood cells and the temporarily permeable platelet plugs ("white thrombus") are converted into an impermeable, insoluble, and irreversible fixed *"red thrombus"* composed of a fibrin mesh enclosing erythrocytes, platelets, and white blood cells (Fig. 2–45).

As a result of release of *tissue thromboplastin* (a microsomal lipoprotein released from injured cells in tissues and blood vessels), fibrin may also be formed through the *extrinsic* pathway of coagulation.

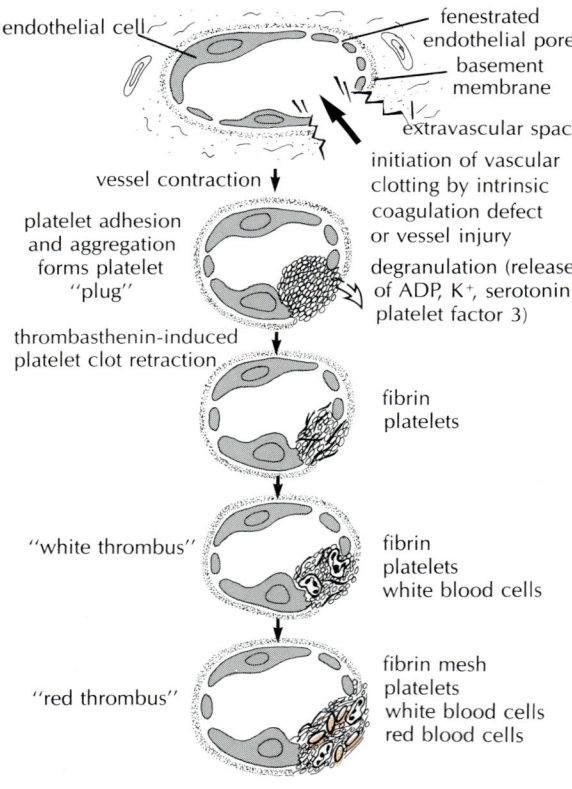

Figure 2–45. Steps in clot formation.

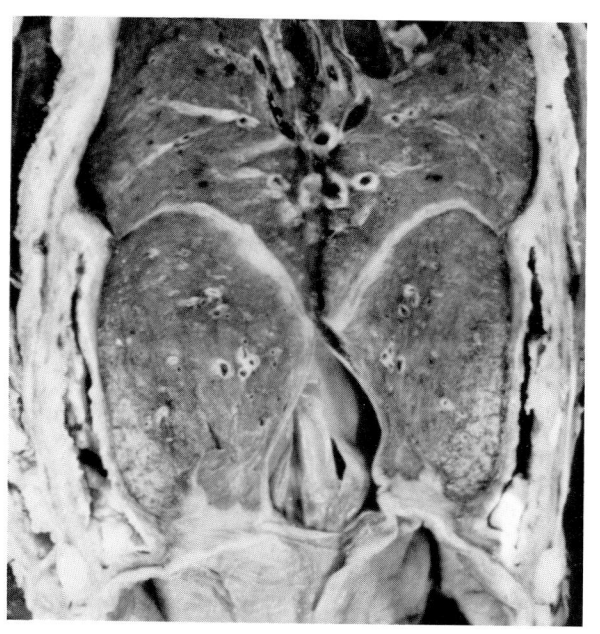

Figure 2–46. Lung with dense pleural scarring. Specimen is bisected through the hilum and reflected.

REPAIR, REGENERATION, AND SCAR FORMATION

The usual repair process results in complete *resolution* of inflammation and restitution of normal tissue structure. There is usually *regeneration* of both mesenchymal and epithelial elements and approximate restoration of the normal architecture.

If tissue is unable to regenerate because of the inherent characteristics of its cell population, or if tissue-associated factors such as nutritional deficiency or hypoxia exist, the normal structures will be replaced by *scar tissue*. Although scar tissue does not have the same functional capacity as the original, differentiated parenchymal cells, it serves to maintain the organization of the tissue and organ and acts as a bridge between the remaining, effectively functioning cells (Fig. 2–46). Ineffective host response to the injurious agent, including failure of destruction, removal, or detoxification, may perpetuate abnormal repair processes in the form of chronic inflammation.

Regeneration of Cells

Different types of cells have different generation times and regenerative capacities. One can discuss cellular responses to injury in terms of cell and organ *hypertrophy* and *hyperplasia*. Another cellular response to injury is *metaplasia*. If, for example, stem cells are injured, they may be stimulated to produce a type of cell different from the indigenous population (metaplasia). A well-known example of metaplasia is the replacement of columnar or transitional epithelium by squamous cells.

If the compensatory responses of hyperplasia and hypertrophy within the cell are ineffective, *death* or *atrophy* of the cell may result. The resulting space is then filled in with ground substance and proliferating fibroblasts that synthesize collagen.

Factors and Mediators in Regeneration

Considerable study has been devoted to factors that influence regeneration (Table 2–24). Generalized *systemic factors* such as age, nutrition, and hormonal states are of no small importance. *Local factors* such as blood supply and location of the injurious lesion determine the rate, extent, and type of regeneration that ensues. Injured or regenerating cells may elaborate factors that influence the regenerative process. For example, early experiments on parabiotic rats suggested that injured and regenerating liver cells produced a substance that could also stimulate injured liver cells in the paired rat to divide.[104]

Table 2–24. *Requirements for Growth of Cells and Tissues*

I. Basic nutrients
   A. Glucose
   B. Amino acids
   C. Minerals and trace elements
   D. Fatty acids
   E. Vitamins

II. Hormones (depending on tissue involved)
   A. Insulin (muscle, liver)
   B. Thyroid-stimulating factor (TSH) (thyroid)
   C. Follicle-stimulating factor (FSF) (ovary, testes)
   D. Luteinizing factor (LH) (ovary, testes)
   E. Growth hormone (GH)
   F. Estrogen and progesterone (endometrium)

III. Other growth factors
   A. Epidermal growth factor (EGF)
   B. Melanocyte growth factor (MGF)
   C. T-cell growth factor (leukokinin)
   D. Angiogenesis factor

IV. Binding proteins for transport
   A. Transferrin (iron)
   B. Ceruloplasmin (copper)
   C. Albumin (fatty acids)

Folkman has partially isolated a factor from tumor cells that he believes stimulates endothelial growth *(tumor angiogenesis factor).*[105] We now recognize the existence of *specific epidermal growth factors,* neural growth factors,[106] and mesenchymal growth factors. Injury may alter epithelial permeability and may allow release of growth inhibitory substances *(chalones).*[107] Intracellular mechanisms of inhibition are thereby removed, permitting injured cells to divide without constraint.

Much of the regulation of cell growth in normal states as well as in regeneration occurs at the level of the plasma membrane. Regulation may be mediated by specific receptors for hormones, specialized cell junctions, and other less well defined mechanisms.

Studies on in vitro tissue cultures have emphasized the role of *contact* and *density inhibition* in controlling growth of mesenchymal cells. Disruption of a tissue culture flask surface that is completely covered with cells stimulates the remaining cells to grow until cellular contact is once again established. At this point, inhibition of growth occurs.

A variety of *lectins* including PHA, as well as *platelet factors,* low-density lipoproteins *(LDL),* and *hypertensive serum factors* stimulate mitosis in vitro. These and other similar substances may control mitosis in vivo.

Stem Cells, Intermitotic, Postmitotic, and Reverting Postmitotic Cells

Many years ago, Cowdry classified cells according to their capacities for division and designated them as either *post-mitotic, intermitotic,* or *reverting postmitotic* (Table 2–25). Some cells remain in the G_0 stationary phase of the cell cycle for long periods, whereas others spend varying periods of time in the G_1, S, and G_2 phases. Generally, cells spend approximately 30 to 60 minutes in the 4 stages of *mitosis: prophase, metaphase, anaphase,* and *telophase.*

Table 2–25. Capacity of Cells to Divide

Postmitotic Cells	Reverting Postmitotic Cells	Intermitotic Cells
(no division)	(capable of division following stimulation)	(stem cells in constant state of division)
Cardiac myocytes	Renal tubular epithelium	Bone marrow
	Hepatocytes	Skin
Neurons	Lung	Gastrointestinal
	Endocrine epithelium	Genitourinary
	Mesenchymal tissue	Reproductive
	Connective tissue	
	Bone	
	Skeletal muscle	

asymmetric division

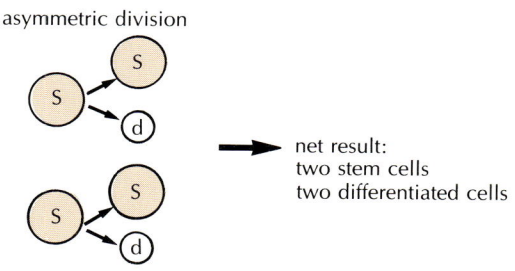

net result:
two stem cells
two differentiated cells

symmetric division

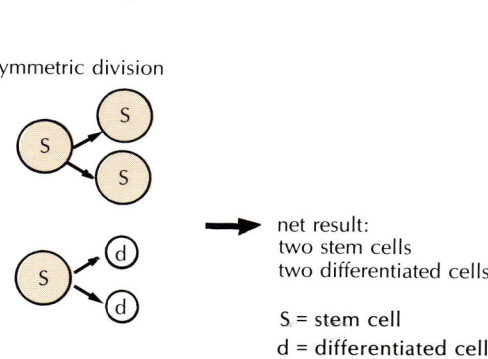

net result:
two stem cells
two differentiated cells

S = stem cell
d = differentiated cell

Figure 2–47. Comparison of results of asymmetric versus symmetric stem cell division. By either mechanism, two stem cells divide to yield two progeny stem cells and progeny differentiated cells. S, stem cell, d, differentiated cell.

Stem Cells.   These cells in the bone marrow are usually large in relation to their nearby differentiated blood cell derivatives. They have high nuclear:cytoplasmic ratios. In other tissues, stem cells lie near the basement membrane and are largely distinguished by their ability to incorporate radioactive thymidine rapidly. Stem cells may undergo *asymmetric division:* the dividing cell produces one daughter cell that remains a stem cell and another daughter cell that becomes a differentiated cell. *Symmetric division,* alternatively, may occur: a stem cell produces two daughter stem cells or two differentiated cells, depending on the stimulus at any one time. The potential results of division of two stem cells by asymmetric or symmetric means are identical, with the generation of two differentiated and two stem cells by either mechanism (Fig. 2–47). The proportion of stem cells to differentiated cells is variable in different tissues, however.

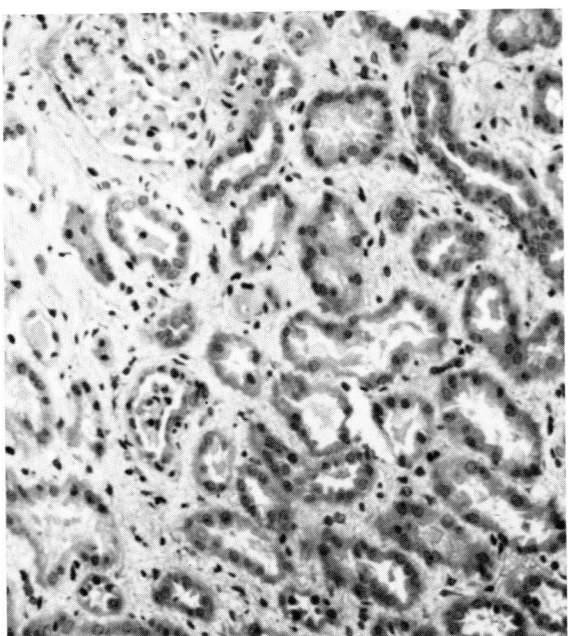

Figure 2–48. Renal tubular epithelium is regenerating following acute tubular necrosis. (Courtesy of Dr. Conrad L. Pirani, College of Physicians & Surgeons, Columbia University, New York.)

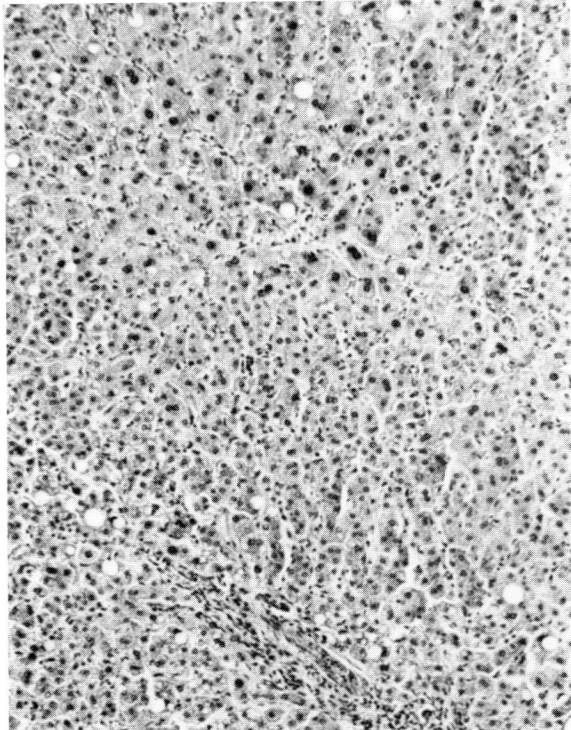

Figure 2–49. In resolving hepatitis, large regenerating hepatocytes are present in the liver cell plates. The sinusoids still contain inflammatory cells; there is mild residual portal inflammation (bottom).

Intermitotic Cells. Intermitotic ("labile") cells, in a continual state of division, include cells in the *skin, bone marrow,* and *gastrointestinal, genitourinary, respiratory,* and *reproductive tracts.* The stem cells in these sites may be difficult to detect. They divide, differentiate, and sometimes migrate at varying intervals of time. A partly differentiated daughter cell emigrates to its principal anatomic site of function before, during, or after maturation. Bone marrow B-lymphocyte stem cells migrate to spleen and lymph nodes, whereas T cells from the bone marrow migrate to the thymus, where further differentiation takes place.

Stem cells of the skin and gastrointestinal, genitourinary, respiratory, and reproductive tracts mature and are sloughed off the tissue surface, thereby allowing replacement by other daughter cells. Completely differentiated cells of these organs have the advantage of being able to suffer injury without serious consequences, because their half-lives are short and they usually have no daughter cells. Some authors believe that differentiated cells of the bowel and bronchial wall are capable of division, however.[108]

Postmitotic Cells. Postmitotic ("permanent") cells are at the opposite end of the spectrum. These include *nerve cells*[109] and *adult cardiac muscle cells.* In the heart, although hyperdiploid chromosomal states exist as a result of DNA repair and replication and can be demonstrated by uptake and incorporation of tritiated thymidine, cardiac myocytes cannot divide, that is, they cannot undergo hyperplasia. The response to injury of cardiac muscle cells is variable and may result in atrophy, hypertrophy, or death. Both small and large myocardial muscle infarcts feature muscle replacement by scar tissue.[110] Smooth muscle, in contrast, may undergo hyperplasia as well as hypertrophy, as in the uterine muscle in pregnancy, or medial muscle in the walls of arteries in atherosclerosis and hypertension. Skeletal muscle may also regenerate by means of satellite cells.[111]

Reverting Postmitotic Cells. The final class, reverting postmitotic *("stable")* cells are found in tissues in which regeneration is variable. These cells are probably in a low, continual state of division, but when injured, they have the capacity to divide rapidly and to regenerate their tissue architecture.

Mature, differentiated *liver, kidney, lung,* and *endocrine cells* are capable of such division which, in certain of these organs, may involve proliferation from reserve stem cells or mature cells. For example, after acute tubular necrosis, renal tubular epithelium may regenerate from remaining differentiated cells[112] (Fig. 2–48).

Liver cell division, again demonstrated by incorporation of tritiated thymidine, allows regeneration following injury depending on various factors[113,114] (Fig. 2–49). Epithelial and endothelial cells in pulmonary alveoli may regenerate, for example, following lobar pneumonia. Infection in the prostate may be followed by hyperplasia and hypertrophy of both the muscle and epithelial glandular elements. Pan-

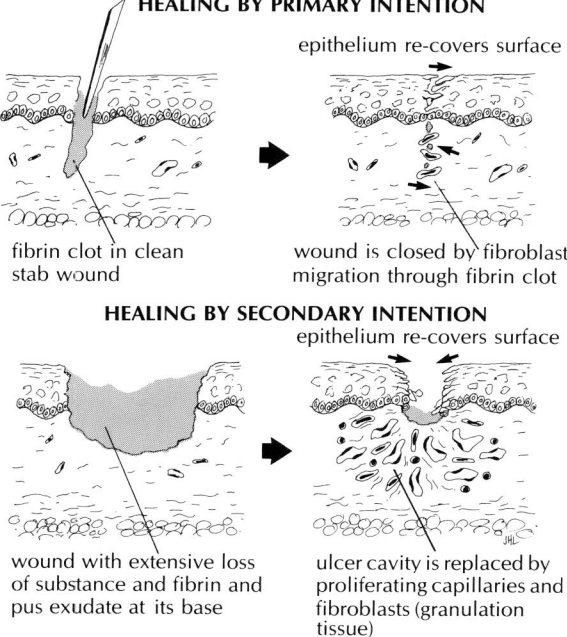

HEALING BY PRIMARY INTENTION

epithelium re-covers surface

fibrin clot in clean stab wound

wound is closed by fibroblast migration through fibrin clot

HEALING BY SECONDARY INTENTION

epithelium re-covers surface

wound with extensive loss of substance and fibrin and pus exudate at its base

ulcer cavity is replaced by proliferating capillaries and fibroblasts (granulation tissue)

Figure 2–50. Two mechanisms of wound healing are shown here.

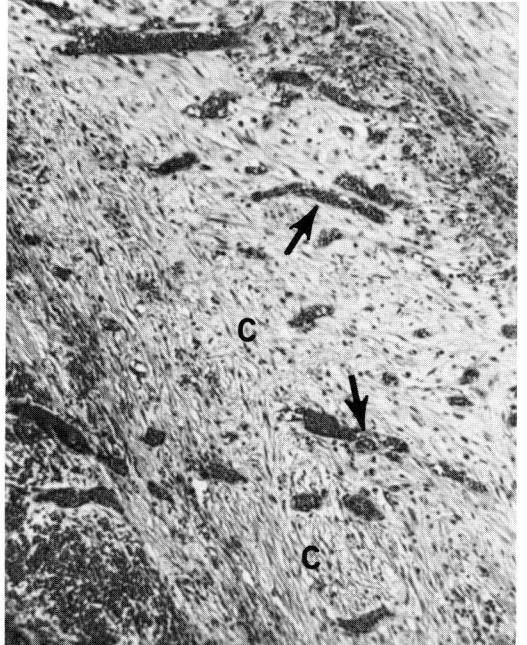

Figure 2–51. Granulation tissue features proliferating capillaries (arrows), inflammatory cells, new collagen (C), and ground substance.

creatic beta cells may also undergo division after injury and may be seen as hyperplastic islets of Langerhans.[115]

Among the mesenchymal tissues, the *fibroblast* is the best example of a reverting postmitotic cell, one with multipotentiality.[116] Following injury, it may divide, may synthesize collagen, and may become a lipid-storing and synthesizing cell or a tissue histiocyte capable of phagocytosis.

Regeneration of Tissues

The principal requirement for normal regeneration of epithelial cells of the lung, kidney, and endocrine glands is an *intact basement membrane.* A glomerulus cannot be reformed following destruction of the basement membrane. A pulmonary infarct with basement membrane destruction always results in scar tissue. Regeneration of liver cells along collapsed reticulin fibers depends on other factors such as blood supply and critical baseline residual cell mass. In all these instances, *if regeneration is impossible, scar tissue usually develops* instead of restitution of the previous, organized structure.

Healing by Primary Intention

Animal experiments, verified by observation of human clinical trauma cases, have shown that simple, clean wounds with apposable edges that can be closed with sutures are quickly filled with fibrin and platelet clot in the space between millions of destroyed cells. During the first two days after injury, this clot is rapidly infiltrated by PMN, followed by mononuclear cells during the second and third days. Proliferating fibroblasts are seen during the third and fourth day, and by the fifth day, loose, newly synthesized collagen is present in the injured area (Fig. 2–50). This process is called healing by *primary intention.*

Healing by Secondary Intention

If appreciable amounts of tissue are destroyed and the wound of skin surface or internal viscera is unable to be approximated with sutures, the area will heal by *secondary intention* (Fig. 2–50). Once the injurious agent is overcome and scavenger monocytes have removed dead organisms, granulation tissue is formed. *Granulation tissue* (Fig. 2–51) is composed of (1) infiltrating, proliferating fibroblasts, which lay down collagen on the fibrin scaffold; (2) infiltrating proliferating capillary endothelial buds, which provide new vessels for transport of nutrition and oxygen; and (3) monocytes and lymphocytes to continue phagocytosis, local immune reaction, and maintenance of a sterile wound.

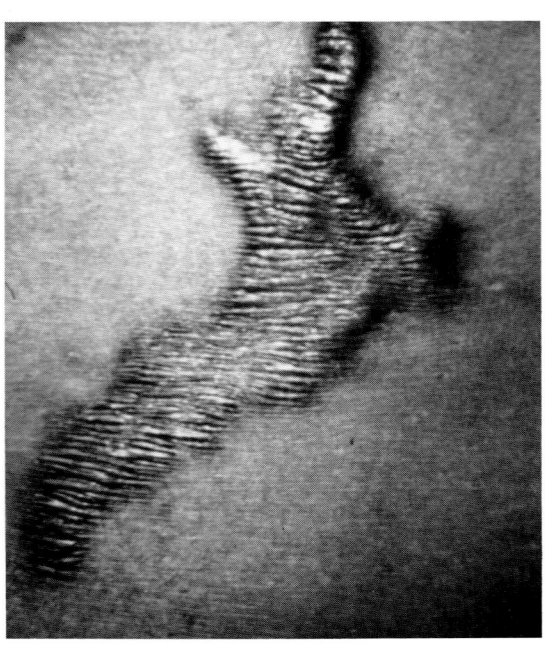

Figure 2–52. Hypertrophic scar tissue forms an irregular, large keloid on the skin surface. (Courtesy of Dr. David Silvers, College of Physicians & Surgeons, Columbia University, New York.)

As indicated previously, following injury of organs in which tissue restitution is impossible, granulation tissue is eventually replaced by collagen scar. On the skin or organ surfaces, granulation tissue progresses from deeper areas below the surface at the same time that epithelial proliferation and migration takes place on the surface itself. Overproduction of granulation tissue on the skin surface results in *"proud flesh."* In order to remove this superfluous granulation tissue, chemical means or surgical debridement is necessary. Eventually, a scar results, with an epithelial covering. It retracts to 5 to 10% of its original size in a few months. Occasionally, unabated proliferation of underlying connective tissue occurs, producing a mass of flesh called a *keloid* (Fig. 2–52), which is prominent in blacks.

Controversy exists over the *tensile strength* of scars in healed wounds. Originally, it was believed that the contraction of a scar was due to *contraction* of *collagen bundles.* Scar contraction is now thought to be due to *actin-like proteins* in fibroblasts and other cells. Gabbiani and Majno were among the first to point out that the majority of the fibroblasts in granulation tissue possess contractile structures; hence, the researchers named these cells *myofibroblasts.*[117]

Following suturing, the tensile strength of a wound is approximately 70% of the tissue's original strength. This figure may vary after removal of the sutures, yet 8 weeks later, it still does not exceed the original 70%. Scar tissue, in critical organs such as the heart, rapidly gains tensile strength after the first 10 to 14 days and reaches a plateau at the end of 3 months.[118] Infection, stress, increased age, and poor nutrition retard the entire process.[118]

Organization of Exudates and Thrombi

Some inflammatory reactions, particularly at free surfaces of cavities (pleura, peritoneum, pericardium, and respiratory, gastrointestinal, and genitourinary mucosal surfaces and skin) may result in the escape of fluid, proteins, and cells in the form of transudates or exudates. *Transudates* are low-protein extravascular fluids with a specific gravity under 1.012. *Exudates,* in contrast, are high-protein fluids containing cells and with a specific gravity above 1.020. Several types of exudates are recognized and may be associated with specific inflammatory conditions. Serous (clear, light yellow) exudates occur in congestive heart failure. Purulent or suppurative (pus-containing) exudates are present in kidneys infected with bacteria in pyelonephritis. Hemorrhagic exudates are associated with infarcts or neoplasms of organs such as the lung. Fibrinous exudates of the epicardium characterize rheumatic fever (Table 2–26).

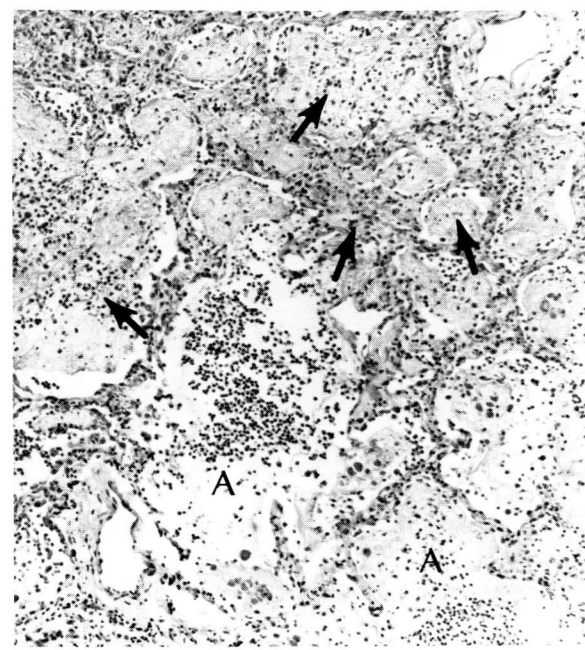

Figure 2–53. Autopsy lung section of patient with organizing pneumonia. Several alveoli (A) contain neutrophilic leukocytes. Areas of early organization (arrows) show alveoli filled with fibrin and inflammatory cells. Subsequent proliferation of fibroblasts and capillaries would result in scar formation.

Table 2–26. *Classification of Exudates and Effusions*

Description	Disease and Site of Involvement
Serous effusion	Cirrhosis (ascites in peritoneal cavity)
	Acute cardiac failure (hydrothorax)
Serosanguinous effusion	Chronic cardiac failure (pleural cavity)
Purulent exudate	Abscess (empyema of lung)
Hemorrhagic effusion	Klebsiella pneumonia (lung)
	Carcinoma (pleural cavity)
Fibrinous exudate	Uremia (pericardium)
	Rheumatic fever (pericardium)

Although *reabsorption* occurs to a large extent with transudates or serous exudates, purulent, hemorrhagic, and fibrinous exudates are usually subsequently "organized." Organization implies infiltration by monocytes, proliferating capillaries, and fibroblasts with granulation tissue formation, synthesis of new collagen, and eventual scar formation (Fig. 2–53).

Scar Tissue

Scar tissue consists of *collagen,* few *blood vessels,* sometimes *elastic tissue,* and variable amounts of *ground substances* (hyaluronic acid and proteoglycans). It is sometimes "*hyalinized,*" with a glassy appearance, and usually contains a few dormant fibroblasts and round cells (monocytes and lymphocytes). Collagen, elastin, hyaluronic acid, and proteoglycans are synthesized by fibroblasts; other glycoproteins, found extracellularly and in plasma, are synthesized in the liver and other components of the lymphoreticular system and are delivered to sites of scar formation.[119]

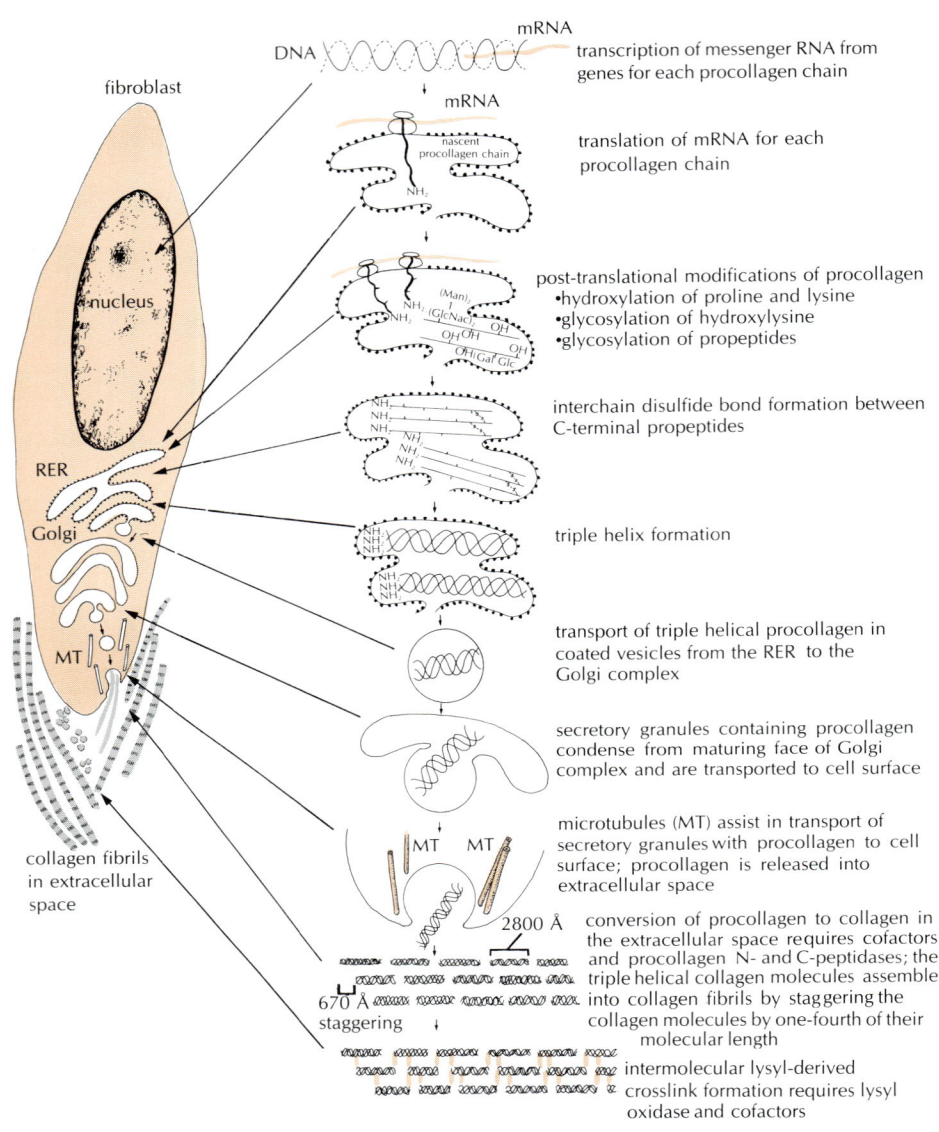

mRNA

DNA

transcription of messenger RNA from genes for each procollagen chain

mRNA

nascent procollagen chain

NH₂

translation of mRNA for each procollagen chain

NH₂
NH₂
(Man)ₙ
(GlcNac)₂
OH OH   OH
OH(Gal Glc)ₙ OH

post-translational modifications of procollagen
•hydroxylation of proline and lysine
•glycosylation of hydroxylysine
•glycosylation of propeptides

NH₂
NH₂
NH₂
NH₂
NH₂
NH₂

interchain disulfide bond formation between C-terminal propeptides

NH₂
NH₂
NH₂
NH₂
NH₂
NH₂

triple helix formation

transport of triple helical procollagen in coated vesicles from the RER to the Golgi complex

secretory granules containing procollagen condense from maturing face of Golgi complex and are transported to cell surface

MT   MT

microtubules (MT) assist in transport of secretory granules with procollagen to cell surface; procollagen is released into extracellular space

2800 Å

670 Å
staggering

conversion of procollagen to collagen in the extracellular space requires cofactors and procollagen N- and C-peptidases; the triple helical collagen molecules assemble into collagen fibrils by staggering the collagen molecules by one-fourth of their molecular length

intermolecular lysyl-derived crosslink formation requires lysyl oxidase and cofactors

fibroblast

nucleus

RER

Golgi

MT

collagen fibrils in extracellular space

Figure 2–54. Schematic representation of collagen synthesis, processing, secretion, deposition, and stabilization.

Collagen

Collagen is a protein containing three peptide chains (α chains), each of approximately one thousand amino acids with a total molecular weight of approximately one million.[120]

The 3 α chains are twisted into a 300 × 1.5 nm right-handed triple *helix*. The triple helices are in turn assembled into *microfibrils*, which are covalently bonded into the mature collagen *fibrils* of tissue (Figs. 2–54 and 2–55).

Five separate types of collagen are now known. *Type I* collagen consists of two different types of α chains (two α_1 (I) and one α_2), whereas *Types II, III,* and *IV* are each composed of three identical chains, α_1 (II), α_1 (III), and α_1 (IV), respectively. *Type V* consists of polypeptides called $[\alpha_1(V)]_2\alpha_2(V)$ (αA and αB) chains. Nearly every third amino acid of collagen α chains is glycine, and other frequent amino acids include proline, hydroxyproline, lysine, and hydroxylysine. The various types of collagen are characteristic of certain tissues (Table 2–27).

Each of the three peptide chains of collagen is synthesized on the ribosomes of the rough endoplasmic reticulum. The three chains are first assembled in the cisternae of the endoplasmic reticulum as *procollagen* (pro-α) chains. Iron and ascorbic acid are necessary for the posttranslational modifications of hydroxylation of proline and lysine as well as glycosylation of hydroxylysine.

The general sequence of events is: hydroxylation of the pro-α chains, synthesis of interchain disulfide bonds, and formation of the triple helix. Procollagen passes from the rough endoplasmic reticulum through the Golgi complex, and the triple-helical procollagen then passes to the extracellular space with the help of microtubules.

The extracellular conversion of procollagen to collagen occurs by degradation of the molecule with procollagen amino- and carboxyproteases. The collagen molecules produced by cleavage of procollagen spontaneously assemble

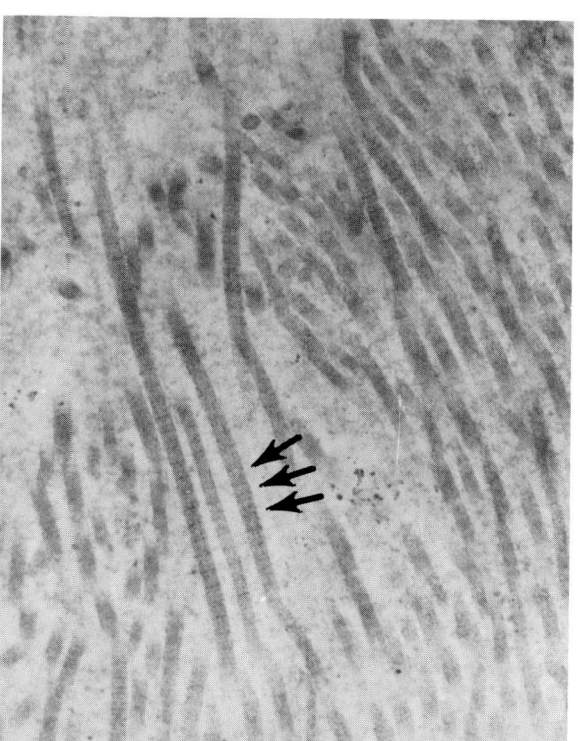

Figure 2–55. In this electron micrograph of collagen bundles in the uterus, note the characteristic periodicity in the banding of these fibrils (arrow).

Table 2–27.   *The Collagen Isotypes*

Collagen Type	Composition	Tissue Location	Cell Types that Synthesize Various Collagen Types
I	$[\alpha_1(I)]_2\alpha_2(I)$	Skin, bone, tendon, cornea, dentin, ligament, fascia, arteries, uterus	Fibroblasts, osteoblasts, smooth muscle cells, epithelium
II	$[\alpha_1(II)]_3$	Cartilage, cornea, vitreous body	Chondrocytes, neural retinal cells, notochord cells
III	$[\alpha_1(III)]_3$	Fetal skin, blood vessels, organs, uterus	Fibroblasts, myoblasts
IV	$[\alpha_1(IV)]_3$ $[\alpha_2(IV)]_3$	Basement membrane lens, glomeruli	Endothelial and epithelial cells
V	$[\alpha_1(V)]_2\alpha_2(V)$ (formerly αA and αB chains)	Blood vessels, smooth muscle, skin, placenta	Smooth muscle cells, chondrocytes under certain conditions

(Modified from Kleinman, H.K., Klebe, R.J., and Martin, G.R.: Role of collagenous matrices in the adhesion and growth of cells. J. Cell Biol., *88*:473, 1981.)

into collagen fibrils, which gain tensile strength by cross-linking through covalent bonds. The first step in cross-linking involves oxidative deamination by lysyl oxidase, a copper-containing enzyme.[121]

Once collagen microfibrils are assembled into fibrils, a cross-striated pattern becomes apparent. The distance or periodicity of *670Å* between cross striations on electron microscopy (Fig. 2–55) is due to the staggering of the *300-nm* collagen molecules by about one quarter of their length. Both intramolecular cross-links of α chains and intermolecular cross-links through Schiff base interactions stabilize tissue collagen fibrils (Fig. 2–54). New collagen formed following injury may be reabsorbed following collagenase degradation.

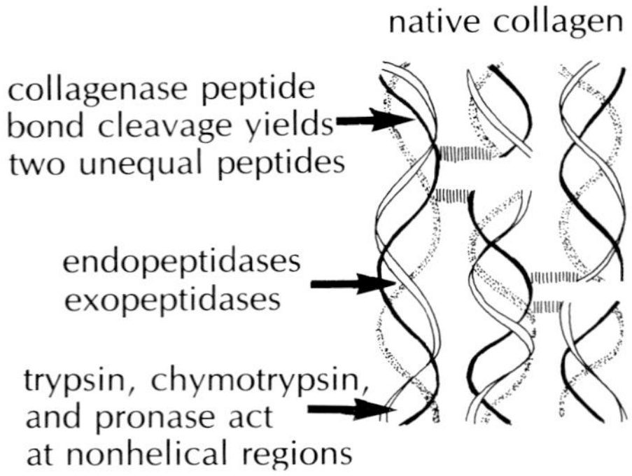

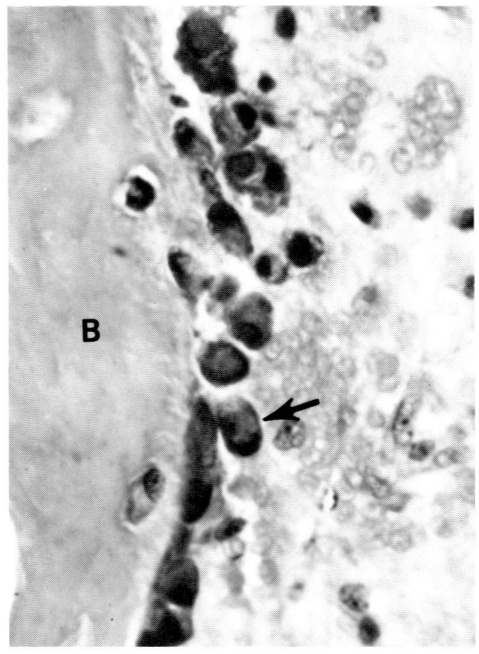

native collagen

collagenase peptide bond cleavage yields two unequal peptides

endopeptidases exopeptidases

trypsin, chymotrypsin, and pronase act at nonhelical regions

Figure 2–56. Collagen degradation.

Figure 2–57. Portion of remodeling bone, with osteoblasts (arrow) lining the edge of the bone (B) as it undergoes active remodeling.

Collagenase

Collagenase is the major collagenolytic enzyme in the body. Numerous examples of enzymes with this activity exist. The enzyme cleaves native soluble collagen at a single peptide bond along the helical part of the molecule generating two unequal peptides. The kinetics of the degradation process depend on the extent of the cross-linking. A variety of endo- and exopeptidases then further degrade the collagen molecule. Other collagenolytic enzymes include proteases, trypsin, chymotrypsin, and pronase. They interact with the molecule at nonhelical regions[122] (Fig. 2–56).

Macrophages can be stimulated to produce collagenase by endotoxin or lymphokines. Eosinophils are known to be collagenolytic, and their presence in increased numbers as scar tissue is being formed and remodeled suggests a role for these cells in connective tissue metabolism.[123]

Increased collagenase activity occurs in many conditions, including postpartum uterine involution, granuloma formation, pulmonary fibrosis,[124] periodontal disease, rheumatoid arthritis, wound healing, and invasion by tumor. *Decreased collagenase activity* has been identified in cirrhosis, scleroderma, and osteopetrosis.

Deficiencies in collagen synthesis, secretion, cross-linking, and degradation impair wound healing, especially with age, poor nutritional status, and genetic defects.

Bone Repair

Bone repair is a specialized example of mesenchymal repair. Functional cells include the short-lived *osteoclast*, which produces dissolution of the mineral phase and lysis of the bone matrix. The *osteoblast*, a cell with an intermediate life span, deposits osteoid matrix that is subsequently mineralized into bone. The *osteocyte* is a long-lived, mature cell sequestered in bony lacunae awaiting transformation into osteoblastic form when repair is necessary (Fig. 2–57).

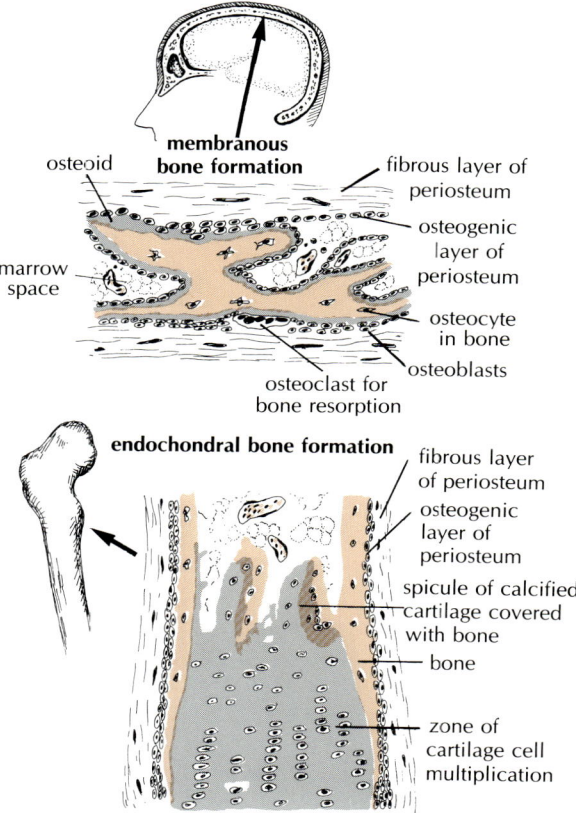

Figure 2–58. Comparison of membranous and endochondral bone formation.

Following fracture, osteoblasts secrete soluble collagen which, when polymerized, makes up 95% of the bone matrix. The other 5% of the matrix includes polysaccharide, glycoprotein, and phospholipid. After initial phosphate binding, mineralization takes place, with calcium phosphate and calcium hydroxide forming *hydroxyapatite crystals*. Small amounts of potassium, calcium, magnesium, and zinc are deposited in the matrix during the first few days after injury.

Fractures may be healed by one of two processes. Solid bones, such as the skull, are healed by *intramembranous ossification* arising from osteoblasts in the periosteum, and long bones are healed by *endochondral ossification* arising from the cartilaginous plate (Fig. 2–58). The initial stage of healing involves organization of the hemorrhage associated with the fracture and the formation of a *procallus*. The procallus is formed by invading fibroblasts and capillary buds.

Osteoblasts are derived from nearby periosteum and perhaps from fibroblasts; in the first few days, new cartilage and osteoid are laid down, converting the *procallus* to *fibrocartilaginous callus*. This is then converted to *osseus callus*. Extensive remodeling depends on the site of fracture, weight-bearing, and stress, and takes place over a period of weeks or months until repair is complete and new bone has been formed. Osteoclasts play an important role in this process.

COMPLICATIONS OF INFLAMMATION

If the repair of mesenchymal and epithelial damage does not lead to resolution, abnormal repair processes, which may persist for months or years, may ensue. These include abscesses, chronic inflammatory reactions, or granulomata.

Abscess

An abscess represents a failure of repair. It is a localized collection of pus containing dead tissue cells, dead white blood cells, and often dead organisms, usually surrounded by a fibrous capsule infiltrated by acute and chronic inflammatory cells (Fig. 2–59). The classic example of an abscess is a *"boil"* of the skin. Initially, there is infection of a hair follicle by staphylococci. The infection may spread through underlying tissue along fascial planes as *cellulitis* or may give rise to multiple *furuncles* at the skin's surfaces.

Abscesses may also be found in internal organs including the tonsils, liver, lung, brain, kidney, and gastrointestinal, genitourinary, and reproductive tracts. Localized collections of pus in the peritoneum *(peritoneal abscesses)* are seen in the greater or lesser omental sacs, the right and left colic gutters, and Douglas's pouch between the urinary bladder and the rectum. An abscess in the pleural cavity is known as *empyema*.

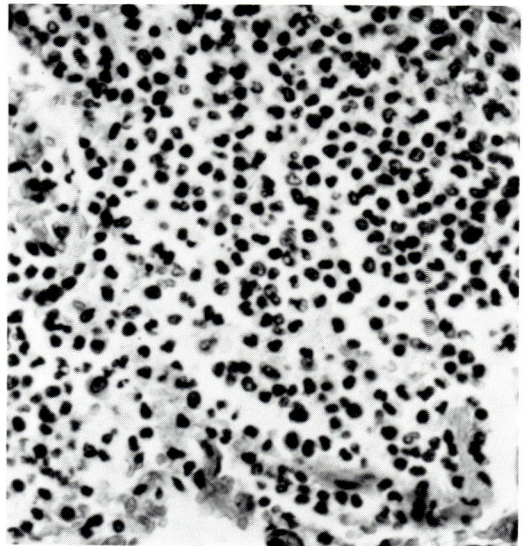

Figure 2–59. Abscess; note the large number of neutrophils admixed with mononuclear cells.

Communications between an abscess and a surface such as the skin or the gastrointestinal tract are known as *sinuses,* whereas communications between two hollow viscera are known as *fistulas.*

Microabscesses may heal by reabsorption of fluid, once phagocytosis and removal of all the organisms and tissue debris has taken place. Some abscesses may be effectively sterilized with extensive chemotherapy, after which *organization* of the exudate with scar formation, or reabsorption with *cyst* formation, may occur.

If spontaneous rupture and drainage do not occur, a common treatment for larger abscesses is surgical drainage and sterilization of the infectious agents by either systemic or local antibiotics. This treatment is often effective with abscesses in the peritoneal and pleural cavities or meningeal surfaces. Persistent abscesses in sites such as bone often contain viable organisms that provide a nidus of infection with septicemia over a period of many years, despite extensive antibiotic therapy and repeated drainage. The only effective treatment for such persistent abscesses is complete surgical removal.

Chronic Inflammation

Autopsy of individuals over 50 years of age shows some minimal scarring in all organs and tissues. One presumes from this finding that there has been previous damage by a variety of injurious agents or that these are perhaps the results of wear-and-tear aging processes. If the fibrous stroma of tissues is infiltrated with substantial numbers of chronic inflammatory cells (that is, lymphocytes, monocytes, and plasma cells), it may indicate that an injurious agent is still present or that an autoimmune reaction has developed.

Granulomata

Granulomata were originally believed to be tumors of granulation tissue or neoplastic growths composed of granules. In the development of a granuloma, the initial response to injury (within the first 24 hours) may include an infiltration of PMN followed by a chronic inflammatory cellular infiltration of lymphocytes, macrophages, and sometimes plasma cells.[125] Vascular endothelial budding is often present in early phases. The tissue changes progress to a mature granuloma, composed of epithelioid cells (macrophages) often in the form of giant cells and lymphocytes (T and B cells), as well as a collagenous fibrous reaction, which may become hyalinized or calcified[126] (Fig. 2–60).

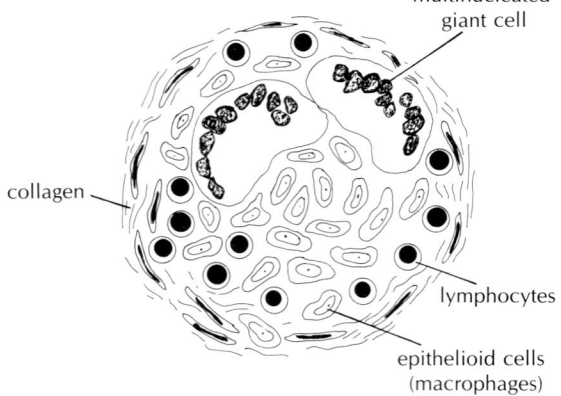

multinucleated giant cell

collagen

lymphocytes

epithelioid cells (macrophages)

Figure 2–60. Components of a granuloma.

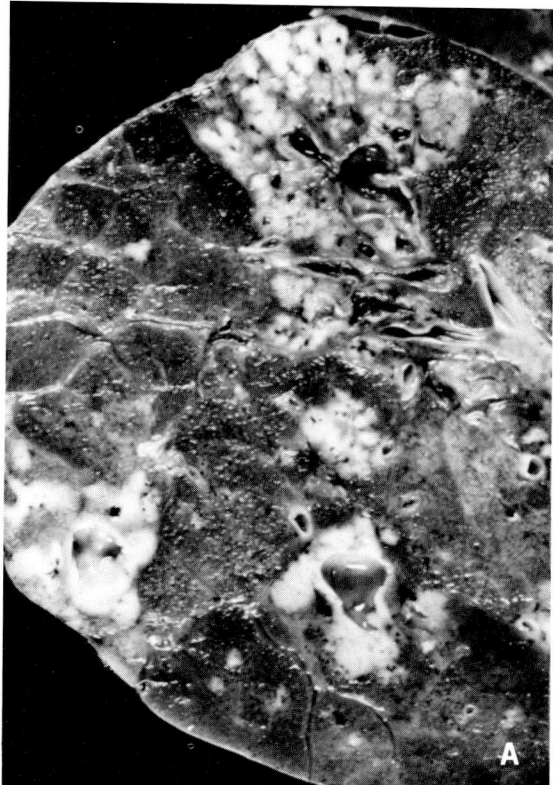

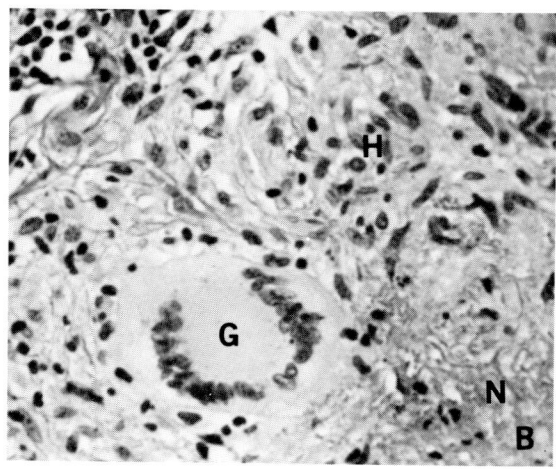

Granulomata may be produced by bacteria (listeriosis, brucellosis), fungi (histoplasmosis, coccidiomycosis), and parasites (leishmaniasis, schistosomiasis, toxoplasmosis). Sarcoidosis (Boeck's sarcoid) is a prominent granulomatous disorder of uncertain origin.

The classic granuloma-associated disease is *tuberculosis.* Tuberculous granulomata contain central *caseous necrosis,* consisting of dead tissue cells, dead white blood cells, and mycobacterial organisms (Fig. 2–61). This necrosis is surrounded by a palisading wall of *epithelioid cells* derived from macrophages, some of which fuse together to form *Langhans giant cells.* The partially hyalinized fibrous tissue surrounding the caseous necrosis also contains numerous macrophages and lymphocytes (mostly T cells) and a few plasma cells.[127]

Figure 2–61. Portion of lung in a patient with tuberculosis. *A,* The cut surfaces of the lung show many caseous and cystic whitish granulomas. *B,* Histologically, the granulomas have central necrosis (N) surrounded by histiocytic cells (H) and giant cells (G).

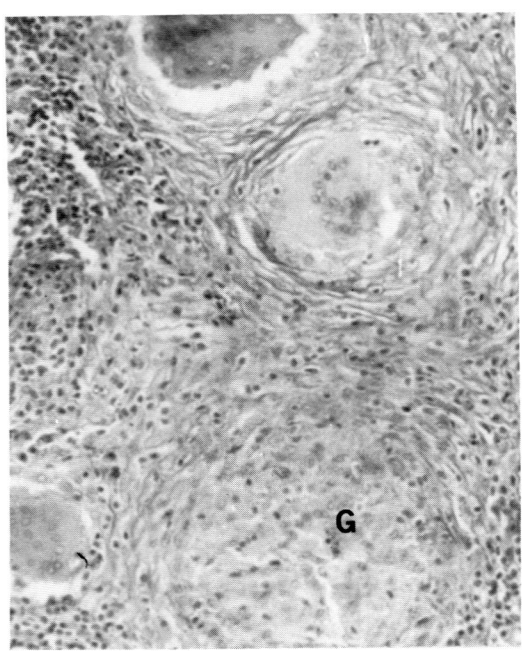

Figure 2–62. A small, end-stage granuloma (G) with giant cells but without central necrosis.

Other granulomata may resemble those of tuberculosis, but conspicuously lack central caseation (Fig. 2–62). Sarcoid granulomata may show *Schaumann bodies* (calcium and protein concretions) and stellate *"asteroid" inclusion bodies.*

The granuloma is a host response to an injury that cannot be handled by neutrophils, mononuclear cells, and immune reactions by the usual mechanisms of inflammation. Experimentally, granulomata can be produced in as few as nine or ten days. The cells that play the most prominent and characteristic roles in granuloma formation are macrophages and T lymphocytes, cells generally involved in cell-mediated immunity.

T cells

The first cell of importance in granulomata is the T cell. One of its prominent functions is the production of *lymphokines*, including four classes of chemotactic factors for white blood cells. The T cell also produces *lymphotoxins, mitogenic factors,* and *interferon.* An additional factor, macrophage-inhibitory factor (MIF), retards macrophage movement away from the area of injury (see Fig. 2–40). The macrophage-activating or arming factor (MAF) increases the macrophage's mobility and enhances its effectiveness in phagocytosis.

Monocytes and Epithelioid Cells

Precursor stem cells in the bone marrow are converted to *monoblasts,* then to *promonocytes,* and are released into the blood stream as *monocytes.* Upon leaving the vascular system and entering the tissue, the monocyte becomes a macrophage. It cannot be distinguished morphologically from the resting tissue histiocyte. The tissue macrophage becomes transformed so that it morphologically resembles an epithelial cell; it is thereafter called an *epithelioid cell.*

Epithelioid cells may fuse to become either *foreign body giant cells* or *Langhans giant cells.* Macrophages may appear as early as the first 24 hours of the inflammatory response when neutrophils are present, but they usually appear in 3 to 7 days. Shortly after this appearance, the mature granuloma with epithelioid cells may be found.

Macrophages are involved in the production of interferon, endogenous pyrogens, complement components, lysosomal hydrolases, and plasmin activator substances.[128] Macrophages usually have a half-life of four days, epithelioid cells may persist for three to four weeks, and the giant cell lives only a few days. The macrophage is obviously capable of division in vivo and in vitro if grown in a conditioned medium with proper growth stimulatory factors.

On transformation into an epithelioid cell or on fusion with other macrophages to form a giant cell, the macrophage has the capacity to destroy, segregate, or inactivate infectious agents or injurious foreign proteins.[129]

Phagocytosis of tubercle bacilli by macrophages may alter the macrophage's surface membrane so that it appears "foreign" to host killer T cells, which then participate (by unknown membrane-membrane interactions) in its lysis. Such a mechanism may be involved in the *"hypersensitivity necrosis"* that is said to occur in certain granulomatous responses. Macrophages may respond in this setting because of prior sensitization to the antigen and by movement directed by lymphocyte products.

Senile Granulomata

Most granulomata seen at autopsy are old (Fig. 2–62). They consist of whorls of hyalinized connective tissue infiltrated with a few epithelioid cells and lymphocytes. Thus, the final result of an earlier exposure to *histoplasmosis* or *tuberculosis* is often hyalinized, burnt-out granulomata in which calcium deposits occupy the previously necrotic region. Individuals may also enter into symbiosis with dormant granulomata containing viable organisms in various sites (lung, lymph nodes), however. Such granulomata may be later activated in the immunosuppressed or immune-deficient host, and the previously successful isolation of organisms may lead to local or disseminated disease.

Large amounts of alpha-1-antitrypsin *(AAT)* are detectable in granulomata. This substance is the major protease inhibitor in serum. It inhibits many enzymes released from lysosomes of inflammatory cells including collagenase, elastase, leukocyte protease, plasmin, thrombin and, of course, trypsin. *Alpha-1-antitrypsin,* therefore, acts as an important regulator in the inflammatory reaction.[130]

It is often impossible to make a specific etiologic diagnosis based on the histologic picture of a burnt-out granuloma, and in these situations it is necessary to rely on the patient's medical history, the physical examination, x-ray studies, skin tests, serologic tests, tissue culture, and special histologic stains in attempts to elucidate the cause of these lesions.

FACTORS AFFECTING INFLAMMATORY AND REPAIR MECHANISMS

Inflammation, repair, and growth are cardinal features of all disease. These processes depend on many substances in the plasma (coagulation factors, chemotactic agents, blastogenic factors, hormones, and humoral factors), vascular function and integrity, and the number, characteristics, and capacities of the cells involved in the inflammatory and repair reactions. The diversity of responses seen in cell and tissue injury is due to the various inflammatory cells we have considered earlier and to the unique reactions of the mesenchymal and epithelial cells present at the sites of injury.

Congenital Immunodeficiency Diseases

In man and experimental animals, *immunodeficiency* diseases affecting nearly every component of the immune system have been recognized[131,132] (Table 2–28). These disorders vary from gross absence or deficiency of immune cells or circulating proteins to subcellular alterations in cell morphology, metabolism, and synthetic mechanisms involved in immune responses. Such defects often involve abnormalities in cell-mediated responses, antibody synthesis, and phagocytosis. Diagnosis of these disorders may be made by assays of levels of the component under question, pathologic examination of pertinent tissue, or tests for adequacy of function.

Table 2–28. *Classification of Immunodeficiency Diseases*

I. *Antibody (B cell) immunodeficiency diseases*
   X-linked hypogammaglobulinemia (congenital hypogammaglobulinemia)
   Transient hypogammaglobulinemia of infancy
   Common, variable, unclassifiable immunodeficiency (acquired hypogammaglobulinemia)
   X-linked immunodeficiency with hyper-IgM
   Selective IgA deficiency
   Selective IgM deficiency
   Selective deficiency of IgG subclasses

II. *Cellular (T cell) immunodeficiency diseases*
   Congenital thymic aplasia (DiGeorge's syndrome)
   Chronic mucocutaneous candidiasis (with or without endocrinopathy)

III. *Combined antibody-mediated (B cell) and cell-mediated (T-cell) immunodeficiency diseases*
   Severe combined immunodeficiency disease (autosomal recessive, X-linked, sporadic)
   Cellular immunodeficiency with abnormal immunoglobulin synthesis (Nezelof's syndrome)
   Immunodeficiency with ataxia telangiectasia
   Immunodeficiency with eczema and thrombocytopenia (Wiskott-Aldrich syndrome)
   Immunodeficiency with thymoma
   Immunodeficiency with short-limbed dwarfism
   Immunodeficiency with enzyme deficiency
   Episodic lymphocytopenia with lymphotoxin
   Graft versus host disease

IV. *Phagocytic dysfunction*
   Chronic granulomatous disease
   Glucose-6-phosphate dehydrogenase deficiency
   Myeloperoxidase deficiency
   Chediak-Higashi syndrome
   Job's syndrome
   Tuftsin deficiency
   "Lazy leukocyte syndrome"
   Elevated IgE, defective chemotaxis, eczema, and recurrent infections

V. *Complement abnormalities and immunodeficiency diseases*
   C1q, C1r, and C1s deficiency
   C2 deficiency
   C3 deficiency (type I, type II)
   C5 dysfunction

The adequacy of T-cell function can be assessed by examining quantitative proliferative responses following the exposure of these cells to mitogens such as *PHA* and the development of delayed hypersensitivity to ubiquitous antigens such as streptokinase-streptodornase (SK-SD), mumps, candida, and trichophyton (Table 2–29).

Adequacy of B-cell function may be ascertained by quantitation of levels of the major immunoglobulin classes by immunodiffusion, immunoelectrophoresis, or radioimmunoassay *(RIA)*, as well as by response to a variety of widely distributed antigens.[133]

Adequacy of granulocytic function may be assessed by the nitroblue tetrazolium (NBT) test for white blood cell phagocytic activity.

Immunodeficiency states are often primary congenital diseases or are secondarily associated with a variety of systemic illnesses[134] (Table 2–28). Many examples exist of the latter: Low levels of IgG develop in some patients with lymphoma or chronic lymphocytic leukemia, thereby predisposing these patients to bacterial infections. Delayed hypersensitivity (allergic) reactions have also been associated with lymphomas, often with opportunistic fungal or mycobacterial infection. Diminished leukocyte mobilization is seen with alcohol ingestion, steroid administration, and diabetic acidosis.

The classic congenital immunodeficiency diseases include *Bruton's disease* (sex-linked agammaglobulinemia), *DiGeorge's syndrome, combined Swiss immunodeficiency, Wiskott-Aldrich syndrome,* and *ataxia-telangiectasia* (Table 2–30).

Table 2–29. *Diagnostic Tests for Immunodeficiency Disorders*

Assay	Test	Results
Serum antibody	Protein electrophoresis Radial immunodiffusion Radioimmunoassay	Hyper- hypo gammaglobulinemia Quantitative IgG, IgA, IgE Quantitative IgE determinant
Number of WBC	WBC count and differential Absorption to cotton or glass wool	Increased in infection Decreased in immunodeficiency
Number of B and T cells	Cytofluorometry	Decreased in immunodeficiency
Classes of T cells	Monoclonal membrane antigens assay	Determines number of helper/inducer/suppressor/cytotoxic T cells
Macrophage phagocytosis	Nitroblue tetrazolium (NBT) test	Measures metabolic function Decreased in chronic granulomatous disease
Macrophage chemotaxis	Boyden chamber test Rebuck window test	Decreased in severe infection
General movement of WBC	Random migration test	Decreased in lazy leukocyte syndrome

Table 2–30. Selected Immunodeficiency Diseases

Disease	Inheritance	Deficiency	Characteristic Features
Congenital agammaglobuline-mia (Bruton's syndrome)	X-linked recessive	IgG, IgM, IgA absent Plasma cells absent Lymphocytes present	Predisposition to pyogenic infections Rejection of grafts
Swiss-type severe combined immunodeficiency (SCID)	Autosomal recessive (also an X-linked form)	IgG, M, A absent No plasma cells, lymphocytes, or Hassall's corpuscles Vestigial thymus	Predisposition to bacterial, viral, fungal infections Inability to reject grafts
Ataxia-telangiectasia	Autosomal recessive	Thymic hypoplasia Hormonal immune deficiency	Ataxia and telangiectasis Sinus and pulmonary infections Broken chromosomes
Wiskott-Aldrich syndrome	X-linked recessive	Variable cellular and humoral immune deficiency	Thrombocytopenia Eczema Bloody diarrhea Predisposition to infection
Congenital thymic aplasia (DiGeorge's syndrome)	No genetic basis known	Complete absence of thymus and thymus-dependent lymphocytes Normal Ig and plasma cells, but specific antibody responses deficient	Predisposition to viral and fungal infection Hypoparathyroidism with tetany Anomalies of heart, neck, and great vessels

(Modified from Nora, J.J., and Fraser, F.C.: Medical Genetics: Principles and Practices. Philadelphia, Lea & Febiger, 1974.)

Lymphocyte Deficiencies

B Cell (Bruton's Syndrome). Antibody-deficient syndromes involve abnormalities in B-cell lines, and include effects on differentiation or production of B cells, impaired generation of clonal diversity, and accelerated immune elimination of B lymphocytes.

In *Bruton's X-linked congenital agammaglobulinemia*, B-cell deficiency results in recurrent infections with high-grade, encapsulated organisms such as pneumococcus. The disorder appears to be due to a regulatory gene defect that affects pre-B-cell differentiation. It may be treated by frequent and regular injections of gammaglobulin.

Patients with a selective IgA deficiency have normal numbers of B cells containing IgA on their surface.[135] That these cells are unable to differentiate into IgA-secreting cells, however, suggests an abnormal intrinsic control mechanism or abnormal interaction with other cells. In patients with IgA deficiency, three major pathogenetic groups exist: (1) those with excessive numbers of suppressor cells, (2) those with a deficiency of helper T cells, and (3) those with an unknown deficit.[136] Selective IgA deficiencies have been described in which T-cell function appeared intact, but suppression of IgA synthesis occurred when T cells were cultured with normal B cells.[137]

Recently described is a new X-linked *recessive lymphoproliferative syndrome* associated with genetic immunodeficiencies and subsequent infection by agents such as measles and Epstein-Barr virus (EBV). These children with agammaglobulinemia who later have infectious mononucleosis may subsequently develop American Burkitt's lymphoma, histiocytic lymphoma, immunoblastic sarcoma of B cells, or plasmacytoma. The studies by Purtilo et al. suggest that EBV triggered a B-cell proliferation that continued unabated because of a defective immune control mechanism.[138,139]

T Cell (DiGeorge's Syndrome). In the *DiGeorge syndrome* (thymic hypoplasia), in which there is deficiency of T cells, Ig production is adequate, but patients lack cellular immune responses and have increased susceptibility to fungal, viral, and atypical mycobacterial infections.

Severe Combined Immunodeficiency Disease (SCID). *Severe combined (Swiss-type) immunodeficiency* is a fatal disease of infancy in which both cellular and humoral immune functions are compromised. This disorder may be related to an inhibition of T-cell maturation with lesser effects on B-cell development. Clinical symptoms involve recurrent infections that begin in infancy and involve all tissues with exposure to exogenous organisms (skin and gastrointestinal and respiratory tracts).[140]

Wiskott-Aldrich Disease. This X-linked disorder is characterized by thrombocytopenia, eczema, and a higher than expected incidence of lymphomas. Although B cells appear normal in number, low levels of IgM are seen, with absent antibody responses to polysaccharide antigens. Lymphopenia is also present, with depletion of T-cell-dependent areas of lymphoid organs.

Ataxia-Telangiectasia. This multisystem disease is associated with cerebellar ataxia, oculocutaneous telangiectasia, recurrent sinopulmonary infections, and a high incidence of lymphomas.[141] Humoral antibody responses may be abnormal and vary from patient to patient. In this autosomal recessive disease, IgA is absent in 80% of patients, and thymic hypoplasia is present as well.

Therapy of Lymphocyte Immune Deficiency. Transplants of bone marrow, fetal thymus, and fetal liver containing hematopoietic stem cells have been given to patients with immune deficiencies with varying degrees of success.[142] In one report, Buckley gave fetal cell transplants to 2 infants with combined Swiss deficiency. No functional improvement was seen in one infant, but the second had remarkable improvement, even 19 months later. Lymphocytes of the successfully treated patient responded to pokeweed mitogen, although IgA remained low. Transient graft-versus-host disease was seen in both infants and is, in general, a major cause of morbidity and mortality in recipients of bone marrow transplants.[143]

Thymosin has also been given to patients with cellular immunodeficiency.[144] In one patient with thymic hypoplasia, T-cell rosettes increased 15% to 48% after in vitro incubation with thymosin. Tsukimoto, however, showed no appreciable changes when thymosin was incubated in vitro with lymphoblasts from 10 patients. Thymosin therapy apparently had a beneficial effect on B-cell immunity, as evidenced by increasing immunoglobulin production. Thymosin may act by decreasing the population of T-cell suppressors or by stimulating T helper cells; both actions result in increased antibody synthesis by B cells.[144]

In some patients with combined Swiss deficiency, a deficiency of an enzyme important in maturation of white blood cells *(adenosine deaminase)* has been described. Polmar attempted to correct this enzyme deficiency by giving frozen irradiated red blood cells. The rationale is that the substrate for this enzyme diffuses out of the recipient host tissue and is acted upon by adenosine deaminase from donated irradiated human red blood cells. This treatment temporarily restored both humoral antibody and cell-mediated immunity in a few patients.[145]

Mononuclear Cell Deficiencies. Mononuclear leukocyte chemotaxis deficiency has been recognized for years.[146] As both monocytes and granulocytes arise from a single stem cell, deficiencies in the stem cell may affect either or both derivative lines. A classification has been proposed to include various disease groups[147] (Table 2–31).

Table 2–31.   Mononuclear and Phagocytic System

Major Alterations	Type of Disease
Monocytes, granulocytes, RBC, platelets	Acute and chronic nonlymphocytic leukemias, preleukemic states, polycythemia vera, osteomyelofibrosis, aplastic anemia
Granulocytes	Chronic granulomatous disease, Chediak-Higashi syndrome, myeloperoxidase deficiency, different forms of neutropenia

Macrophages	Lipid storage diseases
	Idiopathic histiocytosis:
	    Letterer-Siwe syndrome
	    eosinophilic granuloma
	    histiocytic medullary reticulosis
	    familial erythrophagocytic lymphohistiocytosis

Lymphocytes	Inflammatory, infectious, immunologic, malignant disorders

(Modified from Muenet, G.: Disorders of the mononuclear phagocyte system. An analytical review. (Blut, *34*:317, 1977.)

Granulocyte Deficiencies

Genetic disorders may also affect granulocytes.[148,149] *Congenital neutropenia* is an autosomal dominant disease associated with persistently low levels of circulatory neutrophils in the absence of anemia or thrombocytopenia.[150] Interestingly, infections are usually not a problem in these patients.

Disorders of phagocytic cells include defects in migration and chemotaxis, disorders of membrane attachment or ingestion of particles, and defects associated with lysosomal degranulation and hydrolysis of ingested particles. The two classic genetic leukocyte diseases are *Chediak-Higashi disease* and *chronic granulomatous disease.*

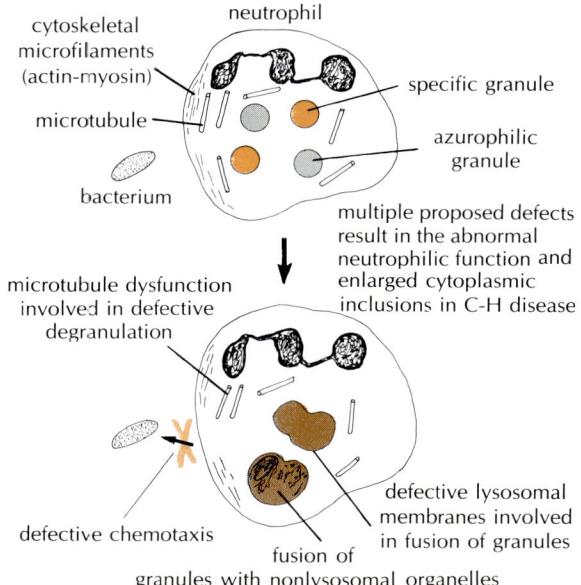

Figure 2–63. Pathogenesis of Chediak-Higashi (C–H) disease. Defective neutrophil bacteriocidal activity results from defects in chemotaxis and lysosomal degranulation.

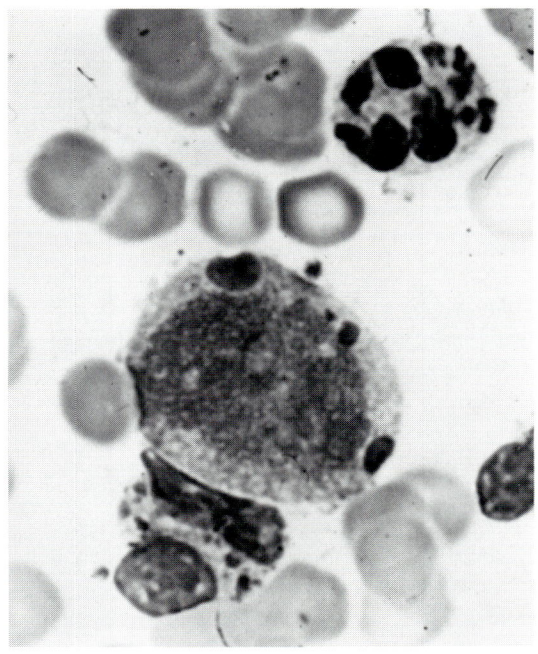

Figure 2–64. An early Chediak-Higashi promyelocyte. (Courtesy of Dr. P. Gregory, Raush Fountain Medical Center, Md.)

Chediak-Higashi Disease. This disease (Fig. 2–63) is associated with hematologic, cutaneous, neurologic, and renal symptoms and involves defective neutrophilic degranulation.[151] Abnormal giant lysosomal granules fuse belatedly with phagosomes (Fig. 2–64), and the cells are sluggish in response to chemotactic factors.[152] In the accelerated phase of the disease, patients die with pancytopenia, fever, and infiltration of many organs with atypical mononuclear cells. Treatment with ascorbic acid has produced marked improvement in the neutrophils' chemotactic ability as well as the normal secretory and bactericidal activity of the lysosomes.[153] The action of ascorbic acid is unknown; it may lower cAMP levels, which are increased in this disorder.[154]

Chronic Granulomatous Disease *(CGD).* This disease is an *x-linked recessive disorder* associated with impaired lysosomal enzyme activity during the early stages of phagocytosis. Patients with this disease have recurrent bacterial or fungal infections associated with defective phagocytic oxidative metabolic responses and impaired intracellular microbial killing. Unlike the cells in Chediak-Higashi disease, the cells in this syndrome are morphologically normal. Various tests are used to assay the differences.

The basic molecular defect here is deficient activity of the enzyme responsible for the conversion of oxygen to bactericidal forms ($O_2\cdot$, H_2O_2, hydroxyl radical or singlet oxygen). The postulated deficient enzymes include nicotinamide adenine dinucleotide (NADH) oxidase, nicotinamide adenine dinucleotide phosphate (NADPH) oxidase, and glutathione peroxidase. Curnutte et al.[155] have quantitated the rate of enzyme degradation and activity and have shown that the net release of lysosomal enzymes was reduced in patients with this disease. Although CGD was formerly considered to be a disease of childhood, with early death, the use of supportive therapy, antibiotics, and careful management has allowed some of these children to live into adulthood, with the disadvantage of potential transmission of the trait to future generations.

Complement Deficiencies

Deficiencies of all components of complement have been reported in experimental animals and in humans,[156] and investigators have linked C2, C4, C6, and C8 deficiency to an HLA locus on chromosome number 6. The close association of four complement genes on chromosome number 6 seems unlikely to be a chance occurrence. The homology between the β-2 microglobulin fraction of the HLA antigens and immunoglobulins has previously been noted.

Genetic deficiencies have been described for C1r, C2, C3, C4, C5, C6, C7, C9, C1 inhibitor, and C3b inactivator.[157,158] The clinical features of homozygous individuals deficient in C1r, C2, C4, and C5 are similar, and autoimmune diseases are more prevalent in these cases[159] (Table 2–32).

Table 2–32. *Human Disorders Associated with Complement Deficiencies*

Complement	Deficiency Disease
C1q	CGN, SLE, hypogammaglobulinemia
C1r	CGN, recurrent infections, rheumatoid disease, SLE
C1s	CGN, SLE
C1 inactivator (C1-esterase inhibitor)	Hereditary angioedema
C2	Arthralgia, MPGN, SLE, susceptibility to infection, Henoch-Schönlein purpura
C3	Repeated infections, MPGN
C3b inactivator	Recurrent infections
C4	Decrease in hereditary angioneurotic edema and immune complex disorders (SLE)
C5	Leiner's disease (present in normal amounts but functionally abnormal), recurrent GC or meningococcal infection, SLE
C7	Raynaud's phenomenon, ankylosing spondylitis
C8	SLE, GC, or meningococcal infection

CGN, chronic glomerulonephritis; SLE, systemic lupus erythematosus; MPGN, membranoproliferative glomerulonephritis; GC, gonococcal infection.

In normal patients or in heterozygous-deficient individuals, monocytes have the ability to synthesize or secrete C2. In homozygous-deficient persons, the monocytes lose this ability, and this loss results in altered phagocytic capacity. This defect is specific for C2 biosynthesis, and the synthesis of total protein is normal. An association between C2 deficiency and inflammatory bowel disease with HLA-A10, B18 has recently been described.

Patients with C3 deficiency have severe clinical symptoms, which are identical to those with C3b-inactivator deficiencies. Although this finding appears to be a paradox, it seems that C3b-inactivator deficiency can result in the hypercatabolism of C3, thus resulting in a relative deficiency of this fraction.

Homozygous C3-deficient individuals cannot mount a leukocytic response even during the most overwhelming bacterial infection. The entire molecule is deficient, but the lack of C3a fraction is critical because this component mobilizes PMN from the bone marrow.[160]

C5-deficient individuals also have a propensity for autoimmune diseases and a susceptibility to bacterial infections. These predispositions may relate to the deficient chemotactic activity of C5a. Because C5b serves as the nucleus of the membrane lysis complex (C5b to C9), these patients have difficulty in handling specific bacteria, such as meningococcus and gonococcus, which require complement-mediated cytolysis rather than the other intracellular bactericidal mechanisms. These features also apply to individuals deficient in C6, C7, and C8 because these fractions also form part of the membrane lysis complex.[161]

Hereditary Angioedema. This disorder results from a genetic deficiency of C1-esterase inhibitor.[162] These patients are subject to recurrent episodes of peripheral swelling and laryngeal and pulmonary edema; the latter two sometimes lead to death. The clinical attacks are associated with the generation of activated C1 and the consumption of other complement fractions. The attacks may be brought about by trauma, but often they are precipitated by no apparent cause.

Two forms of the disease have been identified. In one, C1 inhibitor is absent, and in the other, it is defective. It is believed that the pathway of angioedema involves excessive release of kinins, which promote increased vascular permeability. Patients with C1 inhibitor deficiency are also prone to autoimmune phenomena.

Platelet Deficiencies

Hereditary platelet disorders are found in *Ehlers-Danlos syndrome,* a collagen disease, and *von Willebrand's disease,* in which platelet adhesion is defective.[163] In *Chediak-Higashi disease,* there is a storage pool deficiency of platelets. In *cyclo-oxygenase deficiency,* the platelet granule release mechanism is defective, and in glycogen storage disease, platelet energy metabolism is defective. In *gray platelet syndrome* (GPS), large, vacuolated platelets lacking α granules with thrombocytopenia have been reported.[164]

In addition, a disorder known as *congenital giant platelet syndrome* has recently been described. Platelet abnormalities include abnormal granulation, disrupted and disassembled marginal microtubules, defective membranous structures, retention of rough endoplasmic reticulum, and hypermitochondrionism (Table 2–33).

Table 2–33. *Platelet Abnormalities*

Thrombocytopenia

Defective megakaryocyte stem cells in bone marrow
Specific drug toxicity or unknown cause for reduction of platelets

Thrombopathy

Platelets with insufficient pool of adenine dinucleotide
Normal adenine dinucleotide level, but release incomplete
No reaction of platelets with subendothelium and exhibition of a defect in release reaction

Thrombasthenia

Adequate release of adenine dinucleotide and serotonin, but failure of platelet aggregation

Coagulation Diseases

Genetic defects of one or more of the factors involved in clot formation have been identified[96] (Table 2–34). It is interesting that although Hageman factor XII is critical in reactions concerned with clotting, in the activation of kinins and plasminogen and, indirectly, in the activation of com-

Table 2–34. *Hemorrhagic Diseases*

1. Increased vascular fragility
   A. Infections (bacterial endocarditis)
   B. Drugs (hypersensitivity)
   C. Collagen and basement membrane disorders (Ehlers-Danlos)
   D. Purpura (Henoch-Schönlein)
   E. Aneurysms
   F. Congenital (ataxia-telangiectasia)
   G. Endocrine disturbance (cirrhosis)

2. Decreased platelet function
   A. Thrombocytopenia (inherited or acquired)
   B. Abnormal platelets

3. Decreased clotting factors
   A. Classic hemophilia (VIII, AHF)
   B. von Willebrand's disease (VIII, VWF)
   C. Parahemophilia (V, accelerator globulin)
   D. Christmas disease (IX)
   E. Plasma thromboplastic antecedent (PTA) deficiency (XI)

plement, no in vivo clinical syndrome has been associated with Hageman factor deficiency. Deficiency of prekallikrein (Fletcher factor) similarly has not been associated with a distinct clinical presentation.

Abnormalities of Factor VIII are primarily associated with two disorders: *hemophilia A* and *von Willebrand's disease*. Purification of this protein has led to knowledge of its three biologic functions: (1) procoagulant activity, (2) platelet aggregation and correction of bleeding abnormality in von Willebrand's disease, and (3) antigenic immunoprecipitation by heterologous monospecific antisera.[165]

Hemophilia is an X-linked recessive disease. Antihemophilic factor (VIII-AHF) has two dissociable subcomponents. One contains most of the protein, is of high molecular weight, and sustains ristocetin-induced platelet aggregation. The lower-molecular-weight subcomponent has procoagulant activity. Hemophilia appears in one in 10,000 men in the United States and is carried in the female as an X-linked recessive gene. Rare forms of hemophilia may be associated with a deficiency of PTA (factor XI), SPCF (factor VII), or accelerator globulin (factor V). In certain instances, the carrier state can be detected.[166]

In classic *type "A" hemophilia*, the deficiency of factor VIII-AHF is associated with normal amounts of factor VIII-VWF (von Willebrand's) and factor VIII-AGN (agglutination). Clinically, these patients have multiple hemarthroses and surface tissue hemorrhages.

In *von Willebrand's disease*, there is a deficiency of factor VIII-VWF and factor VIII-AGN and a decrease in factor VIII-AHF.[167] The principal symptoms of this autosomal dominant disease are bleeding in the gums and menorrhagia, rather than the joint bleeding associated with hemophilia A. The platelet abnormalities are a result of the deficiency of factor VIII-VWF necessary for proper platelet function, rather than an intrinsic deficiency in the plate-

Table 2-35. *Distribution of Factor VIII Components in Hemophilia*

	Hemophilia A	von Willebrand's Disease
VIII-AHF (antihemophilic factor)	−	↓
VIII-VWF (von Willebrand's factor)	+	−
VIII-AGN (agglutination factor)	+	−

lets themselves. It is interesting that factor VIII appears to be synthesized in endothelial cells, whereas all other clotting factors are synthesized in the liver[168] (Table 2-35).

Other important genetic coagulative deficiencies include *Christmas disease* (a deficiency of factor IX—hemophilia B) and prothrombin (Factor II) deficiency.

Collagen Defects

Figure 2-65 illustrates the major paths of collagen synthesis and four major genetic defects associated with defective collagen formation.[169] These include *Marfan's syndrome,* associated with defective ground substance in the aorta, *Ehlers-Danlos syndrome,* associated with defective collagen synthesis, *osteogenesis imperfecta,* associated with defective bone matrix formation, and *pseudoxanthoma elasticum,* associated with abnormal structure of the elastic tissue.

The Ehlers-Danlos syndrome is a disorder of connective tissue resulting in weakened tendons, ligaments, joints, muscle insertions, bone, dermis, and blood vessel walls. The disorder is heterogeneous with respect to clinical features as well as molecular defects.[170]

Other congenital defects involve a deficiency of hydroxylysine, which is the enzyme necessary for the hydroxylation of lysine, deficiency of protease, which is necessary for the conversion of procollagen to collagen, and deficiency of lysyl oxidase, which is critical in fibril crosslinking. Certain autoimmune disorders, including SLE, rheumatoid arthritis, and scleroderma show abnormal degradation of collagen.[171]

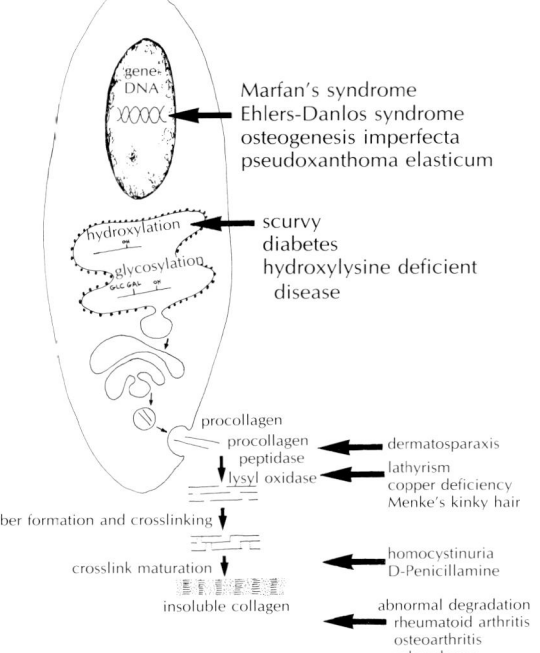

Figure 2-65. Defects in collagen formation.

Nutritional Factors

Poor nutritional status increases susceptibility to injury, retards inflammatory responses, and usually is associated with prolonged healing reactions.[171] Individuals with protein deficiencies usually have an associated vitamin deficiency and, particularly in the aged, the healing process may be prolonged. The prevalence of diabetes in the older-age population, with its hyperglycemia and protein and vitamin imbalances, also complicates healing.

Inflammation and Repair: Multicellular Response to Injury   **93**

Vitamin Deficiencies

Six vitamins play particularly prominent roles in the inflammatory and reparative processes (Table 2–36). *Vitamin C deficiency* is classically associated with *scurvy*. Vitamin C has been found to be essential in the hydroxylation of proline and lysine to hydroxyproline and hydroxylysine[172] (see Fig. 2–54). The lack of this vitamin results in failure to form collagen, osteoid, dentin, enamel, and intercellular cement. When scorbutic cells are studied in vitro, defective collagen fibrils are found. Capillary fragility is a prominent feature of scurvy because the mucopolysaccharides of the intercellular cement are abnormal, as are those of intercellular junctions. Basement membranes are also altered. Experimental models of scurvy show the most severe changes in the synovium.

Table 2–36. *Effect of Vitamin Deficiencies in Inflammation and Repair*

Vitamin	Altered Function
C	Decreased collagen (hydroxylation) synthesis Decreased dentin formation Decreased intercellular cement Decreased bone matrix deposition
D	Decreased mineralization of bone in growth and repair
E	Retarded growth (rats)
A	Stimulation of epithelial metaplasia with keratinization
B_{12}	Lack of maturation of erythrocyte series
K	Deficient synthesis of coagulation factors

Vitamin D deficiency is associated with *rickets*. Vitamin D is critically important in the mineralization of osteoid, with calcium phosphate and calcium hydroxide forming calcium hydroxyapatite crystals. Both vitamin D and parathormone are interrelated in the metabolism of calcium and phosphorus. Fortification of milk with vitamin D has made *"nutritional osteomalacia"* an historical curiosity.[173]

Vitamin A deficiency results in *epithelial metaplasia* with keratinizing stratified squamous epithelium in the mucosa of the gastrointestinal, genitourinary, and respiratory tracts as well as the mucous membranes of the eye. Deficiencies of vitamin A alter the healing and regenerative epithelial process following injury.

Vitamin K is absorbed from the gastrointestinal tract and is critical for the synthesis of clotting factors II, IX, and X in the liver.

Vitamin B_{12} deficiency results in the lack of maturation of the red blood cell series with the resulting production of megaloblasts, which are ineffective in carrying oxygen.

Ion and Metal Deficiencies

Deficiency of trace metals, as previously discussed, leads to often profound effects on inflammation and repair as a result of the important roles of these metals in metabolic reactions[174] (Table 2–37).

Table 2–37. *Effect of Deficiencies of Trace Elements on Inflammation, Repair, and Regeneration*

Trace Element	Effect of Deficiency
Chromium	Decreased growth (rats)
Cobalt	Development of pernicious anemia
Copper	Lack of collagen fibril formation
Manganese	Defective growth (oxidative phosphorylation)
Silicon	Impaired connective tissue formation (chickens)
Tin	Impaired dentition (rats)
Selenium	Cardiomyopathy (man)

Calcium is required for the maintenance of connective tissue and bone as well as for a host of other processes controlling cellular electrical activity, movement, secretion, contraction, and various immune functions necessary in inflammation and repair. The skeleton contains 99% of all body calcium; in deficiency states, it is lost from bone and *osteoporosis* results.[173]

Phosphorus is similarly required for normal bone function. Phosphorus-deficient diets and ingestion of large quantities of phosphorus-binding antacids may produce *hypophosphatemia.*

Excessive fluoride ingestion leads to osteosclerosis, exostoses, and ligamentous calcification.

Physical Factors

Physical, environmental, and occupational factors have a profound influence on increased susceptibility to infection, are sometimes detrimental to repair processes, and occasionally stimulate an uncontrolled regenerative response that results in neoplasia.

Radiation

Ultraviolet radiation causes the common sunburn and may result in varying degrees of *dermatitis*. Massive doses of radiation depress stem cell proliferation in the bone marrow, with a decrease in white blood cell and red blood cell precursors, and result in a poor cellular inflammatory response to injury. Intermediate doses of radiation may stimulate *proliferation of stem cells* and may eventuate in *leukemia*. The use of radiation therapy for a variety of malignant neoplasms may result later in untoward tissue effects such as radiation enteritis.[175] Long-term effects of chronic radiation in humans are presently under intensive investigation.

Oxygen

Hyperoxygenemia in tissue cultures retards growth. However, in vivo it has produced growth stimulation, for example in premature infants with *retrolental fibroplasia*. Severe hypoxia, on the other hand, retards fibroblastic proliferation and collagen formation in scars.

pH and Temperature

Local, marked changes in *pH*, as occur in *acid burns* of the skin or *alkali (lye) ingestion*, may produce coagulative necrosis. Certain biochemical processes involved in inflammation and repair have specific pH requirements and are, therefore, hindered following large pH changes.

Severe temperature changes may also affect the inflammatory reaction. Thermal injuries cause local tissue edema partially by the loosening and disruption of intercellular junctions. Serious damage due to severe cold, on the other hand, as seen in the ischemia and gangrene of frostbite, is due to the constriction of blood vessels. The constricted vessels are unable to carry plasma to the injured cells and are also subject to thrombosis. Milder degrees of "cold" injury, however, have therapeutic uses, as in certain surgical procedures using only local anesthesia and cold packs. The drop in temperature inhibits clotting, depresses sensory stimulation, decreases necrosis, and prevents hemorrhage.

Foreign Bodies

Foreign bodies in surgical wounds, *asbestos* or *beryllium* in the respiratory tract, *urate crystals* in the kidney, and *stones* in the gallbladder may provoke foreign body inflammatory reactions. These reactions may first become manifest as chronic inflammation with fibroblast proliferation and infiltrates of chronic inflammatory cells; they may also induce formation of granulomata consisting of epithelioid cells and giant cells.

Infectious Agents

Injury by most infectious agents is followed either by resolution with restitution of normal tissue structure or by scar formation. Some infectious agents, however, retard healing and provoke *abscess formation, chronic inflammation,* or *granuloma formation*. Certain infectious agents may develop a symbiotic relationship with host cells and may remain latent or dormant for years before becoming active and producing disease.

Bacteria

Most bacteria provoke a polymorphonuclear response followed by a round cell response. *Mycobacteria* (for ex-

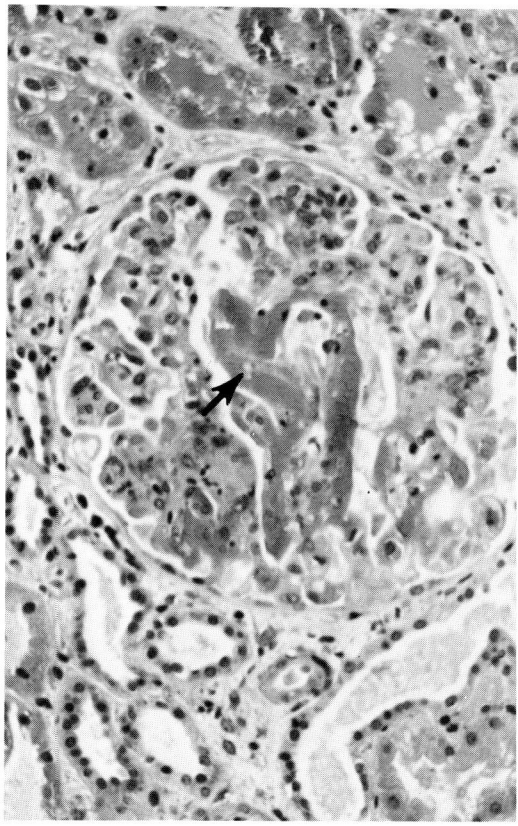

Figure 2–66. Renal glomerulus in patient with disseminated intravascular coagulation; note the central deposition of fibrin (arrow).

ample, the agents of leprosy and tuberculosis), after an initial transitory PMN response, generally provoke a chronic inflammatory response of monocytes and lymphocytes. In addition, they may produce a classic granulomatous response.

Other bacterial organisms are associated with idiosyncratic inflammatory responses. As examples, klebsiella often produces a hemorrhagic pneumonia, Clostridium perfringens produces a liquefaction necrosis enteritis, and *diphtheria* exotoxin produces a membranous exudative pharyngitis. *Spirochetes,* usually primarily infecting the genitalia, may finally come to reside in the cardiovascular system (syphilitic aortitis), the CNS (neurosyphilis), or in various organs as minute necrotic and fibrotic lesions known as *gummas.* In the liver, the scarring of these lesions results in the classic *hepar lobatum.*

An important coagulative disease, *disseminated intravascular coagulation* (DIC), is commonly seen in terminally ill patients with septicemia, especially involving gram-negative bacterial organisms. This disorder is due to the combined effects of generation of degradation products of *fibrin,* the presence of *thrombocytopenia,* and possibly circulating *anticoagulants.* The presence of endotoxin in humans is often accompanied by a rise in bradykinin and a fall in kininogen similar to the effects of endotoxin-associated gram-negative septicemia seen in an animal model, the pig.

Endotoxin introduced in vivo produces endothelial cell damage, thereby exposing collagen and activating both factor XII and the kallikrein system. Small vessels are affected by microthrombi (Fig. 2–66), and the patient suffers from a *diffuse bleeding diathesis.*[176] Gram-negative septicemia may also be associated with *granulocytopenia.*[177]

Viruses

Viruses are often accompanied by a *chronic inflammatory reaction* at the site of infection, and the draining lymph nodes may become hyperplastic. Infections with viruses such as *herpes* and *myxoviruses,* which are released by budding off cell membranes, induce *cell-mediated responses.* The cell-mediated responses are less constant and are of a lower magnitude following infection or immunization with non-membrane-associated viruses such as poliovirus.[178] This is of interest when one considers that the products of the major histocompatibility complex on membranes are important target structures in T-lymphocyte-mediated cytolysis. It is believed that T cells not only recognize virus-specific antigens, but MHC membrane products as well, which are modified by the viral products. Human cells infected with virus, but lacking necessary specific HLA antigens, resist specific T-lymphocyte cytolysis.[179]

Viral infection of the liver *(hepatitis),* in addition to typically producing liver cell lysis and necrosis and stimulating a round cell inflammatory response, interferes with syn-

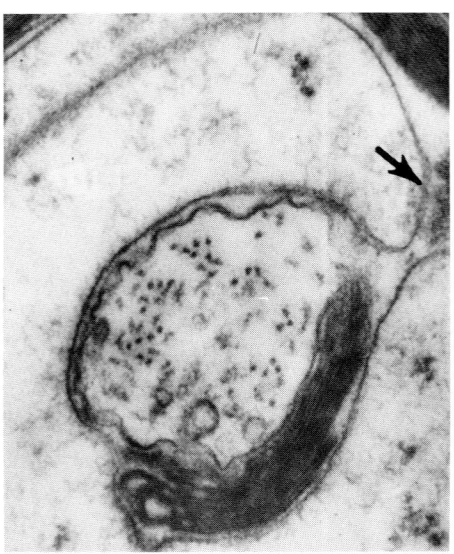

Figure 2–67. An electron micrograph of demyelinating nerve from a rat with allergic encephalomyelitis shows dissolution of meylin sheath (arrow).

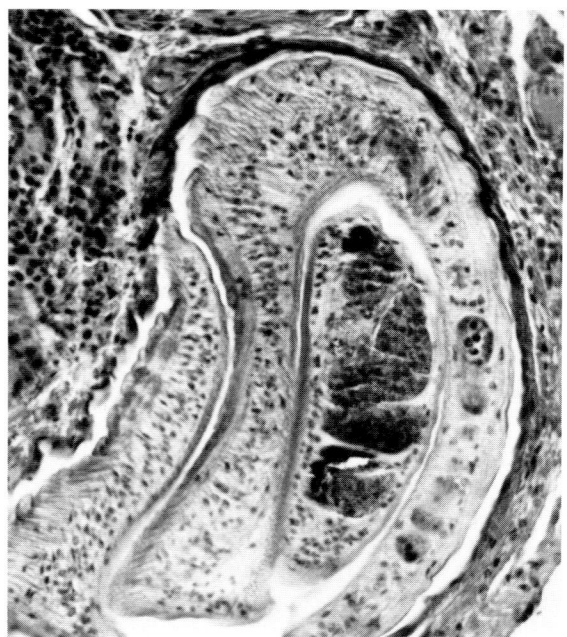

Figure 2–68. A portion of a mature schistosome is found in the soft tissue of a patient with widespread schistosomiasis.

thesis of important plasma proteins, including kinins and coagulation factors.

In some instances, a viral agent may or may not be present at the time a slowly progressive autoimmune-like disorder develops. *Slow virus infections* are examples of this phenomenon. *Multiple sclerosis* (MS) may be another example, as some evidence links MS to previous measles infection. Patients with MS have antibodies to various subcomponents of the measles virus.[180,181]

It is believed that a relationship may exist between measles viral infection and sensitization to myelin basic protein, which then becomes the target of immune attack (Fig. 2–67). An increased cell-mediated response of cerebrospinal fluid lymphocytes to myelin basic protein is seen in primary demyelinating diseases such as MS.[182] Similarly, the disease *subacute sclerosing panencephalitis* (SSPE) has been linked to measles infection.[183] It is characterized by progressive, degenerative neurologic changes. Patients with this disorder also demonstrate sensitivity to myelin basic protein.

Parasites and Fungi

A chronic inflammatory reaction and sometimes florid granulomata are associated with parasites and fungi. Other distinctive features are present, depending on the parasite. Schistosomes are commonly found within blood vessels (Fig. 2–68), and rickettsiae have a predilection for endothelial cells. Vasculitis, petechial hemorrhages, and disseminated intravascular coagulation may be prominent features of Rocky Mountain spotted fever infections. Infection here is associated with activation of the kallikrein-kinin system.[184]

Chemicals, Drugs, and Hormones Affecting Inflammation and Repair

Many chemicals and drugs produce acute *necrosis* (e.g., acids and alkalis), *cell degeneration* (e.g., arsenic, lead,[185] alcohol), local *allergic reactions* (e.g., poison ivy), and autoimmune *cytolytic reactions* (e.g., penicillin). Some drugs indirectly permit neoplasms to develop by suppressing the immune or defense response, prednisone, for instance, and some, such as vinyl chloride, directly stimulate neoplastic transformation.[186]

Anticoagulation and Fibrinolytic Drugs

As we have seen earlier, fibrinolysis is as important as coagulation in maintaining hemostasis. Plasminogen transformation to plasmin is accelerated by drugs such as chloroform, enzymes (streptokinase from beta-hemolytic streptococcus; urokinase, an enzyme in normal human urine), and fractions released from ruptured cells (perhaps microsomal in origin). Many circulating agents (e.g., tes-

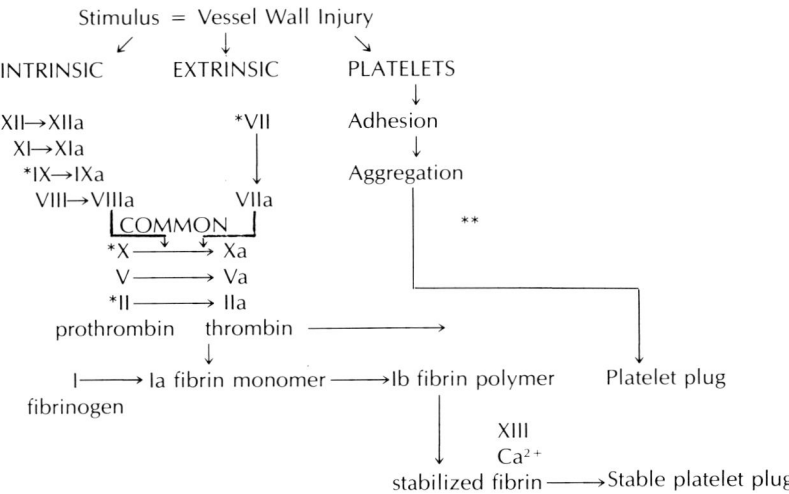

Figure 2–69. The pathology of coagulation is shown here. Synthesis is inhibited by the oral anticoagulants coumarin (*) and aspirin (**).

tosterone, epinephrine, and norepinephrine) and common therapeutic agents (e.g., *aspirin*) act in vivo, but not in vitro, to promote fibrinolysis.[187] Associated platelet abnormalities, as in renal disease, following the use of certain drugs such as aspirin and penicillin, or with injection of macromolecules (dextran), may compound the fibrinolytic effects (Fig. 2–69).

Chemotherapeutic Agents

Some chemotherapeutic agents used in therapy of neoplasia (for example, vinblastine) and for palliation of pain in arthritis (for example, colchicine) also inhibit phagocytosis because of their actions on microtubules. They may also produce lethal leukopenias.

Hormones

Modulation of hormonal activity exerts multiple effects on inflammation and repair.[188] Pituitary growth hormone stimulates repair, whereas its deficiency retards repair. Imbalances of parathormone and calcitonin may alter bone repair. The multisystem actions of insulin on inflammation are only partly elucidated; however, diabetics are known to have increased susceptibility to infections and poor repair processes. Ovarian estrogens play a major role in endometrial repair. Testosterone and erythropoietin are important factors in bone marrow stimulation (Table 2–38).

It has been previously noted that adrenal *glucocorticoids* have depressive effects on protein synthesis. Collagen formation and lymphocyte proliferation, important in repair, may be diminished by corticosteroid activity. Corticosteroids may produce profound lymphopenia and immuno-

Table 2–38. *Effect of Hormones on Inflammation, Repair, and Regeneration*

Hormone	Effect of Increase
Growth hormone	Stimulates repair
Parathormone	Demineralizes bone
Calcitonin	Mineralizes bone
Thyroxin	Stimulates regeneration
Prednisone	Retards inflammation response
Aldosterone	Maintains electrolyte balance
Estrogen	Regenerates endometrium
Progesterone	Promotes secretory phase of endometrial growth
Testosterone	Stimulates growth
Erythropoietin	Stimulates bone marrow growth
Insulin	Stimulates growth of cells (in vitro)

suppression. Certain stages between stem cells and fully committed differentiated B and T lymphocytes are most susceptible to the effects of cortisone. The susceptibility of lymphocytes is related to the number of cortisone receptor sites on their surface membranes. A high density of steroid receptors is present on immature lymphocytes in the thymic cortex, an area extremely sensitive to cortisone. Cortisone also suppresses phagocytic activity and chemotaxis.[189]

Effect of Immune Response and Products on Inflammation and Repair

It is clear that the cells of the immune system including granulocytes, white blood cells, mast cells, and platelets play a large role in helping the host tissue to destroy an infectious agent by antibody and lymphokine production. The release of humoral substances important in vasodilatation and chemotaxis and the direct interaction with injured cells and tissues are also important in the repair process.[190]

The lack of a proper immune response, as in congenital or acquired deficiency states, may have a profound inhibitory effect on inflammation. B-cell deficiencies as well as decreased helper T cells (T_H), suppressor T cells (T_S), and the presence of killer T cells (T_K) hinder a proper response, as do complement, granulocyte, and platelet, and coagulation factor deficiencies.

In certain instances, an uncontrolled immune response may provoke or may aggravate inflammation; a large group of diseases associated with this reaction, classified as immunopathology, will be discussed in the chapter on agents of disease.

REFERENCES

1. Cohen, S.: Cell mediated immunity and the inflammatory system. Hum. Pathol., 7:249, 1976.
2. Cohen, S.: The role of cell-mediated immunity in the induction of inflammatory responses. Am. J. Pathol., *88*:502, 1977.

3. Weissman, I.L., Hood, L.E., and Wood, W.B.: Essential Concepts in Immunology. Menlo Park, CA, Benjamin/Cummings Publishing, 1978.
4. Sell, S.: Immunology, Immunopathology and Immunity. 3rd Ed. New York, Harper & Row, 1980.
5. Gill, T.J., Cramer, D.V., and Kunz, H.W.: The major histocompatibility complex—comparison in the mouse, man, and the rat. Am. J. Pathol., 90:737, 1978.
6. Klein, J., et al.: The traditional and a new version of the mouse H-2 complex. Nature, 291:455, 1981.
7. Benacerraf, B.: The role of MHC gene products in immune regulations and its relevance to other reactivity. Science, 212:1229, 1981.
8. Miller, J.F.A.P., et al.: Histocompatibility linked immune responsiveness and restrictions imposed on sensitized lymphocytes. J. Exp. Med., 145:1623, 1977.
9. Suciu-Foca, N.: The HLA system in human pathology. Pathobiol. Annu., 9:81, 1979.
10. Dausset, J.: The major histocompatibility complex in man. Science, 213:1469, 1981.
11. Terhorst, C., et al.: Further structural studies of the heavy chain of HLA antigens and its similarity to immunoglobulins. Proc. Natl. Acad. Sci. U.S.A., 74:4002, 1977.
12. Motulsky, A.G.: The HLA complex and disease. N. Engl. J. Med., 300:918, 1979.
13. Malissen, M., Malissen, B., and Jordan, B.R.: Exon/intron organization and complete nucleotide sequence of an HLA gene. Proc. Natl. Acad. Sci. USA, 79:893, 1982.
14. Duquesnoy, R.J., et al.: Association of MB compatibility and successful intrafamilial kidney transplantation. N. Engl. J. Med., 302:421, 1980.
15. Sasazuki, T., McDevitt, H.O., and Grumet, F.L.: The association between genes in the major histocompatibility complex and disease susceptibility. Annu. Rev. Med., 28:425, 1977.
16. Ritzmann, S.E.: HLA patterns and disease association. JAMA, 236:2305, 1976.
17. O'Reilly, R.J., et al.: Reconstitution in severe combined immunodeficiency by transplantation of marrow from an unrelated donor. N. Engl. J. Med., 297:1311, 1977.
18. Yoshida, A.: Biochemical genetics of human blood group ABO system. Am. J. Hum. Genet., 34:1, 1982.
19. Fenoglio, C.M.: Antigens, enzymes and hormones. Their roles as tumor markers in gynecologic neoplasia. Diagn. Gynecol. Obstet., 2:33, 1980.
20. Adams, J.M.: The organization and expression of immunoglobulin genes. Immunol. Today, 1:10, 1980.
21. Kabat, E.A.: The structural basis of antibody complementarity. Adv. Protein Chem., 32:1, 1978.
22. Kabat, E.A.: Structural Concepts in Immunology and Immunochemistry. New York, Holt, Rinehart & Winston, 1976.
23. Brandtzaeg, P.: Immunohistochemical studies on various aspects of glandular immunoglobulin transport in man. Histochem. J., 9:553, 1977.
24. Isobe, Y., et al.: Studies on translocation of immunoglobulins across intestinal epithelium. Acta Histochem. Cytochem., 10:161, 1977.
25. Ruddy, S., Gigli, I., and Auster, K.F.: The complement synthesis of man. N. Engl. J. Med., 287:642, 1972.
26. Ochs, H.D., et al.: Linkage between the gene (or genes) controlling synthesis of the fourth component of complement and the major histocompatibility complex. N. Engl. J. Med., 296:470, 1977.
27. Porter, R.R., and Reid, K.B.M.: The biochemistry of complement. Nature, 275:699, 1978.
28. Trabyn-Jensea, J., et al.: Complement lysis: the ultrastructure and orientation of the C5b-9 complex on target sheep erythrocyte membranes. Scand. J. Immunol., 7:45, 1978.
29. Hammer, C.H., et al.: On the mechanism of cell membrane damage by complement: evidence on insertion of polypeptide chains from C8 and C9 into the lipid bilayer of erythrocytes. J. Immunol., 119:1, 1977.
30. Pillemer, C.H., et al.: The properdin system and immunity. I. Demonstration and isolation of a new serum protein, properdin, and its role in immune phenomena. Science, 120:279, 1954.

31. Frank, M.M.: Complement. Scope Current Concepts. Kalamazoo, MI, Upjohn, 1975.
32. Weissman, I.L., et al.: The lymphoid system. Its normal architecture and the potential for understanding the system through the study of lymphoproliferative diseases. Hum. Pathol., 9:25, 1978.
33. Grob, D.: Introduction: myasthenia gravis in perspective. Ann. N.Y. Acad. Sci., 274:1, 1976.
34. Bishop, M.B., and Lansing, L.S.: The spleen: a correlative overview of normal and pathologic anatomy. Hum. Pathol., 13:334, 1982.
35. Goetzl, E.J., Weller, P.F., and Valone, F.H.: Biochemical and functional basis of the regulatory and protective roles of the human eosinophil. In Advances in Inflammation Research. Vo. I. Edited by G. Weissmann, B. Samuelsson, and R. Paoletti. New York, Raven Press, 1978.
36. Dvorak, A.M., and Dvorak, H.F.: The basophil. Its morphology, biochemistry, motility, release reactions, recovery, and role in the inflammatory responses of IgE-mediated and cell-mediated origin. Arch. Pathol. Lab. Med., 103:551, 1979.
37. Kaliner, M.: The mast cell—a fascinating riddle. N. Engl. J. Med., 301:498, 1979.
38. Strober, S.: T- and B-cells in immunologic diseases. Am. J. Clin. Pathol., 68:671, 1977.
39. Clark, R.B., et al.: T-cell colonies recognize antigen in association with specific epitopes on Ia molecules. Nature, 295:412, 1982.
40. Shortman, K., and Jackson, H.: Proliferation genetics and interrelationships of subpopulations of mouse thymus cells. Cell. Immunol., 12:230, 1976.
41. Asofsky, R., and Tregelaar, R.: Graft vs. host activity of mouse thymocytes. J. Immunol., 110:567, 1973.
42. Raulet, D.H., and Bevan, M.J.: A differentiation factor required for the expression of cytotoxic T-cell function. Nature, 296:754, 1982.
43. Friedman, R.M.: Interferons: Basic research, clinical studies, and their support. Arch. Pathol. Lab. Med., 106:259, 1982.
44. Adams, D.O.: Macrophage activation and secretion. Fed. Proc., 41:2193, 1982.
45. deSousa, M.: Lymphocyte maldistribution and immunodeficiency. Hosp. Pract., 15:71, 1980.
46. Polliack, A.: Surface morphology of lymphoreticular cells: a review of data obtained from scanning electron microscopy. Recent Results Cancer Res., 64:66, 1978.
47. Ross, G.D.: Surface markers of B and T cells. Arch. Pathol. Lab. Med., 101:337, 1977.
48. Anderson, R.E., Standefer, J.C., and Scaletti, J.V.: The phospholipid and glycoprotein composition of T and B cells. Lab. Invest., 37:329, 1977.
49. Herberman, R.B., and Ortaldo, J.R.: Natural killer cells: their role in defenses against disease. Science, 214:24, 1981.
50. Pierce, C.W.: Macrophages: modulators of immunity. Am. J. Pathol., 98:10, 1980.
51. Rosenthal, A.S.: Regulation of the immune response: role of the macrophage. N. Engl. J. Med., 303:1153, 1980.
52. Keller, R., et al.: An IgG-Fc receptor induced in cytomegalovirus-infected human fibroblasts. J. Immunol., 116:772, 1976.
53. Sullivan, T.J., and Parker, C.W.: Pharmacologic modulation of inflammatory mediator release by rat mast cells. Am. J. Pathol., 85:437, 1976.
54. Melcher, U., and Uhr, J.W.: Cell surface immunoglobulin. XVI. Polypeptide chain structure of mouse IgM- and IgD-like molecule. J. Immunol., 116:409, 1976.
55. Marchalonis, J.J., Cone, P.E., and Atwell, J.: Isolation and partial characterization of lymphocyte surface immunoglobulins. J. Exp. Med., 135:956, 1972.
56. Binz, H., Kemura, A., and Wigzell, H.: Editorial: idiotype-positive T lymphocytes. Scand. J. Immunol., 4:413, 1975.
57. Woda, B.A., et al.: The lack of specificity of the sheep erythrocyte in lymphocyte rosetting phenomenon. Am. J. Pathol., 88:69, 1977.
58. Milstein, C.: Monoclonal antibodies. Cancer, 49:1953, 1982.
59. Setcanage, T.M., et al.: A novel receptor for secretory component on porcine mononuclear cells. Cell. Immunol., 27:67, 1976.
60. Benacerraf, B.: Suppressor T cells and suppressor factor. Hosp. Pract., 13:65, 1978.

61. Cunningham, B.A., et al.: Structure and activities of lymphocytic mitogens. *In* Mitogens in Immunobiology. Edited by J.J. Oppenheim and D.L. Rosentereich. New York, Academic Press, 1976.
62. Wabl, M.R., Forine, L., and Loor, F.: Switch in immunoglobulin class production observed in single clones of committed lymphocytes. Science, *199*:1078, 1978.
63. Sharon, N.: Lectins as mitogen. *In* Mitogens in Immunobiology. Edited by J.J. Oppenheim and D.L. Rosentereich. New York, Academic Press, 1976.
64. Parker, C.W.: Control of lymphocyte function. N. Engl. J. Med., *295*:1180, 1976.
65. Robertson, M.: The life of a B lymphocyte. Nature, *283*:332, 1980.
66. Zucker-Franklin, D.: The ultrastructure of lymphocytes. Semin. Hematol., *6*:4, 1969.
67. Earp, H.S., et al.: Lymphocyte surface modulation and cyclic nucleotides. I. Topographic correlation of cyclic adenosine 3'5'-monophosphate and immunoglobulin fluorescence during lymphocyte capping. J. Exp. Med., *145*:1087, 1977.
68. Weigle, W.D.: Cyclical production of antibody as a regulatory mechanism in the immune response. Adv. Immunol., *21*:87, 1975.
69. Greaves, M.F.: Membrane receptor-adenylate cyclase relationships. Nature, *265*:681, 1977.
70. Grayson, J., et al.: Immunoglobulin production induced *in vitro* by glucocorticoid hormones. J. Clin. Invest., *68*:1539, 1981.
71. Goodwin, J.S., Bankhurst, A.O., and Messner, R.P.: Suppression of human T-cell mitogenesis by prostaglandin. J. Exp. Med., *146*:1719, 1977.
72. Kabat, E.A., Wu, T.T., and Bilofsky, H.: Evidence supporting somatic assembly of the DNA segments (minigenes), coding for the framework, and complementarity-determining segments of immunoglobulin variable regions. J. Exp. Med., *149*:1299, 1979.
73. Seidman, J.G., and Leder, P.: The arrangement and rearrangement of antibody genes. Nature, *276*:790, 1978.
74. Marx, J.L.: Antibodies (II): Another look at the diversity problem. Science, *202*:412, 1978.
75. Cramer, F.: Somatic mutations. Nature, *273*:423, 1978.
76. Marx, J.L.: Antibodies: getting their genes together. Science, *212*:1015, 1981.
77. Gearhart, P.J.: Generation of immunoglobulin variable gene diversity. Immunol. Today, *3*:107, 1982.
78. Claman, H.M.: T-cell tolerance—one signal? Cell. Immunol., *48*:201, 1979.
79. Dinarello, C.A., and Wolff, S.M.: Molecular basis of fever in humans. Am. J. Med., *72*:799, 1982.
80. Cline, M.J., et al.: Autoimmune panleukopenia. N. Engl. J. Med., *295*:1489, 1976.
81. Ryan, G.B., and Majno, G.: Acute inflammation. A review. Am. J. Pathol., *86*:247, 1977.
82. Marx, J.L.: The leukotrienes in allergy and inflammation. Science, *215*:1380, 1982.
83. Movat, H.Z.: The kinin system and its relation to other systems. Curr. Top. Pathol., *68*:111, 1979.
84. Johnston, M.G., Hay, J.B., and Movat, H.Z.: The role of prostaglandins in inflammation. Curr. Top. Pathol., *68*:259, 1979.
85. Wilkinson, P.C., and Lackie, J.M.: The adhesion, migration, and chemotaxis of leucocytes in inflammation. Curr. Top. Pathol., *68*:47, 1979.
86. Adler, J.: The sensing of chemicals by bacteria. Annu. Rev. Biochem., *234*:40, 1976.
87. Bessis, M.: Studies on cell agony and death: an attempt at classification. *In* Cellular Injury (Ciba Found. Symp.). Edited by A. de Reuck and J. Knight. London, Churchill, 1964.
88. Ward, P.A., Johnson, K.J., and Krentzer, D.L.: Regulatory dysfunction in leukotaxis. Am. J. Pathol., *88*:701, 1977.
89 Brozna, J.P., et al.: Chemotactic factor inactivators of human granulocytes. J. Clin. Invest., *60*:1280, 1977.
90. Scribner, D.J., and Fahrney, D.: Neutrophil receptors of IgG and complement: their roles in the attachment and ingestion phases of phagocytosis. J. Immunol., *116*:892, 1976.
91. Stossel, T.P.: Phagocytosis. N. Engl. J. Med., *290*:761, 774, 833, 1974.

92. Stossel, T.P.: Contractile proteins in phagocytosis: an example of cell surface-to-cytoplasm communication. Fed. Proc., *36*:2181, 1977.

93. Fantone, J.C., and Ward, P.A.: Role of oxygen-derived free radicals and metabolites in leukocyte-dependent inflammatory reactions. Am. J. Pathol., *107*:397, 1982.

94. Badwey, J.A., Curnutte, J.T., and Karnovsky, M.L.: The enzyme of granulocytes that produces superoxide and peroxide. N. Engl. J. Med., *300*:1157, 1979.

95. Papageorgiou, P.S., Sorokin. C.F., and Glade, P.R.: Similarity of migration inhibitory factors produced by human lymphoid cell line and phytohemagglutinin and tuberculin-stimulated human peripheral lymphocytes. J. Immunol., *112*:675, 1974.

96. Mason, R.G., and Saba, H.I.: Normal and abnormal hemostasis—an integrated view. A review. Am. J. Pathol., *92*:775, 1978.

97. Polley, M.J., and Nachman, R.: The human complement system in thrombin-mediated platelet function. J. Exp. Med., *147*:1713, 1978.

98. Shainoff, J.R., and Dardik, B.N.: Fibrinopeptide B and aggregation of fibrinogen. Science, *204*:200, 1979.

99. Owen, C.H., and Bowie, E.J.W.: The Intravascular Coagulation-Fibrinolysis Syndromes in Obstetrics and Gynecology. Kalamazoo, MI, Upjohn, 1976.

100. White, J.G.: Current concepts of platelet structure. Am. J. Clin. Pathol., *71*:363, 1979.

101. Cusack, N.J.: Platelet-activating factor. Nature, *285*:193, 1980.

102. Nishikawa, M., and Hidaka, H.: Role of calmodulin in platelet aggregation. J. Clin. Invest., *69*:1348, 1982.

103. Huang, T.W., and Benditt, E.P.: Mechanisms of platelet adhesion to basal lamina. Am. J. Pathol., *92*:99, 1978.

104. Bucher, N.L.R.: Regeneration of mammalian liver. Int. Rev. Cytol., *15*:245, 1963.

105. Taylor, S., and Folkman, J.: Protamine is an inhibitor of angiogenesis. Nature, *297*:307, 1982.

106. Heumann, R., Schwab, M., and Thoenen, H.: A second messenger required for nerve growth factor biological activity? Nature, *292*:838, 1981.

107. Barnes, D.W.: Epidermal growth factor inhibits growth of A431 human epidermoid carcinoma in serum-free cell culture. J. Cell Biol., *93*:1, 1982.

108. Becci, P.J., McDowell, E.M., and Trump. B.F.: The respiratory epithelium. II. Hamster trachea, bronchus, and bronchioles. J.N.C.I., *61*:551, 1978.

109. Marx, J.L.: Regeneration in the central nervous system. Science, *209*:378, 1980.

110. Mallory, G.K., Hite, P.O., and Salcedo-Salgar, J.: The speed of healing of myocardial infarction: a study of the pathologic anatomy in 72 cases. Am. Heart J., *18*:647, 1931.

111. Lipton, B.H., and Schultz, E.: Developmental fate of skeletal muscle satellite cells. Science, *205*:1292, 1979.

112. Kempczinski, R.F., and Caufield, J.B.: A light and electron microscopic study of renal tubular regeneration. Nephron, 5:249, 1968.

113. Becker, F.F., and Lane, B.P.: Regeneration of the mammalian liver. Am. J. Pathol., *47*:783, 1965.

114. Yee, A.G., and Revel, J.P.: Loss and reappearance of gap junction in regenerating liver. J. Cell Biol., *78*:554, 1978.

115. Creutzfeldt, W.: Endocrine tumors of the pancreas: clinical, chemical and morphological findings. *In* The Pancreas. Edited by P.J. Fitzgerald and A.B. Morrison. Baltimore, Williams & Wilkins, 1980.

116. Martin, G.M., et al.: Clonal selection, attenuation and differentiation in an *in vitro* model of hyperplasia. Am. J. Pathol., *74*:137, 1974.

117. Majno, G., et al.: Contraction of granulation tissue *in vitro*: Similarity to smooth muscle. Science, *173*:548, 1971.

118. Carpenter, N.H., Gates, D.J., and Williams, H.T.G.: Normal processes and restraints in wound healing. Can. J. Surg., *20*:314, 1977.

119. Sporn, M.B., and Harris, E.D.: Proliferative diseases. Am. J. Med., *70*:1231, 1981.

120. Wozney, J., et al.: Structure of the pro α2(I) collagen gene. Nature, *294*:129, 1981.

121. Prockop, D.J., et al.: The biosynthesis of collagen and its disorders. N. Engl. J. Med., *301*:13, 77, 1979.

122. Perez-Tamayo, R.: Pathology of collagen degradation: a review. Am. J. Pathol., *92*:509, 1978.

123. Basset, E.G., Baker, J.R., and deSouza, P.: A light microscopical study of healing dermal wounds in rats incised with special reference to eosinophil leukocytes and to the collagenase fibers of the peri-wound areas. Br. J. Exp. Pathol., 58:581, 1977.

124. Gadek, J., et al.: Collagenase in the lower respiratory tract of patients with idiopathic pulmonary fibrosis. N. Engl. J. Med., 301:737, 1979.

125. Spector, W.G.: The granulomatous inflammatory exudate. Int. Rev. Exp. Pathol., 8:1, 1969.

126. Adams, D.O.: The granulomatous inflammatory response. Am. J. Pathol., 84:164, 1976.

127. Schmitt, E., Meunet, G., and Stix L.: Monocyte recruitment in tuberculosis and sarcoidosis. Br. J. Haematol., 35:11, 1977.

128. Papdimitriou, J.M., and Wee, S.H.: Selective release of lysosomal enzymes from cell populations containing multinucleate giant cells. J. Pathol., 120:193, 1976.

129. Papadimitriou, J.M., and Kington, K.J.: The locomotory behavior of the multinucleate giant cells of foreign body reactions. J. Pathol., 121:27, 1976.

130. Ishibashi, H., et al.: Distribution of α 1-antitrypsin in normal granuloma and tumor tissues in rats. J. Lab. Clin. Med., 91:575, 1978.

131. Johnston, R.B., Jr.: Defects of neutrophil function. N. Engl. J. Med., 307:434, 1982.

132. Siegal, F.P., Siegal, M., and Good, R.: Role of helper, suppressor and B-cell defects in the pathogenesis of the hypogammaglobulinemias. N. Engl. J. Med., 299:172, 1978.

133. Gelfand, E.W., et al.: Abnormal lymphocyte capping in a patient with severe combined immunodeficiency disease. N. Engl. J. Med., 301:1246, 1979.

134. Strober, S.: T- and B- cells in immunologic diseases. Am. J. Clin. Pathol., 68:671, 1977.

135. Strober, W., et al.: Secretory component deficiency. N. Engl. J. Med., 294:351, 1976.

136. Waldmann, T.A., et al.: Disorders of suppressor immunoregulatory cells in the pathogenesis of immunodeficiency and autoimmunity. Ann. Intern. Med., 88:226, 1978.

137. Atwater, J.S., and Tomasi, T.B., Jr.: Suppressor cells and IgA deficiency. Clin. Immunol. Immunopathol., 9:379, 1978.

138. Purtilo, D.T., et al.: Variable phenotypic expression of an X-linked recessive lymphoproliferative syndrome. N. Engl. J. Med., 297:1077, 1977.

139. Purtilo, D.T., et al.: Immunodeficiency to the Epstein-Barr virus with X-linked recessive lymphoproliferative syndrome. Clin. Immunol. Immunopathol., 9:147, 1978.

140. Hitzig, W.H., Dooren, L.J., and Vossen, J.M.: Severe combined immunodeficiency diseases. Springer Semin. Immunopathol., 1:283, 1978.

141. Saxon, A., et al.: Helper and suppressor T-lymphocyte leukemia in ataxia telangiectasia. N. Engl. J. Med., 300:700, 1979.

142. O'Reilly, R.J., et al.: Reconstitution in severe combined immunodeficiency by transplantation of marrow from an unrelated donor. N. Engl. J. Med., 297:1311, 1977.

143. Buckley, R.H., et al.: Correction of severe combined immunodeficiency by fetal liver cell. N. Engl. J. Med., 294:1076, 1976.

144. Tsukimoto, I., and Lampkin, B.C.: Effects of thymosin on lymphoblasts. N. Engl. J. Med., 293:455, 1975.

145. Polmar, S.H., et al.: Enzyme replacement for adenosine deaminase deficiency and severe combined immunodeficiency. N. Engl. J. Med., 295:1337, 1976.

146. Snyderman, R., et al.: Defective mononuclear leukocyte chemotaxis: a previously unrecognized immune dysfunction. Ann. Intern Med., 78:509, 1973.

147. Meunet, G.: Disorders of the mononuclear phagocyte system. An analytical review. Blut, 34:317, 1977.

148. Boxer, L.A., Hedley-Whyte, T., and Stossel, T.P.: Neutrophil actin dysfunction and abnormal neutrophil behavior. N. Engl. J. Med., 291:1093, 1974.

149. Oliver, J.M.: Cell biology of leukocyte abnormalities—membrane and cytoskeletal function in normal and defective cells. Am. J. Pathol., 93:221, 1978.

150. Lalezari, P., et al.: Chronic autoimmune neutropenia due to anti-NA2 antibody. N. Engl. J. Med., 293:744, 1975

151. Clawson, C.C., White, J.G., and Repine, J.E.: The Chediak-Higashi syndrome. Evidence that defective leukotaxis is primarily due to an impediment by giant granules. Am. J. Pathol., *92*:745, 1978.
152. Oliver, C., and Essner, E.: Formation of anomalous lysosomes in monocytes, neutrophils and eosinophils from bone marrow of mice with Chediak-Higashi syndrome. Lab. Invest., *32*:17, 1975.
153. Clawson, C.C., Repine, J.E., and White, J.G.: The Chediak-Higashi syndrome. Quantitation of a deficiency in maximal bactericidal capacity. Am. J. Pathol., *94*:539, 1979.
154. Boxer, L.A., et al.: Correction of leukocyte function in Chediak-Higashi syndrome by ascorbate. N. Engl. J. Med., *295*:1041, 1976.
155. Curnutte, J.T., et al.: Defect in pyridine nucleotide dependent superoxide production by a particulate fraction from the granulocytes of patients with chronic granulomatous disease. N. Engl. J. Med., *293*:628, 1975.
156. Lackmann, P.J., and Rosen, F.S.: Genetic defects of complement in man. Springer Semin. Immunopathol., *1*:339, 1978.
157. Muller-Eberhard, H.J.: Complement abnormalities in human disease. Hosp. Pract., *13*:65, 1978.
158. Jackson, C.G., et al.: Immune response of a patient with deficiency of the fourth component of complement and lupus erythematosus. N. Engl. J. Med., *300*:1124, 1979.
159. Hall, R.E., and Colten, H.R.: Genetic defect in biosynthesis of the precursor form of the fourth component of complement. Science, *199*:69, 1978.
160. Day, N.K., Moncada, B., and Good, R.A.: Inherited deficiencies of the complement system. *In* Comprehensive Immunology. Biological Amplification Systems in Immunology. Vol. 2. Edited by N.K. Day and R.A. Good. New York, Plenum Publishing, 1977.
161. Lint, T.F., et al.: Hereditary deficiency of the ninth component of complement (C) in man. Clin. Res., *26*:714A, 1978.
162. Rosen, F.S., and Austen, K.F.: Androgen therapy in hereditary angioneurotic edema. N. Engl. J. Med., *295*:1476, 1976.
163. Ts'ao, C-H., Rossi, E.C., and Lestina, F.C.: Abnormalities in platelet function and morphology in a case of thrombocythemia. Arch. Pathol. Lab. Med., *101*:526, 1977.
164. White, J.G.: Ultrastructural studies of the gray platelet syndrome. Am. J. Pathol., *95*:445, 1979.
165. Gralnick, H.R., et al.: Factor VIII. Ann. Intern. Med., *86*:598, 1977.
166. Lusher, J.M., et al.: Efficacy of prothrombin-complex concentrates in hemophiliacs with antibodies to factor VIII. N. Engl. J. Med., *303*:421, 1980.
167. Weiss, H.J., et al.: Pseudo-von Willebrand's disease. N. Engl. J. Med., *306*:326, 1982.
168. Jaffe, E.A.: Endothelial cells and the biology of factor VIII. Semin. Med. Beth Israel Hospital, Boston, *296*:377, 1977.
169. Vogel, A., et al.: Abnormal collagen fibril structure in the gravis form (type I) of Ehlers-Danlos syndrome. Lab. Invest., *40*:201, 1979.
170. Pope, F.M., and Nicholas, A.C.: Molecular abnormalities of collagen. J. Clin. Path., *12*(Suppl.):95, 1978.
171. Hegster, D.M.: Protein-calorie malnutrition. Sci. Am., *66*:61, 1978.
172. Levene, C.I., Ockleford, C.O., and Barber, C.L.: Scurvy: a comparison between ultrastructural and biochemical changes observed in cultured fibroblasts and the collagen they synthesize. Virchows Arch. (Cell Pathol.), *23*:325, 1977.
173. Gallagher, J.C., and Riggs, B.L.: Nutrition and bone disease. Vitamin D. N. Engl. J. Med., *298*:193, 1978.
174. Ulmer, D.D.: Current concepts. Trace elements. N. Engl. J. Med., *297*:318, 1977.
175. Kasarett, G.W.: Radiation Histopathology. Vols. I and II. Boca-Raton, FL., CRC Press, 1980.
176. McKay, D.G., and Shapiro, S.S.: Alterations in the blood coagulation system induced by bacterial endotoxin. J. Exp. Med., *107*:353, 1958.
177. Bergman, M.J., et al.: Interaction of polymorphonuclear neutrophils with Escherichia coli. Effect of enterotoxin on phagocytosis, killing, chemotaxis and cyclic AMP. J. Clin. Invest., *61*:227, 1978.
178. Rytel, M.W., and Neibojewski, R.A.: The role of membrane association of antigens in induction of cell-mediated immunity to viruses. Clin. Exp. Immunol., *32*:302, 1978.
179. Tursz, T., et al.: Human virus-injected target cells lacking HLA antigens resist specific T-lymphocyte cytolysis. Nature, *269*:806, 1977.

180. Rola-Pleszczynski, M., et al.: Lymphocyte-mediated cytotoxicity to viruses in patients with multiple sclerosis: presence of a blocking factor. Clin. Immunol. Immunopathol., 5:165, 1976.

181. Sheremata, W., Sazant, A., and Wattens, G.: Subacute sclerosing panencephalitis and multiple sclerosis: *in vitro* measles immunity and sensitization to myelin basic protein. Can. Med. Assoc. J., *118*:509, 1978.

182. Lisak, R.P., and Aweiman, B.: *In vitro* cell-mediated immunity of cerebrospinal-fluid lymphocytes to myelin basic protein in primary demyelinating diseases. N. Engl. J. Med., *297*:848, 1977.

183. Makino, S., et al.: Isolation and biological characterization of a measles virus-like agent from the brain of an autopsied case of subacute sclerosing panencephalitis (SSPE). Microbiol. Immunol., *21*:193, 1977.

184. Yamada, T., et al.: Activation of the kallikrein-kinin system in Rocky Mountain spotted fever. Ann. Intern. Med., *88*:764, 1978.

185. Klein, M.Y., Buse, M., Louria, D.B.: Lead cardiomyopathy in mice. Arch. Pathol. Lab. Med., *101*:89, 1977.

186. Marther, J.F., et al.: Vinyl chloride in associated liver disease. Ann. Intern. Med., *84*:717, 1976.

187. Ratnoff, O.D.: A new property of an old remedy: fibrinolysis and aspirin. N. Engl. J. Med., *296*:566, 1977.

188. Simon, L.S., and Mills, J.A.: Nonsteroidal anti-inflammatory drugs. N. Engl. J. Med., *302*:1179, 1980.

189. Craddock, C.G.: Corticosteroid-induced lymphopenia, immunosuppression, and body defense. Ann. Intern. Med., *88*:564, 1978.

190. Mackowiak, P.A.: Microbial synergism in human infections (first of two parts). N. Engl. J. Med., *298*:21, 1978.

Chapter 3

AGENTS OF DISEASE

Which can as well inflame as it can kill.

—Pericles, II, ii

It is well accepted that most diseases are not the result of a single etiologic agent. Even when a single agent is identified, multiple host factors determine the degree of injury, the repair process, and the final outcome of the disease.

Nevertheless, for purposes of classifying disease by origin, we have reviewed the general effects of injury on cells and tissues of six major classes of etiologic agents or factors. These are: (1) genetic factors; (2) nutritional factors; (3) physical agents; (4) infectious agents; (5) environmental disorders associated with exogenous drugs, chemicals, and hormones; and (6) immune reactions and products resulting in injury to cells and tissues and immunopathology. At the end of each section we have discussed in more detail a prototype of disease associated with each class of injurious agent. A clinical disease exhibiting a multifactorial origin, diabetes mellitus, concludes the discussion.

GENETIC FACTORS

In this section we discuss genetic diseases of three principal categories: *inborn errors of metabolism, cytogenetic abnormalities,* and *teratology*. This field has such broad ramifications, however, that genetic diseases are discussed in several other chapters. These include the immune deficiency diseases and defects in coagulation and collagen metabolism (discussed under inflammation in Chapter 2), the storage diseases (discussed under lysosomes in Chapter 6), and several genetic deficiencies such as hemochromatosis (discussed under inclusions in Chapter 6).

Methods of Studying Genetic Diseases

All human disease has a genetic component, but in only about 12% is its effect readily apparent (Fig. 3–1). A gross chromosomal abnormality is present in 1% of all live births, in 10 to 20% of aborted fetuses, in 57% of stillbirths, and in 45% of mentally retarded children.[1]

Classic *pedigree* studies on large families with genetic disorders (for example, color blindness and glucose-6-phosphate dehydrogenase (G6PD) deficiency) provided early significant information about particular gene sites on sex chromosomes. Many genetic diseases are associated with a change in a specific gene or group of genes. This may involve additions, deletions, or substitutions in the nucleotide sequence of the genome. Several hundred inborn errors of metabolism are known.[2] Since the average gene is only nanometers in length, no gross karyotypic chromosomal abnormality is usually seen in single or group gene mutations.

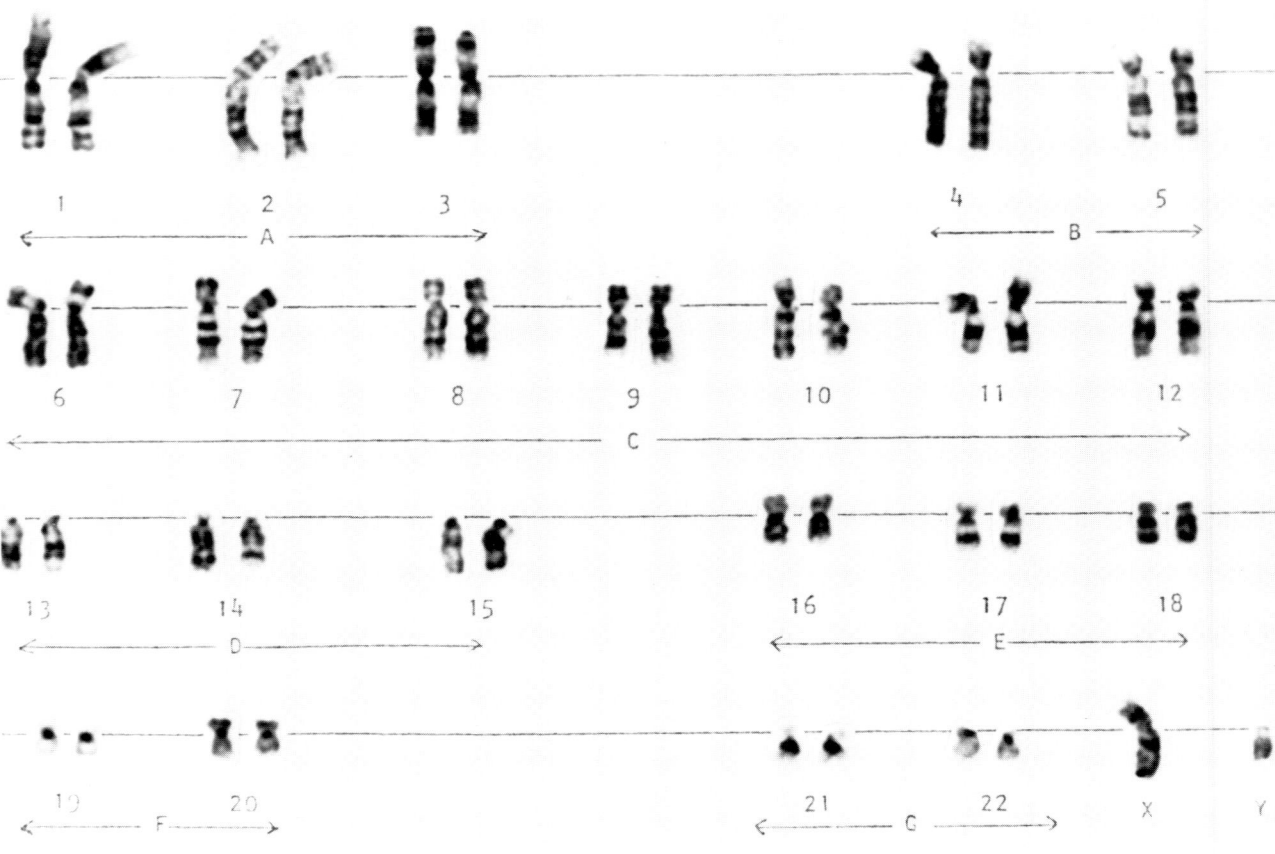

Figure 3–1. A normal human male karyotype (banded). (Courtesy of Dr. T.T. Puck, University of Colorado, Denver.)

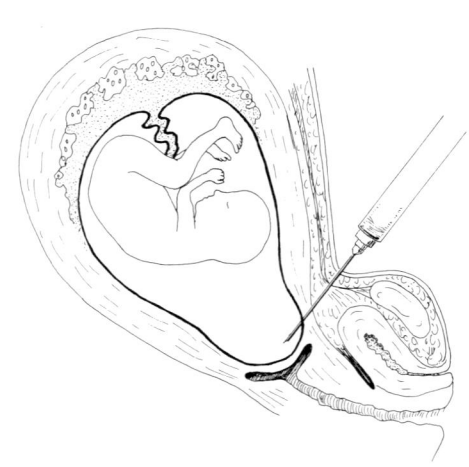

Figure 3–2. Assessment of amniotic fluid withdrawn in amniocentesis is a means of evaluating prenatal status, including many genetic disorders.

Modern *molecular hybridization* techniques and *banding reactions* based on the chemical structure of the chromosomes provide methods for detecting nucleotide alterations at specific sites of specific chromosomes.[3] *Cell fusion* studies, with loss of marker chromosomes during subsequent growth and division of hybrid cells in tissue culture, have already provided mapping information on many genes in mammalian cells, such as localization of a particular enzyme activity to a specific chromosome.[4] *Cellular hybridization* studies with radioautographs are not sufficiently sensitive at present to detect genes located on a particular chromosome, except for genes with multiple copies (for example, DNA for rRNA and *satellite DNA*).[5]

Amniocentesis may be performed in the fifteenth or sixteenth week of gestation, allowing studies and culture of the cells obtained. Over 100 inborn errors of metabolism and numerous chromosomal abnormalities have been detected in this way.[6,7] Better-informed physicians and families may then consider abortion of such an affected fetus where a viable existence seems unlikely (Table 3–1 and Fig. 3–2).

Table 3–1. Inborn Errors of Metabolism Diagnosable Before Birth

Lipidoses

Cholesterol-ester storage disease
Fabry's disease (angiokeratoma corporis diffusum)
Farber's disease (disseminated lipogranulomatosis)
Gaucher's disease
Generalized gangliosidosis (GM$_1$ gangliosidosis type I)
Juvenile GM$_1$ gangliosidosis (GM$_1$ gangliosidosis type 2)
Tay-Sachs disease (GM$_2$ gangliosidosis type 1)
Sandhoff's disease (GM$_2$ gangliosidosis type 2)

Juvenile GM$_2$ gangliosidosis (GM$_2$ gangliosis type 3)
GM$_3$ sphingolipodystrophy
Krabbe's disease (globoid-cell leukodystrophy)
Metachromatic leukodystrophy
Niemann-Pick disease type A
Niemann-Pick disease type B
Niemann-Pick disease type C
Refsum disease (heredopathia atactica polyneuritiformis)
Wolman disease (primary familial xanthomatosis)

Mucopolysaccharidoses

MPS I—Hurler's
MPS I — Scheie's
MPS—Hurler/Scheie
MPS IIA—Hunter's
MPS IIB—Hunter's

MPS III—Sanfilippo's A, B
MPS IV—Morquio's syndrome
MPS VIA—Maroteaux-Lamy syndrome
MPS VIB—Maroteaux-Lamy syndrome
MPS VII—β-glucuronidase deficiency

Amino Acid and Related Disorders

Argininosuccinic aciduria
Aspartylglucosaminuria
Citrullinemia
Congenital hyperammonemia
Histidinemia
Hypervalinemia
Iminoglycinuria
Isoleucine catabolism disorder
Isovaleric acidemia
Maple-syrup-urine disease (ketoaminoacidemia)
Methylmalonic aciduria
Cystathionine synthase deficiency (homocystinuria)

Cystathioninuria
Cystinuria
Hartnup's disease
Methylenetetrahydrofolate reductase deficiency
Ornithine-α-ketoacid transaminase deficiency
Propionyl CoA carboxylase deficiency
Succinyl CoA: 3 ketoacid CoA-transferase deficiency
Vitamin B$_{12}$ metabolic defect

Disorders of Carbohydrate Metabolism

Fucosidosis
Galactokinase deficiency
Galactosemia
Glucose-6-phosphate dehydrogenase deficiency
Glycogen-storage disease (type II)
Glycogen-storage disease (type III)

Glycogen-storage disease (type IV)
Mannosidosis
Phosphohexose isomarase deficiency
Pyruvate decarboxylase deficiency
Pyruvate dehydrogenase deficiency

Miscellaneous Hereditary Diseases

Acatalasia
Acute intermittent porphyria
Adenosine deaminase deficiency
Chédiak-Higashi syndrome
Congenital erythropoietic porphyria
Congenital nephrosis
Lysosomal acid phosphatase deficiency
Lysyl-protocollagen hydroxylase deficiency
Myotonic muscular dystrophy
Nail-patella syndrome (arthro-onychodysplasia)
Orotic aciduria

Cystinosis
Familial hypercholesterolemia
Glutathionuria
Hypophosphatasia
I-cell disease (mucolipidosis II)
Leigh's encephalopathy
Lesch-Nyhan syndrome
Protoporphyria
Saccharopinuria
Sickle cell anemia
Testicular feminization
Thalassemia
Xeroderma pigmentosum

(Modified from Milunsky, A.: Prenatal diagnosis of genetic disorders. N. Engl. J. Med., 295:378, 1976.)

Inborn Errors of Metabolism

Garrod introduced the concept of *inborn errors of metabolism* in 1908.[8] In general, each inborn error of metabolism is associated with a specific protein deficiency, often an enzyme.[9] This deficiency may result in an accumulation of an ineffective, sometimes toxic, metabolic product or the diversion of an intermediary product to an alternative pathway, resulting in synthesis of other products in unusual amounts. Storage diseases are often associated with altered cellular structure, sometimes with altered cellular function, and with the appearance of unusual amounts of certain metabolic products in cells, extracellular fluid, the vascular space, urine, sweat, and other secretions.

Genetic diseases are often classified according to their principal effects on protein, carbohydrate, lipid, or polysaccharide metabolism.[10] Disorders with defective proteins are well known, as exemplified by the hemoglobinopathy *sickle cell anemia*, the coagulation defect in *hemophilia* (factor VIII deficiency), or the β and γ hemoglobin gene deficiencies in *thalassemia*.[11] Many of the genetically induced carbohydrate defects are the result of protein (enzyme) deficiencies. An example is the glycogen storage disorder *von Gierke's disease* in which deficient glucose-6-phosphatase activity results in marked accumulation of glycogen in cells.

Abnormalities in lipid metabolism are seen in a wide spectrum of genetic diseases. A deficiency of sphingomyelinase results in an accumulation of sphingomyelin *(Niemann-Pick disease)*. The various forms of *familial hyperlipidemia* have been widely implicated in an increased incidence of atherosclerosis and myocardial infarction.[12]

In the *adrenogenital syndrome*, an abnormality in steroid metabolism, a deficiency of 21-hydroxylase, results in the diversion of normal adrenal hormone precursors into a pathway leading eventually to testosterone. Disorders related to deficient enzymes involved in polysaccharide metabolism include *Hurler's* and *Hunter's diseases* (mucopolysaccharidosis type I and type II). The enzyme deficiency in Hurler's disease is iduronidase, and in Hunter's disease it is iduronidate sulfatase.

In *Wilson's disease* (hepatolenticular degeneration), low levels of the serum copper-binding protein ceruloplasmin result in excess storage of copper in the cornea, liver, and basal ganglia of the central nervous system.[13] Another metal, iron, is accumulated in *idiopathic hemochromatosis*. Iron is deposited in the liver, pancreas, and other organs and may interfere with function.[14,15] The large group of inborn errors also includes little known enzyme deficiencies in connective tissue metabolism (for example, *Marfan's syndrome*) and muscle structure (for example, *muscular dystrophy*).[16]

Cytogenetic Abnormalities

With the advent of new chromosomal banding techniques using Giemsa staining and quinacrine fluorescence,

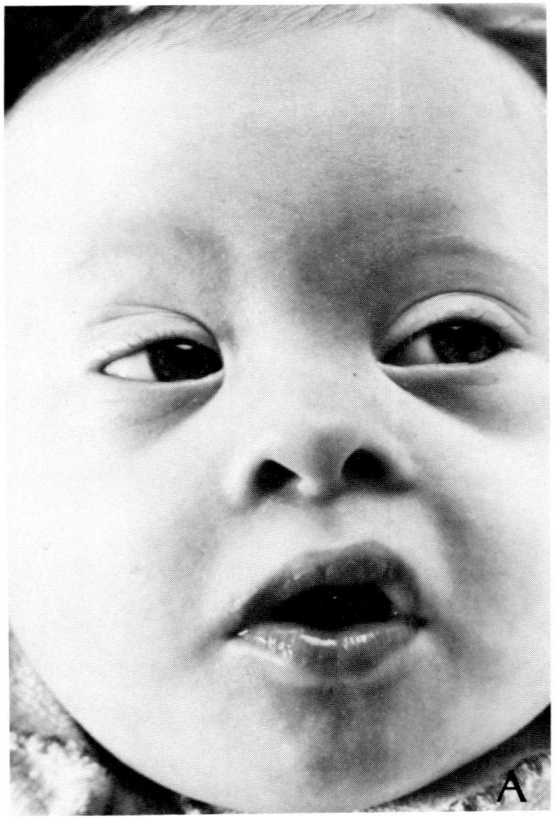

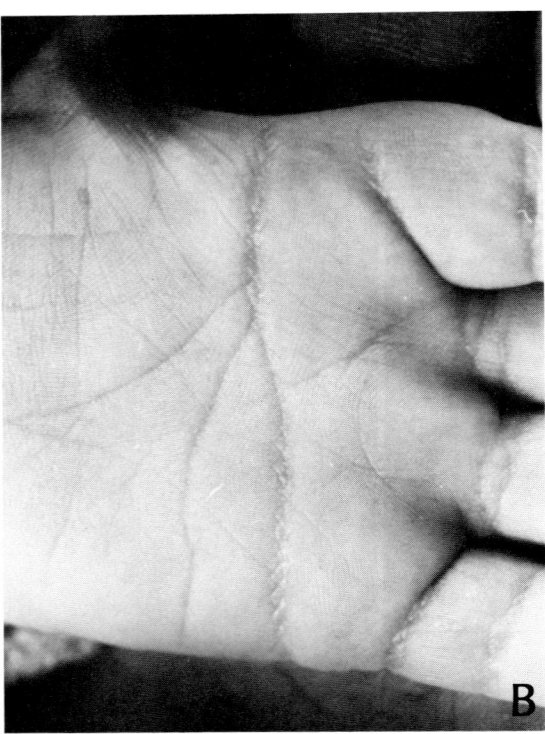

Figure 3–3. Down's syndrome. *A,* Facial view with typical features. *B,* Palmar crease. (Courtesy of Dr. J. Priest, Department of Pediatrics, Division of Medical Genetics, Emory University, Atlanta.)

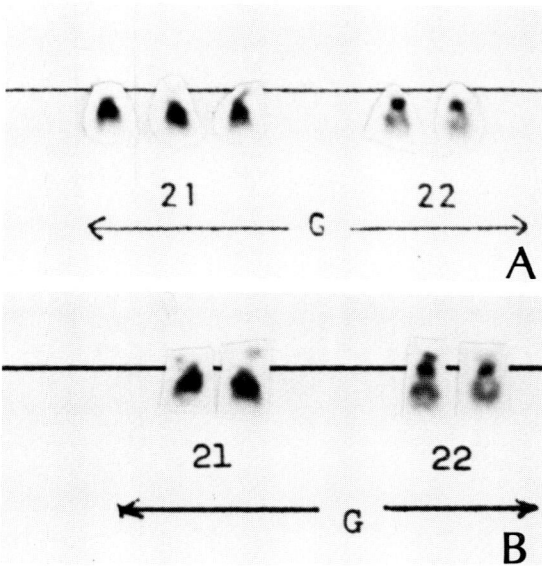

Figure 3–4. Compare the karyotype of Down's syndrome with a trisomy 21 *(A)* with the normal karyotype (B). (Courtesy of Dr. T.T. Puck, University of Colorado, Denver.)

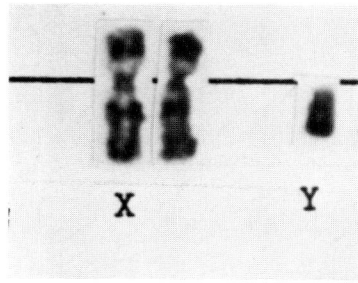

Figure 3–5. The karyotype of Klinefelter's disease. (Courtesy of Dr. T.T. Puck, University of Colorado, Denver.)

an intensive search has been undertaken to link chromosomal abnormalities with specific diseases, including cancer.[17] Increased sophistication in chromosome identification techniques, potentially computer assisted, may elucidate specific abnormalities in banding patterns that may allow one to diagnose at birth various diseases or the increased probability of developing certain diseases. This advance will require finer resolution of structural components of the chromosome and the evaluation of minor abnormalities.[18]

Although chromosomal karyotypes of 0.5 to 1.0% of all individuals show abnormalities, most of these are unassociated with any discernible phenotypic changes. Exceptions include the well-documented physical and functional abnormalities of *Down's syndrome* (trisomy 21)[19] (Figs. 3–3 and 3–4), the congenital malformations associated with trisomies 13 and 15, and the *cri du chat syndrome* (translocation of the short arm of chromosome 5).[20]

The classic syndromes associated with alterations in the sex chromosomes include *Klinefelter's disease* (XXY karyotype or modifications thereof) (Fig. 3–5) and *Turner's syndrome* (XO karyotype).

These chromosome abnormalities are believed to result primarily from nondisjunctions or translocations during meiosis or mitosis.

Although most malignant diseases are associated with chromosome abnormalities, usually aneuploidy and particularly hyperdiploidy, few consistent chromosomal changes are associated with neoplasia. One exception is the *Philadelphia chromosome* (translocation of one arm of chromosome 22 to chromosome 9 or sometimes to chromosome 6).[21] More recent chromosomal changes have been recorded in retinoblastoma (chromosome 13), Wilms's (chromosome 11), Burkitt's (translocation of 8 to 14), and other tumors (see Chap. 4).

Congenital Malformations and Teratology

In addition to inborn errors of metabolism and cytogenetic diseases, another large class of congenital diseases exists. These disorders are a heterogeneous group associated with single genes or chromosomal abnormalities and are sometimes caused by known environmental factors *(teratogens).*[22] Congenital disorders caused by teratogens are usually not heritable and affect only somatic cells or their progenitors. The agents causing the injury are particularly damaging during organogenesis in the first trimester of pregnancy. The best-known teratogens in man are viruses, radiation, and drugs.[23] Among the many environmental factors implicated as etiologic agents in the production of congenital defects in many organ systems are several well-recognized examples, including rubella virus (congenital heart defects, cataracts, deafness), cytomegalovirus,[24] and the drug thalidomide (phocomelia) (Table 3–2). Other changes have also been recognized (Fig. 3–6).

Table 3–2. Teratogens Known to Cause Human Malformations

Teratogens	Malformations
Androgenic agents Ethisterone Norethisterone	Masculinization of female fetuses (e.g., labial fusion and clitoral hypertrophy)
Antitumor agents Aminopterin Busulfan (Myleran) alternating with 6-mercaptopurine	Skeletal defects, malformations of CNS (anencephaly) Stunted growth, skeletal abnormalities, corneal opacities, cleft palate, hypoplasia of various organs
Methotrexate	Multiple malformations (e.g., skeletal)
Thalidomide	Meromelia and other limb malformations
Infectious agents Cytomegalovirus Rubella virus Toxoplasma gondii	Microcephaly, hydrocephaly, mental retardation Cataract, deafness, congenital heart defects Microcephaly, microphthalmia, hydrocephaly, chorioretinitis
Therapeutic radiation	Microcephaly, skeletal malformations

(Modified from Moore, K.L.: Before We Are Born. Basic Embryological and Birth Defects. 2nd Ed. Philadelphia, W.B. Saunders, 1982.)

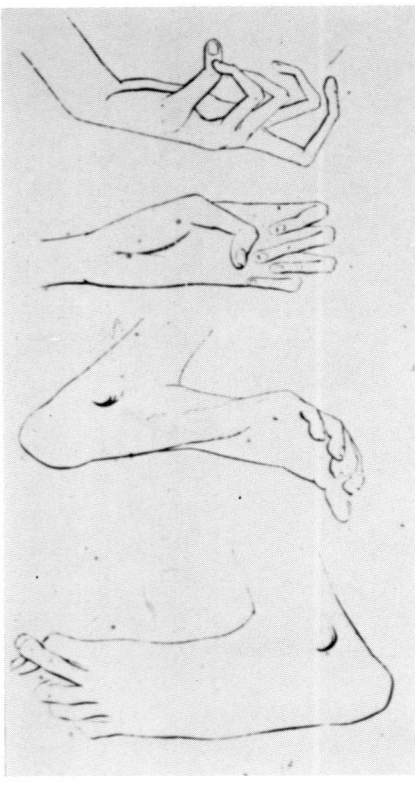

Figure 3–6. Arachnodactyly. (Courtesy of Dr. A. Johnston, College of Physicians & Surgeons, Columbia University, New York.)

During embryogenesis and throughout an individual's lifetime, minor mutations and alterations in the genome may be found, either in the germ cell line from preceding generations or acquired in somatic cells during life. These mutations are not generally discernible by the usual karyotypic analysis, do not result in specific overt phenotypic changes, and may only be present in one copy of a structural gene.

These minor genetic changes result in decreased cellular reserve and might allow deficiencies to develop with age, thereby resulting in degenerative changes. Minor alterations in the genome could conceivably be related to a host of age-associated changes; they might aggravate hyperlipidemia associated with heart disease, influence the development of spondylitis associated with arthritis, accelerate the adult onset of diabetes mellitus, or increase vasospasm associated with essential hypertension. They could also influence host susceptibility to various infectious agents. More important, they could be a major factor concerned with the rate of the aging process itself as well as the control mechanisms of cell division.

Sickle Cell Anemia

Sickle cell anemia occurs in large parts of Africa and India, and is estimated to affect 50,000 blacks in North America. It is inherited as a single mendelian dominant gene and may result in a severe hemolytic anemia. The homozygous form is known as sickle cell disease. The disease gets its name from the characteristic shape of the red blood cells. These cells acquire a sickled shape in situations of reduced oxygen tension due to the polymerization of deoxygenated hemoglobin S (HbS) to form helical rods that distort the cell shape. Generally, the cells resume their nor-

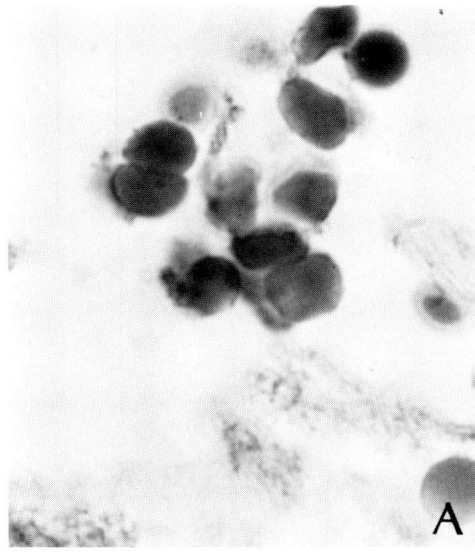

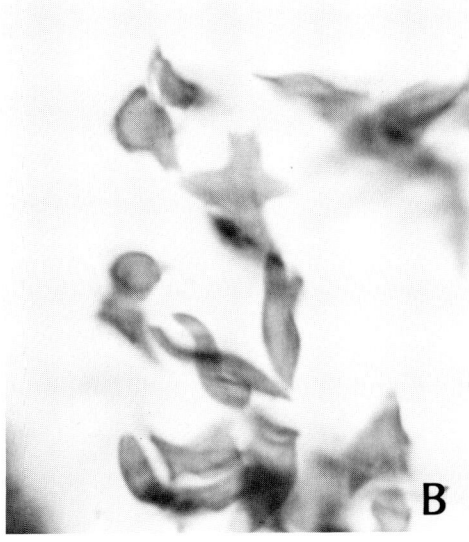

Figure 3–7. Light micrographs of red blood cells: *A*, normal and *B*, sickled.

mal shape when normal oxygen levels are restored; however, irreversibly sickled cells do not resume their normal shape even if the oxygen concentration is returned to normal.[25]

Structure of Normal Red Blood Cell Membrane

The normal red blood cell membrane contains surface antigens, sialic acid groups, sodium-potassium-adenosine triphosphatase (Na-K-ATPase) (on the internal face), glycolytic enzymes, acetylcholinesterase, spectrin, hemoglobin, and membrane-bound IgM antibodies.[26] The resting shape of the red blood cell appears to be an excellent probe of membrane structure, since its morphology is determined by the membrane characteristics (Fig. 3–7).[27]

As outlined in the chapter on membranes, the red blood cell membrane is a fluid mosaic structure that has integral proteins that pass through it. The best characterized of these proteins is glycophorin. The internal face of the plasma membrane is associated with actin and spectrin; these substances form a self-supporting, fibrillar lattice-like network on the cytoplasmic membrane surface. Spectrin is a red blood cell membrane protein, believed to help control erythrocyte shape and deformability. The human red blood cell membrane also contains a cyclic adenosine monophosphate (cAMP)-dependent protein kinase and another protein kinase which can use adenosine triphosphate (ATP) or guanosine triphosphate (GTP) as its phosphoryl donor so that autophosphorylation of the membrane occurs.[28] As will be seen in the following sections, severe abnormalities of the red blood cell membrane are found in sickle cell disease. Some of these are inherent membrane defects associated with the disease; others are secondary to the presence of the polymerized hemoglobin molecules.

Hemoglobin Structure and Synthesis

Hemoglobin is one of the best-characterized proteins in the biologic world.[29] We know that each globin molecule is

Table 3–3. *Various Hemoglobins*

	Normal		
	$A = \alpha_2\beta_2$		
	$A_2 = \alpha_2\delta_2$		
	$F = \alpha_2\gamma_2$		

Variants			
Hemoglobin	Abnormal Chain	Number of Sequence	Change
S	β	6	Glutamic acid → Valine
C	β	6	Glutamic acid → Lysine
D Punjab	β	121	Glutamic acid → Glutamine
E	β	26	Glutamic acid → Lysine

coded for by a distinct structural gene. These genes are grouped as α and non-α (δ and β). The non-α genes are expressed either in fetal or adult life, whereas α genes are expressed during both. If structural mutants of each globin molecule are present in a single individual, they are transmitted independently to the progeny (Table 3–3).

Heme and globin synthesis appear to be coordinated during erythropoiesis. The heme is synthesized in mitochon-

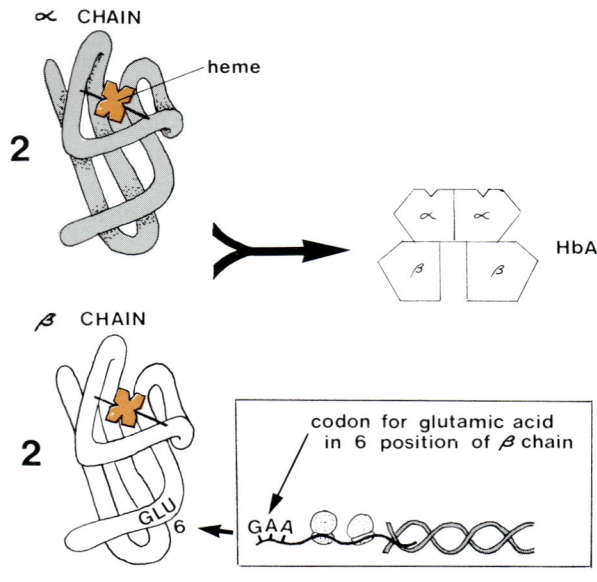

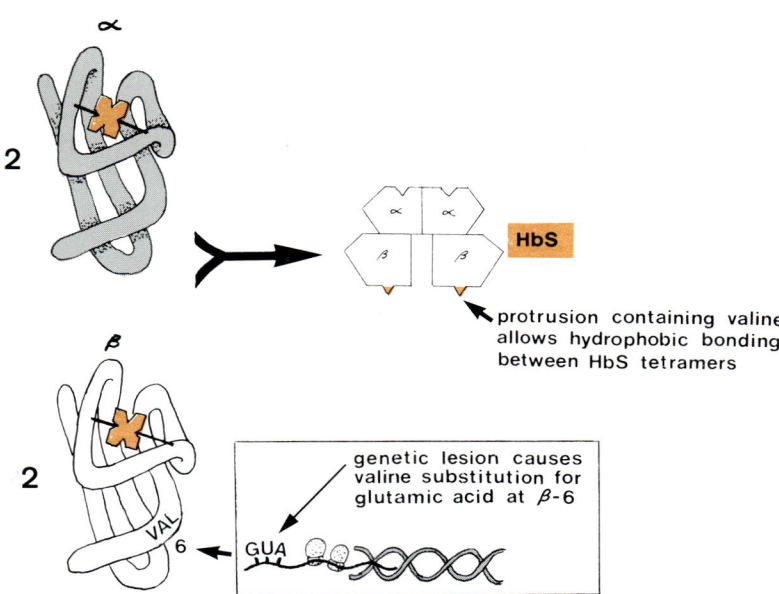

Figure 3–8. This figure compares the structure and amino acid substitution in hemoglobin S (HbS) to that of hemoglobin A (HbA).

dria and the globin by polysomes, and they are then assembled into the molecule we recognize as hemoglobin.

The latter has a molecular weight of 65,458 daltons and consists of 4 heme groups (protoporphyrin IX) linked to a globin molecule of 4 chains. The globin molecule has 142 amino acids in the α chain and 146 in all other chains. Of these, 7 amino acids are invariant in all species. Embryonic hemoglobin (HbE) consists of 4 ϵ chains or 2 α and 2 ϵ chains ($\alpha_2\epsilon_2$).

When the embryo reaches 10 cm, fetal hemoglobin (HbF) is formed, which consists of 2 α and 2 γ chains.[30] Shortly after birth, the fetus synthesizes adult hemoglobin of 2 types. HbA, 2 α and 2 β chains ($\alpha_2\beta_2$), and HbA$_2$, 2 α and 2 δ chains ($\alpha_2\delta_2$). The normal adult red blood cell contains about 96% HbA, 2.5% HbA$_2$, and 1% HbF. Sickle hemoglobin (HbS) contains 2 α and 2 β chains, in which a single amino substitution takes place in the β chain: glutamic acid is replaced by valine (Fig. 3–8).

A number of mutational events can alter the hemoglobin molecule. The resultant changes have been classified by Nagel and Bookchin as structural mutations that induce a hemoglobin instability, changes in oxygen affinity that induce polymerization or crystallization, changes that interfere with synthesis of globin chains, or changes that induce methemoglobin formation.[31]

Biochemistry of Sickle Cell Disease

Sickle cell disease falls into the group of hemoglobinopathies with a mutation that induces polymerization of the molecule. Red blood cells from patients with sickle cell disease (homozygous SS) have a change in the solubility and configuration of hemoglobin molecules under reduced oxygen tension. The hemoglobin becomes a semisolid tactoid.[32,33] This tactoid is characterized by an orderly grouping of long, thin, rod-like particles that are parallel and equidistant to each other. Tactoid formation appears to be through tetramer interactions via the hydrophobic residues of β-6 valine between complementary binding sites in the

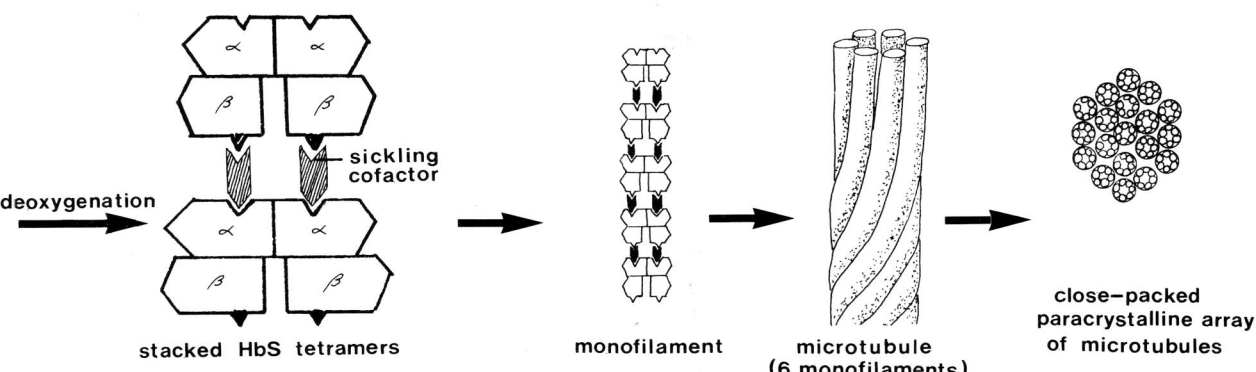

Figure 3–9. Abnormal structural configurations resulting from deoxygenation of sickle hemoglobin.

adjacent chains (Fig. 3–9). A sickling cofactor (nonprotein) is thought to mediate this formation. The complementarity in binding is lost with oxygenation since the chains move 7 Å closer together. Upon reoxygenation, the hemoglobin redissolves, and the cells assume their normal shape.

Ultrastructurally, the sickled RBC contain 17.6-nm fibers (HbS polymers), which are arranged hexagonally to form bundles of varying size and compactness.

By high-resolution electron microscopy (EM), each polymer consists of 6 monofilaments of linearly stacked Hb molecules measuring 6.5 nm in thickness and helically wound around a core. The reticulocytes in the bone marrow also show these arrays, but they are fewer in number.[34,35]

Studies on sickling and unsickling show that the earliest event after deoxygenation is the aggregation of Hb into the fibers previously described. These polymers are distributed in a loose network. Depolymerization without oxygenation involves a shortening of the fibers with aggregation similar to that seen early in the polymerization process. Polymerization precedes the appearance of the sickle cell shape, and after reoxygenation, the return to a disc shape follows the disappearance of the polymers. In addition to containing HbS microfilaments in the cytoplasm, the cell membrane binds large concentrations of hemoglobin to the cell surface. This process does not apparently contribute to the sickled shape.

Each cell in heterozygous (SA) patients contains approximately 40% HbS and 60% HbA. The heterozygous cell containing HbS and HbA is not highly sensitive to reduced oxygen tension and will not sickle until the oxygen tension goes below 10 mm of mercury. The heterozygous patients usually have no symptoms, regardless of exercise and oxygen lack.

Sickle cell disease or sickle cell trait can be easily diagnosed by placing red blood cells under anaerobic conditions and observing the sickling phenomenon. The general type of hemoglobinopathy can be identified by electrophoretic mobility and the exact type determined by sequencing the polypeptide chains. Use of restriction enzyme DNA analysis to detect mutant sickle genes is part of the newer technology for prenatal diagnosis.[36]

Red Blood Cell Membrane Abnormalities

The abnormal shape of the RBC in sickle cell disease has been known for some time, but not the membrane alterations. We now know that in this disease widespread abnormalities are found in many membrane components. These abnormalities include increased rigidity and decreased deformability, and associated changes in phospholipids, proteins, and glycoproteins as well as in the actin, spectrin, and the cytoskeletal lattice of the cells[37] (Fig. 3–10).

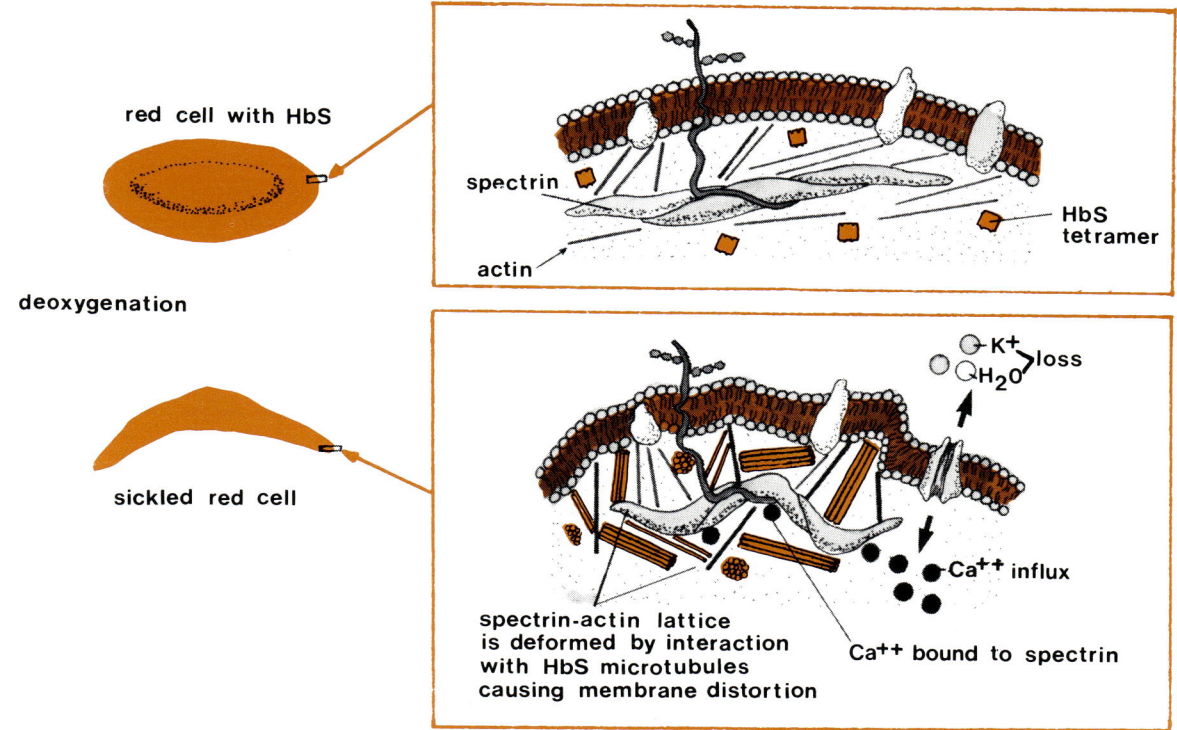

red cell with HbS

spectrin

actin

HbS tetramer

deoxygenation

sickled red cell

K^+
H_2O } loss

Ca^{++} influx

spectrin-actin lattice
is deformed by interaction
with HbS microtubules
causing membrane distortion

Ca^{++} bound to spectrin

Figure 3–10. Erythrocyte membrane alterations in the sickling phenomenon.

The repetitive sickling and unsickling of erythrocytes from patients with sickle cell disease results in the formation of irreversibly sickled cells, independent of the state of the HbS.

By scanning electron microscopy (SEM), these cells manifest a variety of bizarre shapes with long, filamentous spicules. When the sickled cells are reoxygenated, they lose their long filaments and develop terminal sphericles that fragment and are lost from the central part of the cell. The cell loses part of its membrane by this process, leading to cellular crenation, increased cell density, and decreased resistance to osmotic and mechanical stress. As more membrane is lost, these cells cannot resume their normal disclike shape (Fig. 3–10).

These cell membranes are also excessively permeable to cations (especially calcium) when deoxygenated. Sickled cells appear to contain excessive amounts of calcium intracellularly and associated with their membranes. They also have low potassium and moderately increased sodium levels.

Changes in cation concentration, as well as a marked decrease in ATP, may fix the actin-spectrin lattice of these cells in a permanently sickled shape.

As previously indicated, membrane-associated protein phosphorylation activities take place in the RBC. These protein kinase-dependent protein phosphorylations are one mechanism for post-transcriptional modifications of protein structure and enzyme activity.

The red blood cell contains both protein kinase and protein phosphatase activity and exhibits reversible phosphorylation of membrane proteins. An abnormality of this system is present in the red blood cells of patients with muscular dystrophy, hereditary spherocytosis, stomatocytosis, and sickle cell disease. This abnormal autophosphorylation in sickle cell anemia may contribute to the marked decrease of ATP. Erythrocyte deformability is strongly dependent on ATP concentrations within the cell. Furthermore, ATP-depleted cells are accompanied by increased hemolysis when exposed to shear stress. Therefore, this phenomenon may be important in the pathogenesis of the disease.

Moreover, with the decrease in oxygen concentration, the hemoglobin molecules aggregate within the red blood cell and form microfilaments of HbS; this process leads to distortion of the cell shape by passively deforming the actin-spectrin latticework and cell rigidity as discussed in the following section. All these factors alter the shape of the red blood cell. The most commonly seen distortion is the sickled shape, but the red blood cells may also assume a variety of other shapes, including those of *thorn cells, burr cells,* and *helmet cells.*

Clinicopathologic Correlations

The fundamental pathophysiologic disturbance in sickle cell disease is secondary to the blood abnormalities. The deoxygenated HbSS is associated with a high viscosity secondary to an increased globulin concentration and the reduced deformability of the erythrocyte.

The structural peptide chain abnormality results in the altered configuration of hemoglobin under reduced oxygen tension and produces an altered, sickled red blood cell shape with increased hemolysis that correlates well with the clinical signs and symptoms of anemia and microinfarction.

When these fragile, bizarrely shaped cells come into contact with the reticuloendothelial cells of the spleen and liver, they are erythrophagocytosed, and hemolysis follows. Hepatic erythrophagocytosis is associated with deposition of needle-like crystalloids in the mitochondria. Hemolysis of red blood cells with aggregation may result in stasis and blockage of the capillaries. An acute vaso-occlusive reaction may result and is called a *"sickle cell crisis"* (Fig. 3–11).

The erythrocytes may contain characteristic intracellular inclusions resembling *Heinz bodies* secondary to the presence of denatured, precipitated hemoglobin.

The primary cause of the hemostatic disturbance appears to be endothelial damage from prolonged local anoxia. The loss of cells exposes the underlying basement membrane and collagen and culminates in platelet adhesion and fibrin deposition.

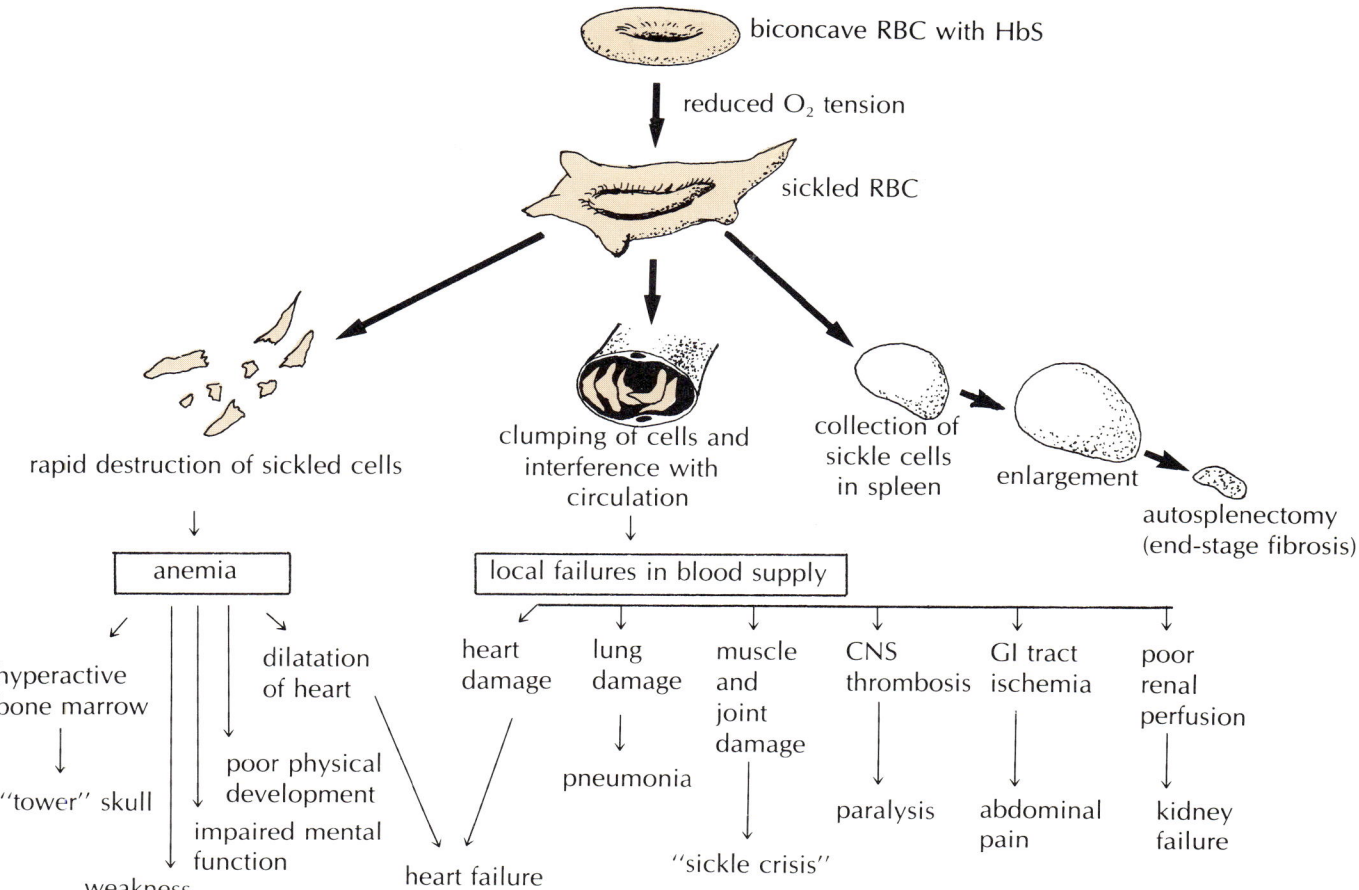

biconcave RBC with HbS

reduced O₂ tension

sickled RBC

rapid destruction of sickled cells

clumping of cells and interference with circulation

collection of sickle cells in spleen

enlargement

autosplenectomy (end-stage fibrosis)

anemia

local failures in blood supply

hyperactive bone marrow

dilatation of heart

"tower" skull

poor physical development

impaired mental function

weakness

heart damage

lung damage

muscle and joint damage

CNS thrombosis

GI tract ischemia

poor renal perfusion

pneumonia

paralysis

abdominal pain

kidney failure

heart failure

"sickle crisis"

Figure 3–11. Systemic changes in sickle cell disease.

Common organs affected by sickle cell disease include *bone* (ring infarcts in skull) (Fig. 3–12), *muscle* (cramps), *spleen* (infarcts in the cortical region), and *kidney* (nephrotic syndrome and infarcts).[38]

The most prevalent renal change in adults is papillary necrosis. The pathogenesis of these changes can be explained by conditions of low oxygen tension, acid pH hypertonicity, which occur in the medulla and which are all conducive to sickle cell formation and vaso-occlusive events.

Jaundice is a frequent problem in patients with sickle cell disease. Chronic hyperbilirubinemia may lead to the formation of gallstones with or without obstructive symptoms. Such patients have elevated levels of unconjugated bilirubin secondary to the hemolysis.

Patients with sickle cell disease are especially prone to infections, particularly by salmonella. However, they are also more resistant than the normal population to malaria. This resistance is believed to represent a genetic selection advantage with a better survival for the HbAS heterozygotes, since they have fewer parasites than the patient who is homozygous for HbA. One suggested mechanism for the

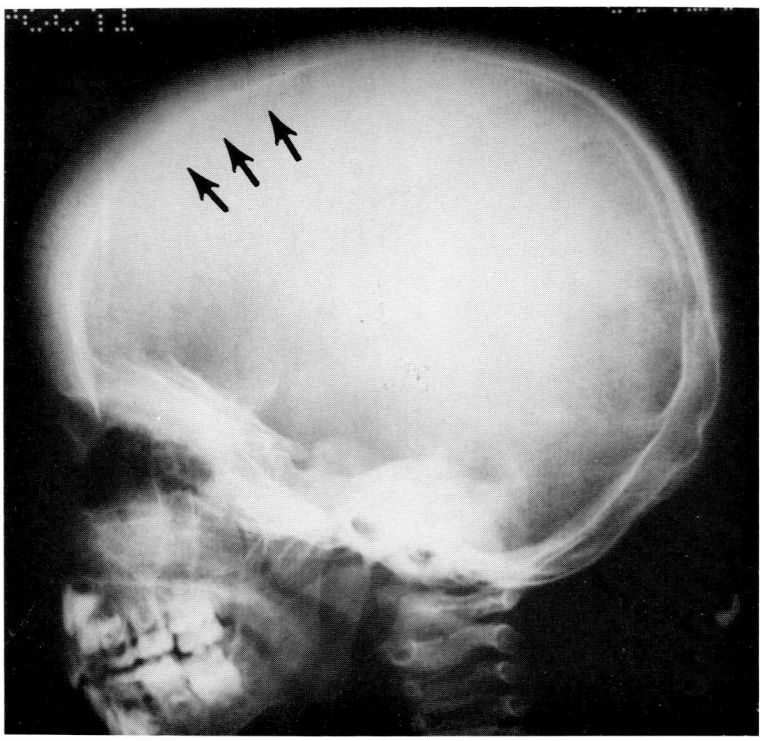

Figure 3–12. Roentgenograms of the skull of patients with sickle cell disease frequently show a characteristic alteration in the bone of the skull, which gives the appearance of minute hairs standing on end (arrows). (Courtesy of Dr. W. Berdon, Department of Radiology, College of Physicians & Surgeons, Columbia University, New York.)

protection is that with the malarial infection comes fever, which causes increased sickling of the cells. The cells are then phagocytosed at an increased rate, and the erythrocytes with their parasites are eliminated by the reticuloendothelial (RE) system.[39]

In the heterozygote (AS), "burr" cells are trapped in capillaries. The resultant anoxia produces sickling, and with a leakage of K^+ from the cell, the parasite dies because it requires a high level of K^+ for survival. In the homozygous state (SS), the microtubular aggregates of aggregated hemoglobin tetramers actually puncture the parasites and cause their death.

Therapy

Trials are in progress to treat this disease by carbamylating the hemoglobin molecules. Carbamylphosphate irreversibly reacts with the amino terminal valine residues. This reaction increases the O_2 affinity of the RBC and keeps them from sickling and increases their lifespan. Other attempts to develop antisickling materials are in progress.[40,41] Compounds that have an aromatic group with a pendant aliphatic polar moiety are the most effective in increasing solubility by inhibiting HbS gelation. This approach is based on an attempt to supplant the protein-protein interaction with a protein-small molecule interaction with the same complementarity.

Certain classes of aspirins also have demonstrable anti-sickling effects by acylating the intracellular hemoglobin and thereby inhibiting gelation of cell-free deoxy-HbS.

NUTRITIONAL FACTORS AND ENDOGENOUS INTERMEDIARY METABOLISM

Disease states are often the result of *nutritional deficiencies*. *Metabolic imbalance* may result from a number of causes, including genetic abnormalities,[42] diet and medications, and a large group of homeostatic factors, both intrinsic and extrinsic (Table 3–4).

Table 3–4. *Essential Nutrients for Humans*

Elements	
Major	Sodium, potassium, calcium, magnesium, phosphorus, chloride, sulfur, carbon, hydrogen, oxygen, nitrogen
Minor	Iron, zinc, copper, manganese, cobalt, iodine
Probably essential	Chromium, nickel, vanadium, tin, molybdenum, selenium, fluorine
Vitamins	
Water-soluble	Thiamine, riboflavin, vitamin B_6 (pyridoxal) nicotinic acid, folic acid, pantothenic acid, cobalamin, biotin, ascorbic acid
Fat-soluble	Vitamin A-carotene, vitamins D, E, and K
Essential amino acids	Lysine, threonine, leucine, isoleucine, methionine, tryptophan, valine, phenylalanine, histidine
Essential fatty acids	Linoleic, arachidonic

(Modified from Thorn, G.W., et al. (Eds.): Harrison's Principles of Internal Medicine. 8th Ed. New York, McGraw-Hill, 1977. Used with the permission of McGraw-Hill Book Company.)

In many parts of the world, *nutritional excesses* are etiologically as important as deficiencies in the pathogenesis of cellular abnormalities and disease. *Obesity* may act as a serious, superimposed, detrimental factor in hypertension, pregnancy, maturity-onset diabetes mellitus, osteoarthritis, osteoporosis, and other diseases. Control by diet and exercise is critical in increasing an individual's longevity.[43]

Gastrointestinal disturbances such as gastritis resulting from alcoholism or excess salicylate intake, vomiting with staphyloccal food poisoning, or diarrhea with dysentery, can cause nutritional and electrolyte imbalances. *Malabsorption* resulting from cholelithiasis, cystic fibrosis, celiac disease, and gastrointestinal tract obstruction may also produce severe *nutritional deficiencies* separate from actual *starvation* states.[44]

Protein and Amino Acid Metabolism

Proteins (Table 3–5) constitute the largest component of the cell by dry weight. They are synthesized on ribosomes in the cytoplasm following translation of mRNA that was previously transcribed by nuclear or mitochondrial DNA. The essential amino acids are lysine, threonine, leucine,

Table 3–5. *Classification of Proteins*

Enzymes
Structural protein (vinculin, collagen)
Storage and transport protein (ferritin)
Contractile protein (actin)
Immune protein (globulin)
Coagulation protein (factor VIII)
Hormone (insulin)

isoleucine, methionine, tryptophan, valine, phenylalanine, and histidine. Proteins stand as the major structural unit of the cells. As a functional constituent they exhibit many enzymatic and hormonal activities. Serum proteins (for example, albumin, globulin, antibody, antigen, complement, and coagulation factors) previously mentioned in Chapter 2 are often tied to lipid or carbohydrate as lipo- or glycoproteins. Proteins also play a large role in the extracellular ground substance (collagen, elastin, reticulin, and proteoglycans).

Deficiencies and Excesses

Abnormal pathways of amino acid metabolism can produce cellular damage either by synthesis of abnormal metabolites or by the accumulation of excessive amounts of normal metabolites that organs cannot metabolize. A number of these pathways involve defects in tyrosine and phenylalanine metabolism (Fig. 3–13). *Phenylketonuria,* a severe genetic disorder with mental retardation if untreated, results from the absence of phenylalanine hydroxylase. Excess ketone bodies (phenylacetate, phenylpyruvate, and phenyllactate) produce systemic toxicity.[45] Absence of the tyrosine pathway to melanin in skin melanocytes causes *albinism.*

Hypothyroidism may also result from defective tyrosine metabolism. Homogentisic acid, a normal intermediate in the metabolism of phenylalanine and tyrosine, is oxidized to acetoacetic acid, fumaric acid, and maleylacetoacetic acid by homogentisic acid oxidase. In *alkaptonuria,* homogentisic acid oxidase deficiency causes excessive urinary excretion of homogentisic acid (with characteristic darkening of the urine), deposition of a dark pigment in connective tissue *(ochronosis)* (a polymer derived from homogentisic acid), and a degenerative form of arthritis.

In systemic amino acid deficiencies *(starvation* or *malnutrition),* compensatory regulatory mechanisms direct amino acids from plasma proteins and muscle to the liver and heart to ensure their continued nourishment. When these fail, as in kwashiorkor, the patient dies (Table 3–6).

Amino acid transport may also be defective, with resulting injury to the cell. In certain kidney diseases, for example, *Fanconi's syndrome,* renal tubular cells may contain large droplets of protein that have been absorbed, but cannot be transported or degraded rapidly.

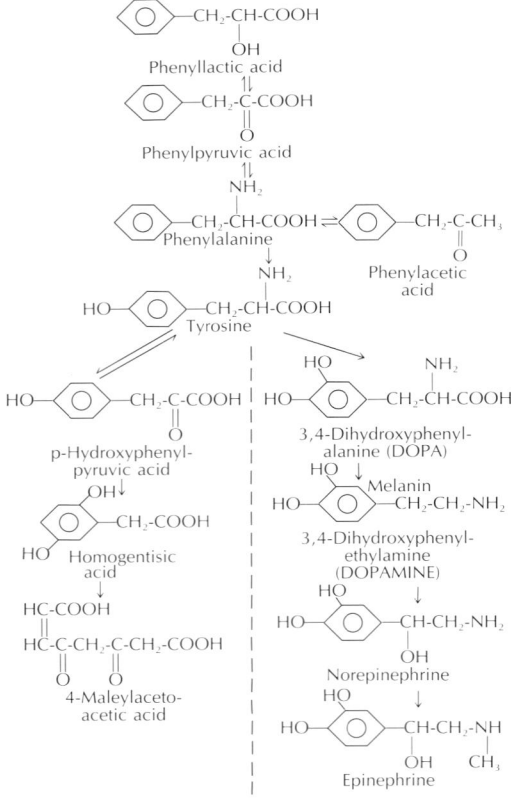

Figure 3–13. Steps in tyrosine metabolism.

Table 3–6. *Protein-Calorie Deficiencies*

Protein-calorie malnutrition (kwashiorkor-marasmus)	Psychomotor change
	Thin, sparse, straight hair
	Dyspigmentation
	Moon face
	Diffuse depigmentation with flaky-paint dermatosis
	Edema, muscle wasting
	Hepatomegaly
Semistarvation (older children and adults)	Marked loss of subcutaneous fat
	Muscle wasting, weakness
	Dirty-brown patchy skin, pigmentation
	Bradycardia at rest

(Modified from Thorn, G.W., et al. (Eds.): Harrison's Principles of Internal Medicine. 8th Ed. New York, McGraw-Hill, 1977. Used with the permission of McGraw-Hill Book Company.)

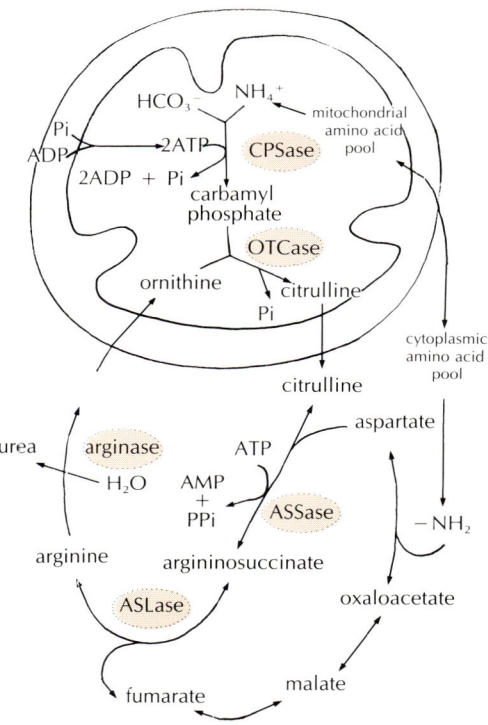

Figure 3–14. Ammonia metabolism by the five enzymes of the urea cycle (indicated in color): arginase, carbamyl phosphate synthetase (CPSase), ornithine transcarbamylase (OTCase), argininosuccinic synthetase (ASSase), and argininosuccinic lysase (ASLase). (Modified from Brown, T., et al.: Transiently reduced activity of carbamyl phosphate synthetase and ornithine transcarbamylase in liver of children with Reye's syndrome. N. Engl. J. Med., *294*:861, 1976.)

Nitrogenous end products of amino acid metabolism are measured clinically as "blood urea nitrogen" (BUN). Excess or overproduction of nitrogen in different disease states involves different organs and results in *uremia*. In the gastrointestinal (GI) tract, generation of nitrogen in the form of ammonia may be due to ingested foods (protein), degraded blood from GI hemorrhage, drugs, or bacterial action. Ammonia is metabolized by the normal liver to *urea*. In *cirrhosis*, damaged hepatocytes cannot convert ammonia to urea and are unable to handle large amounts of protein breakdown products. The resulting elevation of the levels of ammonia and circulating amines causes damage to the central nervous system (CNS), liver, and kidney (Fig. 3–14).

Lipid Metabolism, Hypo- and Hyperlipidemia

Lipids (Table 3–7) serve second to carbohydrates as a principal reserve energy source and produce 9 cal/g when required. The essential fatty acids are linoleic and arachadonic acids. Lipid cells may contain large amounts of neutral fat *glycerides* (one molecule is formed from glycerol plus three fatty acid molecules).

Lipoproteins, for example, chylomicrons, high-density lipoprotein (HDL), and low-density lipoproteins (LDL), play an important role in serum transport systems. As *glycerolphosphatides*, lipoproteins act as both carriers and structural units of cell membranes. Special lipids (*sphingosines*) tied to carbohydrate as cerebrosides or sphingomyelin have specific functions in the CNS. *Steroids* are not lipids, but are often grouped in this classification. The most important

Table 3–7. *Examples of Lipids*

Essential fatty acids
Cholesterol
Triglycerides (neutral fat)
Phosphoglycerides
Sphingolipid (sphingomyelin)
Cerebrosides
Lipoprotein (chylomicrons, low-density lipoprotein)

Agents of Disease **127**

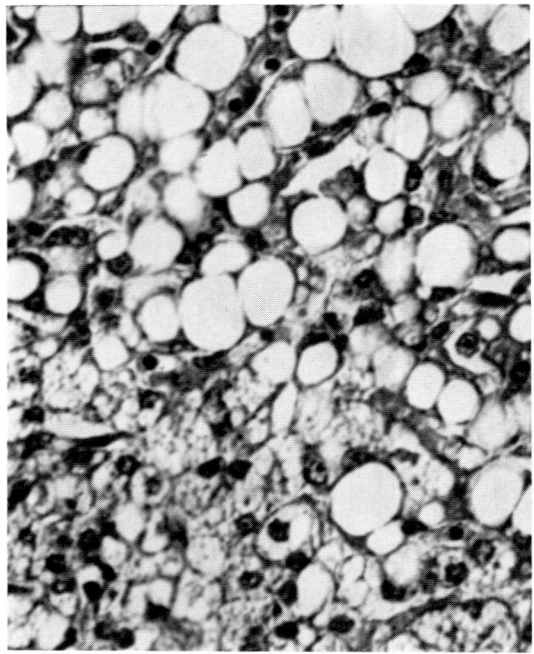

Figure 3–15. In fatty liver, fat droplets displace the nuclei to the side in many of the hepatocytes.

are cholesterol and the steroid hormones, estrogen, androgen, and corticosteroids. The most important prostaglandins are E_1, F_{1A} and F_{2A}.

Defects in lipid metabolism may also result from problems in nutrition, excess activation of normal pathways, or defects in elimination of end products.

In lipid deficiency, particularly in patients too ill to take food orally, *hypolipidemia* is compensated for by the mobilization of fatty acids from the adipose tissue of the body. Attempts to synthesize fat from glucose and amino acids are usually only partially successful. Partial-replacement parenteral therapy for nutritional lipid deficiencies has been moderately successful.[46]

The converse of low lipid levels, *hyperlipidemia,* is often associated with increased levels of lipoproteins in the blood stream and deposits of fat in the heart, liver, and muscle (Fig. 3–15). Many types of metabolic disturbances can cause *hyperlipidemia.* In some diseases, especially in the aged, elimination of end products of lipid metabolism is defective. Under such circumstances, *lipofuscin* or *ceroid* (containing unsaturated fatty acids) is deposited in the form of *residual bodies* in the adrenal, heart, and liver.

Carbohydrate Metabolism

Carbohydrates (Table 3–8) supply the major source of energy (4 cal/g) for the organism. The major carbohydrate is glucose, obtained from the breakdown of polysaccharides, for example, starch. The energy is stored as high-energy phosphate compounds (ADP and ATP) that are derived from glycolysis in the soluble cytoplasm and oxidative phosphorylation in the mitochondria. As *glycoproteins,* they act as structural and functional units of all cell membranes, being part of some receptors, transport carriers, antigens, and all antibodies. They contribute substantially to the structural units of the extracellular matrix as collagen, elastin, and proteoglycans. They also have important functions as precursors to nucleic acid (for example, deoxythymidine) and as regulators (uridine-diphosphoglucose) (UDPG) of carbohydrate metabolism.

Low levels of glucose in the cell may result from a serum deficiency of carbohydrate, as in starvation, or from lack of use, as in diabetes.

Glucose is normally taken into the liver cells and stored as glycogen, or it is metabolized to pyruvic acid, lactic acid, or active acetate. Active acetate is oxidized in the Krebs cycle to CO_2 and water. We have previously discussed var-

Table 3–8. *Classification of Carbohydrates*

Monosaccharide (glucose)
Disaccharide (sucrose)
Polysaccharide (glycogen)
Acid mucopolysaccharide (hyaluronic acid)
Glycoprotein (proteoglycans)

ious genetic diseases that produce an accumulation of glycogen due to a deficiency of one of the many enzymes in the glucose-glycogen metabolic pathways.

Normal end products of carbohydrate metabolism can also be injurious when they are produced in excess. In diabetes and starvation, excess *ketone bodies* are produced, owing to metabolism of body deposits of fat and ketogenic amino acids. Overproduction of ketone bodies causes systemic acidosis. Local overproduction of normal end products of carbohydrate metabolism can also be seen during heavy exercise when lactic acid accumulates in muscle. This response is partially compensated for by pyruvate stimulation of oxidative phosphorylation as well as by the conversion of lactic acid to glucose by recycling through the liver.

Serum *hyperglycemia,* associated with excess carbohydrate in the diet, may lead to *obesity.* Hyperglycemia and hyperglycosuria occur in diabetics unable to transport and to use glucose normally within the cell.

Nucleic Acid Metabolism

Nucleic acids (Table 3–9) are composed of two major purines (adenine and guanine) and one of three major pyrimidines (cytosine and either uracil in RNA or thymine in DNA). These bases are linked to a sugar as a nucleoside and form a nucleotide when a phosphate group is added. The nucleotides form the core of the chromosome as a double helix along with basic proteins (histones in the form of nucleosomes) and acidic proteins.

Synthesis in the nucleus occurs in the S phase regularly in intermitotic cells, rarely in reverting postmitotic cells, and as a reparative, rather than replicative, process in postmitotic cells. Although DNA is largely concerned with storage and transcription of genetic material and RNA is involved in translation, nucleotides function as reservoir sites for high-energy donors (adenosine diphosphate [ADP] and ATP) and as control factors (cAMP and cGMP) for many

Table 3–9. *Classification of Nucleic Acids*

Nucleoside (adenine + ribose = adenosine)	
Nucleotide (adenine + ribose + PO_4 = adenosyl 5′ phosphate)	
High-energy phosphate donor	—Adenosine 5′ monophosphate —Adenosine 5′ diphosphate —Adenosine 5′ triphosphate
Cyclic nucleotides	—Cyclic AMP (cAMP) —Cyclic GMP (cGMP)
Types of RNA	—Messenger RNA (mRNA) —Transfer RNA (tRNA) —Ribosomal RNA (rRNA)
Types of DNA	—Nuclear (chromosomal) —Mitochondrial (mDNA) —Epigenetic

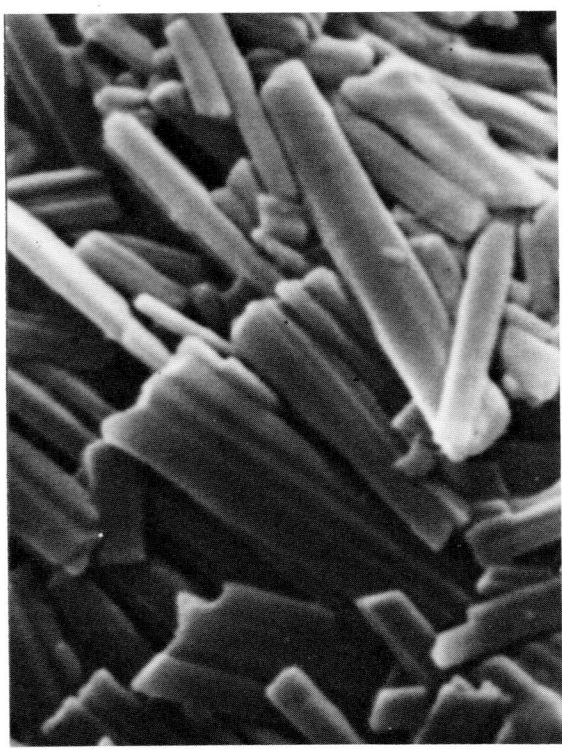

Figure 3–16. Scanning electron micrographs of sodium urate crystals. (Courtesy of Dr. K.P.H. Pritzler, The Mount Sinai Hospital, Toronto, Canada.)

kinase reactions. Nucleotides also combine with flavines (flavine mononucleotide [FMN] and flavine adenine dinucleotide [FAD]). Nucleotides bound to nicotinamide (NAD, NADP, and NADPH) act in oxidation-reduction reactions. The hexose monophosphate shunt is partially controlled by UDPG, whereas adenyl S-methionine acts as a methyl donor in a variety of reactions.

A deficiency in purine and/or pyrimidine bases may inhibit synthesis of RNA or DNA. Cellular repair processes in the heart and brain presumably require appreciably less new synthesis of nucleic acids than is necessary in the bone marrow, mucosa of gastrointestinal and genitourinary tracts, and skin, which are rapidly dividing and passing through multiple regeneration cycles. In bacteria, and in some mammalian cells, a phenomenon called *"thymine-less death"* results from blocked synthesis or a deficiency of thymine that prevents DNA synthesis.[47] In this deficiency state, cells normally in a rapid state of division, as in bone marrow, are unable to complete the cell cycle, grow larger, and finally die.

Overproduction of purine and pyrimidine metabolites may result in disease. *Gout* is a well-known example in which overproduction of uric acid (an end product of purine metabolism) results in deposition of *urate crystals* in the kidney, with the development of acute or chronic nephropathy, and in joints with resultant arthritis (Fig. 3–16).

Enzyme control mechanisms are available for modifying overproduction of DNA and RNA during replication, repair, and transcription processes (for example. DNAase, RNAase, endonuclease, exonuclease, ligase). Nuclear aneuploidy in neoplasia probably results from uncontrolled DNA synthesis.

Vitamins

Vitamins are generally classified as either fat-soluble (A, D, E, and K) or water-soluble (thiamine, pyridoxal, cobalamin, ascorbic acid, riboflavin, nicotinic acid, and folic acid). They are involved in multiple reactions including the metabolism of visual pigments (vitamin A), calcium and phosphate metabolism (vitamin D), prothrombin synthesis (vitamin K), and antioxidation reactions (vitamin E). Thiamine, FMN, and FAD, as well as nicotinamide adenine dinucleotide (NAD), participate in hydrogen atom (electron transfer) reactions. Pyridoxal (vitamin B_6) affects amino transfer reactions, folic acid one carbon transfer reactions, and vitamin B_{12} acts on the 1,2 shift of hydrogen atoms. Vitamin C is necessary for a variety of hydroxylation reactions, especially in the synthesis of collagen.

Cellular disorders may result from a deficiency of vitamins (Table 3–10). *Vitamin C* plays an important role in wound healing and is deficient in scurvy (discussed in detail in Chapter 2). Normal Vitamin D metabolism is essential to health.[48] Vitamin D deficiency classically associated with

Table 3–10. *Vitamin Deficiencies*

Vitamin or Deficiency State	Coenzyme or Active Form	Function	Symptoms of Deficiency
Vitamin A	11-*cis*-retinal	Visual cycle	Bitot's spots, conjunctival skin, corneal xerosis
Vitamin D (rickets)	1,25-dihydroxycholecalciferol	Calcium and phosphate metabolism	Hypercalcemia (incr.), epiphyseal enlargement, painless beading of ribs, persistently open fontanelle, muscular hypotonia
Vitamin E (α-tocopherol)	—	Antioxidant	Growth retardation (rats)
Vitamin K	—	Prothrombin biosynthesis	Hemorrhage
Thiamine (B_1) (beri-beri)	Thiamine pyrophosphate (TTP)	Aldehyde-group transfer	Hyperesthesia and paresthesia, cardiac enlargement, tachycardia and coronary congestion, peripheral edema
Riboflavin (B_2) (ariboflavinosis)	Flavin mononucleotide (FMN), flavin adenine dinucleotide (FAD)	Hydrogen-atom (electron) transfer	Angular stomatitis, cheilosis, Magenta tongue, blepharitis
Nicotinic acid (pellagra)	Nicotinamide adenine dinucleotide (NAD), nicotinamide adenine dinucleotide phosphate (NADP)	Hydrogen-atom (electron) transfer	Scarlet and raw tongue, atrophic lingual papillae, tongue fissuring, malar and supraorbital pigmentation, pellagrous dermatosis
Vitamin B_6 (pyridoxal)	Pyridoxal phosphate	Amino-group transfer	Nasolabial seborrhea, glossitis, peripheral neuropathy, drug-resistant convulsions in infants
Vitamin C (scurvy)	Ascorbic acid	Proline and lysyl hydroxylase	Spongy and bleeding gums, petechiae-ecchymoses-subperiosteal hematoma, follicular hyperkeratosis, painful epiphyseal enlargement
Folic acid	Tetrahydrofolic acid	One-carbon group transfer	Pallor, glossitis, aphthous stomatitis
Vitamin B_{12} (cobalamin) (pernicious anemia)	Coenzyme B_{12}	1,2 shift of hydrogen atoms	Pallor, mild icterus ("lemon-yellow"), anorexia, flatulence, diarrhea, paresthesia-ataxia-areflexia, optic neuritis

(Modified from Thorn, G.W., et al. (Eds.): Harrison's Principles of Internal Medicine. 8th Ed. New York, McGraw-Hill, 1977. Used with the permission of McGraw-Hill Book Company.)

rickets (types I and II) is exaggerated during pregnancy.[49] Vitamin D is also of great importance in renal stone formation and in the healing of fractures.[50]

Vitamin A deficiency results in the loss of the outer-segment photoreceptors in the retina. Vitamin A toxicity is usually only seen following excessive therapeutic ingestion (Table 3–11). It is associated with increased levels of free serum retinal esters, unbound to specific retinal binding protein. These esters become available for lytic action on cell membranes, including the release of lysosomal enzymes. The water-soluble vitamins are also essential in nutrition, and their deficiencies are associated with numerous disease states.

Metals and Trace Elements

Trace elements function in many aspects of cellular and extracellular metabolism. These include glucose metabo-

Table 3–11. *Vitamin Toxicity (Excess Vitamin Ingestion)*

Fat-Soluble Vitamins

Vitamin A	Acute toxicity	Headache, vertigo, diarrhea
	Chronic toxicity	Cirrhotic-like liver symptoms, hypercalcemia, premature epiphyseal union
Vitamin D	Acute toxicity	Hypercalcemia, weakness, lassitude, headache, nausea, vomiting, and diarrhea
	Chronic toxicity	Renal impairment, polydipsia
Vitamin E		Various toxicities reported in animals, minimal toxicity in man
Vitamin K		Hemolysis, antagonism of coumarin anticoagulants

Water-Soluble Vitamins

Niacin (nicotinic acid)	Flushing, pruritus, skin rash, heartburn, nausea, vomiting, diarrhea, activation of ulcer, hypotension, syncope, tachycardia, jaundice
Pyridoxal (vitamin B_6)	Convulsive disorders
Folic acid	Decreased efficacy of phenytoin, renal cell hypertrophy
Ascorbic acid (vitamin C)	Diarrhea, urinary acidification, urinary stones, uric acid, nephropathy, lowered prothrombin time, megaloblastic anemia

Table 3–12. *Trace Element Deficiencies*

Element	Biochemical Function	Signs of Deficiency
Chromium (Cr)	Glucose metabolism (mediation of insulin effect on membranes)	Impaired glucose clearance (many species); impaired growth, reproduction, and life span (rats and mice)
Cobalt (Co)	Biologic methylation (e.g., methionine synthesis)	Pernicious anemia (man); methylmalonic aciduria (man)
Copper (Cu)	Mitochondrial function; collagen metabolism; melanin formation	Menke's syndrome (man); anemia, leukopenia, neutropenia (animals and man)
Fluorine (Fl)	(?) Iron absorption	Anemia (mice); impaired growth and reproduction (rats)
Iodine (I)	Cellular oxidation processes	Thyroid diseases (animals and man)
Manganese (Mn)	Oxidative phosphorylation; fatty acid metabolism; synthesis of proteins, mucopolysaccharides, and cholesterol	Defective growth, bony anomalies, reproductive dysfunction, and central nervous system abnormalities (many species)
Molybdenum (Mo)	Xanthine and hypoxanthine metabolism	Growth retardation, impaired urate clearance (chicks)
Nickel (Ni)	(?) Nucleic acid stabilization; (?) membrane structure and function	Impaired reproduction (rats); deranged liver lipid and phospholipid metabolism (chicks)
Selenium (Se)	Degradation of intracellular peroxides; oxidation of glutathione	Liver necrosis (rats); white muscle disease (lambs); exudative diabetes (chicks)
Silicon (Si)	(?) Connective tissue structure	Impaired growth and connective tissue formation (chicks)
Tin (Sn)	(?) Redox catalysis	Growth and dentition (rats)
Vanadium (V)	Oxygen transport; (?) redox catalysts	Impaired growth, reproduction, bone and lipid metabolism (chickens, rats)
Zinc (Zn)	Metabolism of lipids, protein, carbohydrates, and nucleic acids	Parakeratosis (swine); acrodermatitis enteropathica (man); (?) hypogonadal dwarfism (man)

(Modified from Ulner, D.D.: Trace elements. N. Engl. J. Med., 297:320, 1977.)

lism (Cr), biologic methylation (Co), collagen synthesis (Cu), heme synthesis (Fe), thyroglobulin synthesis (I), synthesis of protein (Mn) xanthine metabolism (Mo), nucleic acid stabilization (Ni), degradation of cellular peroxides (Se), connective tissue structure (Si), redox catalysis (Sn), oxygen transport (V), and metabolism of lipids (Zn).

Excesses or deficiencies of metals may lead to diseases (Table 3–12).[51] Deficiencies of trace metals, such as *zinc*, may result in coenzyme inactivation. Prolonged *iodine* deficiency will produce goiter. *Copper* deficiency, occasionally seen following extensive surgery of the duodenum, may result in severe anemia because copper is necessary for the incorporation of glycine into the heme molecule of hemoglobin. Excessive deposits of metals may also be injurious. An inherent abnormality in *iron* metabolism in idiopathic *hemochromatosis* leads to damaging accumulations of iron in the liver, heart, pancreas, adrenal, and gastrointestinal tract.[52]

Dietary Fiber

"Dietary fiber" refers to the plant polysaccharides and lignin that are resistant to hydrolysis by the digestive enzymes of man. The colon is the organ most affected by the dietary fiber content. The conjugation of bile acids and oxidation of cholesterol attributable to bacteria may depend on the nature and amount of fiber present in the colon.[53] Colonic motor function is also regulated by fiber content.

The concept that dietary roughage is a determinant of health and disease stems from observations that populations with diets containing large amounts of fiber (greater than 5 oz/day) appear to be relatively free of appendicitis, diverticulosis, polyps, and cancer. They also have a lower incidence of ischemic heart disease, diabetes, and hiatal hernias.

Celiac Disease

Celiac disease, also known as *nontropical sprue* or *gluten-sensitive enteropathy* (GSE) requires the exposure of the small intestine to gluten for disease to occur. In the absence of this common dietary protein, the intestinal mucosa functions normally.[54]

Clinical Symptoms

Clinically, celiac disease is characterized by primary steatorrhea (fatty stools), weight loss, malabsorption, lactose intolerance, and dehydration. It may also be associated with osteomalacia and cerebral lesions secondary to calcium loss. Avitaminosis, particularly of the lipid-soluble vitamins A, D, K, and E, occurs because of the malabsorption of lipids. The water-soluble vitamins are also subject to decreased absorption. In cases of long-standing disease there may be edema, skeletal disorders, paresthesias, tetany, bleeding,

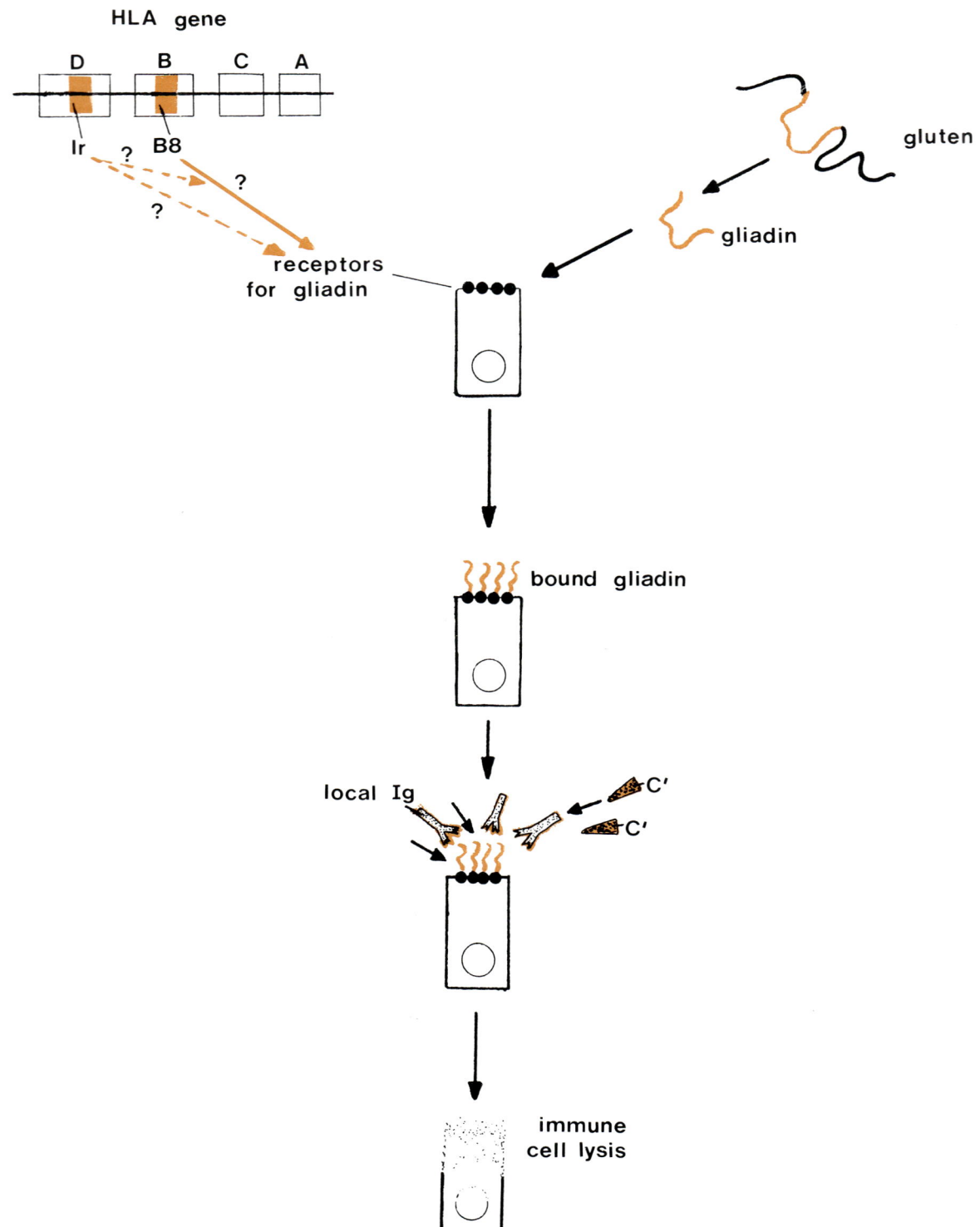

Figure 3–17. Schematic representation of the pathogenesis of celiac disease.

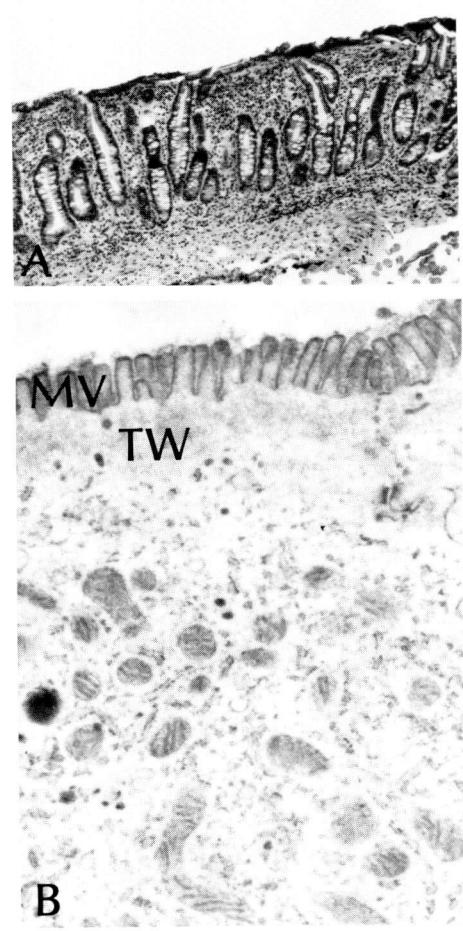

Figure 3–18. Celiac disease. A, Light micrograph demonstrates severe villous atrophy. B, Electron micrograph showing blunted microvilli and poorly developed terminal webs.

muscle tenderness, peripheral neuropathy, and dermatitis.[55,56]

This disorder is also associated with *dermatitis herpetiformis* and with certain neoplasms, especially lymphomas.[57] The reason for these associations is unknown, but may reflect the association of sprue with certain histocompatibility antigens (Fig. 3–17).[58]

Pathogenesis

Gluten, a protein found in grains such as wheat, barley, rye, and buckwheat, contains a molecule called *gliadin* that has a high content of proline and glutamine. When the glutamine components are deaminated to glutamic acid, gliadin is no longer toxic. The exact mechanism by which gluten ingestion results in epithelial cell damage, with the production of a flattened mucosa (Fig. 3–18) and subsequent malabsorption, is still subject to investigation. There are currently two major schools of thought. One suggests that the intestinal absorptive cell is *deficient* in a *peptidase* or *protease* that is capable of breaking down gliadin (Fig. 3–19). Alternatively, gliadin may *inhibit peptidase* activity and may thereby prevent its own degradation to amino acids. *Toxic gliadin peptides* then accumulate and interfere with normal maturation of the intestinal epithelium.[59] A peptidase deficiency has not been successfully demonstrated to date.

The second major theory is essentially immunologic, in which gluten is believed to interact with lymphocytes of the lamina propria and to lead to their sensitization. This process results in the formation of various immune products, including antibodies specifically directed against gluten attached to intestinal cells and sensitized lymphocytes producing lymphokines. These immune products, alone or in combination, are believed to interact with the intestinal cells and to lead to the cytolysis and death of those cells. This loss results in crypt cell proliferation, flat mucosal lesions, and malabsorption (see Fig. 3–18 and Fig. 3–19).[54]

Support for the latter theory has been provided by the demonstration that the intestinal mucosa in patients with sprue reacts immunologically when challenged with gluten. *Antigluten antibodies* have been demonstrated in both the serum and intestinal secretions in patients with GSE.[60] The immune system is further implicated by the demonstration that *levels of complement* fall during challenges with gluten and immune complexes are deposited within the mucosal epithelium.

An increased number of immunoglobulin-secreting cells are identifiable in the jejunal mucosa. Antibodies from these cells are directed both against the whole gluten molecule and to its by-product, gliadin. Antibodies to gluten appear to be sensitive markers for gastrointestinal diseases and are present in Crohn's disease, ulcerative colitis, cystic fibrosis, and "recurrent diarrhea." *Gluten antibodies* are of the *IgA, IgM,* and *IgG* classes.[61]

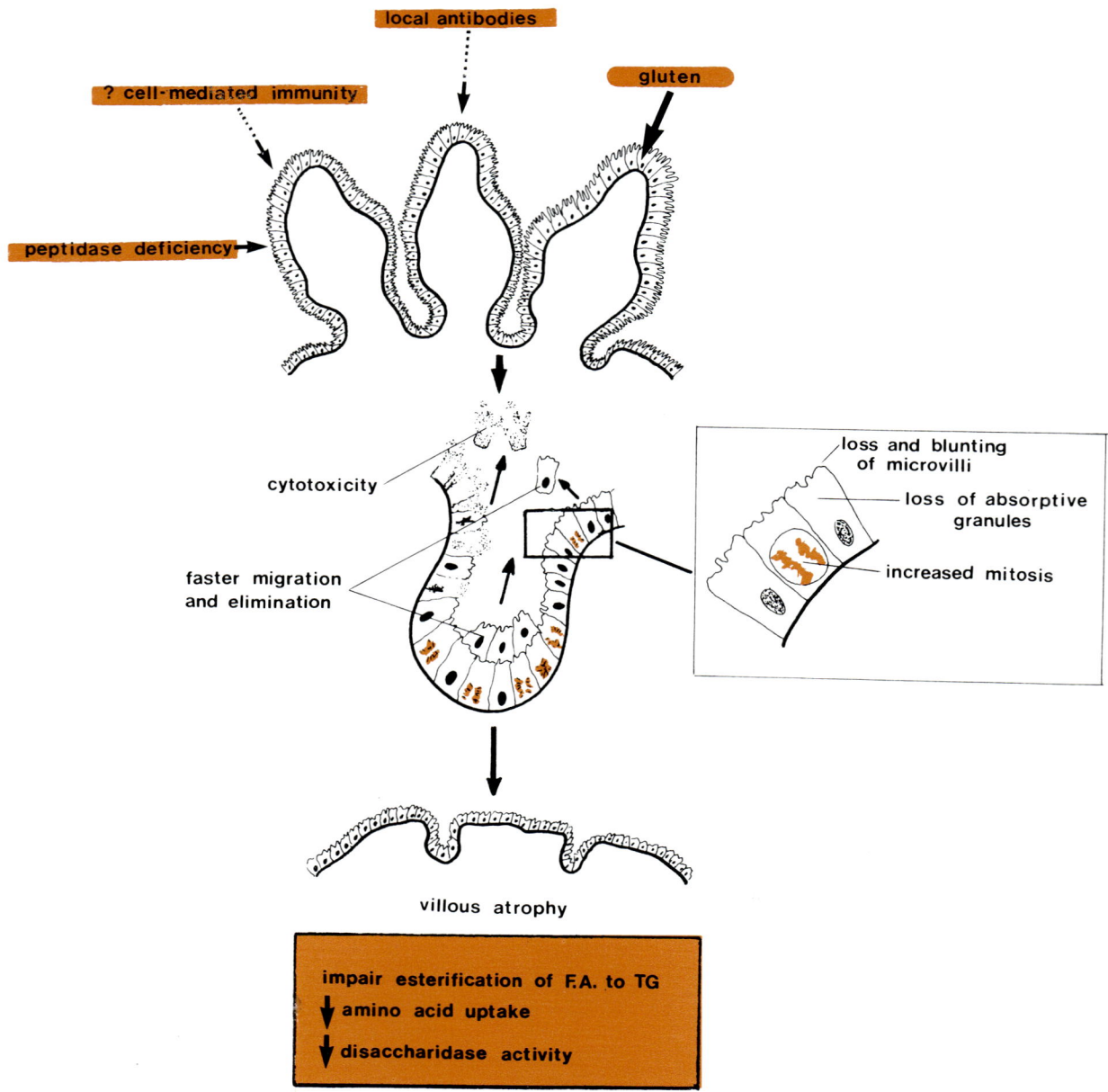

Figure 3–19. The effects of the immune system on epithelial cell turnover in celiac disease.

Finally, specific, cell-mediated responses to gluten fraction III have also been found.[62] Biopsies obtained from GSE patients contain *macrophage inhibitory factor*, a substance made by sensitized lymphocytes when exposed to gluten.[63] Intestinal cell death may result from the reaction of *null* (N_K) *cells* to gluten attached to the cell membrane; this attachment makes the membrane appear as a foreign protein. Null cells may also react in the antibody-dependent cellular cytotoxicity system (ADCC) resulting in cell death. *T lymphocytes* also may secrete macrophage-activating factors stimulating *killer macrophages* or may act directly as *cytotoxic T lymphocytes.*

Analyses of histocompatibility antigen types show that a high frequency of HLA-B8 antigens exists in this disease. The DW3 gene of the major histocompatibility complex is also frequently found. It controls responses in mixed leukocyte reactions. In mice, it is known that histocompatibility antigens are directly linked to immune response genes. It is tempting to believe that genetic associations seen in patients with GSE may in some way alter their immune responses.

In addition to their association with immune response genes, histocompatibility genes also code for certain cell surface receptors. The recognition phenomenon for these receptors may be similar to those responsible for viral susceptibility.

These observations are compatible with the theory that two genes are involved in the pathogenesis of *GSE.* One gene is associated with the HLA region, specifically *HLA-B8* and *-DW3 haplotypes.* The second gene is not in the HLA complex and therefore can be inherited independently. It is believed that the presence of both genes, as well as certain environmental factors, may be required for the manifestation of the disease symptoms.

The chance occurrence of both these genes in a given patient produces a cell surface configuration that is capable of serving as a receptor for gluten proteins. The binding of gluten to this receptor allows the interepithelial lymphocytes of the lamina propria to interact with the gluten in such a way that gluten becomes immunogenic and leads to the production of antibody, sensitized lymphocytes, and lymphokines.[54]

Morphology

In the normal small intestine, slender villi project above the surface, so that the luminal surface is extensively folded, resulting in a large increase in the absorptive area. In nontropical sprue, the *finger-like villi* are *flat* and *blunted,* the crypts are elongated, and the number of villi is reduced,[64] resulting in a decreased absorption area and loss of absorption granules (see Fig. 3–18). The epithelial cells, which are usually columnar in shape, become cuboidal; the basement membrane and the "terminal web" composed of microfilaments becomes thicker; a mononuclear infiltrate is present in the lamina propria. The increase in the number of enterochromaffin cells in the mucosa of these patients becomes greater when patients are given a gluten challenge.[65]

When the number of lymphocytes containing IgA, IgG, and IgM is quantitated, elevations above the numbers seen in normal mucosa are found. IgG-bearing cells are the most numerous.[66] The only significant alteration found in serum Ig levels, however, is an elevated IgA.[67]

Pathophysiology

This disease has been studied in organ cultures by exposing intestinal biopsies from sprue patients to gluten. The proliferative zone of the crypt is expanded, the migration of epithelial cells from this expanded proliferative zone is increased so that immature cells appear on the villi, and the normal digestive enzymes of the brush border are decreased. If biopsies of patients with sprue are cultured in the absence of gliadin, the cellular morphology and the brush-border enzymes revert to normal.[68]

These biochemically immature epithelial cells demonstrate decreased uptake of amino acids, impaired esterification of fatty acids to triglycerides, and decreased disaccharidase activity. For many years, it was believed that impaired nutrient absorption in GSE was considered to be the direct result of the reduction in the absorptive surface and its associated brush-border enzymes.

It is now known, however, that this is not the sole explanation for the malabsorption, and secondary hormonal and secretory abnormalities may profoundly alter the normal digestive mechanisms. Evidence is accumulating that the malabsorption of fat is multifactorial in nature and involves *defects* in *lipolysis* and *micelle formation* as well as in *mucosal absorption.* Biliary dynamics are altered, and enterohepatic circulation is sluggish, with a decreased jejunal concentration of bile salts that impairs the micellar phase of intestinal fat digestion. The intestinal cell depletion and damage compromise the brush-border hydrolysis of small peptides and oligosaccharides and the membrane transport of di- and tripeptides, amino acids, monosaccharides, water-soluble vitamins, and cations.

Because the proximal small intestine is the most severely involved portion of the GI tract, many of these patients malabsorb iron, folate, pyridoxine, and calcium (the small intestine is their most avid site of absorption). *Diminished cholecystokinin* and *pancreozymin secretion* has been demonstrated and leads to secondary abnormalities in bile acid and pancreatic lipase secretion. *Abnormalities* in *water* and *electrolyte transport* also occur, so that water accumulates in the bowel lumen and further dilutes the bile acids and intestinal enzymes below their critical concentrations.

Clinicopathologic Correlations

The clinical presentation of these patients reflects the degree of their malabsorption (Table 3–13). *Diarrhea* and *weight loss,* the most common presenting symptoms, usually develop during the first year of life at the time cereal is introduced into the diet. Many of these children undergo a spontaneous remission in their disease, only to have it recur during their young adulthood. Another group of patients is essentially normal during childhood and develops symptoms only as adults.

Table 3–13. *Clinicopathological Correlation of Malabsorption Deficiencies*

Organ System Affected	Deficiency	Symptoms
Hematologic	Iron Vitamin B_{12} Pyridoxal (B_6)	Hemorrhage, hemolysis
Musculoskeletal	Calcium Vitamin D	Osteomalacia, bone pain, compression fracture
Visual	Vitamin A	Night blindness
Dermatologic	Vitamin A	Follicular hyperkeratosis
Neural	Vitamin B	Neuropathy
Endocrine	Pituitary and adrenal hormones	Hypofunction

The degree of weight loss is a function of the severity of the steatorrhea and the individual's ability to compensate for the malabsorption by increasing caloric intake. In children, *growth retardation* is a frequent sign reflecting generalized malabsorption. These children may be *emaciated* and may have muscle wasting, dehydration, and electrolyte imbalances, including hypokalemia and acidosis.

Hematologic symptoms may be seen secondary to an iron-deficiency anemia, depending on the extent of the mucosal damage. Anemia may be complicated by the *malabsorption of vitamin B_{12}* and *pyridoxine.*

Musculoskeletal symptoms, if present, result from the abnormal metabolism of calcium secondary to the *defective transport* of *calcium* in the abnormal mucosa, coupled with the *impaired absorption* of *vitamin D* and the binding of intraluminal calcium to unabsorbed fatty acids, thereby forming soaps. This defect can result in severe bone calcium depletion and osteomalacia. *Bone pain* is a common symptom, and compression fractures may be present.

Night blindness results from the malabsorption of vitamin A. *Peripheral neuropathies* occur secondary to nutritional deficiency, especially of the B vitamins. *Endocrine dysfunction* can occur secondary to long-standing malabsorption. This includes hypofunctional pituitary and adrenal glands.

Skin manifestations of the disease may include a follicular hyperkeratosis secondary to vitamin A deficiency. Petechiae may be present secondary to hypoprothrombinemia, which may also be seen secondary to a deficiency of vitamin K. The incidence of dermatitis herpetiformis in sprue is high, perhaps 90% or more. The diagnosis of this disease is usually helped by demonstrating the presence of small-intestinal lesions that respond to the removal of gluten from the diet.

Therapy

Because the clinical and morphologic features of this disorder depend solely on the presence of gliadin for their expression, therapy consists simply of removing gliadin

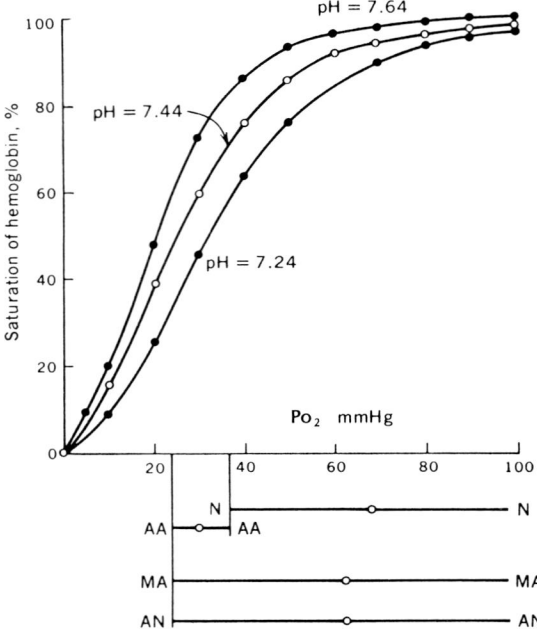

Figure 3–20. This figure depicts the relationship between oxygen tension and oxygen saturation of the hemoglobin of the blood. The heavy line is for blood at pH 7.44. The curves to the right and left are for bloods of pH 7.24 and 7.64, respectively, and indicate quantitatively the magnitude of the Bohr effect for hydrogen ion concentration changes of these magnitudes.

During vigorous muscular effort, the increase in acidity of the blood causes the dissociation curve to shift to the right, raises the tissue oxygen tension for any given degree of saturation of the hemoglobin, and thus makes oxygen more available to the muscles. On the other hand, any condition, such as high altitude, that causes respiratory alkalosis moves the dissociation curve to the left. This change facilitates oxygen uptake in the lungs by increasing the oxygen saturation at a given level of alveolar oxygen tension.

Beneath the abscissas are plotted the calculated arteriovenous oxygen differences, upon the presumption that the right-heart venous oxygen content is normally 5 vol % less than the arterial content, and with constant cardiac output in the following states: N = normal person, arterial oxygen content 20 vol %; AA = same person suffering from arterial hypoxia sufficient to lower the arterial oxygen content to 14.6 vol % (= 73% saturation), but with oxygen consumption unaltered; MA = same person with 100% increase in oxygen consumption; AN = anemic patient, arterial oxygen content 10 vol %, with arterial saturation and oxygen consumption same as in a normal person. The heavy dots indicate the mean oxygen tension in each instance. (From Wintrobe, M.M., et al.: (Eds.): Harrison's Principles of Internal Medicine. 6th Ed. New York, McGraw-Hill, 1970. Used with the permission of the McGraw-Hill Book Company.)

from the diet. In general, this regimen works well, with a return to a more-or-less normal morphology of the small intestinal mucosa. The villous atrophy does not usually totally revert, however. When the skin lesions of dermatitis herpetiformis are also present, these too may regress.

When the flat intestinal lesion typical of celiac disease fails to respond to a gluten-free diet, and it is certain that the patient has adhered to this diet, then other conditions that may minic the morphologic features of sprue must be considered. These conditions include hypogammaglobulinemic sprue and underlying lymphoma or carcinoma. Occasionally, corticosteroids may help in the therapy of refractory GSE. Rarely, the disease pursues a relentless and ultimately fatal course.

PHYSICAL AGENTS

Many disease states result from physical agents of injury. Diseases may involve disturbed gas homeostasis, especially of oxygen and CO_2. These gases, with Na^+, K^+, and Cl^-, are also intimately involved with water and electrolyte regulation and are significant in the control of pH. Alterations in fluid and electrolytes are seen in edema and shock. Alterations in pH are associated with acidosis and alkalosis. Temperature, radiation, and mechanical injury, the last usually resulting from accidents, are other major physically injurious agents.

Cellular Gas Equilibrium

The most important gas in the cell is *oxygen* (Fig. 3–20). It is critical in *cellular respiration* and in the *oxidative phosphorylation* process, which produces ATP. This high-energy phosphate donor molecule is generated in the cytosol as a result of glycolysis and in the mitochondria by oxidation. ATP is stored as *creatine phosphate*. When used, it is broken to ADP and inorganic phosphate, releasing approximately 12,000 calories per molecule.

Hypoxia

Absolute cellular *anoxia* is probably never present in a cell during life because tissues are usually supplied by some degree of collateral circulation ensuring oxygen delivery and because some local oxygen diffusion occurs in all forms of injury. Severe cellular *hypoxia* and the reduced oxygen supply with or without adequate perfusion is common, however.

Ischemia implies a decrease in blood supply associated with vascular obstruction or disease. Hypoxia results in changes in mitochondria, plasma membranes, endoplasmic reticulum, and nuclei and eventually causes a marked decrease in all cellular metabolic processes (Fig. 3–21). If an external oxygen source is supplied soon after hypoxic injury, the cellular changes may be reversible, depending on the cell type. *Neurons, cardiac myocytes,* and *renal tubular* cells appear to be most vulnerable to permanent, irreversible hypoxic damage (Fig. 3–22).

Trump and co-workers have studied hypoxic states in the kidney extensively in vitro and in vivo, especially in cells of the proximal tubule. They have shown swelling of the inner compartment of mitochondria, of endoplasmic reticulum (ER) canaliculi, of microvilli, as well as chromatin clumping and Golgi disorganization.[69]

Cerebral hypoxia may be associated with vascular thrombosis, embolism, and atherosclerosis, or with excessive amounts of compounds such as serotonin, dopamine, and norepinephrine, which may act as cerebrovascular spasmotics.[70]

Experimental obstruction of vascular channels in the myocardium usually produces hypoxia. Release of the obstruction results in the return of blood to the hypoxic area with reversal of previously induced structural alterations.

Experimental hypoxia of the pancreas results in moderate to severe cellular damage, which is related to intracellular zymogen granule activation rather than to extracellular lysosomal release.

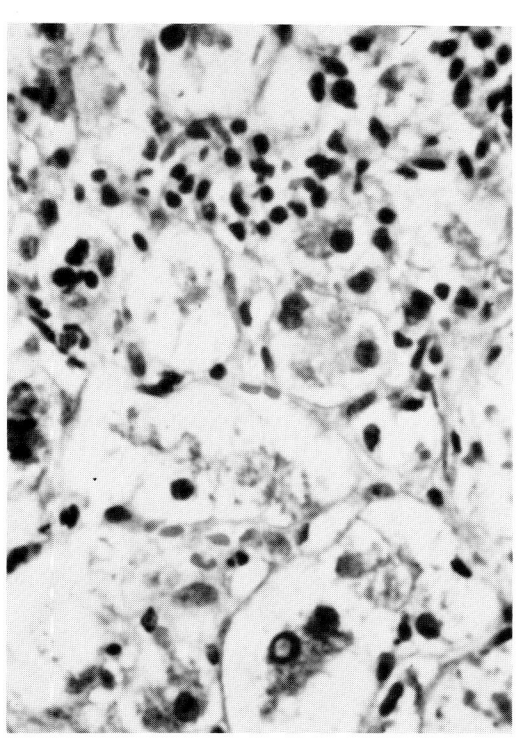

Figure 3–21. Swollen hepatocytes showing hydropic degeneration.

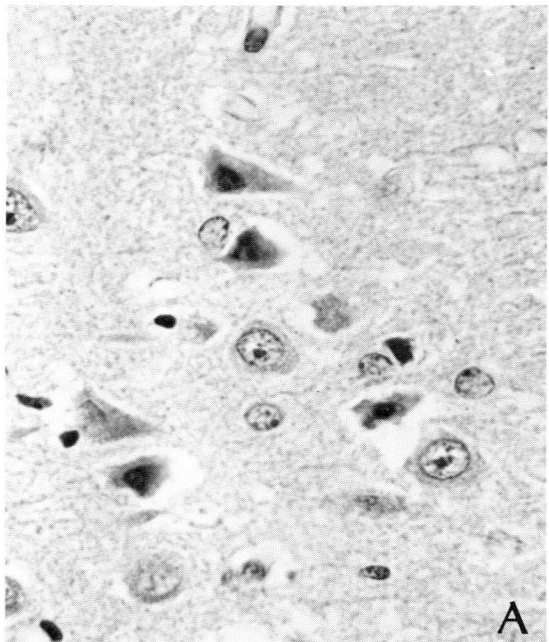

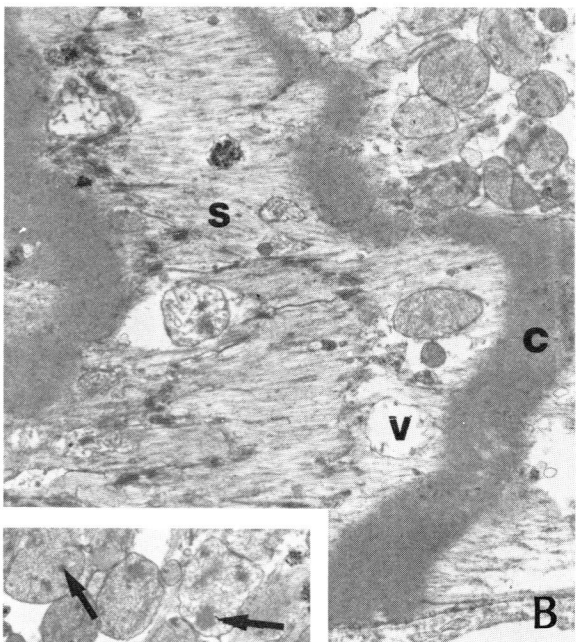

Figure 3–22. *A,* Section of brain demonstrating pyknosis of some of the cells following cerebral anoxia. *B,* In this electron micrograph of ventricular muscle after ischemia, the contraction band (C) is prominent and an area of sarcomere overstretch and disruption (S) is present. A vacuolated mitochondrion (V) is seen, and in the inset, mitochondria with amorphous matrix densities and dense granules (arrows) are illustrated. (Courtesy of Dr. P. Duffy *(A)* and Dr. J. Fenoglio *(B),* College of Physicians & Surgeons, Columbia University, New York.)

An unusual disorder, *"high-altitude pulmonary edema,"* has been reported in individuals from Leadville, Colorado, and in locations with altitudes above 15,000 to 20,000 feet, where there is a significant decrease in available oxygen.[71] Despite physiologic and molecular modifications that are adaptive phenomena, such as increased hemoglobin affinity for oxygen and increased numbers of red blood cells in secondary polycythemia, the high altitude may invoke peripheral vasoconstriction with shunting of blood to the viscera and lungs, with the development of acute pulmonary edema.

Oxygen Toxicity

Excess oxygen can be as harmful as anoxic or hypoxic conditions.[72] Cells in tissue culture fail to grow in an atmosphere containing 100% oxygen.[73] Years ago, when pure oxygen was given as therapy to premature babies, it resulted in *retrolental fibroplasia* and blindness.[74]

Carbon Monoxide Toxicity

According to recent reports, carbon monoxide causes more deaths than any other single toxic agent except alcohol. Individuals who smoke may have as much as 15% of their hemoglobin in the form of *carboxyhemoglobin.* Exposure also occurs in automotive vehicles, garages, and fires; its use in suicide attempts is well known. The net effect of carbon monoxide on tissues (hypoxia) is due to three factors: (1) its increased affinity over oxygen for hemoglobin, (2) induced conformational change in hemoglobin that results in tighter binding of oxygen, and (3) interference with cellular respiration by binding to other heme proteins such as myoglobin and the cytochromes.

Nitrogen Toxicity (Caisson Disease)

Deep-sea divers and workers in tunnels require oxygen under pressure because hemoglobin combines with oxygen in proportion to the atmospheric pressure. Following a deep-sea dive, reduction of the atmospheric pressure *(decompression)* occurs, and nitrogen that was dissolved in the blood comes out of solution. If this process is too rapid, nitrogen bubbles collect, particularly in joints and skeletal muscle ("the bends"). Treatment of *caisson disease* involves gradual decompression, which allows nitrogen to redissolve in the blood.

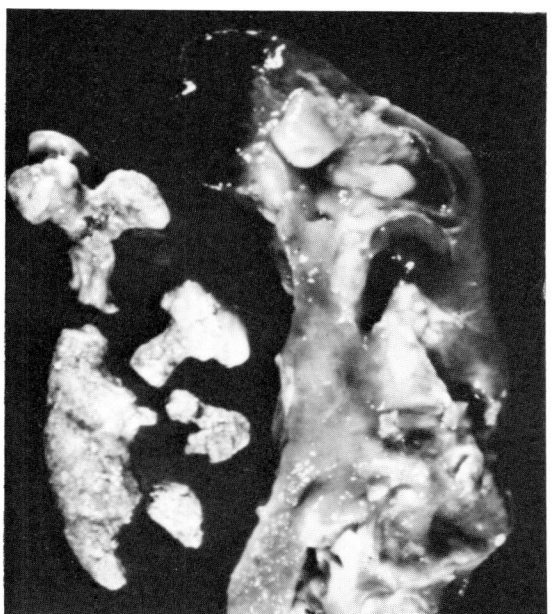

Figure 3–23. Staghorn calculi of kidney. The calculi have been extracted from the renal collecting system and are lying to the left of the atrophic, hydronephrotic kidney.

Ion and Water Balance

The principal cations of the cell are *hydrogen* (H^+), *potassium* (K^+),[75] and *sodium* (Na^+). The principal anions are *chloride* (Cl^-) and *bicarbonate* (HCO_3^-). They are responsible for maintaining both the osmotic equilibrium of the cell and the pH of tissues. The multivalent cations *calcium, phosphorus,* and *magnesium* are involved in many energy-generating and coenzyme-related reactions.

Calcium plays important roles in hormone secretion, nerve excitation, and bone metabolism; serum and tissue calcium levels are controlled by *parathormone* and *calcitonin*. Calcium is also controlled by its receptor protein, *calmodulin,* which activates cyclic nucleotides and scores of cellular membrane enzymes including the kinases.[76] In molecular complexes with phosphate or carbonate, calcium may be deposited intracellularly, particularly in mitochondria, or extracellularly as stones in the kidney or biliary tree (Fig. 3–23). Magnesium, another important extracellular ion, participates in active transport reactions across the cell membrane.

Edema

We have previously discussed extracellular edema as one of the cardinal signs of inflammation and described the transudation and exudation associated with changes in capillary permeability. These changes may be independent, initially, of intracellular water and ion changes (Table 3–14).

Local causes of edema include inflammation from a variety of causes. Common physical agents include burns and mechanical injury. The release of vasodilatory agents associated with allergic conditions, various infectious agents, hypoxia, and obstruction of the venous and lymphatic drainage all may produce a local edematous state. More generalized edema is seen with nutritional protein deficiency with subsequent lowering of serum oncotic pressure, cardiac edema as a result of pump failure, uremic edema associated with kidney failure, various CNS lesions, and the condition *myxedema* associated with hypothyroidism.[77]

Table 3–14. *Causes of Edema*

Local
Burns
Allergy
Obstruction
Infection
Hypoxia
Generalized
Nutritional status
Decreased osmotic pressure
Pump failure (cardiac edema)
Kidney failure (uremia)
Hypothyroidism (myxedema)

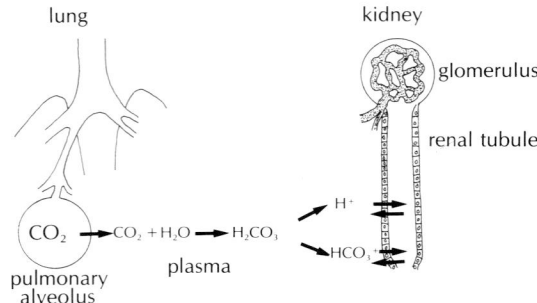

lung

kidney

glomerulus

renal tubule

$CO_2 \rightarrow CO_2 + H_2O \rightarrow H_2CO_3$

H^+

HCO_3^-

pulmonary alveolus

plasma

The lung and kidney play key roles in the generation of and compensation for acid-base disorders. Some of these are indicated below:

Type of acid-base disorder	Type of primary change	Resultant blood pH	Type of compensatory change
metabolic acidosis	↓ HCO_3^-	low	↓ PCO_2
metabolic alkalosis	↑ HCO_3^-	high	↑ PCO_2
respiratory acidosis	↑ PCO_2	low	↑ HCO_3^-
respiratory alkalosis	↓ PCO_2	high	↓ HCO_3^-

Figure 3–24. Pulmonary and renal physiology in acid-base disorders.

pH

The pH of the cell is regulated by the $H_2CO_3/NaHCO_3$ ratio and is normally 7.37 (range 7.1 to 7.5). This intracellular, and subsequently extracellular, balance may be upset by a variety of diseases. Carbon dioxide, a normal product of cellular metabolism, is carried in the blood and is usually released in the lungs. The retention of carbon dioxide, with conversion to and accumulation of carbonic acid (H_2CO_3), leads to *respiratory acidosis*. An excessive accumulation of normal metabolites such as lactic acid, pyruvic acid, and ketone bodies leads to *metabolic acidosis*.[78,79]

Hyperventilation states with increased release of CO_2 result in *respiratory alkalosis*. Vomiting and diarrhea, which are associated with a loss of cations (particularly sodium and potassium), result in *metabolic alkalosis* (Fig. 3–24). These acid-base disorders are injurious to various tissues. Prolonged changes in pH mediate alterations (usually detrimental) in the metabolic machinery and organelles of the cell.

Shock

Shock (Table 3–15) results from alterations in cell metabolism, alterations in the cardiovascular system, a massive loss of fluid, or a vasodilatory phenomenon associated with overwhelming infection. Shock often results from circulatory failure with inadequate perfusion and tissue hypoxia. It should be distinguished from shock-like states, such as those associated with overdose of insulin, and coma associated with CNS lesions.

Table 3–15. *Causes of Shock*

Infection—sepsis
Cardiogenic failure
Hemorrhage
Extensive fluid loss
Renal failure
Anaphylaxis

Cardiogenic shock, as a result of pump failure, is often associated with arrhythmias, severe infarct, and long-standing congestive failure. The backup of fluid in lungs, liver, and peripheral extremities depletes blood volume once available for other organs, particularly the CNS.

In *septic shock,* particularly associated with gram-negative organisms, the lipid A component of the endotoxin activates factor XII, which mediates the kinin reaction and releases the vasodilator bradykinin. The endotoxin may also stimulate coagulation and may produce *disseminated intravascular coagulation (DIC).*[80] The endotoxin may stimulate adrenergic receptors in vessels to produce vascular spasm, but the endothelial anaerobiosis resulting soon leads to hypoxia and dilatation.

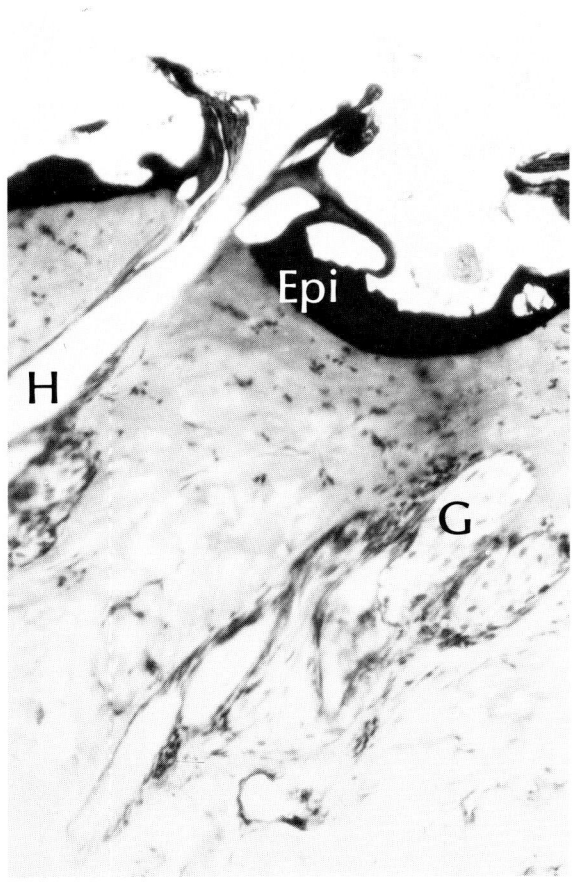

Figure 3–25. In burn injury involving the skin, note the lack of cellular detail in the epidermis (Epi). The hair is absent from what should have been the hair shaft (H), and the adnexal sebaceous glands (G) are beginning to atrophy.

One of the most common causes of shock is loss of fluid often associated with massive *hemorrhage*. Precipitating factors include bleeding peptic ulcers and diverticula, trauma, or ruptured aneurysms. Shock may also be seen with severe burns, extensive vomiting or diarrhea, or severe loss of fluid associated with renal failure.

Temperature Changes

Heat Injury

The normal temperature of the human body is approximately 98.6°F (37.5°C), but ranges from 88 to 113°F have been known to occur for short periods of time. High environmental temperatures may lead to *heat stroke*, with cellular hypermetabolism, vasodilatation, and unconsciousness.[81]

Burns result from contact with excessive heat (or sometimes cold), and they may involve outer layers of the skin or the full thickness of the epidermis (Fig. 3–25). Massive burns of the body surface are often fatal, but newer therapeutic procedures have increased recovery rates. In addition to coagulation of cellular and extracellular protein and aggregation of platelets with secondary thrombosis, burns usually cause microcirculatory changes associated with edema and later secondary infection.

Cold Injury

Injury due to exposure to *cold* initially results in vasoconstriction with ischemia, hypoxia, and a decrease in cellular metabolism. Vascular stasis may lead to local thrombosis. Exposures to extreme cold in vitro, however, may not necessarily be harmful to individual cells. When rewarmed, cells that have been stored at −70°C for years and that were previously incubated with glycerol or dimethyl sulfoxide (DMSO) retain characteristics of viability, including growth.[82]

Robinson reported that in vitro cells frozen to −196°C and rewarmed showed good recovery in conditioned medium, but did not divide immediately. It was seen that in the recovery phase of restitution there was a drop in membrane phosphatidylinositol. The delay in cell division therefore appeared to be related to a time period necessary for activation of glycosyl transferase-mediated repair of the damaged membrane oligosaccharides. In vivo transfer of corneas, sperm, and blood cells to human subjects has also demonstrated the viability of cells following freezing.

Radiation

It is often difficult to assess the effects of radiation on a given individual. This inherent problem exists because, as

Table 3–16. *Electromagnetic Spectrum*

hf Photon Energy (eV)	f Frequency (sec^{-1})	x Wavelength (cm)	
4×10^{17}	10^{32}	3×10^{-22}	
4×10^{15}	10^{30}	3×10^{-20}	Cosmic ray photons
4×10^{13}	10^{28}	3×10^{-18}	
4×10^{11}	10^{26}	3×10^{-16}	
4×10^{9}	10^{24}	3×10^{-14}	
4×10^{7}	10^{22}	3×10^{-12}	
4×10^{5}	10^{20}	3×10^{-10}	Gamma rays
4×10^{3}	10^{18}	3×10^{-8}	x rays
40	10^{16}	3×10^{-6}	Ultraviolet
0.4	10^{14}	3×10^{-4}	Infrared
4×10^{-3}	10^{12}	3×10^{-2}	
4×10^{-5}	10^{10}	3	Microwaves Radar Ultra high frequency (UHF)
4×10^{-7}	10^{8}	300	Very high frequency (VHF) Frequency modulation (FM) Shortwave
4×10^{-9}	10^{6}	3×10^{4}	Amplitude modulation (AM) radio
4×10^{-11}	10^{4}	3×10^{6}	Longwave radio

(Modified from Ford, K.S.: Basic Physics. Waltham, MA, Blaisdell Publishing, 1968.)

in experimental models, it is nearly impossible to compare the effects of different forms and dosages of radiation (Table 3–16) administered under different environmental conditions in different species.

Types of Ionizing Radiation

Radiations are forms of energy traveling through space without the aid of a material medium. *"Ionizing radiations"* are highly energetic radiations with the ability to eject electrons from atoms in the matter through which they pass; this ejection leads to the production of positively and negatively charged ions.

Ionizing radiations fall into two classes, *particulate and electromagnetic*. Particulate radiations are streams of atomic

Table 3–17. *Particulate and Electromagnetic Radiation*

Particulate Radiation	Charge
β-particle (e$^-$)	-1
proton	$+1$
neutron	0
deuteron	$+1$
α-particle (He nucleus)	$+2$

Electromagnetic Radiation

radiowaves
infrared waves
visible light
x rays (ionizing)
gamma rays (ionizing)

or subatomic particles with high velocities and kinetic energy (Table 3–17). Lighter particles, such as electrons, may approach the speed of light. Their kinetic energy, however, is unlimited. Electromagnetic radiations are vibrating electromagnetic fields traveling through space and include radiowaves, infrared, visible light, x, and gamma rays. The last two are the only ionizing radiations. These radiations consist of continuously distributed waves, but when involved in energy interchanges with matter, they are composed of discrete and characteristic packages of energy called *photons*. Electromagnetic radiations sufficiently energetic to produce ionizations are called x rays if produced by machines, or gamma rays if emitted by radioactive elements. Apart from their origin, no major difference exists between x and γ rays.

Interactions Between Radiation and Matter

Ionizing radiations differ in their ability to penetrate matter. Electromagnetic radiations, such as x rays and photons, penetrate deeply and transfer a large proportion of their energy to the electrons encountered; these electrons acquire high velocity and form widely spaced ion clusters. Charged particle radiations, on the other hand, rarely penetrate more than a few centimeters and transfer small proportions of their total energy to a large number of orbital electrons that can produce secondary ionizations.

The unit of absorbed ionizing radiation dose is the *"rad"* (that amount of radiation that deposits 10^{-2} joule of energy/kg). One can also measure the output of an x-ray machine or source of gamma rays by the *"exposure dose."* The unit of exposure dose is the *"roentgen" (r)*; conveniently, a dose of one roentgen to living matter results in energy absorption of approximately one rad.[83]

Effects on Cells and Their Constituents

The cell is the primary site of biologic radiation damage. Low radiation doses, on the order of 500 rad, are sufficient to destroy the dividing cell and, consequently, the organisms themselves. The coded information defining a cell's growth, structure, and function is contained in the DNA of its chromosomes. Work by Sparrow, Cole, Von Borstel, and Rogers and others has clearly indicated *DNA* to be the major target affected by radiation, although effects on other cellular constituents must also be acknowledged[84] (Fig. 3–26).

DNA is the only component of the cell that is not freely replaceable, although it is probably constantly being repaired; any change leading to its faulty replication when the cell divides may potentially cause inherited abnormal-

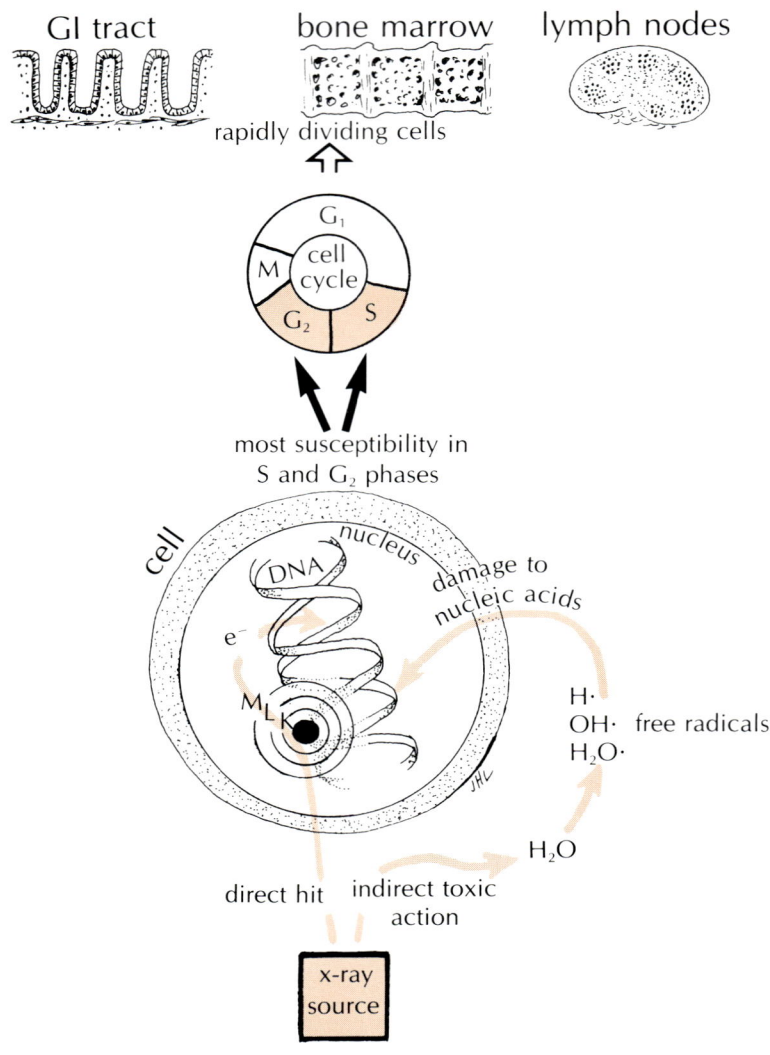

Figure 3–26. Effects of radiation on cells.

ities, cellular malfunction, and cell death.[85] Effects on other macromolecules are doubtless also important in radiation-induced cell injury, as for example, in the damage to proteins and phospholipids on the cell membranes of nondividing cells. Radiation can damage macromolecules in two ways: by *direct action*, whereby the macromolecules themselves are ionized; and by *indirect action*, in which water or solute molecules are ionized and produce free radicals that secondarily damage macromolecules.

Radiolysis of water, which comprises 75% of living tissue, forms reactive species including hydrated electrons, hydrogen atoms, *hydroxyl radicals*, and, in the presence of dissolved oxygen, *hydroperoxyl radical ions*. Indirect effects of these free radicals, as well as direct effects of ionizing radiations, result in alterations in cellular macromolecules including carbohydrates, proteins, lipids, and nucleic acids.

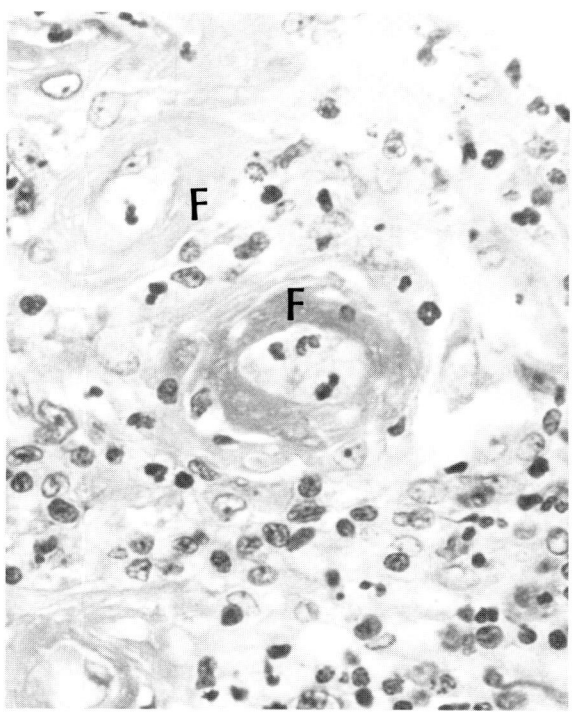

Figure 3–27. Blood vessels demonstrating fibrinoid necrosis (F) in their walls following the administration of external radiation.

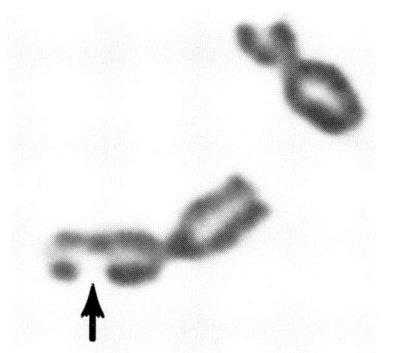

Figure 3–28. Chromosome demonstrating a break (arrow) in one of the long arms following exposure to radiation. (Courtesy of Dr. T.T. Puck, University of Colorado, Denver.)

Effects on Organ Systems

The cells composing tissues show different radiation sensitivities, depending on a number of factors including normal cell turnover time, cell-cell interactions within the tissue, the tissue's ability to replace or repair damaged cells, and the cell's reserve capacity. Designation of cells as intermitotic, postmitotic, and reverting postmitotic has already been discussed.

Intermitotic cells are *radiosensitive,*[86] and *postmitotic cells* are *radioresistant.* Most vascular and connective tissue cells are intermediate in sensitivity. Early radiation effects on radiosensitive cells are based on destruction or mitotic inhibition of parenchymal cells. Replacement of these cells occurs rapidly, so that there may be early damage and quick recovery. Postmitotic cells such as muscle and brain require high radiation doses for their removal, although their associated vasculature may be damaged with only moderate doses (Fig. 3–27). Vascular damage may also occur in organs composed of reverting postmitotic cells such as liver and kidney. It follows, therefore, that the major changes in postmitotic and reverting postmitotic parenchymal cells are late effects secondary to vascular tissue damage.

There are three main phases of radiation-induced damage. In the *first,* mitotically active cells show immediate *inhibition of division, chromosomal aberrations* appear in cells engaged in mitosis, and degenerative changes are seen in other cells. In the *second* phase, vascular damage leads to *hemorrhage* and *edema,* whereas relatively radioresistant phagocytic cells actively remove remnants of destroyed radiosensitive cells. In the *third* phase, *regeneration,* the first abortive mitoses lead to degenerative cells. Complete or nearly complete tissue regeneration follows the high mitotic activity, which may be greater than normal (Fig. 3–28).

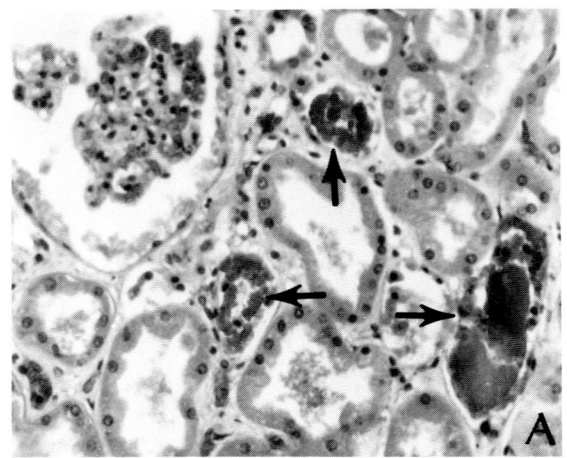

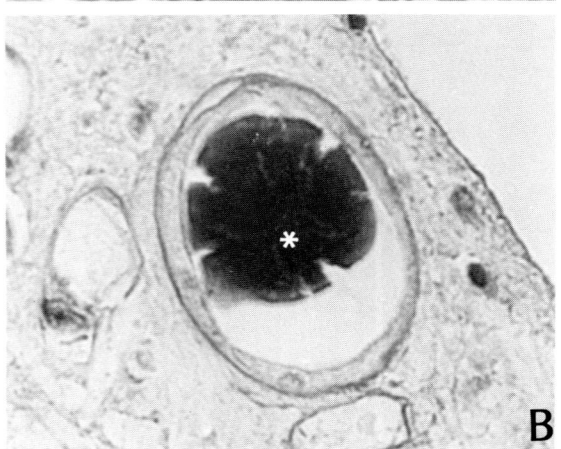

Figure 3–29. Myoglobin casts from a patient suffering from myoglobinuria following an automobile accident. Note the presence of myoglobin in the renal tubules *(A)*. *B* shows an immunoperoxidase reaction using an antimyoglobin antibody. The dark reaction product (*) represents myoglobin.

Mechanical Injury

Different forms of mechanical injury may result from *accidents,* including *falls, knife* and *gunshot wounds,* or *crushing injuries* associated with automobile accidents (Fig. 3–29). *Pressure phenomena* may rupture hollow viscera, for instance, of the gastrointestinal or genitourinary tracts, may fracture bones, or may lacerate solid organs such as liver, kidney, heart, or brain. This primary tissue damage is often then extended by hemorrhage, thrombosis, and hypoxia. In the absence of severe hemorrhage, shock, or irreparable disorganization of tissue and organ structure, prompt surgical repair may allow recovery. Advanced age, poor nutrition, and secondary infection are significant complicating factors in the final outcome.

Myocardial Ischemia

Incidence and Risk Factors

Ischemic heart disease is a common serious health problem. In the United States alone, more than 675,000 people die each year from ischemic heart disease and its complications. Approximately 1,300,000 patients per year have myocardial infarctions, and many more suffer from congestive heart failure secondary to ischemic myocardial damage. Over 50% of individuals above the age of 50 have cardiovascular disease. Thus, ischemic heart disease and its complications are by far the most common cause of death in the United States and in the developed world.[87] *Risk factors* that predispose a person to myocardial ischemia include *hypertension, diabetes, atherosclerosis, hypercholesterolemia,*[88] increased *age, obesity,* and *smoking*[89] (Table 3–18).

Myocardial infarcts (MI) are more common in men than in women, particularly between 40 and 60 years of age. Postmenopausal women have an incidence of myocardial infarction that approaches that for men. This incidence is concurrent with an increased incidence of atherosclerosis.

Myocardial infarcts are often preceded by *angina pectoris* (pain in the chest radiating to the left arm). Warning signals either may be absent or may be manifested by crushing pain in the chest, which may be referred to the epigastrium, left shoulder, or vertebral column. The frequency of a second myocardial infarct is 20 times that of the first. The average length of life following the first attack is 2.5 years.

Table 3–18. *Risk Factors in Myocardial Infarction*

Hypertension
Atherosclerosis
Hypercholesterolemia
Increased age
Obesity
Diabetes mellitus
Smoking

With coronary bypass surgery, newer statistics suggest that this period of survival may be lengthening, dependent on the severity of the lesion when the bypass procedure is performed. The major determinant of the subsequent clinical course in a patient with an acute MI is the extent of irreversible myocardial injury.

Pathogenesis

Myocardial infarction results from ischemia secondary to reduced blood flow in the coronary arteries. This flow may be temporarily reduced as the result of coronary thrombosis, atherosclerotic plaques, or vessel spasm. Indeed, single local areas of narrowing in the coronary arteries may play a role in triggering episodes of coronary artery spasm.[90]

The terms *"acute myocardial infarction"* and *"acute coronary thrombosis"* are often used interchangeably, but the validity of this usage has been challenged. Studies of isotopically labeled fibrinogen within coronary thrombi have suggested that thrombi may be propagated following muscle damage, rather than preceding it.[91] Maseri et al.[92] monitored patients at risk for developing MI using hemodynamic monitoring, thallium myocardial scintigraphy, or angiography during anginal attacks. These investigators suggest that the temporal sequence of events may initially involve vasospasm, followed by platelet aggregation and coronary thrombosis.[92]

Coronary spasm can precipitate an infarct and can occur in a number of situations. Platelets, which play a role in thrombosis, may provide an additional stimulus for coronary artery spasm. When circulating platelets are aggregated by thrombin or by an endothelial injury, *thromboxane A_2*, a powerful local coronary arterial vasoconstrictor, may be released.[93]

Ischemia can also occur in the absence of occlusive or spasmodic events under conditions in which myocardial oxygen supply and demand relationships are altered. Depressed postoperative myocardial performance (low-output syndrome) is caused most often by ischemic cardiac damage occurring during surgical procedures. The left ventricular subendocardial muscle is the most severely affected part of the heart.

Coronary artery embolism is a rare cause of myocardial infarction. The underlying diseases predisposing a person to coronary emboli include valvular heart disease, cardiomyopathy, coronary atherosclerosis, and chronic atrial fibrillation.[94]

Atherosclerosis

Lesions. Shortly after one year of life in humans, lipid deposits appear in the intima of the aorta, particularly around the cusps of the heart valves. These streaks soon disappear. Starting somewhere near the end of the first decade, lipid deposits are again seen; these deposits continue to accumulate for the rest of one's life. The lipid initially appears to be in macrophages of the intima under the endothelial lining. Some investigators insist that even at this stage, lipid is in *myointimal cells* that have migrated into the intima from the media, and proliferation of myointimal cells precedes the lipid infiltration. No tissue reaction is apparent.

The intermediate state of atherosclerosis with a typical intimal plaque contains lipid, principally cholesterol, both within macrophages and myointimal cells and lying free in the extracellular space. Free fatty acids combine with calcium to form calcium soaps. There is a marked proliferation of myointimal cells migrating from the media; these cells are apparently able to synthesize collagen. Electron-microscopic observations show that these cells also contain a few myofibrils. Chronic inflammatory cells, principally lymphocytes and monocytes, are present. The internal elastic membrane is disrupted with reduction of the elastic fibrils in the media. Injury is usually present in the overlying endothelial cells.

The late stage of atherosclerosis shows massive intra- and extracellular deposits of lipid associated with calcium visible both grossly and microscopically. The thickened intimal plaque is infiltrated by many chronic inflammatory cells, proliferating myointimal cells, and extensive fibrous deposits (often hyalinized). The overlying endothelial surface is grossly ulcerated, often with a superimposed mural thrombus lying on the encrusted edges of the plaque. The media is thin, is composed of a few elastic fibrils and some replacement collagen, and is susceptible to aneurysm formation (Fig. 3–30).

Etiology. Most everyone agrees that the *plaque* is a response to an "injurious agent" in its broadest sense, including chemical, mechanical, immune agents, and perhaps viral mutagens, that it is progressive, and that it is influenced by a multitude of factors. Considerable effort has been expended to elucidate the initial factor(s) or agent(s) causing the disease.

Over the years, it has been proposed that the plaque represented (1) an organized thrombus secondary to endothelial injury, (2) a reaction to injury due to abnormal lipoproteins that had infiltrated the area, and (3) an autoimmune reaction following injury by toxic substances in the circulation.

Ross and others believe that the initial injury is to the endothelium[95] (Fig. 3–31). If it does not heal, there is focal desquamation of endothelial cells and aggregation of platelets with the release of a *platelet mitogenic factor*. Passage of plasma constituents into the underlying arterial wall, migration and proliferation of medial smooth muscle cells into the intima, and later synthesis of a connective tissue matrix are followed by lipid accumulation.

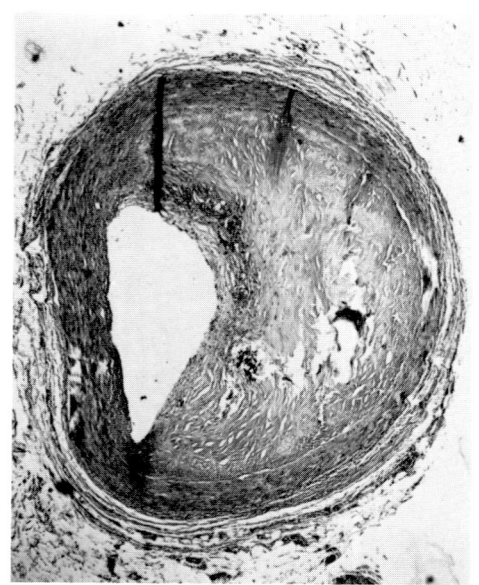

Figure 3–30. A coronary artery nearly completely occluded by atherosclerotic plaque. A small, eccentrically located lumen remains.

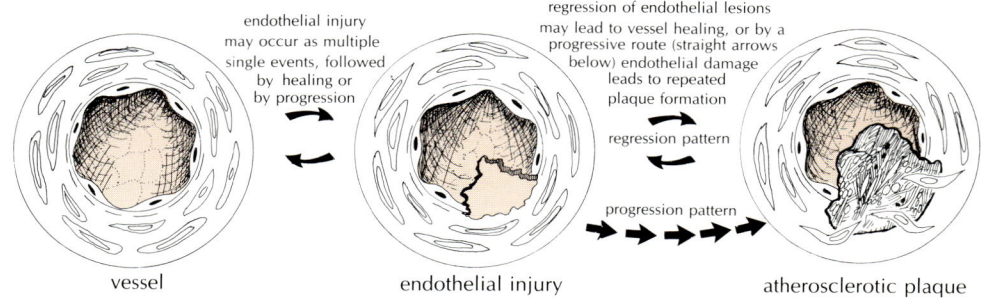

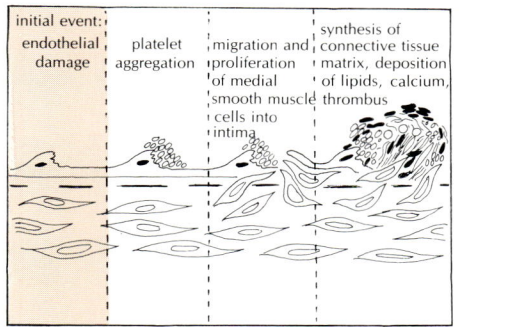

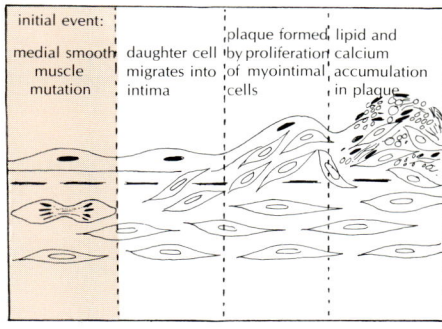

Two theories of atherogenesis

Figure 3–31. Schematic representation of concepts currently believed to play a role in the development of atherosclerosis.

Benditt believes the initial injury (perhaps a *mutagenic event*) occurs in a single myointimal cell followed by proliferation of a single clone,[96] as shown from studies of G6PD on plaques from black heterozygous females. Other groups of investigators suggest that whereas old plaques selectively overgrow from one cell, early plaques contain two cell types.[97] The accompanying lipid and calcium deposits, overlying thrombotic reactions, and chronic inflammatory cells are then present because of the proliferation of the myointimal cells and are only prominent because of the unique site in the circulation.

Factors Affecting Atherosclerosis. These include genetic, nutritional, physical, chemical, hormonal, infectious, and immune factors.

Genetic Factors. Certain families have a propensity to develop coronary or cerebral atherosclerosis and a history of death by myocardial or cerebral infarction. Primary *hyperbetalipoproteinemia* is a genetic disorder associated with

Table 3–19. *Characteristics of Familial Hypercholesterolemia*

	Heterozygotes	Homozygotes
Frequency	1/500	$1/1 \times 10^6$
Serum levels LDL	Increased × 2.5	Increased 6×
Average age of myocardial infarction	35–45	5–15

Table 3–20. *Alleles Responsible for Receptor Defect in Familial Hypercholesterolemia*

Allele	Defect
R^{b0}/R^{b0}	No binding of LDL to receptor
R^{b-}/R^{b-}	Reduced binding to receptor
$R^{b+}/R^{b+,i0}$	Normal binding, no internalization

premature heart disease. One form of this is *familial hypercholesterolemia,* which is inherited as an autosomal dominant disorder (Table 3–19). Homozygotes for the disease have a deficiency of cell surface receptors for LDL, defective LDL receptors, or an inability to internalize receptors[98] (Table 3–20). This disease leads to defective regulation of cholesterol metabolism.

A genetic susceptibility to atherosclerosis and hypertension also exists. Although the *"A"* and *"B" somatic genetic phenotypes* have not been completely accepted, the psychologic factors associated with stress appear to have an important effect on the incidence of heart attacks.

In baboons, *chronic homocystinuria* can produce atherosclerotic lesions. Patients with homocystinuria usually die of atherosclerosis before 30 and have decreased platelet survival time (thus more prevalent mitogenic factor), 50% lower than control subjects.[99] This decrease in platelet survival time was not seen, however, in other studies.

Nutritional Factors. Although abnormal lipoproteins may not be the initiating factor, the presence of increased lipids in the serum, especially *low-density particles,* and most particularly cholesterol, is well documented in patients with atherosclerosis. The normal components of lipoproteins in serum are shown in Table 3–21. *High-density lipoprotein* fractions appear to have a protective effect. Aggravation of myocardial infarcts in humans and initiation of atherosclerosis in experimental animals has been noted with high-lipid diets containing unsaturated fatty acids.

Wissler and co-workers showed a reversal of atherosclerotic lesions in swine and monkeys, respectively, once the lipid levels were lowered.[100] Wissler's group has also shown that *LDL* and *serum* from *hypertensive patients* promote

Table 3–21. *Characteristics of Chylomicrons and Lipoprotein*

	Chylomicrons	VLDL	LDL	HDL
Diameter (Å)	10^3–10^4	250–750	200–225	80–120
Molecular weight	10^9	10^7	2.3×10^6	3.8×10^5
Composition (%)				
Protein	2	10	22	40
Total glycoprotein	85	56	8	5
Cholesterol ester	4	10	40	15
Cholesterol	2	7	10	5
Phospholipid	7	17	20	35

VLDL, very low density lipoprotein; LDL, low-density lipoprotein; HDL, high-density lipoprotein.

division of smooth muscle cells in a manner similar to Ross's platelet mitogenic factor.[100]

Several investigators have produced early sclerotic lesions in monkeys given a hyperlipid diet with destruction of endothelium by a catheter. De Duve believes that lipoproteins are taken up by smooth muscle cells deficient in numbers of lysosomes, and the amount of cholesterol esterases is ineffective in their hydrolysis.[101] Thus, intra- and extracellular cholesterol accumulates, with progression of the plaque.[102]

Ross and co-workers have also produced endothelial desquamation (5% of the surface in thoracic abdominal elastic arteries) in lipid-fed monkeys. He postulates that susceptibility to mechanical shear forces may be increased in these portions of the aorta.[103]

Physical Factors. Atherosclerosis is present prominently on the posterior aspect of the aorta and at vessel intersections where intravascular pressure is greatest. In pulmonary vessels atherosclerosis is rare and is almost always restricted to patients with pulmonary hypertension. This finding documents the role that increased vascular pressure plays in potentiating, if not initiating, atherosclerosis. Benditt suggests that hypertension increases the susceptibility to mutagens. It has also been suggested that the lack of vasa vasorum in the intima and the increased thickening of the intimal plaque result in hypoxia, further cell damage, and subsequent inflammatory response.

Chemicals, Drugs, and Hormones. Premenopausal women have appreciably less atherosclerosis than men, whereas in postmenopausal women, atherosclerosis proceeds more rapidly than in men. It is difficult, however, to implicate estrogens directly as the principal factor, although the attractive *"estrogen-effect"* theory demands further study.

The toxic chemicals in cigarette smoke accelerate the appearance of atherosclerosis in coronary vessels. Many believe that benzpyrene and methylcholanthrene in cigarettes cause cancer of the lung after conversion to an *ultimate carcinogen* by *aryl hydrocarbon hydroxylase*. Benditt hypothesized that a similar growth stimulation, although not malignant, might occur in a vessel myointimal cell and might thereby produce an atherosclerotic plaque.[96]

Infectious Agents. It is doubtful that an infectious agent is either an initiating or a potentiating factor, as no organisms have been reliably associated with sclerotic plaques despite the tens of thousands of sections that have been examined in electron-microscopic studies. It is known that *endotoxin* is capable of producing atherosclerosis in experimental animals, however.

More disturbing is that in animal tumors produced by *DNA viruses*, that is, polyoma virus and simian virus 40 (SV40), the virus cannot be identified in the proliferative phase unless special attempts at *"rescue"* are made. In tumors produced by cell-free lysates of adenovirus, the virus has never been seen or rescued in animals, presumably because only a small portion of the viral genome is necessary for integration in the host genome. Similarly, failure to isolate virus is not incompatible with Benditt's theory of stimulation of plaque growth by a mutagenic virus.

Immune Reactions. It is suspected that atherosclerosis is partially an autoimmune injury. The presence of immunoglobulins in walls of vessels with arteriosclerosis suggests that they may be contributing factors. Following arterial injections of antigen in rabbits, Minick and co-workers showed *antigen-antibody complexes* and lesions resembling a form of arteriolosclerosis.[104] Lipid deposits are seen in similar arteriolar lesions of dermatomyositis, systemic lupus erythematosus (SLE), rheumatoid arthritis (RA), scleroderma, and periarteritis, all diseases involving immune reactions.

Summary. Most investigators agree that atherosclerosis is a progressive disease starting early in life. It is associated with mechanical forces including increased pressure, is restrained by estrogen, and is accelerated by hyperlipidemia, principally of cholesterol, smoking, and obesity. Many continue to hope that if a single, initial, injurious agent is identified, it may be possible to mitigate the effects of multiple contributing factors. Consequences of atherosclerosis include infarction, stroke, aneurysm, and accentuation of lesions associated with diabetes and hypertension.

Structure and Function of Myocardium

The myocardium consists of a syncytium of cells with branching fibers, 5 to 10 μ in length. *Sarcomeres* in the cells are regular, repeating structural units containing myofilaments (actin and myosin filaments) found within myofibrils (also see Chap. 6).

Myofibrils are surrounded by a membranous structure called the sarcolemma, which also gives rise to tubular invaginations into the myofiber known as the transverse tubules or *T system*. The ends of cardiac fibers are joined by modified surfaces of the cell membrane, the *intercalated discs*. These discs are responsible for carrying the electrical activity. Electrical activity is initiated by the release of calcium from the sarcoplasmic reticulum (SR). Secondary recapture of calcium into the SR and the mitochondria turns off the electrical activity.

Initial events in resting cardiac muscle demonstrate that pacemaking action potentials are transmitted along the surface of the sarcolemma and thereby trigger the release of calcium from the SR to act on the sarcomere. ATPase on the head of the myosin filament is activated in the presence of *calcium, magnesium, actin,* and *troponin*, with resultant cleavage of ATP.[105] The calcium bound to the *troponin complex* releases inhibition of actin-myosin interaction, allows their electrostatic interaction, and results in contraction. Calcium later dissociates and diffuses back into the SR.

Energy is generated aerobically and anaerobically.

Mitochondria provide aerobic energy, and glycolysis in the cytosol provides anaerobic energy in the form of ATP. Myocardial cells contain many mitochondria for generating the large amounts of ATP necessary for continual contraction of heart muscle (see Chap. 6).

In the aerobic pathway, amino acids, fatty acids, glycogen, and glucose enter the Krebs cycle through acetyl coenzyme A (acetyl CoA) and generate 16 moles of ATP per mole of glucose. This process is accompanied by the production of carbon dioxide and water following hydrogen transfer through the electron transport system of cytochromes and flavoproteins. Fats are more efficient energy producers than are carbohydrates; that is, gram for gram, more ATP may be formed from fatty acids than from glucose.

Effects of Ischemia on Myocardial Contractility

Transient episodes of myocardial ischemia during angina pectoris may also cause transient episodes of left ventricular failure. Initially, it was postulated that ischemic regions do not contract because of loss of excitability secondary to changes in ion flux between the intra- and extra-cellular spaces.

The second major postulate was that ischemia reduced myocardial contractility by depleting intracellular stores of high-energy phosphate compounds. This postulate was modified to state that the concentration of high-energy phosphate compounds in certain critical areas, such as the SR, were reduced.

The third major theory related contractile failure to structural changes in cardiac contractile protein;[106] however, biochemical analyses have failed to demonstrate changes in cardiac actin, myosin, and actomysosin or in myofibrillar ATPase.

The fourth possibility, becoming increasingly popular, is that ischemia interferes either with the release of calcium ions from the SR or with the interaction of calcium ions with the contractile proteins. In severe ischemia, all the foregoing conditions obtain.[107]

Hemodynamic evidence of left ventricular failure becomes apparent when contraction ceases, or is seriously impaired, in 20 to 25% of the left ventricle. With a loss of 40% or more of the left ventricular myocardium, severe *pump failure* develops, and if not reversed, cardiogenic shock may ensue. *Cardiogenic shock* is usually defined as a relentless form of cardiac failure with severe hypotension, usually as the result of a massive infarct.[108]

Morphology of Myocardial Infarction

In 1939, Mallory et al. defined the histologic changes that occur in infarcts of differing ages.[109] This field has also been reviewed by others.[110] Edema, intra- and extracellu-

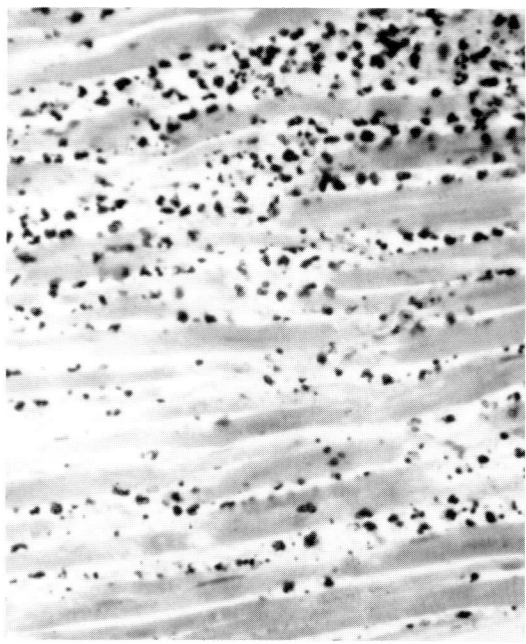

Figure 3–32. Light micrograph from an area of infarct of heart demonstrating muscle cell degeneration and inflammatory cells between the muscle fibers.

lar, may be present as early as 2 hours from the time of infarction, and coagulative *eosinophilic clumping* of myofibrils is also seen within this period. The earliest definitive signs of an infarct seen using the light microscope are manifest in 4 to 6 hours, with nuclear changes in the muscle cells. *Polymorphonuclear leukocytic infiltration* occurs in 6 to 12 hours and reaches a maximum in 36 to 48 hours (Fig. 3–32). Frank *necrosis* is seen in 6 to 24 hours. *Macrophages* arrive in 3 to 4 days, *lymphocytes* and *plasma cells* in 5 to 7 days, and eosinophils in 7 to 14 days. *Fibroblasts* are seen in 4 to 5 days, with production of collagen starting at the end of the first week and reaching its maximum in 1 to 2 months.[111,112]

These findings approximate the description by Trump et al. of cell injury.[113] In their review, cardiac edema is said to occur in 7 to 15 hours. In 24 to 36 hours, the infarct is defined with a yellow, hemorrhagic border and an opaque center. PMN come at 6 hours, with a maximum at 36 to 48 hours. At this time, cells degenerate with *pyknosis* and *karyolysis*, and lymphocytes and macrophages appear on the fourth day. In a week, the center of the infarct is rubbery, less yellow, and the hemorrhagic border is less distinct. Granulation tissue is seen at 1 week, and fibroblasts with collagen appear at 4 to 8 days. At 3 months, a white, firm scar has formed.

Biochemical and Ultrastructural Changes

It is believed that the essential initiating factor in ischemia is the deprivation of blood flow, which leads to hypoxia and lack of metabolic substrates. This deprivation leads to the accumulation of the end products of anaerobic metabolism such as lactate and hydrogen ions.

Four phases have been described in experimental ischemic injury. The *initiation phase* is the first event and involves the cessation of respiration and substrate depletion, so that the oxygen content of the tissue drops and mitochondrial function ceases. ATP is needed in membrane transport and myofilament contraction. Calcium becomes redistributed following mitochondrial injury. The

Table 3–22. *Organelle Changes in Myocardial Ischemia*

Stage 1.	Normal cell condition
Stage 1a.	Clumped nuclear chromatin, reduced cell glycogen, disappearance of mitochondrial granules
Stage 2.	ER dilated, blebbing of plasma membrane, cell sap swollen
Stage 3.	Stage 2 changes and contraction of mitochondrial components
Stage 4.	Swelling of inner compartment of mitochondria, condensation of mitochondrial matrix

(Modified from Trump, B.F., et al.: Recent studies on the pathophysiology of ischemic cell injury. Beitr. Pathol., *158*:363, 1976.)

altered metabolic pathways lead to a reduction in cellular pH. The *reversible phase* extends from initiation to the *"point of no return."* This latter phase occurs in several stages (Table 3–22).

In the infarcted myocytes, a conversion to anaerobic metabolism takes place, lactic acid is increased, and a drop in pH is seen, as well as a drop in ATP and the availability of calcium.[114] ADP, AMP, and adenosine accumulate while creatinine phosphate disappears and tissue creatine increases. Tissue carbon dioxide drops with the decrease in mitochondrial respiration. Electrocardiographic (ECG) changes appear with changes in the cell membrane potential. Myocardial temperature drops as the energy obtained from aerobic oxidation decreases.

The *irreversible phase* is heralded by high-amplitude swelling of the mitochondria. The appearance of large, flocculent densities is one of the most characteristic indicators of this phase. The membrane systems (with the ATPase) are severely altered in the mitochondria as well as in the ER and Golgi complex. The increased myocardial damage results in an absent or reduced respiration, a 3 to 4% capacity to completely oxidize labeled pyruvate to CO_2 and water, an 11.8% capacity to decarboxylate pyruvate, and a 30% decrease in ability to metabolize succinate. This deficiency may be reversed in vitro by the addition of cofactors such as magnesium, reduced CoA, NAD, and malate.[115]

The *reflow phase* is the restoration of blood flow in a previously ischemic tissue and is one in which increased damage can nevertheless occur. The sudden reflow of blood is accompanied by arrhythmias secondary to ionic shifts.

Experimentally in dogs, investigators found an increase in cellular sodium, chloride, and water and a decrease in potassium and phosphorus that could be completely reversed with reflow of blood within 20 minutes; after 1 to 2 hours, irreversible electrolyte changes took place. In addition to the loss of potassium and magnesium, calcium may leak in. Within an hour, glutamic oxaloacetic transaminase leaks out, followed in 2 hours by loss of lactic dehydrogenase (LDH). The loss of cellular creatine phosphokinase (CPK) with the increased serum level of CPK_2 is a further indication of irreversible myocardial damage.

The *recovery phase* is that sequence of events that only follows reversible injury. The cell commonly shrinks. Mitochondrial restitution ensues, and membrane remodeling occurs, with increased numbers of residual bodies. With renewed protein synthesis, amounts of polysomes and RER are increased.

Trump believes that the critical cellular factors involved in the loss of reversibility following ischemia are the mechanisms involved in membrane functions of energy transfer. These membrane functions are associated with increased leakiness and permeability of the membranes that accompany changes in lipid content and alterations in proteins and, presumably, in lipid-protein interactions.[113]

Recovery and Repair

Temporary ischemia can be reversed without any apparent residual, structural, or functional alterations. Repair starts at the edge of the infarct at 30 minutes. Permanent ischemia, resulting in irreversible death of cells, is followed by replacement of myocardium with scar tissue. This process is usually associated with hypertrophy of the remaining muscle cells in an attempt to maintain the contractility of the heart.

Hyperplasia is rarely seen in infants over the age of 2 months, although mitotic figures have been seen in children up to 20 months of age with congenitally enlarged hearts.

Although thymidine uptake has been seen in autoradiographs of myocytes, the increased total heart DNA is generally attributed to interstitial fibroblastic cellular proliferation rather than to increased DNA in muscle cells. The increase in RNA and protein synthesis and the drop in the DNA:RNA ratio point to hypertrophy of the myofibrils as the principal compensatory response.

Complications of Acute Myocardial Infarction

Arrhythmias constitute perhaps the major life-threatening complications of an acute infarct in the early period (hours to several days) following the event, and for several weeks later as well. Approximately 10% of patients *rupture* the ventricular wall at the site of the infarct. Of course, *congestive heart failure* is one of the more common long-term effects of infarction (Fig. 3–33).

Left ventricular *mural thrombi* have been detected at autopsy in 30 to 60% of patients with transmural infarctions.[116] These thrombi may be diagnosed using the noninvasive technique of echocardiography.[117]

Anterior transmural infarcts may undergo a regional expansion that results in further deterioration, cardiac dilatation, the development of congestive heart failure, and an increased mortality rate. The generalized dilatation of the left ventricle may leave regional myocardial oxygen demands unfulfilled, making it impossible to contain the infarct size.[118] Risk of ischemic expansion begins 3 days after infarction and continues through the first 14 days, when infarcts are structurally weakest and necrotic, and when little scar tissue is present. Most cardiac ruptures occur at this time and may be associated with *cardiac tamponade*. *Ventricular aneurysm* formation may develop as an alternative to rupture.

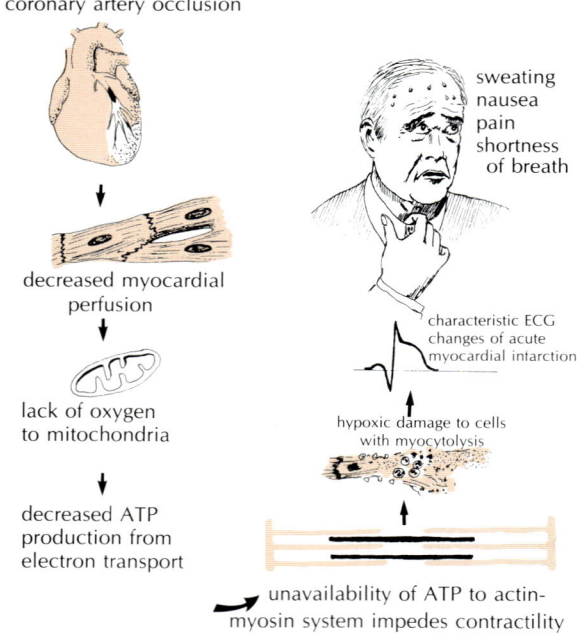

coronary artery occlusion

decreased myocardial perfusion

lack of oxygen to mitochondria

decreased ATP production from electron transport

unavailability of ATP to actin-myosin system impedes contractility

sweating
nausea
pain
shortness
of breath

characteristic ECG changes of acute myocardial infarction

hypoxic damage to cells with myocytolysis

Figure 3–33. Cellular injury results in a dynamic spectrum of changes from the molecular level up to clinical signs and symptoms.

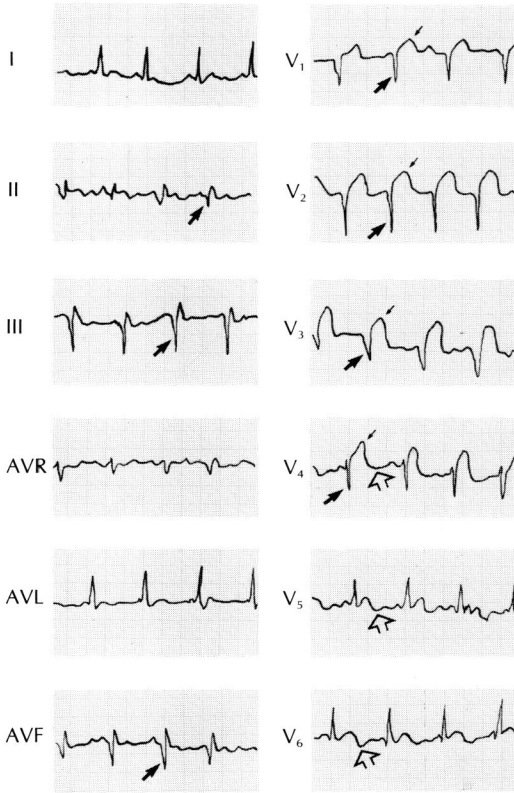

Figure 3–34. Electrocardiogram taken from a patient with acute inferior infarction resulting from occlusion of the left anterior descending coronary artery. Note the significant Q waves in leads II, III, AVF, V₁, V₂, V₃, and V₄ (arrows). ST segments are elevated in V₁ to V₄ (small arrows) and inverted T waves are present in V₄, V₅, and V₆ (open arrows).

Diagnostic Tests

Electrocardiographic Evidence. In general, abnormalities in the *Q, ST,* and *T waves* are taken as the only reliable indicator of an acute MI (Fig. 3–34); in general, the degree of the *ST segment elevation* correlates with the degree of decreased blood flow in the underlying myocardium,[87] and also myocardial metabolism. If rigid criteria are applied in the evaluation of these ECG changes, then only 62 to 82% of acute infarcts are diagnosed. Transmural infarcts that are small and are located in areas not usually discerned by the precordial leads may escape detection.

Biochemical Enzymes. Injured myocardial cells release enzymes, and their levels gradually rise in the hours following acute myocardial infarction, reach a peak, and then fall progressively (Table 3–23). The three enzymes usually measured are serum glutamic oxaloacetic transaminase *(SGOT), LDH* (especially LDH_1), and *CPK.* The LDH and SGOT levels may be elevated in a variety of other disorders, especially those affecting the liver, skeletal muscle, and blood. Therefore, they are not specific for myocardial ischemia.

Table 3–23. *Increased Serum Enzyme Changes in Myocardial Infarction*

Serum glutamic oxaloacetic transaminase (SGOT)
Lactic dehydrogenase (especially LDH_1)
Creatine phosphokinase (especially CPK_2)

The MB fraction of *CPK (CPK_2)* in recent years has become especially helpful in assessing acute infarction and in interpreting elevations of the less specific SGOT and LDH enzymes. An excellent correlation exists between the size of the infarct measured by CPK disappearance and other methods of quantifying the infarction.[119] A number of radionuclide and radiologic techniques can also be used to quantify the degree and effects of cardiac ischemia.

Therapy

The origin of myocardial infarcts is important when considering therapy (Table 3–24). If thrombosis is considered to be the principal cause of infarction, then *anticoagulation* prophylaxis and treatment appear to be logical approaches. Recent studies indicating beneficial effects of aspirin anticoagulation therapy in these regimens have been challenged.

Table 3–24. *Therapy in Myocardial Infarct*

Drugs
Dopamine
Nitroglycerin
Propranolol
Digitalis
Quinidine
Streptokinase

Surgical Procedures
Coronary artery bypass
Thrombectomy-embolectomy
Pacemaker implantation
Intra-aortic balloon pump implantation (with failure)

If coronary artery spasm superimposed on an existing atherosclerotic plaque is critical, then other therapeutic techniques emerge, such as the administration of *coronary vasodilators* (for example, nitroglycerin). The benefits of pharmacotherapeutics in infarction must be weighed against normally operative physiologic factors in repair. For example, propranolol, a drug used in the therapy of infarcts, may also block β-2 receptors that induce vasodilatation and thereby further reduce oxygen tension.

Coronary artery bypass has been used to treat the symptoms and objective findings of myocardial ischemia (angina pectoris). Angina may be relieved and myocardial ischemia reversed by this technique, but its effect on myocardial infarction, ventricular function, and survival is still controversial.[120]

Use of *cardiac pacemakers* in patients with continued conduction abnormalities often improves cardiac performance. In the immediate postinfarction period, oxygen and metabolic regulation of production of lactic acid and other by-products of ischemia, by administration of glucose and carefully titrated electrolytes, are frequently crucial.

Improved cardiac output through newer methods such as *intra-aortic balloon pump* and maintenance of systemic blood pressure through pressor agents, such as *dopamine*, are indicated in individual cases.

INFECTIOUS AGENTS

General Effects of Infection

The major group of infectious agents includes *bacteria, viruses, fungi, protozoa, metazoa* (worms), *chlamydiae,* and *rickettsiae* (Fig. 3–35A, B, C). They are associated with inflammatory (acute and chronic), hyperplastic, hypertrophic, and atrophic reactions. Latent effects may occur many years after the initial infection. Passenger symbiotic relationships may also be established with the host cells.

Most infections are subclinical, inapparent, and never result in any overt signs or symptoms. The ability of an

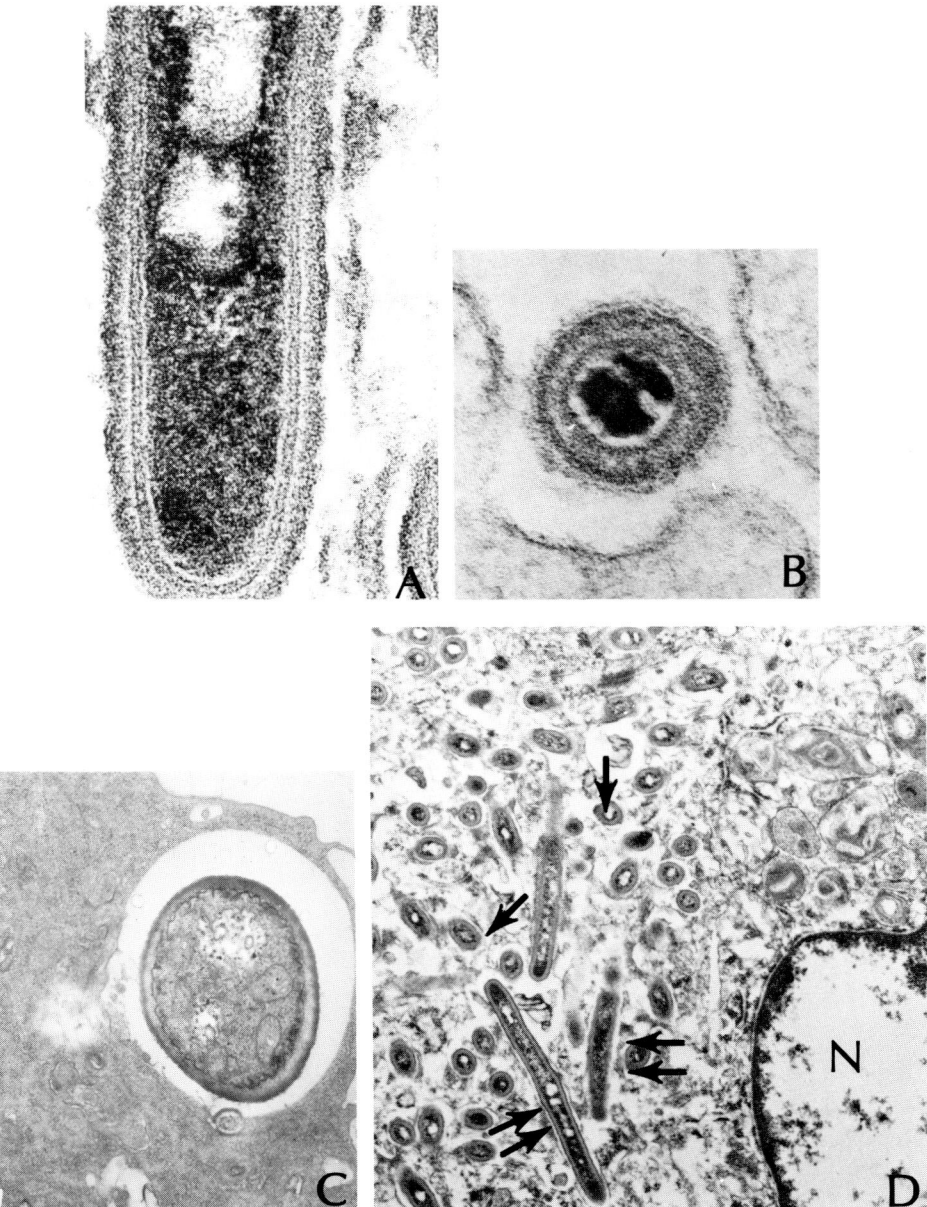

Figure 3–35. Three classes of infectious agents. *A,* Rod-shaped bacillus. *B,* Herpes virus particle. *C,* Yeast. *D,* Intracellular bacilli fill the cytoplasm of this cell. The nucleus (N) is free of organisms. The bacilli are cut in longitudinal (double arrows) as well as cross section (single arrows). (*B,* Courtesy of Dr. C. Morgan, National Research Council, Washington, D.C., and *D,* from Mansbach, C.M., II, Shelburne, J.D., Stevens, R.D., and Dobbins, W.O., III: Lymph-node bacilliform bodies resembling those of Whipple's disease in a patient without intestinal involvement. Ann. Intern. Med., *89:*64, 1978.)

agent to infect the host is determined by the number *(dosage),* *virulence (pathogenicity),* and *portal of entry* of the organism. *Local host factors,* including pH, oxygen concentration, nutrition, and resistance status are also important. More general determinants of *host resistance* include age, the presence of other diseases or infectious agents, climate, geography, social mores, and the general psychologic status of the patient.[121]

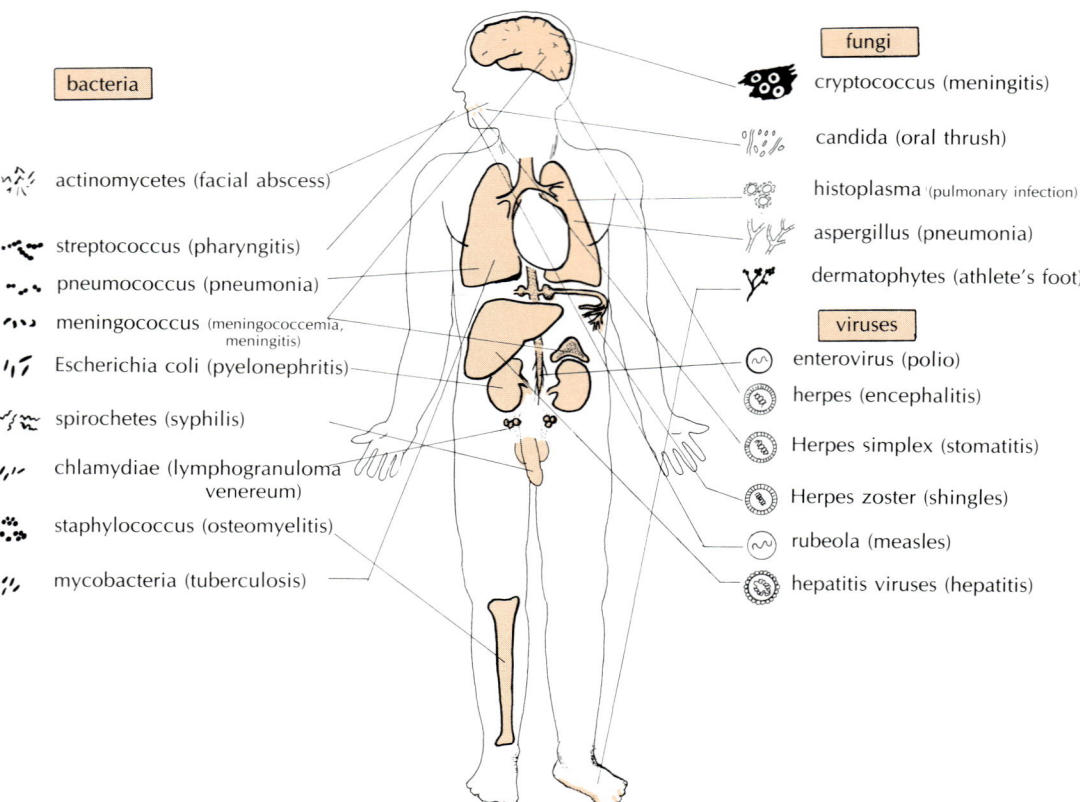

bacteria

⚡ actinomycetes (facial abscess)

🔸 streptococcus (pharyngitis)

🔹 pneumococcus (pneumonia)

🔹 meningococcus (meningococcemia, meningitis)

⚡ Escherichia coli (pyelonephritis)

⚡ spirochetes (syphilis)

⚡ chlamydiae (lymphogranuloma venereum)

⚡ staphylococcus (osteomyelitis)

⚡ mycobacteria (tuberculosis)

fungi

⚫ cryptococcus (meningitis)

⚫ candida (oral thrush)

⚫ histoplasma (pulmonary infection)

Y aspergillus (pneumonia)

Y dermatophytes (athlete's foot)

viruses

◯ enterovirus (polio)

◉ herpes (encephalitis)

◉ Herpes simplex (stomatitis)

◉ Herpes zoster (shingles)

◯ rubeola (measles)

◉ hepatitis viruses (hepatitis)

Figure 3–36. Tropism of infectious organisms in human disease.

Site of Infection

Infectious agents may be present on the skin surface, in vascular and extracellular spaces, or within the cell. They enter through natural body orifices, traumatic breaks in the skin surface, or iatrogenic routes such as through catheters, intravenous infusions, or surgical incisions.

All viruses, protozoa, rickettsiae, and chlamydiae are *obligate intracellular organisms* (Fig. 3–35D) and must be present inside the cell in order for infection to occur. Mycobacteria are found predominantly intracellularly. Many bacteria, fungi, and metazoa are found in both extra- and intracellular sites however. Many infectious agents are *organotropic.* For example, hepatitis viruses have a predilection for infecting the liver, and polio- and rabies viruses infect the central nervous system[122] (Fig. 3–36).

Host Responses: Cellular

Host defenses against infectious agents are many and varied. Initial barriers to infection include the skin and *epithelial linings* of the gastrointestinal, respiratory, and reproductive tracts. Within these barriers, local *IgA antibodies* may be present, especially in the mucous membranes. Many organisms have capsules or membranes that induce the formation of *humoral antibody* by the host. These antibodies may lyse bacteria and viruses, inhibit their entrance into host cells, enhance their phagocytosis by white blood cells, and neutralize bacterial toxins. In addition to stimulating production of humoral antibodies, many of the organisms provoke a cellular immune response.

Phagocytosis, that ubiquitous defense mechanism against intrusion of foreign substances, is assisted by *opsonins* in the plasma (C1, IgG, IgM) that coat the surfaces of invading organisms. Following transfer of the organism into the phagolysosomes of macrophages and PMN, the infectious agent is degraded by hydrolytic enzymes or by *myeloperoxidase reactions* generating hydrogen peroxide and free radicals.

Host Responses: Tissue

Acute and chronic inflammatory reactions are associated with transudation of plasma proteins, emigration of PMN and, later, monocytic cells, and production of antibodies. The activation and release of cellular lysosomal and plasma proteolytic enzymes, critical in the destruction of infectious agents, depend on local tissue factors such as the vascular and oxygen supply and indigenous populations of lymphoreticular cells.

Host Responses: Systemic

Depending on the severity of the infection, many compensatory systemic reactions occur that may also aid in the diagnosis of an infection. Hematologic examination may show an increase in white blood cells *(leukocytosis).* Increased numbers of *PMN* are commonly seen in most bacterial infections, except those caused by mycobacteria. Increased numbers of *monocytes* and *lymphocytes* are prominent with viral, fungal, parasitic and metazoal infections. *Basophilia* in the peripheral blood is seen rarely. *Eosinophils* are increased in parasitic infections and in allergic responses.

The walls of many dead organisms contain lipopolysaccharide *endotoxins* that may stimulate a *pyrogenic* response (fever). Altered host metabolism or bacterial pyrogens may cause an increase in cardiac output with *tachycardia.* A patient's dietary intake is often reduced in infection, and the resultant *hypoglycemia* may be accentuated by altered host metabolism and altered transport mechanisms among various body compartments. For example, the blood-brain barrier may be altered in meningitis and may influence handling of infectious organisms by tissue as well as delivery of antimicrobial agents to tissue. Infection may provoke a *negative nitrogen balance* that is prominent in, and contributory to, the debilitation seen in many chronic diseases.

Bacterial Infection

General Characteristics

Bacteria are usually divided into two groups by their staining reaction with the Gram stain and are described as *gram-positive* and *gram-negative* organisms. They are also classified by their growth characteristics and shape: *bacilli* (rod-shaped) and *cocci* (spherical). Other classification schemes depend on the ability of bacteria to metabolize certain substrates and to undergo specific fermentation reactions (Table 3–25). Their growth can be characterized in regard to requirements of temperature and concentrations of oxygen and different types of media, as well as in their ability to produce endospores.

Table 3–25. *Principal Groups of Pathogenic Bacteria*

	Genera
Flexible, thin-walled cells, motility with axial filament	
Spirochetes	Treponema
	Borrelia
	Leptospira
Rigid, thick-walled cells with flagella	
Mycelial (actinomycetes)	Mycobacterium
	Actinomyces
	Nocardia
	Streptomyces
Simple unicellular	
Lacking cell walls	Mycoplasma
Possessing cell walls	
Obligate intracellular parasites	Rickettsia
	Chlamydia
Free-living	
Gram-positive	
Cocci	Streptococcus
	Diplococcus
	Staphylococcus
Nonsporulating rods	Corynebacterium
	Listeria
Sporulating rods	
Obligate aerobes	Bacillus
Obligate anaerobes	Clostridium
Gram-negative	
Cocci	Neisseria
Nonenteric rods	
Spiral forms	Spirillum
Straight, small rods	Pasteurella
	Brucella
	Haemophilus
	Bordetella
Enteric rods	Escherichia
	Salmonella
	Shigella
	Klebsiella
	Proteus
	Vibrio
	Pseudomonas

(Modified from Jawetz, E., Melnick, J.L., and Adelberg, E.A.: Review of Medical Microbiology. Los Altos, CA, Lange Medical Publications, 1976.)

Damage to the Host Cell

Bacteria may be *virulent* or *avirulent* and *pathogenic* or *nonpathogenic,* depending on host and environmental factors. A bacterium is considered to be virulent and pathogenic when it has at least one of two properties, *invasive capacity* and *toxicity.* Bacteria release a variety of extracellular enzymes that, depending on strain and virulence, enable them to invade host tissue. Enzymes released include hemolysin, hyaluronidase, collagenase, fibrinolysin, coagulase, and various kinases. In addition, bacteria may have resistant capsules (for example, pneumococcal polysaccharide or coat protein of group A streptococcus) that prevent phagocytosis and destruction by host cells.

Toxins

Endotoxin. Bacterial toxicity, as alluded to earlier, is often associated with an *endo-* or *exotoxin. Endotoxins,* derived from the polysaccharide capsule of the organism, are generally less toxic than exotoxins, but may induce fever and occasionally endotoxic shock with DIC.[123]

Exotoxin. *Exotoxins* are synthesized intracellularly, are secreted extracellularly, are often extremely toxic, and are sometimes lethal in small quantities.[124] Most organisms that produce potent exotoxins are not capable of invasion; an exception is the streptococcus.

Some exotoxins are capable of causing serious damage to cells at great distances from the site of the initial infection (Table 3–26). These include lecithinase from Clostridium perfringens, which produces its cytolytic effect by binding membrane phosphorylcholine. The exotoxin of Corynebacterium diphtheriae prevents the elongation of peptide chains by binding elongation factor (EF_2). Tetanus toxin of Clostridium tetani binds gangliosides of nerve cells, is anticholinergic, and blocks inhibitory synapses; these actions result in uncontrolled, generalized muscle spasm. The toxin of Clostridium botulinum is also anticholinergic either at

Table 3–26. *Bacterial Exotoxins*

Organism (Disease)	Toxin	Action
Corynebacterium diphtheriae (Diphtheria)	Diphtheria toxin	Inhibits protein synthesis
Vibrio cholerae (Cholera)	Enterotoxin	Fluid loss from intestinal cells
Clostridium botulinum (Botulism)	Neurotoxin	Paralysis
C. tetani (Tetanus)	Neurotoxin	Paralysis
C. perfringens (Gas gangrene, food poisoning)	Lecithinase	Hemolysis
	θ-toxin	Cardiotoxin
	κ-toxin	Collagenase
	λ-toxin	Protease
Staphylococcus (Pyogenic and respiratory infections)	α-, β-, λ-, δ-toxin	Hemolysis, leukolysis
(Enteritis)	Enterotoxin	Induces vomiting, diarrhea
Streptococcus pyogenes (Pyogenic infections, tonsillitis, scarlet fever)	Streptolysin	Hemolysis
	Erythrogenic toxin	Scarlet fever rash

(Modified from Brock, T.: Biology of Microorganisms. Englewood Cliffs, NJ, Prentice-Hall, 1974.)

myoneural junctions or at spinal cord synapses. It prevents secretion of acetylcholine by ganglion cells. These effects inhibit deglutition and respiration, with resultant asphyxiation. Vibrio cholerae toxin activates adenylcyclase and stimulates the intestinal secretion of Na^+, Cl^-, and water into the lumen of the gut; these actions cause severe dehydration. It is interesting that although the final inhibitory step of each toxin may be different, the intermediate effect of Corynebacterium diphtheriae, pseudomonas, V. cholerae[125] and E. coli toxin is through an ADP ribosylation stage.

Diphtheria

This disease, principally of children, is caused by the gram-positive, club-shaped Corynebacterium diphtheriae (Fig. 3–37). It is not an *invasive organism* and is rarely found in the blood or intestinal tract, but produces a *fibrinous, pseudomembranous exudate* in the upper respiratory passages associated with edema and sore throat. Occasionally, it causes obstruction and asphyxia. The organism produces a powerful *exotoxin* that affects the heart, liver, kidney (occasionally resulting in failure), CNS, and peripheral nerves.

Exotoxin. Nontoxigenic strains of corynebacterium exist, and Freeman discovered that toxigenicity is correlated with infection of the bacterium by a certain temperate phage. Toxin is only produced in those bacteria that have

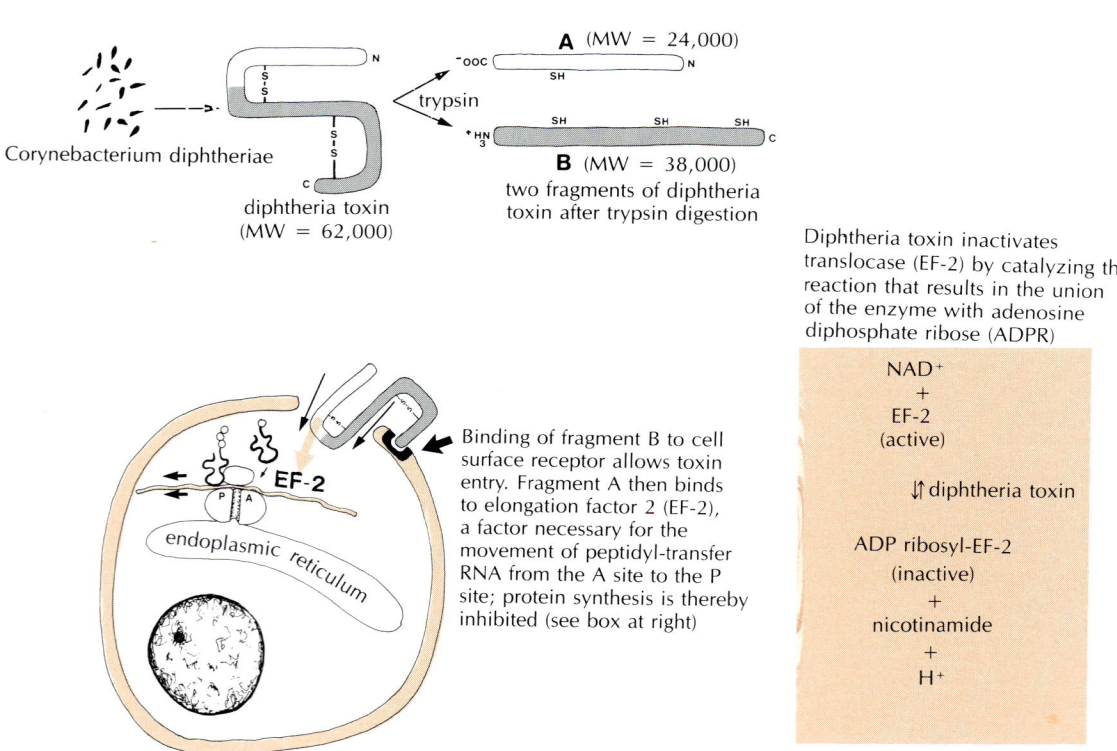

Figure 3–37. Structure and function of diphtheria toxin in inhibition of protein synthesis.

been infected and lysogenized by this β prophage, as only it contains the "tox" gene for the toxin. *Lysogenization* of non-tox-bacterial strains with phage that carry *tox+* gene convert them to toxigenic strains, thereby proving that the structural gene for diphtheria toxin is in the phage genome.

The toxin is a phage protein consisting of a single peptide chain with a molecular weight (MW) of 62,000 daltons, portions of which are linked by 2 disulfide bonds. Fragment A is a peptide of 24,000 MW and carries the toxic portion. Fragment B, a peptide of 38,000 MW, is necessary for attachment of the molecule to the target cell membrane.

Action of Toxin on Target Cells. Diphtheria toxin is transported throughout the body by the blood and lymph, where it attacks most of the cells exposed to it. The *toxin B* portion attaches to *specific receptors* on the cell surface and is transported into the cell by endocytosis. The toxin is broken into fragment A and fragment B is "nicked" when it reaches the cell and binds to the membrane. Alternatively, the nicking may occur intracellularly, perhaps in the endocytic vesicles by lysosomal proteases. *Fragment A* is then released into the cytoplasm, an event promoted by gluthathione. Fragment A *inactivates* the free form *of* EF_2 required for the translocation of peptidyl-tRNA from the acceptor to the donor site on the ribosomes and the subsequent movement of mRNA by one nucleotide triplet. Fragment A catalyzes the transfer of the adenosine diphosphate ribosyl moiety of NAD to itself and thereby inactivates EF_2[126] (Fig. 3–37).

The modified form of EF_2 can still attach to ribosomes and bind GTP, but the toxin interferes with the translation mechanism (Fig. 3–37). EF_2 is usually not the rate-limiting factor for protein synthesis, but when large amounts of EF_2 are inactivated, protein synthesis is inhibited and cell necrosis occurs. One molecule of diphtheria toxin may kill a cell. There is a latent period before maximum toxic activity of approximately five to six hours. In tissue culture, the lethal activity of the toxin can be inhibited by antitoxin given up to an hour following infection. *Ammonium salts abolish* the *toxin's* cytopathologic effects by appearing to block the interaction of the toxin and the cell surface. *Inhibitors* of *energy* metabolism also *block* the effect of the toxin, but cellular proteases do not.

Effects of Toxin on Organism. Multiple *physiologic effects* occur as the result of toxin release into the systemic circulation. These include decreased muscle phosphorylation, decreased ability to metabolize lactic acid, decreased synthesis of carbohydrate, increased resistance to insulin, decreased cardiac capacity, and increased blood potassium levels. The most profound abnormality, however, is the *defect* in *protein synthesis* by the mechanism already explained.

Cellular Morphologic Changes. The structural abnormalities of a cell in which protein synthesis is inhibited depend on the cell's metabolic activity and its ability to degrade the toxin. The heart and CNS both have high rates of metabolism, have highly differentiated cells, and do not have large numbers of lysosomes; however, continual synthesis of protein is essential for effective functioning of the cell. With exposure to the toxin, disaggregation of the ribosomes and hydropic swelling of the ER are noted. The myofibers are distorted in muscle cells, and Nissl substance is lacking in the CNS. The adrenal may be hemorrhagic. The hemorrhage seems to be secondary to endothelial damage with accumulation of glycogen and an increase in endocytic vesicles.

Legionnaire's Disease

Legionnaire's disease came to light during the Bicentennial summer of 1976 when those attending a state American Legion convention at a Philadelphia hotel experienced an epidemic of a respiratory illness with a high mortality rate. The disease, which involved the lungs, kidneys, and CNS, was postulated to be secondary to the production of a toxin. The causative organism is a gram-negative bacillus, *Legionella pneumophila,* and can be readily identified by direct immunofluorescent staining of sputum smears. It has also been identified using standard staining methods for acid-fast bacilli.[127,128]

Viral Infection

Structure

Complete infective viruses *(virions)* consist of a single- or double-stranded nucleic acid core (RNA or DNA *nucleoid)* and an associated capsid protein *(nucleocapsid)* arranged in an *icosahedral* or *helical* form. Nucleocapsids may be surrounded by a *membrane envelope* or may remain as a *"naked"* nucleoprotein molecule (Fig. 3–38). They vary in size from 10 to 300 nm, contain RNA (Table 3–27) or DNA (Table 3–28), and often have associated enzymes necessary for replication. Genetic material in viruses may code for few proteins (5 to 10 in picornavirus) or for many (400 in poxvirus) (Table 3–28).

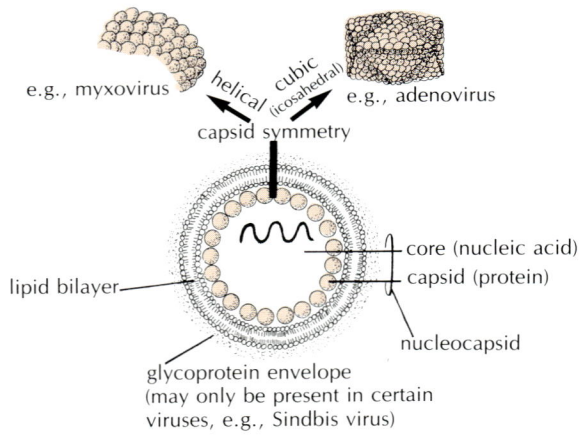

Figure 3–38. Viral particle (virion) components.

Table 3–27. Major RNA Viruses

Generic Name	Strand Nucleic Acid	Number of Genes	Capsid Symmetry	Virion Enveloped or Naked	Size of Viral Particle (nm)
Picornavirus	SS	12	Icosahedral	Naked	20–30
Reovirus	DS segmented	40	Icosahedral	Naked	60–80
Arbovirus Group A Group B Group C Ungrouped	SS	15	Icosahedral	Enveloped	40–70
Myxovirus and Paramyxovirus	SS	30	Helical	Enveloped	150–300
Rhabdovirus	SS	20	Helical	Enveloped	70–175
Coronavirus	SS	30	Unknown or complex	Enveloped	80–130
Arenavirus Tacaribe–LCM	SS	15	Unknown or complex	Enveloped	50–300

(Modified from Jawetz, E., Melnick, J.L., and Adelberg, E.A.: A Review of Medical Microbiology. Los Altos, CA, Lange Medical Publications, 1976; and Thorn, G.W., et al. (Eds.): Harrison's Principles of Internal Medicine. 8th Ed. New York, McGraw-Hill, 1977. Used with permission of McGraw-Hill Book Company.)

Table 3–28. Major DNA Viruses

Generic Name	Strand Nucleic Acid	Number of Genes	Capsid Symmetry	Virion Enveloped or Naked	Size of Viral Particle (nm)
Papovavirus	DS circular	10	Icosahedral	Naked	45–55
Adenovirus	DS	50	Icosahedral	Naked	70–90
Herpesvirus	DS	180	Icosahedral	Enveloped	100
Poxvirus	DS	400	Complex	Complex coats	230–300

(Modified from Jawetz, E., Melnick, J.L., and Adelberg, E.A.: A Review of Medical Microbiology. Los Altos, CA, Lange Medical Publications, 1976; and Thorn, G.W., et al. (Eds.): Harrison's Principles of Internal Medicine. 8th Ed. New York, McGraw-Hill, 1977. Used with the permission of McGraw-Hill Book Company.)

Types of Infection

Two types of viral infection occur. *Productive* infections result in increased numbers of viral progeny, and the cell usually undergoes *lysis*. *Nonproductive (latent)* infection usually occurs only when part of the viral genetic material is replicated in the host cell. *Cytolysis* usually does not occur, and the spectrum of possible host responses is partially dictated by the expression of viral antigens or other functions encoded in the segment of incorporated viral genome.

The normal mechanism of productive viral infection involves: (1) adsorption of virus to membrane, (2) penetration of the membrane, (3) uncoating of virus resulting in release of viral nucleotides in the cytoplasm, (4) synthesis of new nucleoprotein in the cytoplasm or nucleus, (5) assembly of nucleoprotein, and (6) release of the nucleoprotein from the nucleus or cytoplasm.

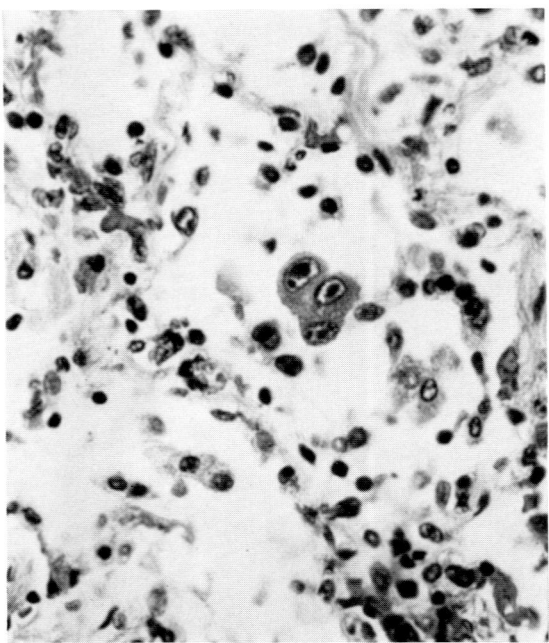

Figure 3–39. Lung of a patient showing viral (influenza) pneumonia. Note the homogeneous intranuclear inclusions in the cells in the center of an alveolar space (center of figure).

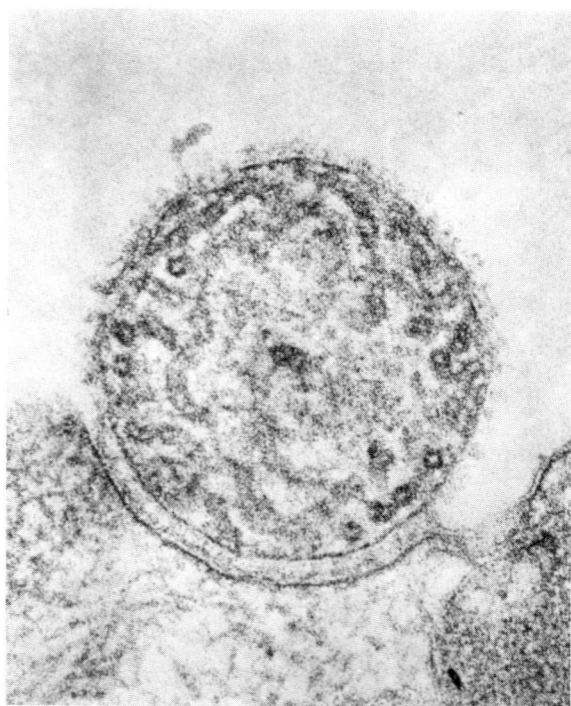

Figure 3–40. In viral attachment, the coat of the virus and the cell (at the bottom of the figure) fuse with each other. (Courtesy of Dr. C. Morgan, National Research Council, Washington, D.C.)

Several methods of viral release are possible. Poliovirus, for example, is released by a sudden burst, whereas in influenza there is a gradual leakage of infectious particles with delayed death of the cell (Fig. 3–39). Measles, herpes-, Sendai, and adenoviruses may promote fusion of cells causing *giant cell* formation.

Influenza Viral Infection

Structure of Virus. One of the best examples of the mechanism of viral infection is demonstrated by influenzal pneumonia caused by a number of influenza viruses, types A, B, and C.[129] The influenza viruses are large (80 to 100 μ in diameter), enveloped viruses containing RNA.

The helical RNA-nucleoprotein core consists of 5 to 7 units, each 1×10^6 in MW, and an associated RNA-dependent RNA polymerase. This core is surrounded by an inner M protein and an outer bilipid membrane. These 3 proteins constitute the complement-fixation antigen. Hydrophobically embedded in the surface bilipid layer are several thousand spikes or projections of 2 types, hemagglutinin (HA) and neuraminidase (NA). The HA spike, an 80,000-dalton-MW trimer (140 × 40 Å), is made up of 3 glycoprotein subunits. Each subunit contains 2 glycopeptides, HA_1 and HA_2, held together by disulfide bonds. The NA spike is a 200,000 to 250,000-dalton-MW polypeptide measuring 85 × 50 Å. It is composed of a centrally attached fiber terminating in a 40-Å tetrameric unit possessing enzymatic activity.[129]

Adsorption and Penetration. Infection is initiated by adsorption (attachment of the viral particle to the cell membrane), which requires an interaction between viral spikes and mucoprotein receptors of the epithelial cell membrane[130] (Fig. 3–40). The analogy between adsorption of virus to erythrocytes in hemagglutination and adsorption of virus to host epithelial cells suggests a similar binding mechanism.

Virus may be bound by sialylation of the HA_1 portion of the HA spike by N-acetyl neuraminic acid residues, terminally attached to the mucoprotein receptor of the host cell membrane. Action of viral neuraminidase may then allow the second stage, penetration, to proceed.

Current evidence suggests two possible mechanisms for viral penetration. The first is viropexis, a process similar to phagocytosis, whereby viral particles are incorporated into pinocytotic vesicles. A second, less likely, alternative is the process of fusion of viral envelope with host cell membrane, followed by injection of ribonucleocapsid into the cytoplasm in a manner similar to phage DNA injection into bacterial cells.

Uncoating, Replication, Assembly, and Release. Following penetration and uncoating, viral RNA is transported to the cell nucleus, where progeny virion RNA are replicated and viral messenger RNA transcribed (Fig. 3–41). Certain nonstructural nucleoproteins associated with viral RNA may be involved in synthesis of new virion RNA. Translation of mRNA for viral envelope and nucleocapsid proteins appears to occur in the cytoplasm in close proximity to the nucleus. Viral envelope proteins, NA and HA, are transported to the cell surface, where they are incorporated into segments of the membrane in preparation for budding of infective viral particles.

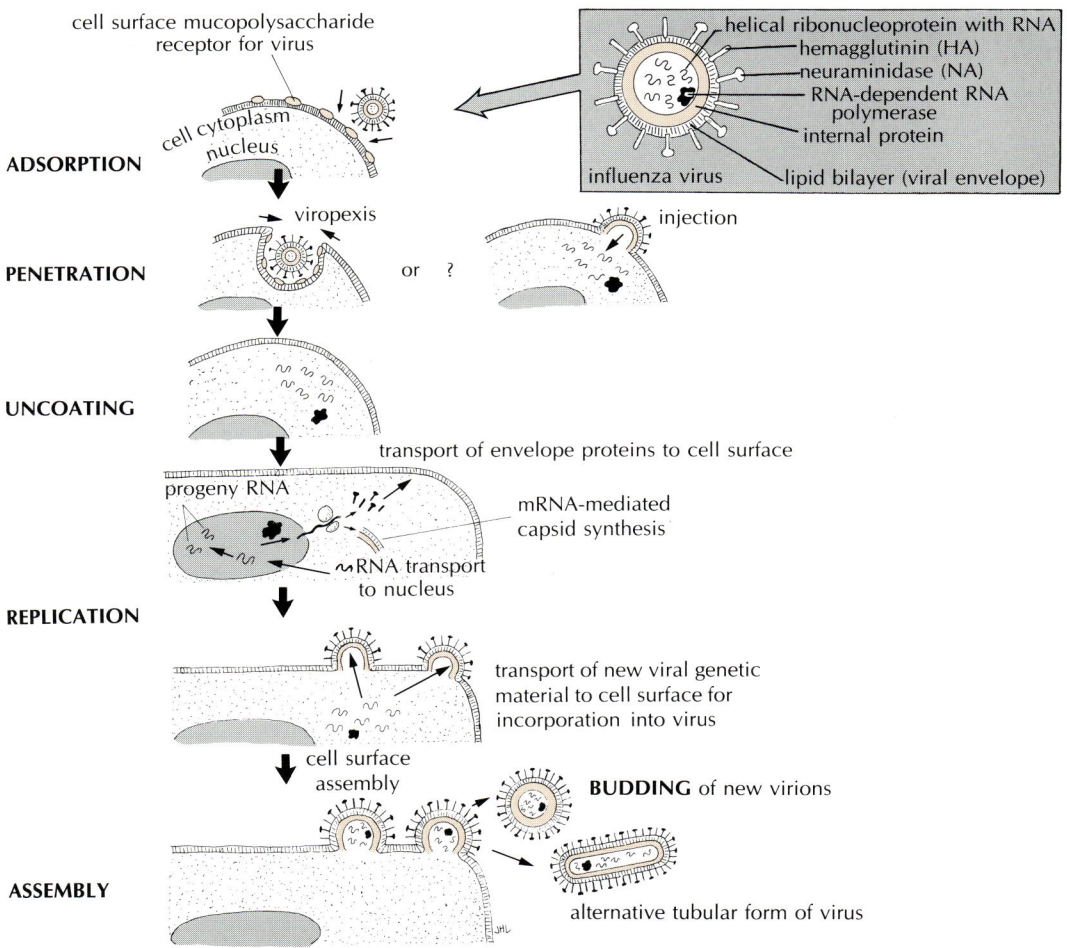

Figure 3–41. Mechanism of influenza viral infection.

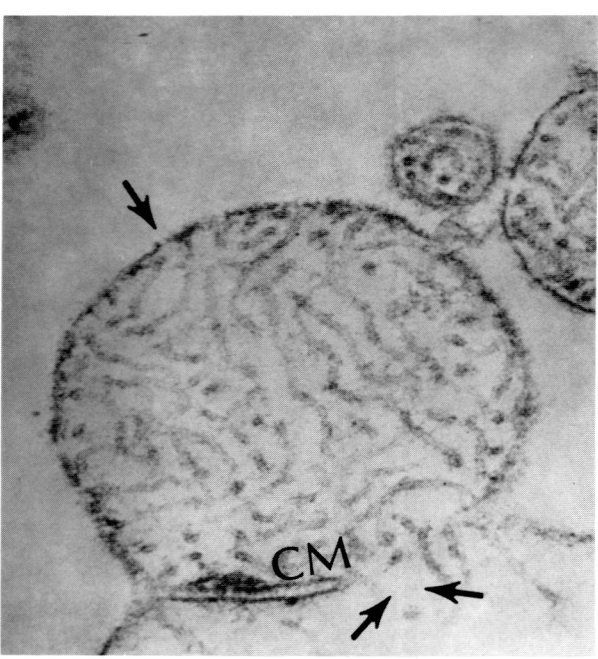

Figure 3–42. The incorporation of influenza virus (long arrow) into tissue culture cell (C) is shown at bottom. Strands of viral genetic material (short arrows) are seen passing through gaps in the cell membrane (CM). (Courtesy of Dr. C. Morgan, National Research Council, Washington, D.C.)

Newly assembled virion RNA nucleocapsids seen initially in the perinuclear cytoplasm are eventually found in proximity to the forming viral envelope at the cell surface, in its five- to seven-subunit segmented form. Budding of spherical infective virions occurs by a pinching off (exocytosis) of RNA-nucleocapsid cores enclosed in viral envelopes. A delay in pinching off the growing virion at the cell surface may result in a filamentous form of virus that may also be infective (Fig. 3–42).

Cell Death

A virus kills a cell by three mechanisms: (1) interfering with DNA, RNA, and protein synthesis of the host (during viral infection; The host often has complete cessation of its DNA synthesis and drastic modification of RNA and protein synthesis); (2) increasing the lability of lysosomal membranes with resultant intracellular hydrolysis; and (3) stimulating formation of viral membrane antigens on host cells that provoke a humoral or cellular immune lytic response.

Incomplete viruses, which may cause abortive infections, may injure cells even though infectious particles are not produced. An example of this type is mumps virus, which possesses a hemolysin capable of lysing chick red blood cells.

Latent and Slow Virus Infection

Although many viruses cause cell death immediately, some cause benign or malignant proliferative lesions in experimental animals. Others persist for a long time in a subclinical state and may or may not cause disease.[131] The group known as *"slow viruses"* causes disease many years after infection (Table 3–29).

Table 3–29. *Slow Virus Infection*

Disease	Host	Target Organ
Kuru	Man	Brain
Subacute sclerosing panencephalitis (SSPE) following measles	Man	Brain
Creutzfeldt-Jakob disease	Man	Brain
Progressive multifocal leukoencephalopathy	Man	Brain
Scrapie	Sheep	Brain
Visna	Sheep	Brain and lung
Maedi	Sheep	Lung
Lymphocytic choriomeningitis (LCM virus)	Mouse/Man	Kidney, brain, and liver
Aleutian mink disease (ADV virus)	Mink	Lymphoreticular system

(Modified from Davis, B., et al.: Microbiology. 2nd Ed. New York, Harper & Row, 1973.)

Two classic examples of slow virus infections are *kuru,* which causes dementia and early death in New Guinea, and *Creutzfeldt-Jakob* disease, which causes encephalopathy many years after infection.

The *herpesviruses* (Table 3–30) also display latency of infection, although these are not classified as slow viruses.[132,133] *Herpes zoster virus,* which causes chickenpox (varicella) in children, may reside for years in ganglion cells[134] and may appear later in life as a painful neuropathy *("shingles").*

Table 3–30. *Herpesvirus Infections*

Virus	Lesion
Herpes zoster	Varicella (chickenpox or shingles)
Herpes simplex 1 (HSV$_1$)	Cold sores in oral cavity ?Nasopharyngeal cancer
Herpes simplex 2 (HSV$_2$)	Infection in genitourinary tract ?Cervical cancer
Epstein-Barr (EBV)	?Burkitt's lymphoma ?Nasopharyngeal carcinoma Infectious mononucleosis
Cytomegalic Inclusion (CMV)	Hepatitis Pneumonitis Chorioretinitis ?Kaposi's sarcoma
Lucké virus	Kidney tumor (frog)
Marek's virus	Lymphoid tumors (chickens)
Herpesvirus saimiri	Tumors (monkeys, rabbits)
Herpesvirus ateles	Tumors (monkeys, rabbits)

Herpes simplex virus 1 *(HSV 1)* (also called Herpesvirus hominis), which primarily infects nongenital sites, especially mucous membranes of the mouth *(cold sores),* and Herpes simplex virus 2 *(HSV 2)* (also called Herpesvirus genitalis), which mainly affects the mucous membranes of the genitourinary tract, especially the cervix, produce infections that may come and go for decades. One-third of the world's population is believed to be infected with HSV 1 and thereby serves as a constant reservoir. *Epstein-Barr virus* (EBV) may produce infectious mononucleosis or may be associated with malignant disease, either nasopharyngeal carcinoma or *Burkitt's lymphoma.*

Cytomegalovirus (CMV), a herpesvirus, causes the most common viral infection of the fetus and the newborn.[135,136] It is estimated that about 40,000 transplacental and 150,000 intrapartum infections are acquired each year in the United States.

Subacute sclerosing panencephalitis (SSPE) has been associated with *measles* virus, possibly following childhood infec-

Table 3–31. *Common Viral Etiologic Agents*

Organ or System Affected	Viral Agent
Upper respiratory tract	Respiratory syncytial, rhino-parainfluenza-, adeno-, entero-, and reoviruses
Lower respiratory tract	Influenza-, adeno-, parainfluenza-, respiratory syncytial-, and rhinoviruses
Pleura	Coxsackie virus
Cutaneous and mucous membranes	Vesicular: smallpox and vaccinia, herpes simplex and varicella/zoster viruses Exanthematous: measles, rubella, and enteroviruses
CNS (acute)	Enterovirus: herpes simplex, mumps, lymphocytic choriomeningitis Arboviruses: western equine encephalitis, eastern equine encephalitis, Venezuelan equine encephalitis; California encephalitis, St Louis encephalitis, Japanese B encephalitis, rabies
CNS (chronic)	Measles (subacute sclerosing panencephalitis), human papovavirus (progressive multifocal leukoencephalopathy)
Parotid glands	Mumps, cytomegalovirus
Multiple organs (congenital anomalies)	Cytomegalic inclusion virus, rubella

tion. There has been considerable discussion as to why, despite adequate humoral antibody titers, infection persists with later clinical sequelae.[137] Similar unanswered questions pertain to herpes, cytomegalic, and rubella viral infections. The spectrum of morbidity and mortality inducible by viruses is vast (Table 3–31).

Diagnosis of Viral Disease

The demonstration of specific viral hemagglutinin antigens adsorbed to red blood cell membranes has proved to be of great diagnostic value in viral diseases. Sera containing antiviral antibodies inhibit viral hemagglutination and form the basis of the hemagglutination tests. A monoclonal fluorescent antibody to particular viral antigens is a further aid in diagnosis. Inclusions, nuclear or cytoplasmic, representing either clusters of virus or remnants related to viral replication, are morphologic aids in diagnosis, as is the electron-microscopic examination.[138]

Fungi

Important fungal infections include candidiasis, aspergillosis, nocardiosis, histoplasmosis, blastomycosis, and coccidioidomycosis.[139]

Fungi exist in both extra- and intracellular sites (Table 3–32). Although they are commonly nonpathogenic saprophytes, they may produce serious infection in debilitated patients. Favorable conditions for these opportunistic infections include increased age of the patient, suppression of normal flora by broad-spectrum antibiotics, compromised host defenses, such as with immunosuppressive drugs, and foreign instrumentation, for example, catheters in the bladder, heart, and vessels.

Table 3–32. *Fungal Infections in Man*

Causal Organism (Disease)	Target Organs
Microsporum audouini (Ringworm)	Scalp of children
Trichophyton schoenleinii (Favus—chronic ringworm)	Scalp
Epidermophyton and other genera (Athlete's foot)	Between toes, skin
Cryptococcus neoformans (Cryptococcosis)	Lungs, meninges
Coccidioides immitis (Coccidioidomycosis)	Lungs
Histoplasma capsulatum (Histoplasmosis)	Lungs
Blastomyces dermatitidis (Blastomycosis)	Lungs, skin
Candida albicans (Candidiasis)	Oral cavity, intestinal tract
Asperigillus fumigatus (Aspergillosis, superficial dermatomycosis)	Bronchi, lung

(Modified from Brock, T.: Biology of Microorganisms. Englewood Cliffs, NJ, Prentice-Hall, 1974.)

Parasites

Parasites include protozoa, metazoa, chlamydiae, and rickettsiae. Common reservoirs of these organisms include pets (cats and dogs), wildlife (rabbits and squirrels), birds (parrots), and insects (fleas, ticks, and mosquitoes).[140,141]

Protozoa

Protozoa are seen throughout the world (Table 3–33), and one of the more pathogenic protozoans, *Entamoeba histolytica*, is responsible for *amebic dysentery.*[142] The infection may be asymptomatic, but dysentery and hepatic abscesses are frequent in non-Western countries.[143] In the United States, another protozoan, *Giardia lamblia*, often found in infected water, causes severe gastrointestinal illness. *Trypanosomiasis*, transmitted by the tsetse fly, affects man *(T.*

Table 3–33. *Protozoan Agents of Infection*

Pneumocystis carinii
Entamoeba histolytica (amebiasis)
Plasmodium species (malaria)
Toxoplasma gondii (toxoplasmosis)
Leishmania species (leishmaniasis)
Giardia lamblia (giardiasis)

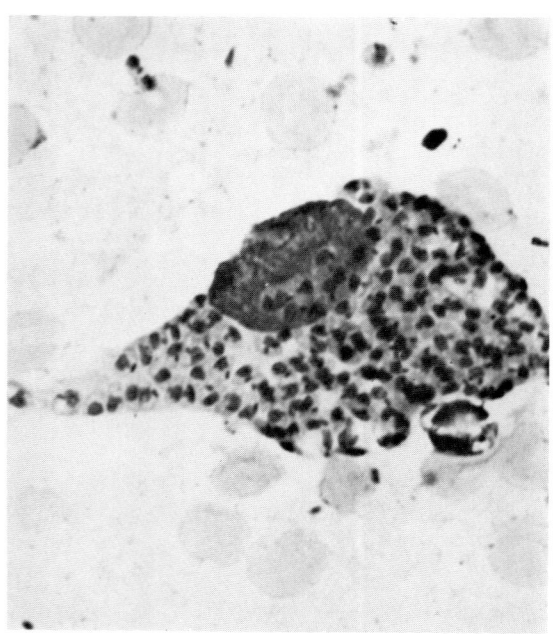

Figure 3–43. Amastigotes of Leishmania tropica in a human macrophage. (Courtesy of Dr. K. Dixon, University of Cambridge, England.)

cruzi) and domestic animals *(T. brucei)* in a devastating manner.[144] Immunocompromised hosts are at particular risk for respiratory infection by the protozoan *Pneumocystis carinii.*

Leishmaniasis. This parasitic disease of man is caused by four principal organisms with specific tissue tropism: *L. donovani,* which causes visceral leishmaniasis involving the reticuloendothelial system including liver, spleen, and bone marrow; *L. braziliensis,* the cause of mucocutaneous leishmaniasis, which involves the skin and mucous membranes; and *L. mexicana* and *L. tropica,* causing cutaneous leishmaniasis involving the integument[146,147] (Fig. 3–43).

Malaria. This common disease affects over 15 million people in the world. It is principally disseminated by the anopheline mosquito. The most serious and malignant type of tertiary malaria is caused by *Plasmodium falciparum.* Two benign types of tertiary malaria are caused by *P. vivax* and *P. ovale.* Quartan malaria is caused by *P. malariae.* Simian malaria, caused by *P. knowlesi,* is the most commonly studied experimental infection (Table 3–34).

Table 3–34. *Malarial Parasites and Their Characteristic Infections*

Agent	Type of Malaria
Plasmodium falciparum	Tertiary, malignant
Plasmodium vivax	Tertiary, benign
Plasmodium ovale	Tertiary, benign
Plasmodium malariae	Quartan
Plasmodium knowlesi	Simian

Malaria is an acute, often protracted disease in which the main symptoms include fever, anemia, and splenomegaly. The febrile paroxysms are preceded by shivering and are followed by sweating. They may often occur at regular intervals on alternate days *(tertiary)*, with an interval of two days *(quartan)*, or daily *(quotidian)*.

Life Cycle. In man, sporozoites are introduced into the blood by the bite of an infected anopheline mosquito. The asexual reproductive phase of the parasite begins in human tissues, especially the liver, where multiplication *(schizogony)* occurs. Following five to seven days of division, the cell ruptures, freeing several thousand merozoites into the circulation. These *merozoites* enter red blood cells and start intraerythrocytic asexual multiplication; the merozoites develop into male and female cells *(gametocytes)*.

Following a subsequent mosquito bite, the gametocytes are ingested by the female mosquito, and the sexual portion of the life cycle starts in the cytocyst on the outer wall of her stomach. Here gametocytes mature and produce a zygote that releases hundreds of *sporozoites* into the body cavity of the mosquito; these sporozoites quickly travel to the salivary gland. When the mosquito bites the skin of a human, the organism is again transmitted (Fig. 3–44).

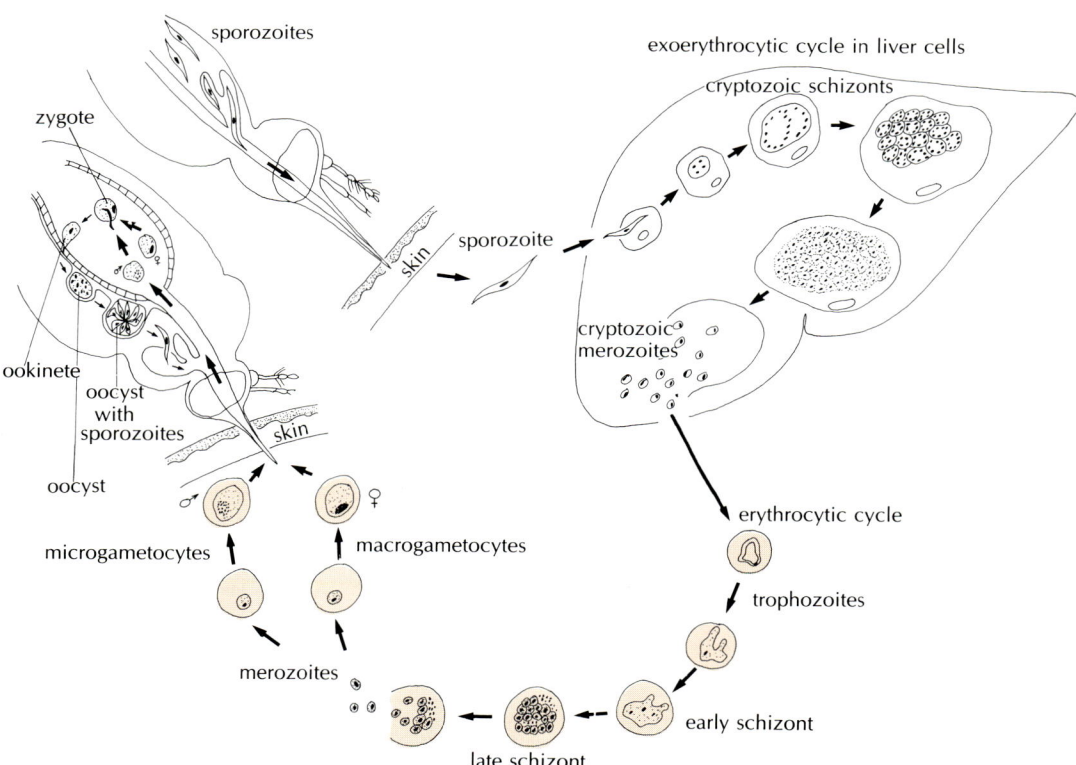

Figure 3–44. Malaria life cycle in man and mosquito. (Modified from Brown, H.W.: Basic Clinical Parasitology. 3rd Ed. New York, Appleton-Century-Crofts, 1969.)

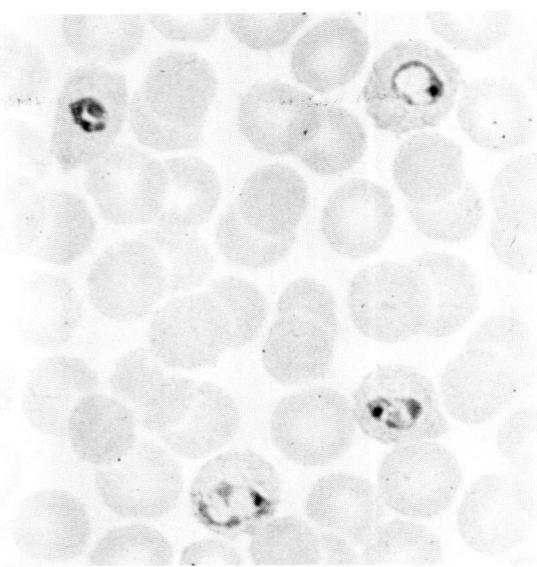

Figure 3–45. The ring stage of Plasmodium vivax in red blood cells. (Courtesy of Dr. D. Despommier, Division of Tropical Medicine, School of Public Health, Columbia University, New York.)

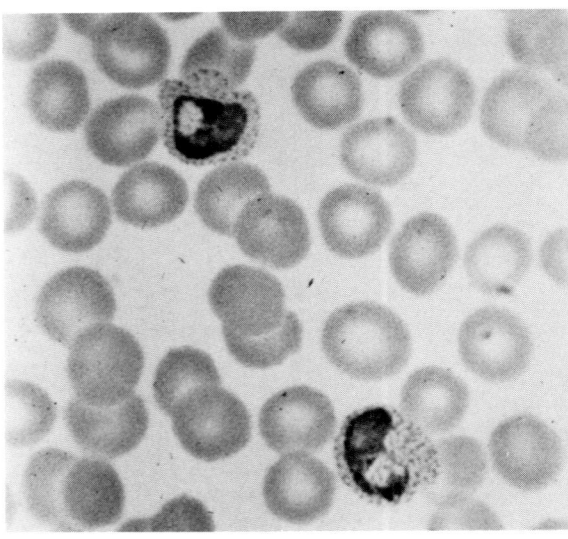

Figure 3–46. Trophozoites of Plasmodium vivax in red blood cells. (Courtesy of Dr. D Despommier, Division of Tropical Medicine, School of Public Health, Columbia University, New York.)

Parasites in Red Blood Cells. Plasmodia (Figs. 3–45 and 3–46) are characterized by their limited host range. Some plasmodia have specificity for certain subpopulations within a species (resistance of blacks to P. vivax) or a preference for a particular age of red blood cell (preference of P. vivax for reticulocytes). It may be that this host specificity is determined by a specific receptor on red blood cell surfaces. That chymotrypsin- and pronase-treated human red blood cells are refractory to invasion by P. knowlesi supports the theory that a specific receptor protein or lipoprotein is destroyed by the enzyme.

Attachment Sites. Dvorak and Miller reported that one group of parasites attaches at one point on the membrane of the red blood cell, but only on human red blood cells that have a *Duffy positive blood* type Fy[a] or Fy[b]. Human red blood cells with a negative Duffy type (FyFy) are resistant to infection of P. knowlesi.[148] The parasite receptor is either identical with, or genetically associated with, the Duffy blood group. This finding may explain malarial resistance in West Africa, where many people have a negative Duffy blood group.

Another factor that influences the fate of the parasite in man is the presence of antimalarial antibodies. These are IgG molecules that coat the exocytic parasites, but not the intracellular ones. Immune serum agglutinates the merozoites of P. knowlesi, and these agglutinated merozoites have the capacity to attach to, but not to invade, red blood cells. This agglutination is immunologically specific and appears to be directed at the surface coat of the parasite.[149]

Change in Membrane Structure. Certain plasmodia alter the surface properties of the parasitized erythrocytes, so that they adhere to venular and capillary endothelial cells. P. falciparum and P. coatneyi are characterized by marked sequestration of the parasitized red blood cells in the venules of heart and other tissues. Ultrastructurally, these red blood cells have 100-nm knob-like protrusions on their membranes that are the points of attachment to the underlying endothelium.

P. malariae and P. brasilianum, which are not characterized by deep vascular schizogony, also have demonstrable knobs on the membranes of the parasitized red blood cells. In addition to the knobs, there are also changes in the membrane-associated enzymes, proteins, and glycoproteins of the infected versus the noninfected red blood cells.[150]

Multiplication of Parasites. Once inside the red blood cells, parasites develop into a multinucleated schizont that contains many merozoites attached to a residual body. These merozoites rupture the cell membrane and invade other red blood cells. This process happens every two to three days and is responsible for the chills and fever. The complication of malaria known as blackwater fever, with jaundice and dark urine, is believed to result from a "crisis" hemolytic state.

Following multiplication in the red blood cell, the parasite is capable of carrying on all the intermediary metabolic reactions of any free-living cell. In the extracellular state, the parasite is unable to synthesize many necessary factors including the coenzymes for metabolic reactions. The plasmodium parasite obtains most of its amino acids by phagocytosing small portions of the red blood cell cytoplasm. It then secretes hydrolytic proteinases into the segregated vacuole that degrade the hemoglobin to amino acids while the iron pigment is converted to malarial pigment.[151]

The knobs of the red blood cell membrane, previously discussed, may enhance attachment to endothelium and may cause sludging of blood flow. Attachment of antibody-coated parasites to the red blood cell may promote phagocytosis. Furthermore, some evidence suggests that the decreased deformability of the parasitized red blood cells may lead to entrapment in the reticuloendothelial system and small capillaries in a manner analogous to that in sickle cell anemia.

Clinicopathologic Correlations. Extensive organelle damage may occur in the cells of the host, especially hepatocytes (Table 3–35). These changes consist principally of mitochondrial damage and the release of acid hydrolases from the lysosomes. The endoplasmic reticulum (ER) becomes disrupted and vesiculated, and the mitochondria are completely destroyed.[152] Red blood cells infected with certain plasmodia enlarge and develop small, reddish dots seen with the *Romanowsky stain.* These are known as *Schüffner's dots.* Ultrastructurally, they appear to be pinocytotic vesicles containing malarial antigens.

Table 3–35. *Clinicopathologic Correlations of Malaria*

Signs or Symptoms	Lesions
Anemia	Decreased erythroid precursors in erythropoietic production
	Extramedullary hematopoiesis
	Intravascular hemolysis by parasites
	Phagocytosis of RBC by lymphoreticular system
	Schüffner's dots
Splenomegaly	Infarcts associated with microthrombi
Fever	Release of parasites from red blood cells

Anemia is associated with decreased erythroid precursors in the bone marrow, increased erythropoietin production, and extramedullary hematopoiesis. The host cannot keep up with the red cell destruction. Anemia, splenomegaly, intravascular hemolysis, hemoglobinuria, and renal complications are especially prominent in acute tertiary malaria.

The kidney lesions are related to circulating soluble immune complexes. Such complexes increase vascular permeability and cause acute vasculitis and glomerulonephritis.[153]

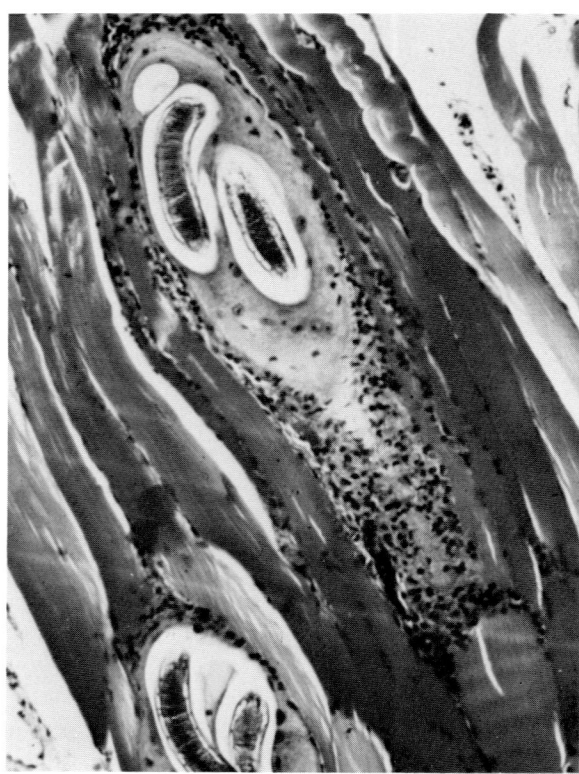

Figure 3–47. Trichinella is shown encysted in skeletal muscle. (Courtesy of Dr. D. Despommier, Division of Tropical Medicine, School of Public Health, Columbia University, New York.)

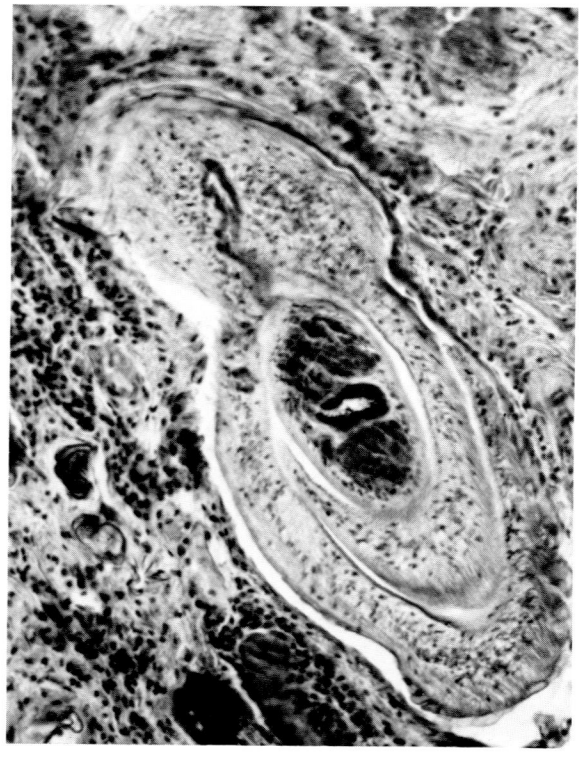

Figure 3–48. Cross section through a schistosome.

Metazoa

Among the metazoans (Table 3–36), the worm *Ascaris* is responsible for malnutrition in several areas of the world. *Trichinosis* (Fig. 3–47) is probably the most important metazoan disease in the United States.[154] *Filariasis* has fascinated parasitologists because of the complex life cycle of filaria and their unusual location in lymphatics.

Schistosomiasis is produced by three major forms of blood flukes.[155] Schistosoma japonicum, S. mansoni, and S. haematobium produce allergic, hepatic, pulmonary, and bladder infections (Fig. 3–48). S. haematobium infection in Egypt is associated with a high incidence of bladder cancer. Shifts in ecology induced by technologic advances, such as altered paths of water flow with the building of dams, have also produced recent changes within populations of schistosome organisms in endemic countries.

Table 3–36. *Types of Metazoa*

Organism (Disease)	Lesions
Ascaris lumbricoides (ascariasis)	Pulmonary, spleen, liver, lymph node
Flukes (e.g., schistosomiasis or bilharziasis)	Intestinal, visceral
Schistosoma mansoni	Intestinal, visceral
S. japonicum	Bladder
S. haematobium	Visceral, intestinal
S. intercalatum	
Wuchereria bancrofti (filariasis)	Lymph vessel and node
Enterobius vermicularis (pinworm) (enterobiasis)	Cecum, ileum, and appendix
Trichuris trichiura (whipworm) (trichuriasis)	Ileum, cecum
Strongyloides stercoralis (strongyloidiasis)	Duodenum, jejunum
Trichinella spiralis (trichinosis)	Muscle, lung, brain
Cestodes (tapeworm) (cestodiasis)	Skin, muscle, heart, brain, liver, lungs, eyes
Taenia saginata (cysticercosis)	
T. solium (pork tapeworm) (cysticercosis)	Intestine
Hymenolepis nana (dwarf tapeworm)	
Diphyllobothrium latum (fish tapeworm)	
Echinococcus granulosus (dog tapeworm)	Liver, lung, bone, brain, intestine

Chlamydiae

The classic *chlamydial* infections (Table 3–37) include *lymphogranuloma venereum, ornithosis, psittacosis,* and *trachoma.*[156] This last disease is a leading cause of blindness in underdeveloped nations, often in an acquired, congenital or childhood infection. The parasites in the adult inhabit the genital tract, with resultant venereal disease.

Table 3–37. Classification of Chlamydia

Species	Disease
C. psittaci	Psittacosis
C. trachomatis	Lymphogranuloma venereum
C. trachomatis (A, B, Ba, C)	Hyperendemic blinding trachoma
C. trachomatis (D, E, F, G, H, I, J, K)	Inclusion conjunctivitis (adult and newborn), nongonococcal urethritis, cervicitis, salpingitis, proctitis, epididymitis, and pneumonia of newborns

(Modified from Schachter, J.: Chlamydial infections. N. Engl. J. Med., 298:428, 1978.)

Characteristics of the Organism. *Chlamydiae* are organisms, with a particle size of approximately 250 to 500 nm, believed by some to be a subspecies of gram-negative bacteria. They are *obligate intracellular parasites* that produce characteristic cytoplasmic inclusions in susceptible host cells. They differ from viruses in their possession of bacterial-type cell walls with muramic acid and mucopeptides, in the presence of ribosomes, and in their susceptibility to many antimicrobial drugs. They possess group-specific complement-fixation antigens and are capable of synthesizing folic acid, lysine, and muramic acid, in contrast to their host. Enzymes capable of synthesizing nucleic acid and protein are present, but energy-generating enzymes are apparently absent.

Rickettsiae

Rickettsiae are also obligate intracellular parasites (Table 3–38). Major diseases such as *Q fever, typhus fever, scrub*

Table 3–38. Diseases of Rickettsiae

Organism	Disease	Area Affected	Insect Vector
Typhus group			
R. prowazekii	Epidemic primary typhus fever	Skin, CNS	Louse
	Brill-Zinsser disease	Skin, CNS (milder)	Louse
R. typhi	Murine typhus	Skin, CNS (milder)	Louse, flea
Spotted-Fever group			
R. rickettsii	Rocky Mountain spotted fever	Skin, brain, muscle, lungs, kidney, testes, heart	Tick
R. tsutsugamushi	Scrub typhus	Skin, brain, muscle, lungs, kidney, testes, heart	Mite
R. burneti (Coxiella burnetii)	Q fever	Lungs, heart (endocarditis), liver (granuloma)	Tick, contaminated dust or milk

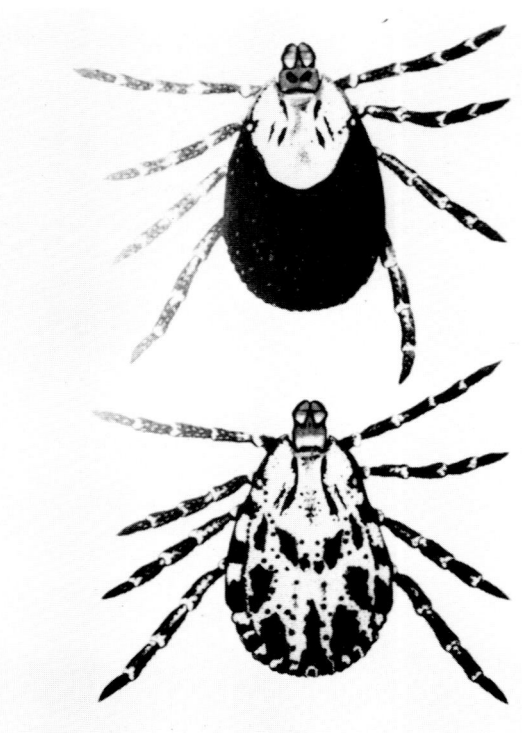

Figure 3–49. Male and female hard ticks, Dermacentor andersoni, vectors of the rickettsial disease Rocky Mountain spotted fever. (Courtesy of Dr. R. Williams, Division of Tropical Medicine, School of Public Health, Columbia University, New York.)

typhus, Rocky Mountain spotted fever, and *trench fever* are associated with several different species of rickettsia. All species, except those producing Q fever, are transmitted by arthropods and are usually organ specific (Fig. 3–49). Rickettsiae may provoke a chronic inflammatory reaction (granuloma), or they may cause acute necrosis and inflammation.

Rocky Mountain Spotted Fever. This disease is found in both North and South America. The vector is a tick; the three most common species are the wood tick *(Dermacentor variabilis),* the Lone Star tick *(Amblyomma americanum),* and *Dermacentor andersoni.* Both the nymphal and adult stages of the tick can transmit the disease.

The disease is characterized by infection of endothelial cells with necrosis of the arterial wall and secondary thrombosis. The vasculitis is an early response and is present before rickettsiae are demonstrable in endothelial cells. The organisms replicate in endothelial cells and cause endothelial cell proliferation, sometimes cell rupture, and secondary hemorrhage.[157]

Symptoms in severe stages include toxemia, vascular collapse, thrombocytopenia, renal failure, and death. The organisms can be isolated from the blood. The diagnosis may be made by the Weil-Felix test or the complement-fixation test.

Viral Hepatitis

The past two decades have seen remarkable advances in the diagnosis of hepatitis caused by viral agents (Table 3–39). Damage to the human liver occurs with many viral infections, including those caused by *cytomegalovirus, Epstein-Barr virus, yellow fever virus, Herpes simplex* and *zoster viruses, Coxsackie virus,* and *rubella virus.* It is in the field of the "hepatitis viruses" that major inroads have been made, perhaps heralding an imminent decline in liver disease due to these agents.

Hepatitis A virus (HAV) and *hepatitis B virus (HBV)* are the infectious agents most commonly responsible for inflammation of the liver (hepatitis). Post-transfusion hepatitis is most often associated with *non-A, non-B hepatitis virus(es) (NANB virus(es)).*

The usual course of acute viral hepatitis involves diffuse parenchymal inflammation with subsequent resolution. Certain patients, however, following HBV and NANB in-

Table 3–39. *Viral Agents of Hepatitis*

Hepatitis A, B, non-A, non-B
Cytomegalovirus (CMV)
Epstein-Barr virus (EBV)
Yellow fever virus
Herpes simplex and zoster virus
Coxsackie virus
Rubella virus

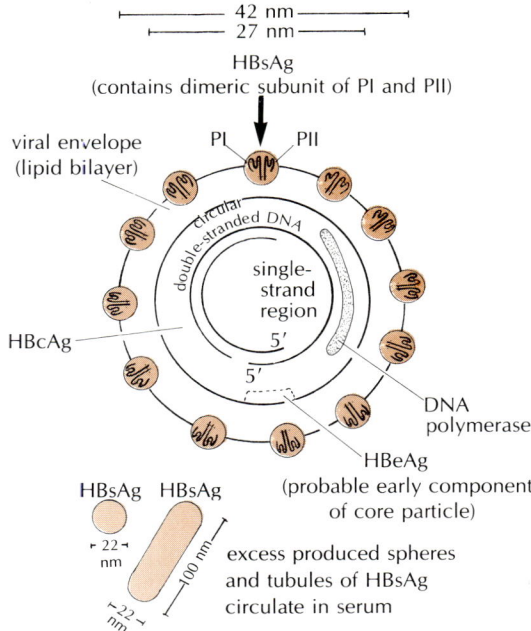

Figure 3–50. Structure of hepatitis B virus (Dane particle). The viral envelope, containing hepatitis B surface antigen (HBsAg) with its component polypeptides PI and PII, surrounds the nucleocapsid containing core antigen (HBcAg). Circular, double-stranded DNA and DNA polymerase are located in the core particle. HBeAg appears to be related to synthesis of the core particle. Components found in the serum include Dane particles, HBsAg (excess spherical and tubular forms), and HBeAg. Antibodies to HBsAg, HBcAg, and HBeAg develop in the normal course of viral infection.

fection, proceed to chronic liver disease of immune or autoimmune pathogenesis, and may further progress to cirrhosis.

Traditionally, *HAV* has been classified as the agent of *"infectious"* ("short-incubation") *hepatitis* and is related to the oral-fecal mode of transmission, to epidemics, and to the ingestion of contaminated shellfish. *HBV*, the classic agent of *"serum"* (*"long-incubation"*) *hepatitis*, was formerly acquired parenterally by blood transfusion and now is more often transmitted by contaminated needles used by drug addicts, and by exposure to contaminated blood among health-care workers and in the male homosexual population.

The discovery of hepatitis B surface antigen by Blumberg in 1965[158] (then known as *"Australia antigen"* because of its discovery in an Australian aborigine) initiated the characterization of this virus. Hepatitis B core antigen (*HBcAg*), e antigen (*HBeAg*), surface antigen (*HBsAg*), antibodies directed against these components, and a core-associated DNA polymerase are serum and tissue markers associated with different phases of HBV infection. These, along with other clinical, biochemical, and histologic features, have allowed the breakdown of hepatitis patients into clinical subgroups with particular prognostic implications. Development of a carrier state, vertical transmission from mother to neonate, chronic liver disease with evolution to cirrhosis, and the association with hepatocellular carcinoma are better understood in light of these markers of HBV infection (Fig. 3–50).

Hepatitis A Virus (HAV)

This virus is a 29 nm-*enterovirus* containing *RNA*.[159] It may be propagated in marmoset monkeys and was also identified as the *MS-1* viral strain transmitted to children of the Willowbrook School in New York City. HAV infection is usually subclinical and has modes of transmission both common to and distinct from hepatitis B virus. There is generally greater exposure to HAV than to HBV, although this varies geographically. Children and young adults are the persons usually affected by an acute disease, typically short in duration and without progression to chronic hepatitis. Infected water, food, and shellfish are important modes of transmission, although intrafamily and institutional spread are known to occur.

HAV can be identified by immunoabsorption assay, immune adherence tests, and immune electron microscopy of feces of infected patients.[160] A solid-phase radioimmunoassay of antigen-antibody complex is being developed. No serum antigenic marker has yet been identified, in contrast to HBV. IgM antibody to HAV always appears in acute infections. The IgG class of antibodies remains detectable years later and confers immunity by its presence.

Hepatitis B Virus (HBV)

The intact HBV, known as the *Dane particle*, measures 42 nm in diameter and is composed of a 28-nm viral core bearing circular, double-stranded *DNA* and DNA polymerase surrounded by the 7-nm thick lipoprotein coat. The hepatitis B surface antigen *(HBsAg)* is present on the outer viral coat, consists mainly of protein, and shares antigenic components with the abundant 22-nm spherical forms and 22 × 100-nm tubular forms found in serum and liver cell endoplasmic reticulum of infected patients. Five antigenic subdeterminants of *HBsAg* have been identified *(a,y,d,w,r)* and in varied combinations are recognized in a number of epidemiologically useful HBsAg subtypes including adw, ady, ayr, ayw.[161] For instance, hepatitis among drug users is usually characterized by the ay subtype, whereas asymptomatic carriers and blood donors show ad subtypes of their surface antigen.

Hepatitis B core antigen *(HBcAg)* makes up the polyhelical viral core, consists of 24- to 27-nm noncoated spheres and is found within nuclei of liver cells and, to a lesser extent, in the cytoplasm. It is antigenically distinct from HBsAg. A third antigen is associated with the presence of circulating Dane particles and serum levels of hepatitis-B-specific DNA polymerase, and is known as *HBeAg*. Three subtypes, e_1, e_2, and e_3, appear to be part of the viral core. This antigen is a marker of chronic infectivity.

Electron-microscopic studies have shown core particles in nuclei, and spheres and tubules of HBsAg in dilated cisternae of endoplasmic reticulum, in liver cells of infected patients. It is believed that HBcAg and HBsAg are produced separately, HBcAg in the nucleus and HBsAg in the cytoplasmic endoplasmic reticulum. It appears that HBcAg migrates from ribosomes through nuclear pores into the nucleus, where it is assembled with viral DNA into core particles. These HBcAg-bearing particles leave the nucleus and become enveloped by HBsAg to form Dane particles within the endoplasmic reticulum. The intact hepatitis B virions are then released from hepatocytes to the extracellular space.[162]

Measurable serum HBsAg, the diagnostic hallmark of HBV infection, is thought to be an excess of viral coat material synthesized and then released from infected liver cells. The three particulate forms identifiable in HBsAg-positive sera include *spheres, tubules,* and *complete Dane particles* (Fig. 3–51).

Within the viral core is double-stranded circular DNA, molecular weight 1.6×10^6 daltons, and DNA polymerase. A portion of the circular DNA is only single stranded.

The temporal development of both antigenic components and antibodies to them following HBV infection has diagnostic and prognostic implications. HBsAg may be first detected at 20 to 30 days preceding a rise in SGOT, whereas the titer drops with the onset of symptoms and jaundice.

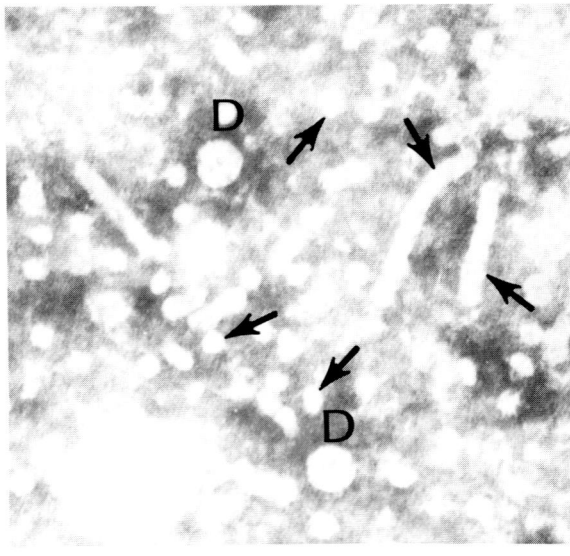

Figure 3–51. Transmission electron micrograph of negatively stained serum of hepatitis B virus carrier shows complete Dane particles (D) and spheres (short arrows) and tubules (long arrows) of hepatitis B surface antigen (HBsAg). (Courtesy of Mrs. E.M. Crawford, Department of Medicine, The Royal Free Hospital, London.)

Anti-HBsAg antibody (anti-HBs) is measurable by radioimmunoassay 3 to 6 months after a self-limited episode of acute hepatitis B. This antibody appears to persist indefinitely and is virtually protective against further episodes of HBV infection. HBcAg, anti-HBcAg antibodies, HBeAg (transiently) and DNA polymerase all appear early in the incubation period before HBsAg and anti-HBs. Anti-HBc antibodies usually disappear more quickly than anti-HBs.

Bianchi and Gudat have proposed four different reaction patterns of HBV expression in liver tissue.[159] The four patterns are: (1) *elimination type* (seen in patients with self-limited acute hepatitis with few or no viral components in liver tissue); (2) *immunosuppression type* (seen in immunosuppressed patients with mild liver disease, HBcAg in liver cell nuclei, and membrane expression of HBsAg); (3) *HBsAg-predominance type* (seen in healthy carriers with tolerance to HBsAg, mild or absent liver disease, and prominent cytoplasmic HBsAg; and (4) *equivalence type* (seen in patients with chronic active hepatitis with variable degrees of immune insufficiency in eliminating HBsAg and HBcAg).

The most common mode of transmission of hepatitis B is parenterally from the transfusion of blood and blood products. The incidence of HBV hepatitis is related to infectious titers in carriers, mode of transmission, and susceptibility of the recipient. Use of illicit drugs by narcotic addicts who also give blood in order to obtain money to support their habit has propagated the association of HBV infection with blood transfusion. Exposure to blood products in settings such as hemodialysis units has put health care professionals at risk of becoming chronic carriers and transmitters of the disease.[163] Hepatitis B surface antigen has been found in almost all secretions tested, including semen, saliva, and vaginal secretions.[164,165]

Non-A, Non-B Hepatitis Virus(es)

The commonest cause of posttransfusion hepatitis in the United States is non-A, non-B hepatitis. This is generally a milder parenteral infection than that caused by HBV. Up to 60% of patients may go on to develop chronic liver disease, however. Both short and long incubation types have been recognized, and recent work has demonstrated preliminary antigen-antibody specificities in serum and liver tissue of patients associated with this form of hepatitis. Viral transmission occurs through administration of contaminated blood and blood products such as fibrinogen and factor VIII and IX preparations or is sporadic.

Pathology of Acute Viral Hepatitis

Acute type A, B, and non-A, non-B hepatitis show generally similar histopathologic features. Full-blown hepatitis is a diffuse process involving the lobular parenchyma and portal tracts. *Liver cell degeneration* and death occur, with disarray of liver cell plates, proliferation of Kupffer cells (*"Kupffer cell hyperplasia"*), and lobular and portal infiltrates of mononuclear cells, including lymphocytes, histiocytes, and sparse plasma cells (Fig. 3–52).

Liver cell degeneration takes two basic morphologic forms: swelling (*"balloon"* cells) and shrinkage (*"acidophilic"* or *Councilman-like bodies*) (Fig. 3–52). These liver cell changes, though seen throughout the lobule, are most severe in centrilobular areas.[166] "Ballooning degeneration" of liver cells results in swollen hepatocytes with rarefied cytoplasm. These swollen cells undergo lytic necrosis by cell membrane breakdown and subsequent cellular dropout. Acidophilic bodies, on the other hand, represent shrunken, *"mummified" liver cells* that, by coagulative necrosis, have

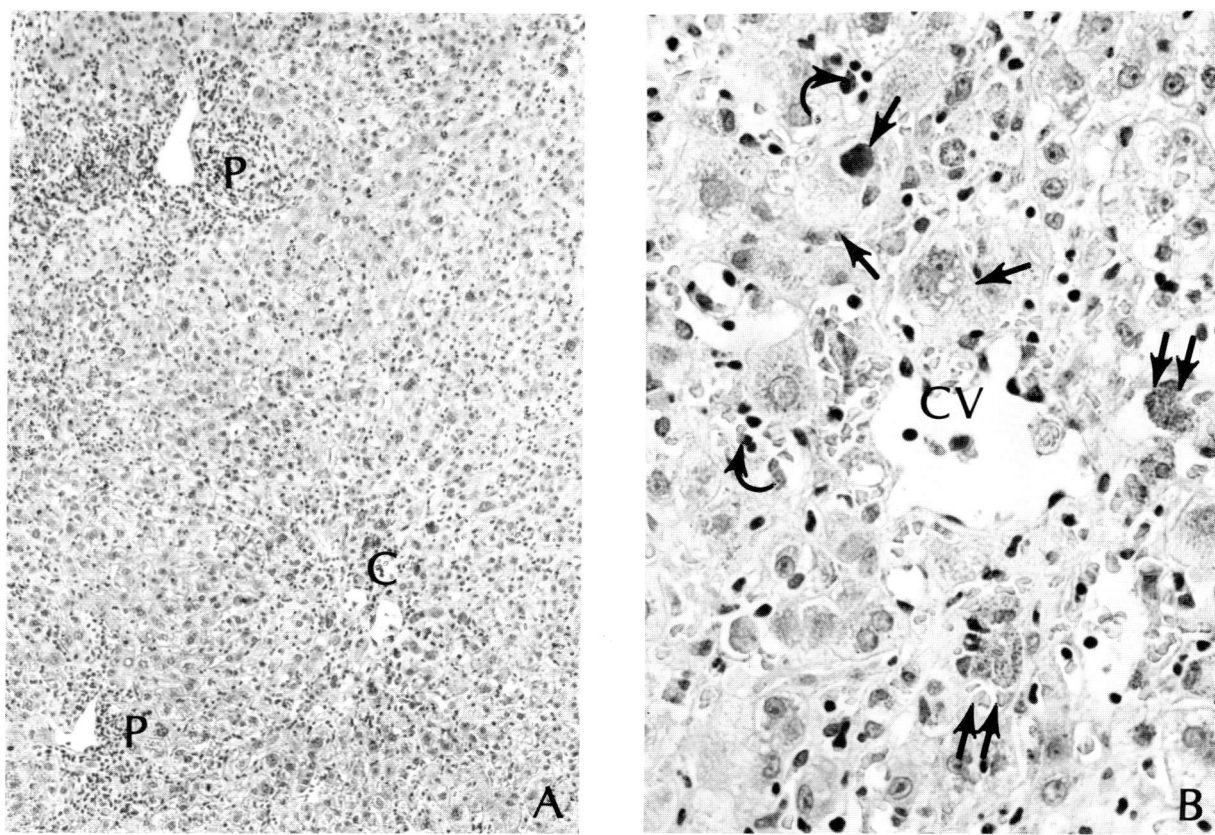

Figure 3–52. *A,* In this low magnification of a liver biopsy in acute viral hepatitis (type B), note the disorganization of liver-cell plates in the centrilobular zone (C) and the spotty necrosis with inflammation in the lobule. Portal tracts (P) are inflamed. *B,* In this higher magnification of a liver biopsy in acute viral hepatitis (type B), hepatocytes around the central vein (CV) are swollen (long arrows) and are surrounded by mononuclear cell inflammatory cells (curved arrows). An acidophilic body is present (short arrow). Kupffer cells containing ceroid debris (double arrows) are prominent.

undergone condensation of cytoplasmic matrix proteins and organelles with loss of water.

Groups of degenerating liver cells surrounded by mononuclear inflammatory cells and proliferated Kupffer cells characterize *"spotty necrosis."* In more severe cases, loss of larger areas of parenchyma bridging between central veins and portal tracts, or between portal tracts, or both, has been termed *"bridging hepatic necrosis."* When accompanied by extensive portal and periportal inflammation, this finding may indicate possible transition to chronic hepatitis.[167]

Multilobular necrosis is the term applied to more extensive fields of liver cell necrosis that extend between lobules. In fulminant hepatitis, necrosis may be marked; Rokitansky in 1842 termed it *"acute yellow atrophy."* It is known today as *massive hepatic necrosis* and involves multiple lobules or even whole lobes of the liver. Certain cases termed *"cholestatic"* viral hepatitis mimic large bile duct obstruction and histologically may show striking bile in liver cells, canaliculi, and ducts. The bile secretory apparatus is damaged in these cases.

As acute hepatitis evolves, a variable degree of collapse and reticulin condensation occurs, and ceroid pigment (formed by liver cell breakdown) accumulates in lobular Kupffer cells engaged in active phagocytosis. Cases of nearly healed hepatitis show liver cell pleomorphism (reflecting liver cell regeneration after necrosis), focal lobular inflammatory infiltrates, and a mild degree of fibrosis involving and extending from portal tracts. In acute type B hepatitis, HBsAg is usually not identifiable on routine light microscopy.

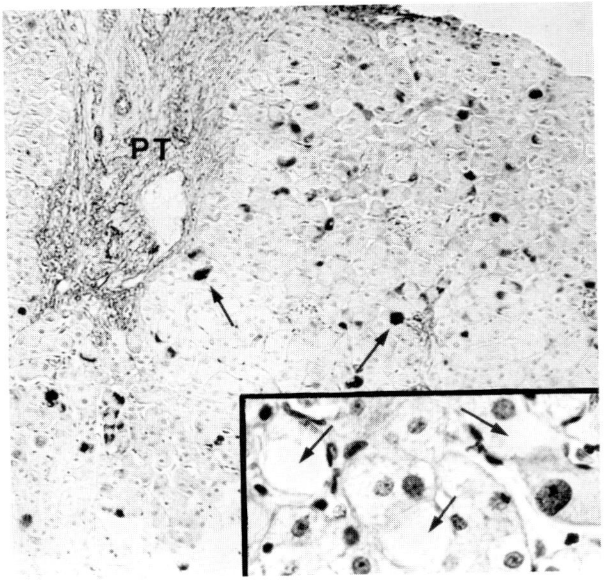

Sequelae of Acute Viral Hepatitis

The possible morphologic outcomes of acute hepatitis include *resolution* (most cases), fatal massive necrosis, chronic hepatitis, cirrhosis, and hepatocellular carcinoma. Five to ten percent of patients do not effectively eliminate hepatitis B virus and become chronic *HBsAg carriers.*

Types of Chronic Hepatitis. Chronic hepatitis has been defined by an international group[168] as "inflammation of the liver continuing without improvement for at least six months." The better defined forms of chronic hepatitis include *chronic persistent hepatitis, chronic lobular hepatitis,* and *chronic active hepatitis.* The entity "chronic active hepatitis" has occasioned much interpretive difficulty because it is a disease process rather than a disease, and as such may have any one of several causes.

Chronic hepatitis does not follow HAV infection, but may complicate both HBV and NANB infection.

Hepatitis B *"carriers,"* with persistence of serum HBsAg four months or more after acute infection, usually have minimal liver inflammation, but may show large numbers of cells bearing cytoplasmic HBsAg (Fig. 3–53). These appear as *"ground-glass"* cells on routine hematoxylin and eosin

Figure 3–53. In this liver biopsy specimen from a hepatitis B-positive patient with chronic active hepatitis, the portal tract (PT) is enlarged and scarred. This orcein stain demonstrates hepatitis B surface antigen (HBsAg) in the cytoplasm of liver cells (arrows). The inset shows "ground-glass" inclusions of HBsAg in the cytoplasm of liver cells (arrows).

staining and have homogeneous, pale pink cytoplasm reflecting their dilated ER, which is filled with HBsAg. Orcein staining strikingly demonstrates the presence of antigen. Ground-glass cells in variable numbers may also be demonstrated in the major forms of HBV-related chronic hepatitis described in the following paragraphs, as well as in cirrhosis.

Chronic persistent hepatitis (CPH) and *chronic lobular hepatitis (CLH)* are forms milder than chronic active hepatitis that have a good prognosis and do not proceed to cirrhosis. CPH is characterized by predominantly lymphocytic inflammation confined within portal tracts. In CLH, foci of inflammation and necrosis exist within the lobular parenchyma, usually with scanty portal inflammation.

The pathognomonic feature of *chronic active hepatitis* (CAH) is *"piecemeal necrosis"* (Fig. 3–53). This term indicates portal and periportal inflammation and necrosis, with erosion of the limiting plate of liver cells lying adjacent to portal tracts. It is prognostically worse than CPH and CLH in that it frequently progresses to cirrhosis. In fact, in more severe cases, piecemeal necrosis may become so extensive as to result in *bridging hepatic necrosis,* strongly favoring the development of *cirrhosis.*

Because some new fibrous tissue is synthesized in conjunction with piecemeal necrosis, a fine line often exists between CAH and cirrhosis. Septa extending from portal tracts may intersect parenchyma and, when associated with bridging hepatic necrosis, may link portal tracts to central veins or other portal tracts.

The combination of diffuse fibrosis and nodules of regenerating liver cells indicates that cirrhosis has developed (Fig. 3–54). Cirrhosis, once it is morphologically acknowledged, may be considered *"active"* if ongoing piecemeal necrosis, inflammatory infiltration of fibrous septa, and continued parenchymal cell loss are demonstrable. With time, fibrous septa become sparsely inhabited by inflammatory cells and surround nodules of varying size (often *macronodular);* then the histologic picture becomes one of *"inactive"* cirrhosis. The complications of cirrhosis, including development of varices, ascites, clotting and protein-synthesis abnormalities, and hepatic failure, may be present.

In the United States, white males over 50 years old who carry HBsAg may have an annual incidence of hepatocellular carcinoma of 6.2%. The relation of this malignant liver tumor to HBV is even more striking in Africa and southeast Asia (Fig. 3–54).

Pathogenesis of Chronic Hepatitis. This field is admittedly controversial. A multifactorial origin of chronic hepatitis is recognized, especially for chronic active hepatitis, and includes drugs, alcohol, Wilson's disease, alpha-1-antitrypsin deficiency, and autoimmune mechanisms in addition to hepatitis B virus. One of the major reasons that HBV-related chronic liver disease receives so much clinical attention must be that the reservoir of worldwide chronic

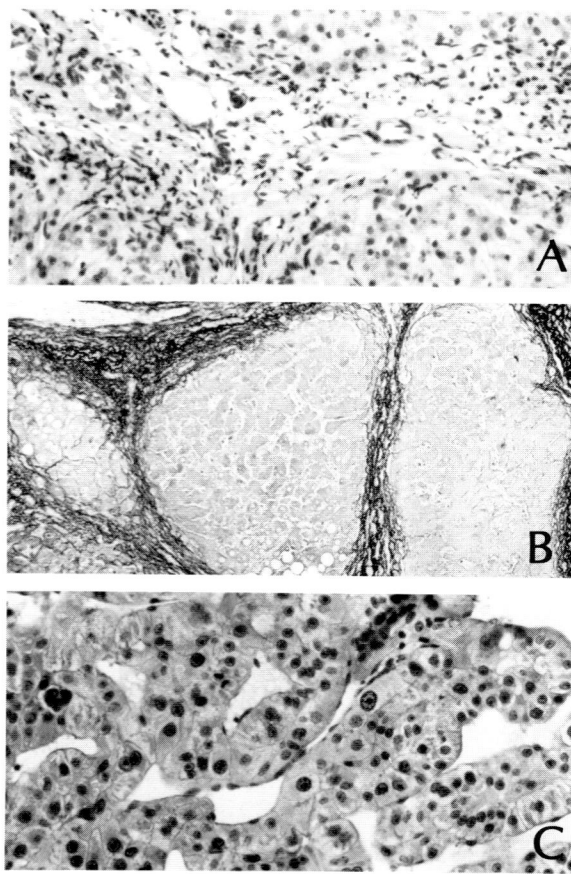

Figure 3–54. Progression from chronic active hepatitis to hepatocellular carcinoma in a hepatitis B-positive patient. *A,* The appearance of chronic active hepatitis with fibrotic portal tract and "piecemeal necrosis" by mononuclear cells at the edges of the fibrous septa. *B,* A subsequent biopsy shows the development of cirrhosis (hepatic-parenchymal nodules surrounded by diffuse fibrosis). *C,* The patient later developed hepatocellular carcinoma. Note the similarity of this malignant tumor of liver cells to normal liver. The tumor grows in microtrabeculae.

HBsAg-positive patients numbers between 120 and 176 million.

Liver cell damage in HBV hepatitis is mediated by autoimmune mechanisms, even though the virus itself initiates the disease. Binding of IgG to liver cell membranes, in addition to cell-mediated immunity against membrane proteins (liver-specific antigen and liver membrane antigen), are involved in HBV-related and other chronic, active liver diseases. A particular form of immune-mediated "self-destruction" may feature prominently in the loss of liver cells *("apoptosis")* in chronic active hepatitis. Several theories generally related to cell-mediated immunity are indicated in Table 3–40.

Table 3–40. *Theories of the Role of Cell-Mediated Immunity in Hepatitis*

Antibodies directed against liver-specific protein antigens in liver cells may bind to liver cells and may thereby sensitize them for destruction by antibody-dependent effector non-T cells with surface receptors for Fc fragments.

Cytotoxic T cells may recognize viral antigens on the surface of infected liver cells.

Inappropriate activity of the liver's macrophages (Kupffer cells) may mediate the liver disease following HBV infection.

Necrosis of liver cells in acute hepatitis liberates *liver-specific lipoprotein,* which activates T and subsequently B cells. Nonelimination of hepatitis B virus perpetuates chronic assault on noninfected liver cells, which bear this liver-specific lipoprotein.

An understanding of the basic roles of antigens, antibodies, and immune cells (B, T, NK cells, macrophages) in mediating disease, along with mechanisms of viral genome expression in host cells, is crucial to the understanding of hepatitis B-related chronic hepatitis. If, for example, during viral proliferation in hepatocytes, liver cell antigens become incorporated into surface coats of HBV, a host antiviral lymphocytic response might also then cross-react with noninfected liver cells.

Formation of lymphocytotoxins[169] and leukocyte-inhibiting factors, lymphoblast transformation, and lymphocyte cytotoxicity against liver cells all point particularly to alterations of cell-mediated immunity. Prevalence of HLA antigens B8 and DRW3 among patients with chronic hepatitis, as in other diseases, suggests the important roles of both genetics and the immune system.

The humoral response to HBV and the formation of hepatitis B antigen-antibody complexes are responsible for the arthritis, polyarteritis,[170] and membranoproliferative glomerulonephritis that may be associated with viral hepatitis.[171]

Involvement of the immune system in the mediation of chronic hepatitis is far from being completely elucidated. Defects in populations of suppressor T cells require further evaluation. It should remain clear that many different clinical groups of patients have chronic hepatitis: those who are antigen-positive or antigen-negative, and those with histories of drug or alcohol ingestion, for example. The pathogenesis of their diseases may not uniformly be linked to autoimmune mechanisms.

Hepatitis B Virus and Hepatocellular Carcinoma (HCC). In contrast to the high-incidence areas of Africa and the Far East, hepatocellular carcinoma (HCC) is rare in North America and Western Europe, where older age groups are affected, cirrhosis is more often associated with it, and α-fetoprotein is less often positive. In high-incidence areas, HCC has been related to environmental factors such as aflatoxins and hepatitis B virus; up to 80% of tumor-bearing patients may show HBsAg in their serum.[172]

Recent studies of patients with HCC from nonendemic areas also show a higher-than-expected association with either past or present HBV infection. Hepatitis B virus may act as a carcinogen (that is, an *"oncogenic" virus*), or as a cocarcinogen in persistently infected liver cells. Hepatitis B viral DNA integration has been demonstrated in HCC of HBsAg-positive patients.[173] The manner in which viral integration and transcription, alone or in concert with already existing factors such as alcoholic cirrhosis, are involved in the development of HCC is currently under investigation.[174] Data from studies of animals infected with viruses similar to HBV (woodchucks, ground squirrels, ducks) should provide further information on the pathogenesis of HCC.

Therapy of Hepatitis

Immune serum globulin (ISG) prevents type A viral hepatitis in 80 to 90% of patients when administered before or within 1 to 2 weeks of exposure. The place of immune globulin prophylaxis of type B viral hepatitis is being recognized, especially in neonates at risk of infection from carrier mothers. A prophylactic HBV vaccine using formalin-inactivated HBsAg is likely to change hepatitis-B-related epidemiology in the future, especially in regard to HCC.[175]

Once acute hepatitis has developed, therapy is generally supportive and does little to alter the course of the disease. The use of corticosteroids in acute type B hepatitis is generally contraindicated because this therapy may inhibit natural elimination of virus and may actually potentiate the development of chronic hepatitis. In contrast, corticosteroids and other immunosuppressive therapy have a known role in the treatment of some forms of chronic active hepatitis and may therein be useful in preventing or forestalling cirrhosis.

Other agents used in treating HBsAg-positive chronic liver disease include *interferon*, the antiviral substance that inhibits viral replication at the level of transcription of viral genome or translation of viral proteins, and *interferon inducers,* for example, a stabilized derivative of polyriboinosinic-polyribocytidylic acid[176] and adenine arabinoside (ara-A), a synthetic purine nucleoside whose main action is to block selectively viral DNA polymerase activity.[177]

In summary, three different viruses, one (HAV) an RNA virus, another (HBV) a DNA virus, and a third (NANB virus(es)) cause the similar clinical and morphologic pictures known as "hepatitis." Type B hepatitis, discussed as a prototype, may resolve completely, indicating a well-functioning immune system, or it may proceed to chronic liver diseases including cirrhosis and primary hepatocellular carcinoma.

The use of effective immunoglobulin therapy of HAV infection is leading to the gradual elimination of this agent as a major cause of acute liver disease. In contrast, HBV infection continues to cause considerable morbidity and mortality through chronic infection. Ominous serum markers indicative of the carrier state (HBsAg, HBeAg, anti-HBc, and DNA polymerase) have been recognized. The nature of non-A, non-B hepatitis virus(es), associated with most cases of post-transfusion hepatitis, is currently being investigated in many laboratories.

PATHOLOGY ASSOCIATED WITH EXOGENOUS DRUGS, CHEMICALS, HORMONES AND ENVIRONMENTAL FACTORS

The cell has multiple intermediary pathways of metabolism by which it synthesizes and degrades macromolecules. These pathways are normally controlled by the demands of the cell and the organism. The rate at which each pathway functions is related to *substrate concentration, pH, ion* requirements, and the presence of cofactors such as *vitamins* and *coenzymes.* The modulation of *receptors* on *endocrine glands* (thyroid, adrenal, pituitary, pancreas, ovary, testes, parathyroid) as well as on *target organs* must be regulated by a complex, at present largely unknown, control system. Other intracellular control factors involve the presence of rate-limiting enzymatic steps, *allosteric regulation, feedback inhibition; modulation of the genes* by these and other mechanisms is a major factor in all disease.

Physiologic changes in metabolism related to sleep, nutrition, stress, and exercise, as well as to the presence of disease, may drastically alter normal metabolic pathways. This alteration may result in either a deficiency or an excess of certain products. The diversion of precursors to other pathways may result in the accumulation, secretion, or absorption of injurious substances. Compensatory responses may ensue and may partially rectify the deficiency or excess states; these responses may also produce added injury.

General Effects of Exogenous Toxic Agents

In addition to endogenous metabolic abnormalities, the organism is bombarded with a variety of injurious agents from the external environment including drugs, chemicals, and hormones.[178] Reports showing the presence of an estimated 60,000 harmful substances in the environment, including 1400 potentially harmful food additives, have made us all aware of this problem[179] (Table 3–41).

Table 3–41. *Environmental Agents Causing Injury*

Home poisons
  Rat poisons
  Cleaning solutions
  Medicines
  Paint (lead)

Air pollution
  Automobile exhaust
  Environmental soot
  Cigarette smoke
  Asbestos

Rural toxic substances
  Pesticides and herbicides
  Fungal spores on grains
  Fertilizers

Industrial toxicity
  Solvents
  Metals
  Chemicals

Food additives
  Oil red dye
  Saccharine
  Cyclamates
  Nitrates

Drugs
  Antibiotics
  Anesthetics
  Analgesics
  Stimulants
  Depressants
  Hormones
  Chemotherapeutic agents
  Ethyl alcohol

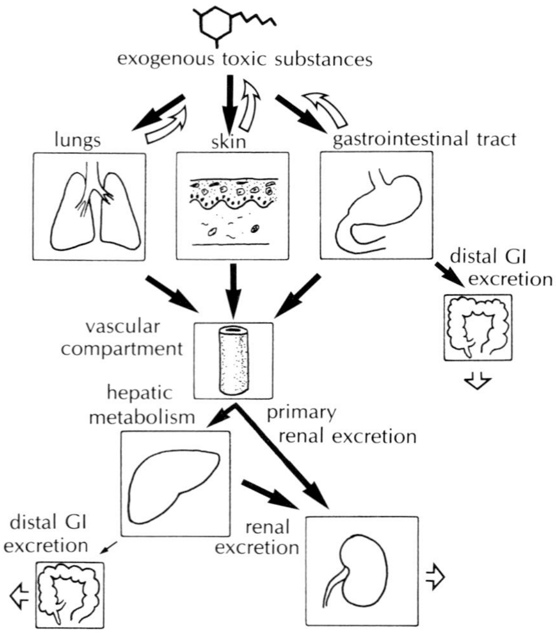

Figure 3–55. The fate of exogenous toxic substances. Toxins enter through the skin, lungs, and the gastrointestinal tract and may, in certain circumstances, be returned to the environment by the same routes or by passing through to the distal gastrointestinal tract. More often, toxins enter the circulation and are excreted through the kidney, or they undergo detoxification and/or metabolism in the liver before renal or gastrointestinal excretion. (Ultimate excretory routes are indicated by open arrows.)

Exogenous toxic agents are usually taken into the organism through the skin or the respiratory or gastrointestinal tracts. If and when they are eliminated, it is by the same systems, as well as by the kidneys. Attempts at detoxification or metabolism of these agents occur in all cells, but particularly in the liver and kidneys (Fig. 3–55). Soluble compounds are transported into cells by active transport and pinocytosis. Large particles may be phagocytized by cells of the lymphoreticular system.

With degradation, hydrolysis, deactivation, or oxidation, some products end up as residual bodies in cells. The cell may be induced to form new lysosomal or metabolic en-

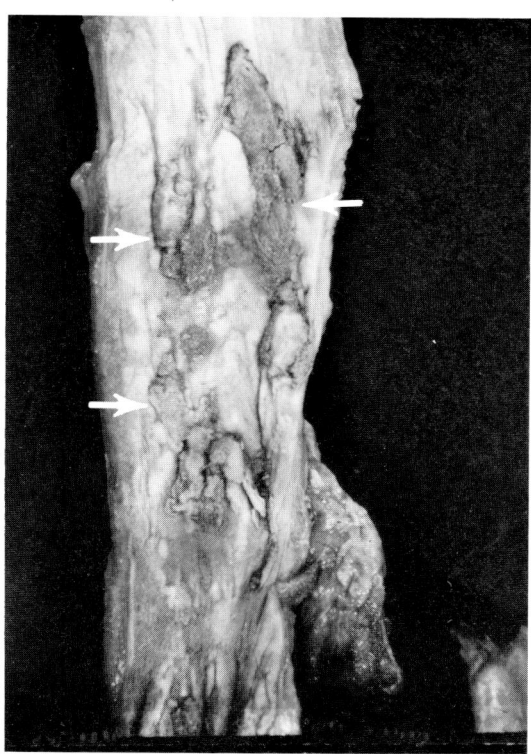

Figure 3–56. In ulcerative esophagitis in a patient who ingested lye, a thick purulent exudate covers the areas of ulceration (arrows).

zymes in an attempt to degrade further or to inactivate undesirable or unused metabolites. Sometimes, metabolic reactions produce toxic intermediary products that have proved to be carcinogenic, for example, nitrosamines. A compound converted to a toxic substance usually has an effect only in the cell in which it is first metabolized.

The effect of injurious agents on cells is determined by route of entry, dosage, and length of exposure, and by the cell's ability to detoxify, metabolize, degrade, or excrete the agent. The presence of advanced age, nutritional deficiency, and disease processes may intensify the effect of the agent and may inhibit the protective defenses of the cell.

Home Poisons

Home poisoning is generally associated with (1) young children who accidentally ingest cleaning and medicinal agents, (2) individuals attempting suicide (Table 3–42), and (3) alcoholics drinking potentially dangerous alcohol-based chemicals. *Methyl alcohol* (a base for perfume), Sterno, and shaving lotions, when ingested, cause neuronal, retinal, and liver cell damage. Cleaning solutions, particularly strong acids or alkalis, ingested orally, produce necrosis of the pharyngeal and esophageal mucosa, with denaturation of cell-membrane proteins (Fig. 3–56). *Rat poisons* often con-

Table 3–42. *Chemical Causes of Suicide 1967— United States*

		Number of Deaths
Poisoning by analgesics and soporific substances		
morphine and other derivatives		6
barbituric acid and derivatives		1694
salicylates		87
others		902
	Total	2689
Poisoning by other solid and liquid substances		
strychnine		12
phenol compounds		5
lye and potash		19
mercury and its compounds		8
arsenic and its compounds		46
fluorides		15
all other unspecific agents		191
	Total	296
Poisoning by gases		
motor vehicle exhaust gas		2049
other motor exhaust gas		1
carbon monoxide		141
other poisonous gases		11
	Total	2202
Poisoning by gases in domestic use		118

(Data from U.S. Vital Statistics, 1967, Vol. II. Mortality. Section 1.)

tain *strychnine*, which paralyzes neuron function, *warfarin*, which blocks thrombin formation in liver cells and results in hemorrhage, or *arsenic*, which binds sulfhydryl groups and causes marked hemolysis of red blood cells and depression of hemoglobin synthesis in the bone marrow.

Lead intoxication has been found in 1 to 2% of children tested in New York and Chicago, apparently as a result of eating lead paint *("pica")* from the walls.[180] The biosynthesis of heme is inhibited by lead, and the resultant anemia is associated with basophilic stippling of red blood cells, vasculitis with increased capillary permeability, and encephalopathy. Mitochondrial abnormalities are prominent in lead poisoning. The severity of change is related to blood levels of lead.

Air Pollution and Chemicals

In western civilizations, the major cause of air pollution is the automobile. Photochemical reactions occur among the hydrocarbons and nitrogen oxides present in the exhaust fumes. The deleterious products of this reaction include *nitrogen dioxide*, an oxidant whose major components are ozone, nitric acid, and nitrates.[181] Automobile exhaust poses a serious threat in closed garages where *carbon monoxide* in small quantities preferentially combines with hemoglobin, inhibiting its ability to carry O_2.

Although commonly associated with suicides, the carbon monoxide levels encountered in highly trafficked city streets often reach dangerous proportions. Carbon monoxide levels are also elevated in smokers. In addition, sulfur dioxide and lead, resulting from degradation of oil products, are toxic. Finally, rubber from tires deposits millions of particles of hydrocarbon in the atmosphere daily.

The population living in the countryside surrounding the Delaware River chemical industry has the highest incidence of bladder carcinoma in the United States. When soot and dust, that is, carbon, are taken into the lungs, deposits form in the reticular system to produce classic pulmonary *anthracosis* (Fig. 3–57). The prohibition of coal burning fireplaces in inner London effectively eliminated much of the smog, which formerly produced emphysema and increased deaths, especially in older patients with lung disease.

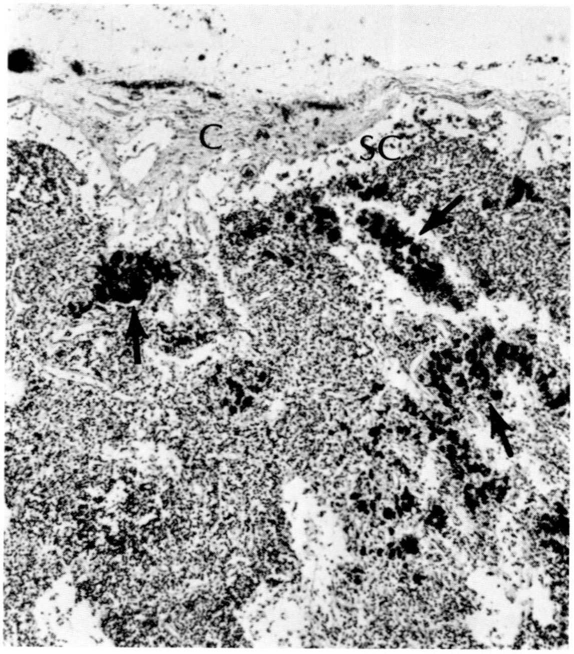

Cigarette smoke, now banned in many schools, elevators, and public places, contains *benzo (a) pyrene* and *methylcholanthrene*, both of which are well known experimental carcinogens. The report from the Surgeon General's Office[182] indicated that about 325,000 people would die prematurely in 1982 from disorders attributable to smoking. Many others would be chronically ill. The risk of developing lung cancer is well known. Auerbach recently compared the histologic features of cancer produced in the last decade with the use of longer cigarettes that are lower in nicotine and have effective filters, and found that the histologic changes

Figure 3–57. In this hilar lymph node from an urban dweller, note the histiocytes in the subcapsular and medullary sinuses (arrows) that contain abundant black carbon pigment (anthracosis). (C, capsule; SC, subcapsular sinus.)

are not as severe as in his earlier study.[183] Nonetheless, significant differences were found between smokers and nonsmokers. In addition to the increased cancer risk, other problems included emphysema, chronic bronchitis, coronary atherosclerosis, heart attacks, gastric and duodenal ulcers, bladder cancer, and risk to unborn children of smoking mothers.

It has recently been discovered that workers in the building industry who have inhaled moderate amounts of *asbestos* have a marked increase in incidence of lung disease (bronchitis, emphysema) and an increased incidence of a rare tumor, *mesothelioma.* There appears to be a significant increase in the proportion of normal lungs containing small numbers of *asbestos bodies.* In one study, a 91.1% incidence was found. The biologic significance of this finding is unknown.[184] The risk of bronchogenic lung cancer is 92% greater for asbestos workers than for the general nonsmoking population. Exposure to asbestos is not confined to industrial workers; it is a hazard in talcum powder, gypsum, and spackling manufacturing plants and is found in over 400 industrial products. Silica toxicity is another hazard for those working in foundries.[185]

The graveyards of western Colorado abound in old gravestones that are testaments to the illnesses of 100 years ago. Many young women died in childbirth, numerous children died of infectious diseases during infancy and early childhood, and miners died in their early thirties from the ravages of lung disease associated with gold, silver, and coal mining. These lung diseases were predominantly *anthracosis* and *silicosis (pneumoconiosis)* aggravated by tuberculosis. More recently, it has been found that *uranium* miners, particularly if they are cigarette smokers, have an increased incidence of cancer of the lung.

Rural Toxic Agents

Many farmers are constantly exposed to various noxious substances, particularly *insecticides* and *fertilizers.*[186] Many insecticides contain arsenic or cyanide, which binds cytochrome oxidase. Other potentially injurious insecticides are

Table 3–43.   *Pesticides in Milk of 1400 Women*

Compound	Percentage Positive
1,1-dichloro-2,2-bis ethylene (DDE)	100
Dichlorodiphenyl trichloroethane (DDT)	99
Dieldrin	81
Heptachlor epoxide	64
Oxychlordane	63
Lindane (BHC)	87
Polychlorinated biphenyls (PCB)	30
Polybrominated biphenyls (PBB)	—

(Modified from Ames, B.N.: Identifying environmental chemicals causing mutations and cancer. Science, 204:587, 1979. Copyright by the American Association for the Advancement of Science.)

used not only in farming, but also are found in toxic concentrations in chemical plants where they are produced. These include *PCB* (polychlorinated biphenyl), *Kepone, endrin,* and *Mirex.*[187,188]

Recent evidence indicates that pesticides and insecticides are polluting our streams, lakes, and rivers, with potentially profound deleterious effects on our water tables in the future (Table 3–43). *Nitrates* in fertilizers, when inhaled in sufficient amounts, are also toxic agents.

Silo fillers' disease results from exposure to oxides of nitrogen generated in poorly ventilated silos filled with freshly fermenting silage. Inhalation of these oxides, chiefly NO_2, may cause pulmonary edema in the acute phase and may later progress to pulmonary fibrosis. Fungal contamination of silos has also caused many infectious diseases among farm workers. When fungal growth is controlled with cyanide gas, occasional accidents with cyanide poisoning have occurred.

Industrial Toxicity

Historically, *coal tar (dibenzanthracene)* was the chemical responsible for scrotal carcinoma in London chimney sweeps. In Denmark, however, chimney sweeps who showered every day did not develop this tumor.

Thousands of manufacturing plants in the United States and the rest of the world are daily using, producing, and discharging toxic agents on land, water, and air under unsafe conditions. The mass media have largely associated this contamination with the chemical industry, but many other industries, including paper mills, steel plants, power plants, automobile parts plants, and almost every field of manufacturing, are involved.

The use of solvents, including acetone, benzene, carbon tetrachloride, diethylene glycol, phenol, kerosene, creosol, alcohol, and many other agents, is dangerous unless they are handled with care. *Polyvinyl chloride (PVC)*, a widely used synthetic plastic, has recently been implicated in an increase in *angiosarcoma* of the liver.[189] In 1964, workers cleaning PVC tanks were found to have a variety of changes including bone lesions and hepatic fibrosis. The toxicity is related to oxidation products produced in the endoplasmic reticulum. PVC also damages the chromosomes and is therefore mutagenic.

Chemical contaminants dumped into water supplies can be ingested by fish and thereby may later cause human disease. *Minamata disease* in Japan, brought about by an accumulation of *mercury* in fish, was an excellent example of this phenomenon.[190] People who consumed contaminated fish developed acute *CNS* and *kidney* damage. Initial sublethal mercury interaction with the *pars convoluta* of the proximal tubule results in decreased sodium resorption. Later, involvement of the *macula densa* invokes *renin* release.

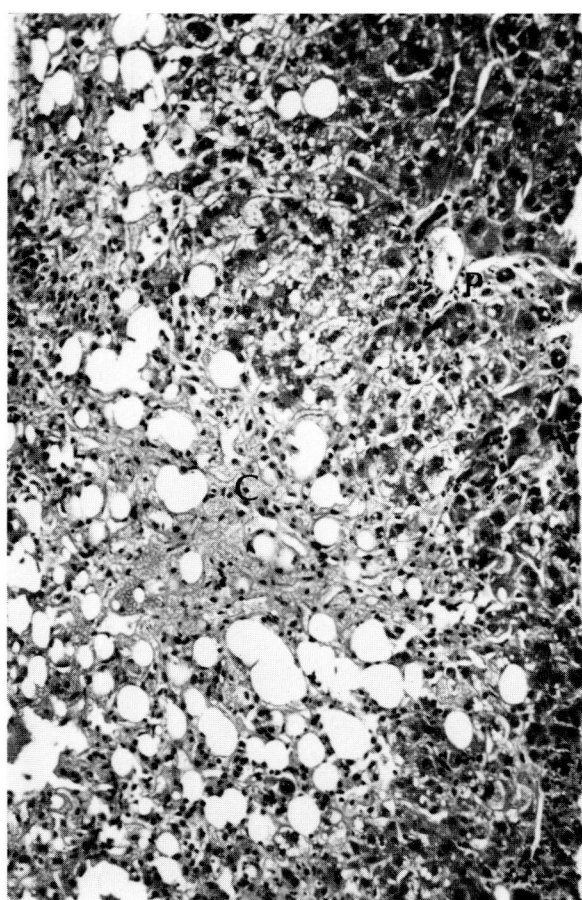

Figure 3–58. Liver biopsy from a patient who survived acute mushroom poisoning. Centrilobular confluent necrosis is evident in this biopsy taken seven days after the ingestion of Amanita. (C, centrilobular; P, portal tract.) (Courtesy of Dr. L. Bianchi, Institut fur Pathologie der Universitat Basel, Switzerland.)

Food Additives

Approximately 1400 food additives are used today in the United States. This list does not include innate toxic substances in food such as *phalloidin toxin* in mushrooms (Fig. 3–58), *cyanide* in peach pits, or *aflatoxin* contaminants in peanuts. The list does include possibly harmful chemicals such as dyes used for color, nitrites used as preservatives in cold meat, and saccharine used as a sweetener in soft drinks (Table 3–44).

Table 3–44. *Examples of Potentially Toxic Food Substances*

Naturally Occurring
Phalloidin toxin (mushrooms)
Cyanide (peach pits)
Aflatoxin (peanuts)
Chemical Food Additives
Dyes for coloring (oil red O)
Preservatives (nitrites in meat)
Sweeteners (saccharine, cyclamates)

The Delaney Amendment states that any drug that produces cancer in any dosage in any species is prohibited from being added to food. It is not economically possible or even feasible to carry out adequate tests on all compounds. Furthermore, that one compound given by an abnormal route (for example, intraperitoneal injection) in grossly abnormal dosage in one species produces tumors (not usually metastasizing) is not proof that it is a human carcinogen. Mutagenic tests developed by Ames, Rosenkrantz, and others have been of great value in detecting carcinogens. Not all carcinogens fulfill the criteria of mutagenicity (for example, experimental viruses and estrogens), however, and not all mutagens are carcinogens.

Drugs and Hormones

We have previously mentioned, in our dicussion of genetics, a large group of environmental drugs that may act as teratogens. It is generally recognized that a drug given in different dosages by different routes may be innocuous, efficacious, or toxic. A small dose under certain circumstances, however, such as in the presence of disease or in interaction with another drug, may produce a hypersensitivity state or serious toxic effects (Table 3–45).

All drugs should only be given when absolutely necessary. They should be monitored closely and discontinued immediately when the desired result is obtained, or when no result appears forthcoming. Synergism among multiple drugs given to patients both in and out of hospital should be recognized in order to avoid accentuated effects. Similarly, the administration of multiple drugs can preclude the efficacy of an individual drug, and this possibility should be considered in patients with multiple drug regimens.

Table 3–45. *Adverse Effects of Drug-Drug Interactions*

Drug A	Interacting With	Drug B	Adverse Effects
Alcohol		Barbiturates Meprobamate Antihistaminics	Increased CNS depression
		Antidiabetic agents such as tolbutamide	Increased effect of drug B; excessive lowering of blood sugar
Anticoagulants such as bishydroxycoumarin		Salicylates (high doses) Quinidine Quinine	Increased bleeding tendency
		Tolbutamide	Excessive lowering of blood sugar
Antidepressant drugs: monoamine oxidase inhibitors such as pargyline or tranylcypromine		Barbiturates Meperidine	Increased CNS depression
Phenylbutazone Sulfonamides Salicylates		Tolbutamide	Excessive lowering of blood sugar
Phenylbutazone Sulfonamides		Bishydroxycoumarin	Increased bleeding tendency
Phenobarbital Glutethimide Meprobamate		Bishydroxycoumarin	Decreased effect of coumarin
Laxatives (prolonged use) Diuretics, such as chlorothiazide		Digitalis	Increased toxicity of digitalis
Antacids		Tetracycline	Decreased antibacterial effect
Salicylates (small doses)		Probenecid	Decreased activity of drug B; decreased excretion of uric acid

(Modified from Levine, R.R.: Pharmacology. Drug Actions and Reactions. Boston, Little, Brown and Company, 1978.)

Antibiotics

Many *antibiotics* have a specific toxic effect only against specific reactions or functions of microorganisms; for example, *penicillin* affects bacterial membrane synthesis, and *sulfathiazine* affects bacterial replication. Penicillin and other antibiotics may sensitize red blood cells, which, in the presence of a specific antibody and complement, produce a *hemolytic anemia.*

Other drugs are directly toxic to some mammalian cells. These include *chloramphenicol* (Chloromycetin), which produces agranulocytosis, and *metronidazole* (Flagyl), an amebocytic drug that causes leukemia in experimental animals[191] (Table 3–46).

Table 3–46. *Examples of Therapeutic Drugs and Toxicity*

Penicillin	Allergy
Chloramphenicol	Agranulocytosis
Sulfa drugs	Kidney tubule necrosis
Metronidazole	Leukemia
Actinomycin	Stem cell mutations
Aspirin	Gastritis
Phenacetin	Kidney tubular necrosis
Digitalis	Heart block
Melphalan	Leukemia

Anesthetics

Procaine hydrochloride, a local *anesthetic*, may produce severe hypersensitivity reactions. General anesthetics, including *chloroform* and *halothane*,[192] may have serious consequences on previously damaged liver cells.

Analgesics

The toxicity of *analgesics*, for example, *salicylates*, in producing peptic ulcers and in inhibiting platelet action, is well recognized. *Phenacetin*, a component of a common analgesic composed also of caffeine and aspirin, may injure renal tubular cells by the formation of the by-product n-acetyl p-aminophenol.

Stimulants, Depressants, and Narcotics

The addictive effects of narcotics such as codeine, a stimulant, and heroin, a depressant, are well documented. Caffeine and amphetamine are examples of stimulatory drugs with toxic effects on the CNS when taken in excess (Table 3–47). The hallucinogens, lysergic acid diethylamide (LSD), mescaline, and marijuana, produce chromosomal changes in cells grown in tissue culture.

Table 3–47. *Common Psychoactive Drugs*

Stimulatory	Cocaine
	Caffeine
	Amphetamine
Hallucinogenic	Lysergic acid diethylamide (LSD)
	Mescaline
	Marijuana

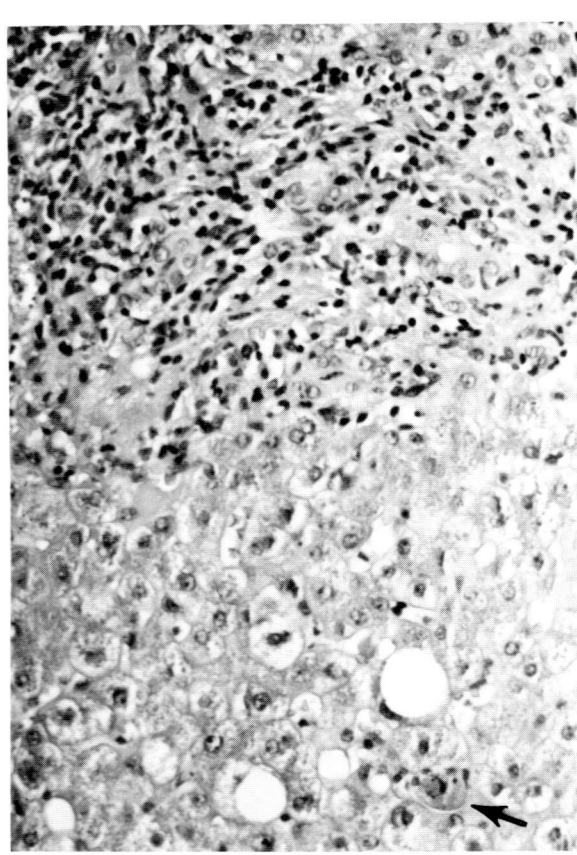

Figure 3–59. In this liver biopsy specimen from a patient with chlorpromazine hepatitis, the portal tract at the top is inflamed and contains prominent numbers of eosinophils. Mild parenchymal fat and an acidophilic body (arrow) are also present.

Sedatives

A common prescription drug in the United States is the sedative diazepam (Valium) (Table 3–48). It is used not only to promote sleep, but is widely taken to induce tranquility during daytime stress. Muscle relaxation and seizure prevention are other uses. Alone or in combination with other chemicals, such as alcohol, diazepam may cause alterations in liver cells by the induction of enzymes of the smooth endoplasmic reticulum (SER). Barbiturates are similarly detoxified by the mixed oxidase enzymes and produce hypertrophy of the SER.

Table 3–48. *Selected Sedative and Hypnotic Agents*

Generic Name	Trade Name(s)
Pentobarbital	Nembutal
Phenobarbital	Phenobarbital
Meprobamate	Equanil, Miltown
Diazepam	Valium
Chlordiazepoxide	Librium

Phenothiazine drugs are commonly used as maintenance therapy for many mental disorders. These agents may occasionally induce liver disease such as chlorpromazine-induced cholestasis, by idiosyncratic mechanisms[193] (Fig. 3–59).

Hormones

Hormones given in excessive amounts may have toxic effects (Table 3–49). An all-too-frequent occurrence is the real or relative *insulin* excess experienced by diabetics, with resultant hypoglycemia. Tolbutamide, an oral hypoglycemic agent used as a substitute for insulin therapy in diabetics, has been implicated in an increased incidence of myocardial infarction.

Table 3–49. *Adverse Effects of Exogenous Hormones*

Hormone	Effect
Insulin	Hypoglycemia
Exogenous estrogens	Vaginal and cervical cancer, endometrial cancer, venous thrombosis, gallbladder disease, hepatocellular adenoma, myocardial infarct
Anabolic steroids	Liver cell adenomas, peliosis hepatis
Thyroid hormone	Increased metabolic rate, anxiety, anorexia
Adrenocorticotropic hormone (ACTH) or cortisone	Lymphopenia, depression of protein synthesis in liver, Cushing's syndrome

Estrogens have been shown to produce endometrial cancer in experimental animals when given in excessive amounts. The addition of estrogen to the food of cattle and chickens to produce growth was banned for this reason. It is socially impossible to eliminate the much larger dosage of estrogen taken daily by millions of women in the form of contraceptive pills. Exogenous estrogens have been implicated in vaginal and cervical cancer,[194] endometrial cancer[195] (Fig. 3–60), venous thrombosis, gallbladder disease,[196] hepatocellular carcinoma,[197] and myocardial infarct. The administration of anabolic steroids has been related to the development of liver cell adenomas and peliosis hepatis.[198]

The treatment of obesity with *thyroid* hormone increases the metabolic rate in all cells and causes loss of weight by reduction of body mass. It also may cause anxiety and anorexia.[199] The treatment of adrenal insufficiency and arthritis with *adrenocorticotropic hormone (ACTH)* or *cortisone* may produce lymphopenia, may depress protein synthesis in the liver, and may cause marked changes in general body habitus *(Cushing's syndrome)*.

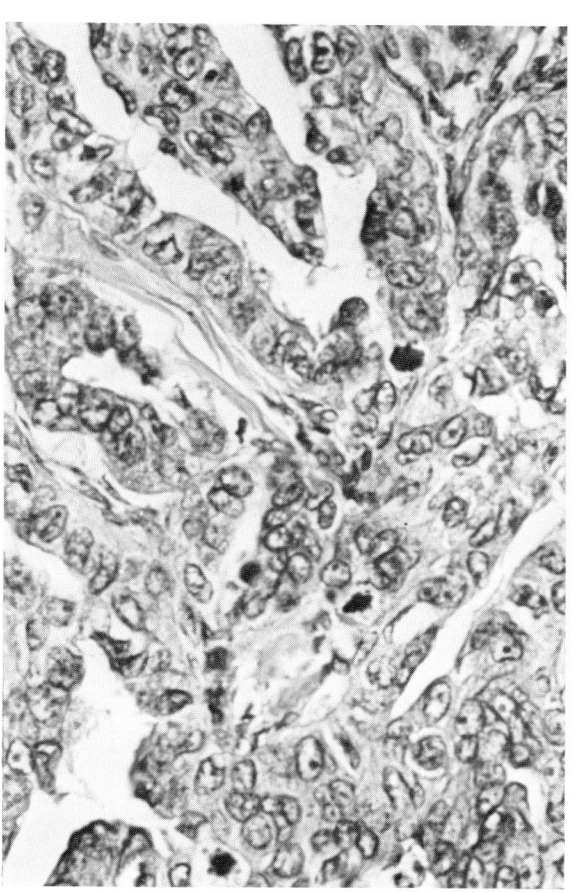

Figure 3–60. Light micrograph showing a moderately differentiated endometrial carcinoma from a patient taking exogenous estrogens.

Chemotherapeutic Agents

Chemotherapeutic drugs produce severe toxicity by design (Table 3–50). Azathioprine *(Imuran)*, an imidazolyl derivative of mercaptopurine, has been used both as a cytotoxic drug in lymphomas and as an immunosuppressive drug of lymphocytes in transplant patients.[200] Cyclophosphamide *(Cytoxan)* and nitrogen mustard destroy malignant as well as normal bone marrow and lymph node cells. *Actinomycin, bleomycin,* and *adriamycin* all may produce severe systemic toxicity.

Table 3–50. *Adverse Effects of Common Cytotoxic Drugs*

Azathioprine (Imuran)	Bone marrow depression, decrease in immune response
Cyclophosphamide (Cytoxan), nitrogen mustard	Depression of bone marrow and lymph node cells, alopecia, nausea, vomiting
Actinomycin, bleomycin, adriamycin	Systemic toxicity, nuclear inhibition
Colchicine, Vinca alkaloids	Cytoskeletal effects

These drugs are not only directly toxic, but they may also induce a variety of autoimmune phenomena. In general, these reactions result from the development of antibodies directed against specific antigenic determinants on the drug. Subsequently, the interaction of antibodies to the drug localized in various cells or tissues leads to release of various allergic mediators such as histamine.

Sometimes a drug may induce the formation of autoantibodies by altering the specific constituents of cells with which it reacts. In this case, the drug acts as a hapten bound to the altered cell component.

Almost every therapeutic agent used in medicine has toxic side effects that, if not carefully monitored, may produce cell injury or cell death. Most of the drugs previously discussed have been used experimentally in vitro, and often in vivo in animals, in order to discover the mechanisms of their toxic action. Other drugs have been used to study effects on organelles and are discussed in a later chapter. These include nuclear inhibitors (for example, actinomycin D), drugs with cytoskeletal effects (for example, cytochalasin D, colchicine), and drugs affecting the cell membrane (for example, phytohemagglutinin (PHA), concanavilin A, and other lectins).

Alcohol Toxicity

Ethyl alcohol (ethanol), a substance that is part of the worldwide social and dietary fabric, is both a beneficial and a harmful chemical. The effects of its ingestion on *central nervous system* functions as well as on physiologic responses of the *liver* and *gastrointestinal tract* are many. Ramifications of its use also are multiple, and alcohol-related traffic *accidents* alone account for 25,000 deaths annually.[201]

It is estimated that over 10 million Americans have serious drinking problems. Alcohol abuse occurs in all age groups and appears in all socioeconomic classes. In urban areas, cirrhosis is the third major cause of death in patients between 25 and 65 years of age.

Nature of Alcoholic Beverages

The basic process for the production of alcoholic beverages is *fermentation*, the conversion of sugar to alcohol by the enzymes of yeasts. There are two major classes of fermented drinks. Wines use their natural sugar content for the conversion. Beers and whiskies require pretreatment with starches to make them fermentable. The major difference in the production of hard liquors (whiskey) is the elimination of some of the unwanted products of fermentation and the increased alcohol content of the final product.

Large quantities of alcoholic drinks are produced yearly in the United States. In 1972, 126 million gallons of whiskey, 1.3 million gallons of rum, 15 million gallons of brandy, and 140 million barrels of beer were produced.[201] The effective blood concentration for loss of function is noted in Table 3–51.

Table 3–51. *Effects of Alcohol*

% Blood Concentration	Effect
0.05	Release of inhibitions and restraints
0.1	Impaired motor function
0.2	Motor function markedly depressed
0.3	Loss of sensory perception
0.4–0.5	Coma
0.7	Respiratory centers affected (death)

Genetic Factors

Genetic factors may be involved in the addiction to alcohol and, of course, they may be modified by cultural, environmental, and psychologic influences.[202] Swedish studies on alcoholism in adopted children who were followed for 25 to 30 years found a 39.4% incidence of alcoholism in their biologic fathers.[203] Other studies have shown a relationship between the severity of the alcoholism in fathers and the incidence of alcoholism in their sons; this finding may reflect environmental influences rather than genetic factors, however.

Studies on twins have suggested that variation in metabolic conversion of alcohol is under genetic control. In addition, genetic factors may determine which organs are specifically affected. Evidence that this may be so was provided by Blass and Gibson, who found an abnormality of fibroblast transketolase in four patients with the Wernicke-Korsakoff syndrome.[204]

Biochemistry

The initial metabolism of ethanol (Fig. 3–61) in the liver occurs by the conversion of ethanol to *acetaldehyde* through the microsomal ethanol-oxidizing system with the conversion of *NADP* to *NADPH*, or in the presence of alcohol dehydrogenase *(ADH)*, the conversion of *NADH* to *NAD* with the release of hydrogen. This hydrogen may be (1) transferred to microsomes later affecting the mitochondrial electron transport system in the citric acid cycle with production of acetyl CoA and CO_2, (2) transferred to fatty acids with the production of ketone bodies and ketosis, (3) transferred to α-glycerophosphate (important in triglyceride fatty acid synthesis) with production of hyperlipidemia, or (4) transferred back to the microsomal ethanol-

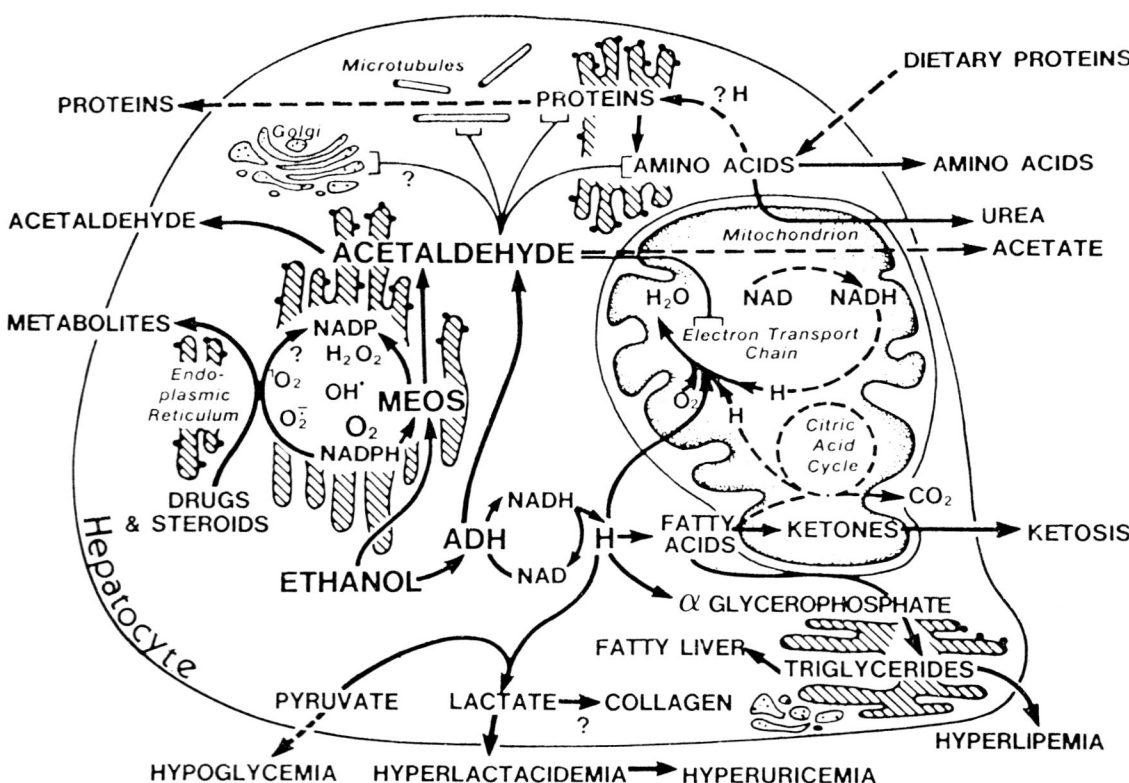

Figure 3–61. Oxidation of ethanol in the hepatocyte and link of the two metabolites (acetaldehyde and H) to disturbances in intermediary metabolism, including abnormalities of amino acid and protein metabolism. *NAD,* nicotinamide adenine dinucleotide; *NADH,* reduced NAD; *NADP,* nicotinamide adenine dinucleotide phosphate; *NADPH,* reduced NADP; *MEOS,* the microsomal ethanol oxidizing system; and *ADH,* alcohol dehydrogenase. The *broken lines* indicate pathways that are depressed by ethanol. The symbol -[denotes interference or binding by the metabolite. (From Lieber, C.S.: Alcohol, protein metabolism, and liver injury. Gastroenterology, 79:375, 1980.)

206   *Agents of Disease*

oxidizing system with conversion of NADP to NADPH. Its effects on carbohydrate, protein, lipid metabolism, and NADH, as well as other metabolic effects, are summarized in Figure 3–61.

The effects of alcohol on lipid metabolism are particularly important. *Chylomicrons* derived from the gastrointestinal tract and adjacent tissues are taken into the liver cell and are degraded to fatty acids, which may be converted to triglycerides or oxidized to CO_2. Triglycerides, cholesterol, and phospholipids, in conjunction with *apoproteins,* form *lipoproteins.* The toxic action of alcohol on the liver may interfere with synthesis, assembly, or release of the protein moiety of the lipid molecule.

Alcohol may also alter the disposition of two carbon precursors, the de-esterification of fatty acids, and fatty-acid oxidation. Effects on protein and lipid metabolism may result in fat in the liver[205] (Table 3–52).

Table 3–52. *Effect of Alcohol Blood Concentrations on Physiologic Function*

Effects on carbohydrate metabolism
 ↓ Gluconeogenesis (hypoglycemia)
 ↓ Galactose oxidation

Effects on protein metabolism
 ↓ Albumin and transferrin synthesis
 ↑ Lipoprotein synthesis

Effects on lipid metabolism
 ↑ Serum triglycerides*
 ↑ Liver triglycerides (fatty liver)

Effects of increased NADH-NAD ratio
 ↑ Lactate production leading to hyperuricemia
 ↑ δ-aminolevulinic acid synthesis leading to ↑ porphobilinogen production
 ↓ Citric acid cycle activity

Other effects
 ↑ Acetaldehyde levels in blood and tissues
 ↓ Serum magnesium and phosphate
 ↑ Catecholamine release leading to ↓ β-adrenergic-receptor sensitivity
 ↑ Oxygen consumption (hypermetabolic state)
 Ketoacidosis

*At blood alcohol concentrations above 250 to 300 mg/dl, the opposite effect may occur. (Adapted from Isselbacher, K.J.: Metabolic and hepatic effects of alcohol. N. Engl. J. Med., 296:612, 1977.)

Morphologic Alterations

The principal organ affected by alcohol is the liver. Following its rapid absorption from the stomach and intestinal tract, alcohol is transported to the *liver*. The severity of changes that one sees in the liver is determined both by the amount and the duration of the intake.[206,207] In chronic alcohol consumption, the liver characteristically shows fat accumulation that is initially readily reversible (Fig. 3–62). The fat derives from several sources.

Alcoholic Hepatitis and Cirrhosis. Heavy drinking results in fatty liver *(steatosis)*, in which the fat is deposited in

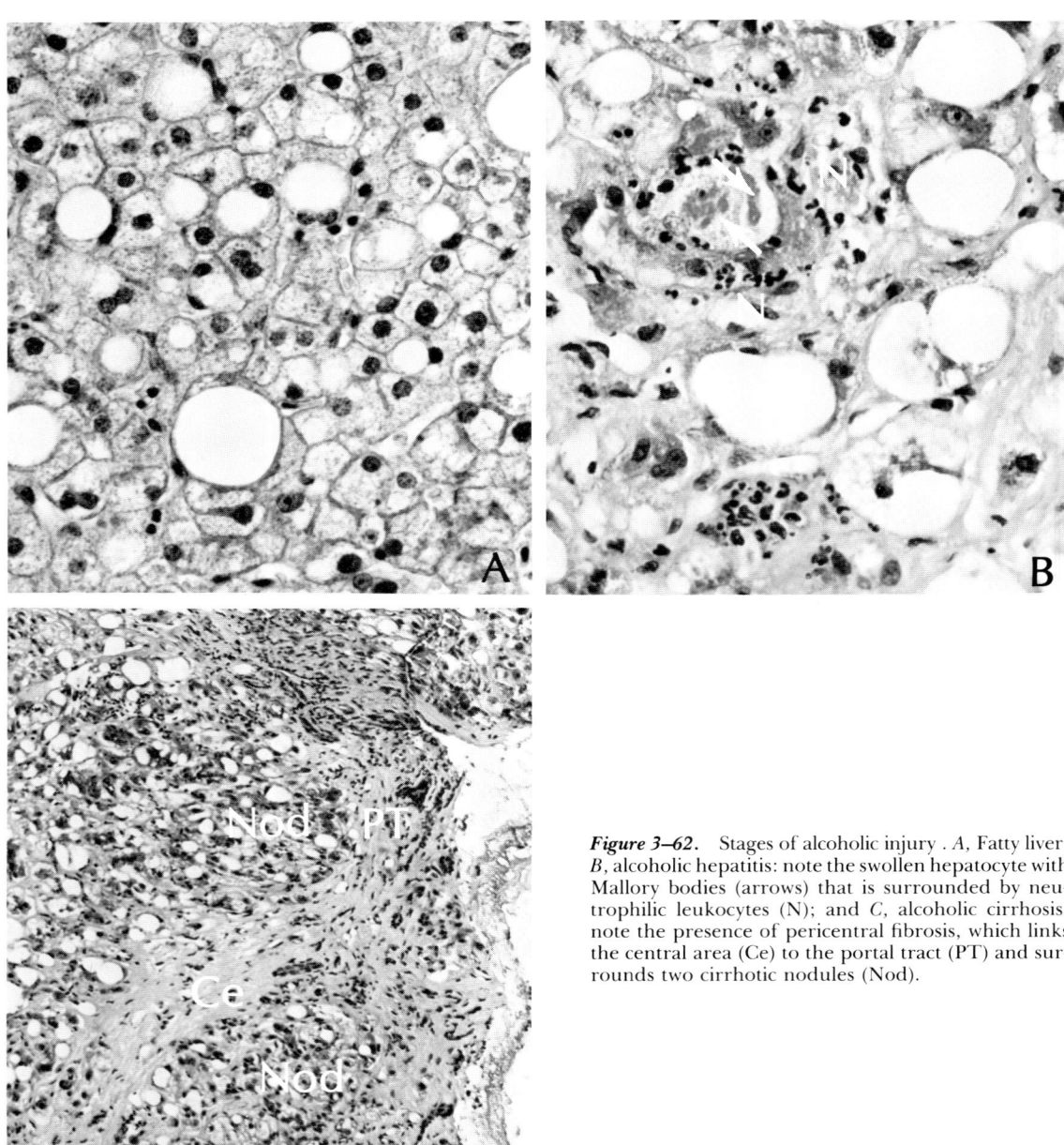

Figure 3–62. Stages of alcoholic injury . *A*, Fatty liver; *B*, alcoholic hepatitis: note the swollen hepatocyte with Mallory bodies (arrows) that is surrounded by neutrophilic leukocytes (N); and *C*, alcoholic cirrhosis: note the presence of pericentral fibrosis, which links the central area (Ce) to the portal tract (PT) and surrounds two cirrhotic nodules (Nod).

a non-membrane-bound form in the liver cell cytosol. This lesion is reversible. Continued drinking maintains the fat in the cells because of increased intracellular transport of free fatty acids, increased cellular production of lipids, and decreased transport out of the cell. Fatty hepatocytes may rupture, discharging their contents into the blood.

More complex acute changes comprising "*alcoholic hepatitis*" follow the continued abuse of alcohol and consist of liver cell death, *Mallory bodies*, and an acute inflammatory response. This response is accompanied by pericentral and pericellular fibrosis. As liver cell death, fibrosis, and regeneration of liver cells continue, architectural landmarks become distorted. The development of widespread fibrosis and regenerative nodules signals the appearance of "*cirrhosis*" (Fig. 3–62).

As previously indicated, maintenance of high-level alcohol intake can lead to alcoholic hepatitis with characteristic *ballooning* of liver cells, centrilobular necrosis, and a leukocytic infiltrate. The prognosis in this stage depends on the extent of hepatocellular necrosis and may be associated with a mortality rate of 10 to 30%.[208]

The development of *cirrhosis* in the alcoholic proceeds as *bridging fibrosis* from central zones (worst affected); then it extends to portal areas with progressive development of portosystemic vascular shunts, and concurrent liver cell regeneration is seen in the form of nodules. These diffuse changes affect most liver lobules and hence lead to a "*regular*," *micronodular cirrhosis*, historically known as "*Laennec's cirrhosis*." This spectrum of changes has been experimentally reproduced in primates following prolonged alcohol ingestion.[209]

The prevalence of cirrhosis in alcoholism is directly proportional to the alcohol consumption. The average-sized man who drinks 170 grams of ethanol (about 0.5 liters of an 86 proof beverage) per day for 25 years has a 50% chance of developing cirrhosis.

Ongoing fibrosis is associated with altered collagen synthesis. Ethanol causes a significant increase in the incorporation of proline and hydroxyproline into collagen[210] as well as an increase in *type III collagen* production. Rubin and Lieber[209] presented evidence that cirrhosis may develop from fatty liver without an intervening state of alcoholic hepatitis. This development may be related to progressive changes of pericentral fibrosis. Production of collagen has been attributed to the *Ito cells (lipocytes* or resting *fibroblasts)* in the *space of Disse,* and perhaps to the collagen-synthesizing capacity of *liver cells* themselves.[210]

Cirrhosis is the tenth leading cause of death in this country, although admittedly not all cirrhotics are alcoholics. Once cirrhosis has developed, abstinence from further alcohol consumption does not restore normal life expectancy.[211] Furthermore, this decreased life expectancy may actually be initiated with alcoholic hepatitis and may proceed even though the patient stops drinking. The morbidity of cirrhosis is associated with its inherent abnormalities of circulation *(portosystemic shunts)*, rupture of *esophageal varices*, as well as with the loss of the multiple synthetic and metabolic functions of the liver, including synthesis of plasma proteins, blood coagulation factors, lipoproteins, and gluconeogenesis.

Alcohol-Induced Liver Cell Subcellular Alterations. The *cytosol* contains increased amounts of fat and proteins that are usually exported *(albumin* and *transferrin)*, all accumulating in the endoplasmic reticulum. That the export proteins are increased in the face of normal levels of constituent proteins has led to the belief that a defect exists in protein secretion from the liver cell. Defective protein secretion has been linked to the decreased number of mi-

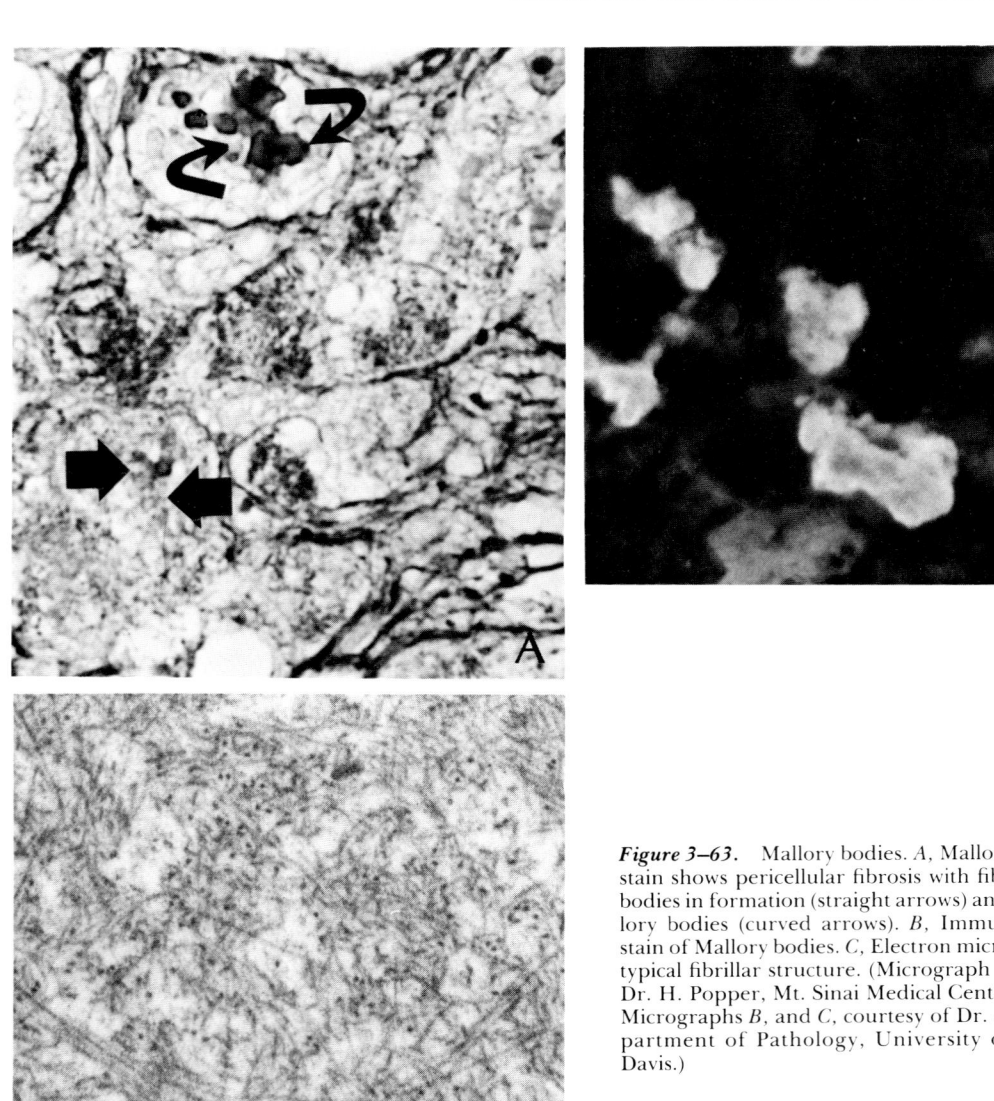

Figure 3–63. Mallory bodies. *A,* Mallory aniline blue stain shows pericellular fibrosis with fibrillar Mallory bodies in formation (straight arrows) and mature Mallory bodies (curved arrows). *B,* Immunofluorescent stain of Mallory bodies. *C,* Electron micrograph shows typical fibrillar structure. (Micrograph *A,* courtesy of Dr. H. Popper, Mt. Sinai Medical Center, New York; Micrographs *B,* and *C,* courtesy of Dr. S. French, Department of Pathology, University of California, Davis.)

crotubules, presumably secondary to altered acetaldehyde or acetate levels, described in chronic alcoholism. The retained proteins lead to a passive retention of water, and the cell undergoes *"ballooning" degeneration* (Fig. 3–62).

One of the morphologic changes in alcoholic hepatitis that has fascinated pathologists for years is *alcoholic hyalin (Mallory bodies)* (Fig. 3–63). These were once considered to be specific for alcoholic liver disease, but we now know that they may be seen in other conditions.[212] It had also been said that their presence indicates a worsened prognosis for the patient, but this idea is controversial. On light microscopy, Mallory bodies appear as masses of clumped, acidophilic material, often horseshoe shaped, within the cytoplasm of swollen liver cells. On electron microscopy, they appear to be *"intermediate filaments."* Recent work by Tinberg et al. has characterized Mallory bodies as *prekeratin-like polypeptides.*[213]

We have already briefly alluded to the adaptive *proliferation* of the membranes of the *smooth endoplasmic reticulum.* Concomitantly, the numbers of associated microsomal enzymes concerned with lipoprotein synthesis and ethanol oxidation are increased. These are beneficial aspects of SER hypertrophy; however, not all enzyme activities are increased.[214]

Perhaps the most striking changes are seen in the *mitochondria* and involve swelling and damage to the *cristae* resulting in a decreased capacity to convert acetaldehyde to acetate. Elevated acetaldehyde levels are toxic and induce secondary organelle damage such as to the microtubules.

Early in alcoholic damage, the mitochondria are typically elongated with aggregated cristae, loose matrix granules, and deposits of large, calcium-like masses. Giant mitochondria may also be seen.[215]

These abnormalities are related to the biochemical alterations noted earlier in Figure 3–61. Mitochondrial-related abnormalities include reductions in (1) the ability to oxidize substrates, (2) energy production with NAD^+-dependent substrates, (3) energy use, and (4) enzyme activities and decreased content of the cytochromes. Energy coupling seems to be particularly sensitive to the effect of alcohol.[216,217]

Complications of Alcohol Toxicity

The effects of alcohol ingestion are systemic, as evidenced by the morphologic changes identifiable at autopsy (Table 3–53).

Gastrointestinal Abnormalities. Thus far, we have only considered the effects of alcohol abuse on the liver, but indeed, chronic alcoholism is a systemic disease (Table 3–53). *Hemorrhagic gastritis* is commonly associated with alcoholism, and an increase of carcinoma of the esophagus has been reported, especially in the Calvados region of France.

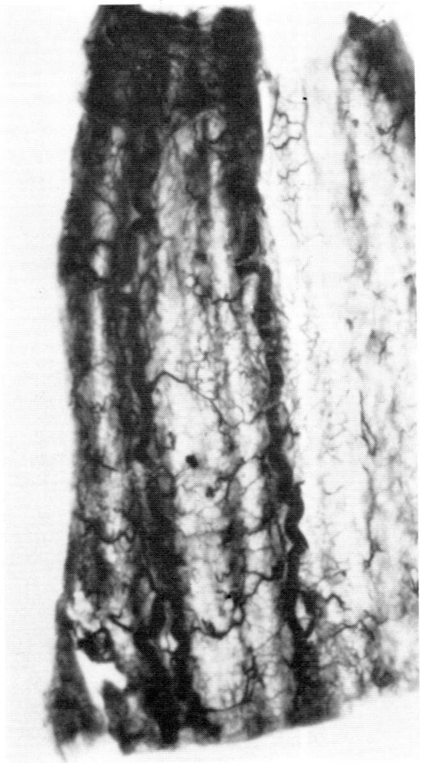

Figure 3–64. Transilluminated portion of esophagus from a patient with esophageal varices.

Table 3–53. *Clinicopathologic Correlations in Alcoholism*

Organ	Lesions
Skin	Pellagra, alcoholic facies, increased vascularity and hair loss
Heart	Alcoholic cardiomyopathy, beriberi disease, fat
Lung	Emphysema
Esophagus	Varices
Liver	Steatosis, alcoholic hepatitis, Laennec's cirrhosis, ascites
Pancreas	Pancreatitis, fibrosis, glandular atrophy
Stomach	Chronic gastritis
Kidney	Glomerulosclerosis, enlargement
Testes	Tubular atrophy
Blood	Anemia and clotting disorders
Brain	Encephalopathy, peripheral neuropathy, cerebral cortex degeneration, cerebellar degeneration, medial mamillary body atrophy
Bone	Idiopathic femoral necrosis, traumatic injury

(Modified from Corrigan, G.E.: Autopsy pathology of alcoholism. Ann. N.Y. Acad. Sci., *273*:385, 1976.)

Esophageal varices are frequently present if cirrhosis and portal hypertension exist. Their rupture can be a serious complication and not infrequently leads to fatal hemorrhage (Fig. 3–64).

The small *intestinal* epithelium may be abnormal and may result in *decreased absorption* of sugars, amino acids, and vitamins (folic acid and B_{12}) and in increased synthesis of triglycerides by the intestine.

Alcoholic Cardiomyopathy. This disorder follows prolonged alcoholic intoxication and leads to severe myocardial dysfunction; heart failure can ultimately occur.[218] Ultrastructurally, the earliest and most severe changes occur in the mitochondria, which increase in both number and size. They eventually fuse together to produce *megamitochondria*. The intercalated discs may dehisce, and eventually severe interstitial edema and fibrosis develop.

Musculoskeletal Abnormalities. Skeletal muscle abnormalities may first be seen as an acute syndrome with muscle aches, tenderness, edema, increased serum glutamic oxaloacetic transaminase activity, and myoglobinuria. The clinical and laboratory features resemble *McArdle's syndrome,* in which there is a hereditary deficiency of phosphorylase.[219] Skeletal abnormalities are identifiable in 57% of patients undergoing alcohol detoxification.[220]

CNS and Peripheral Neuropathies. *CNS* manifestations are associated with the toxic actions of alcohol and general malnutrition, often *avitaminosis B₁₂*. The actions of ethanol on the CNS are of two types: (1) general CNS depression, acting like a general anesthetic, and (2) rapid oxidation in the liver leading to severe cerebral metabolic abnormalities.[221] Sensory perceptions are decreased following intoxicating doses of alcohol as the result of depressed neural transmission.[222] *Astrocytes* drop out, and a *degenerative encephalopathy (Wernicke-Korsakoff syndrome),* manifested by characteristic behavioral abnormalities, is often seen[223] (Fig. 3–65). *Peripheral neuropathies* are more likely to result from *vitamin B deficiency* associated with poor nutrition.

Endocrine Abnormalities. The male alcoholic with cirrhosis frequently shows hypogonadism (testicular atrophy) and gynecomastia. These abnormalities are due, in part, to shunting of blood away from hepatocytes and thereby to

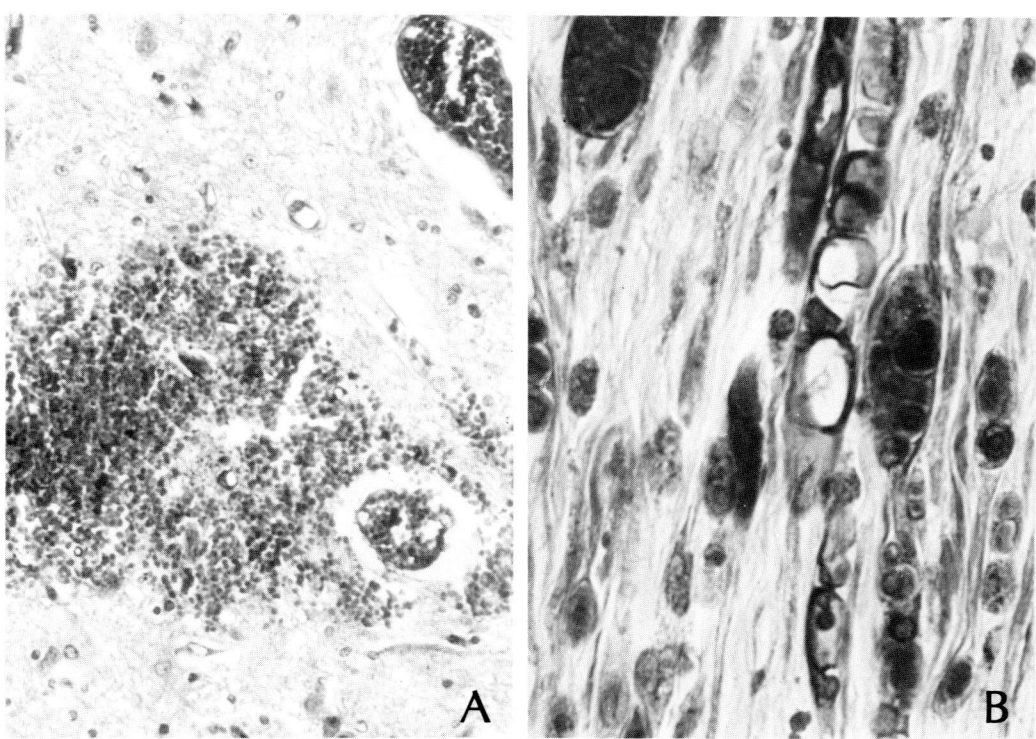

Figure 3–65. Neurologic disorder secondary to alcohol. *A,* Wernicke encephalopathy shows focal hemorrhagic necrosis. *B,* Peripheral nerve stained for myelin shows degeneration of nerve fibers.

altering of steroid metabolism, and not solely to alcohol. Gordon et al. have found that alcohol itself alters endocrine function in males, however. Part of these effects are in the liver, whereas others are in the hypothalamus, pituitary, and testes. Increased binding of testosterone to plasma proteins exists, and other factors serve to reduce the plasma testosterone levels in the male alcoholic.[224]

Recent studies have shown that ethanol has an abnormal effect on retinol. A *deficiency* of *"activated vitamin A"* in the testes has been postulated in the etiology of feminization because it is believed to lead to *aspermatogenesis*.[225]

Immunologic Abnormalities. Patients with alcoholic liver disease often have chronic lymphocytic infiltrates in the liver. Alcoholic liver cell damage of sufficient duration presumably provokes an autoimmune reaction involving both humoral and cell-mediated immunity. *Elevated IgA, IgG,* and *IgM* may be present in the serum of alcoholic patients with cirrhosis. *Lymphocytic* and *plasma cell infiltrates*, even in periportal regions, give the typical appearance of *chronic active hepatitis*. B-cell responses may be abnormal, and the number of blood T cells, as assessed by rosette formation, may be reduced, possibly because of sequestration in the liver where immune reactions against liver cells may occur. Cytotoxicity of lymphocytes may reside in *activated T cells* or in antibody-assisted killer T cells. Both ethanol and acetaldehyde can induce lymphocyte transformation, but only in patients with active hepatitis.[226]

Leevy found that *alcoholic hyalin* or one of its constituents can act as a neoantigen that stimulates synthesis of lymphokines, both macrophage-inhibition factor (MIF) and cytotoxic factors.[227] Hyalin may also increase chemotaxis and hepatocellular necrosis and may stimulate hepatic fibrosis. A *fibroblastic-stimulating factor* isolated from hepatic lymphocytes stimulates collagen formation in all forms of chronic liver disease.

The higher prevalence of HLA-B8 among alcoholic cirrhotics and the absence of HLA-A28 lend credence to the theory that fibrosis in chronic alcoholics may be controlled by interactions of genetic and immune factors.

IMMUNE REACTIONS AND PRODUCTS RESULTING IN INJURY TO CELLS AND TISSUES—IMMUNOPATHOLOGY

In Chapter 2 we discussed the important, supportive role of the immune response in the host inflammatory reaction to cell and tissue injury. We noted the significance of the HLA system in the proper functioning of the immune system and in disease susceptibility in general. The congenital and acquired immune deficiencies associated with white blood cells and complement defects were also reviewed.

Alterations in the immune system involving excessive or deficient immune cells, antigen, antibody, or complement, and formation of immune complexes in appropriately susceptible HLA phenotypes may produce cytotoxic and tissue injury as well as provoking or aggravating an inflammatory response.

Classification of Immune Injury (Hypersensitivity States)

Gell, Coombs, and Lachmann provided a significant contribution to students studying immunopathology by classifying hypersensitivity reactions into four types[228] (Table 3–54). This classification was extended to five groups by Roitt[229] and more recently to six by Sell[230] and others. Unfortunately, the numbered order of types has now been rearranged, and Type I does not always refer to anaphylactic shock. We have kept the four antibody-mediated hypersensitivity reactions together and have left the cellular hypersensitivity reaction as Type V. We have also noted the suggestion of Sell that Type V, delayed hypersensitivity, may be subdivided into two classes (V and VI). This subdivision appears to be at present merely a more progressive state of the cellular response. In graft rejection and in autoimmune and many other diseases, both a humoral and a cellular response appear to exist.[231]

The five types of hypersensitivity diseases are classified as follows:

Type I: Immediate hypersensitivity. This type includes atopic

Table 3–54.   *Comparison of Classifications of Immune Injury*

Gell, Coombs, and Lachmann*	Roitt†	Sell‡	Modification Used in Text
Type I Immediate hypersensitivity (anaphy axis)	Immediate hypersensitivity	Inactivation or activation	Immediate hypersensitivity
Type II Cytotoxic	Cytotoxic	Cytotoxic or cytolytic	Cytotoxic
Type III Immune complex	Immune complex	Atopic or anaphylactic hypersensitivity	Toxic complex
Type IV Delayed (cellular) hypersensitivity—tumor, graft rejection and response to parasites, viruses, and some bacteria	Delayed (cellular) hypersensitivity	Arthus (toxic complex)	Stimulatory or neutralizing activity
Type V —	Stimulatory or neutralizing activity	Delayed (cellular) hypersensitivity—graft and tumor rejection	Delayed (cell-mediated) hypersensitivity
Type VI —	—	Granulomatous (cellular) hypersensitivity	—

Modified from:
*Gell, P.G.H., Coombs, R.R.A., and Lachmann, P.J.: Clinical Aspects of Immunology. 3rd Ed. Oxford, Blackwell Scientific Publications, 1975.
†Roitt, I.M.: Essential Immunology. 2nd Ed. Oxford, Blackwell Scientific Publications, 1975.
‡Sell, S.: Immunology, Immunopathology and Immunity. 3rd Ed. New York, Harper & Row, 1980.

or anaphylactic reactions and IgE-mediated states with a secondary lytic phase.

Type II: Cytotoxic hypersensitivity. This type is mediated by complement lysis or macrophage phagocytosis after antibody interaction.

Type III: Toxic complex hypersensitivity. This includes both precipitation of soluble immune complexes and antibody bound to basement membrane antigens.

Type IV: Stimulatory or neutralizing hypersensitivity. Antibody mimicking hormone binds to structurally similar membrane receptors, and *stimulatory* activity results. Antibody binding to soluble toxins, hormones, or other serum factors produces *neutralizing* activity.

Type V: Delayed (cell-mediated) hypersensitivity. This is concerned principally with *T-cell* or *null-cell* activity. Many delayed hypersensitivity diseases have a significant B-cell activity with production of immune globulins, however.

Type I: Immediate (Anaphylactic) Hypersensitivity

Anaphylaxis is seen as a serious secondary response following initial sensitization to an antigen. Such antigenic stimuli include insect bites, drugs, and a host of environmental agents (Table 3–55). Other diseases with generally similar mechanisms that, however, do not always manifest as crisis situations, include asthma, dermatographia, and urticaria[232] (Table 3–56).

Table 3–55. *Common Causes of Anaphylaxis*

Drugs
  Proteins (presumably complete antigens)
    Foreign serum
    Vaccines
    Allergen extracts
  Nonprotein drugs and some antibiotics (including haptens)
    Penicillin
    Local anesthetics
    Salicylates

Diagnostic compounds
  Sulfobromophthalein
  Sodium dehydrocholate
  Radiographic contrast media

Foods
  Legumes (especially peanuts)
  Nuts
  Berries
  Seafoods
  Egg albumin

Stinging insects
  Honeybees
  Wasps
  Hornets

(Modified from Fudenberg, H.H., et al. (Eds.): Basic and Clinical Immunology. Los Altos, CA, Lange Medical Publications, 1976.)

Table 3–56. *Classification of Atopic or Anaphylactic Reaction*

Anaphylactic shock
Cutaneous (urticaria, poison ivy allergy, hives)
Systemic (bronchial spasm, angioedema)
Atopia (asthma, hay fever, allergic rhinitis, food allergy)

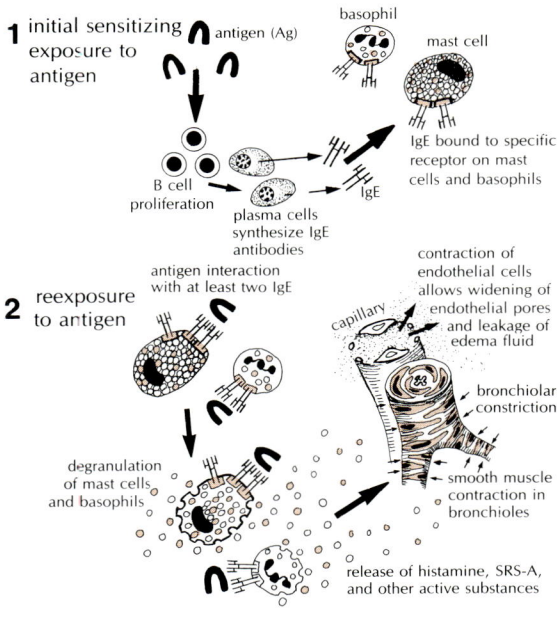

Figure 3–66. Type I immune response: immediate hypersensitivity (anaphylaxis).

The ability of cells to respond in immune hypersensitivity reactions involves the concerted action of mast cells, basophils, and eosinophils in the secondary reaction. The primary processing of antigen involves B and T lymphocytes and macrophages.

Following initial sensitization by an antigen, a clone of B cells may proliferate and may produce IgE. This antibody, largely secreted by plasma cells, is later adsorbed on mast cells in connective tissues and on basophils in the blood. When a person is re-exposed to the original antigen, the antigen combines on mast or basophil cell membranes through the Fab fragment of IgE and provokes the release of *histamine* granules.

Histamine causes contraction of actin in endothelial cells with resultant widening of intercytoplasmic pores and dilatation of capillaries with transudation (Fig. 3–66). The generalized contraction of smooth muscles that may occur is particularly severe in the bronchioles producing anaphylactic shock.

The initial step in mediator release involves the unique IgE receptor on the mast and basophil cell surface. During periods of sensitization, IgE binds to this receptor with affinity. Newmann et al. have found a cell-surface receptor for IgE composed of 2 polypeptide chains with an apparent molecular weight of 130,000.[233] This receptor is univalent and differs from other immunoglobulin receptors on cells. Once IgE attaches to its receptor, it can complex with antigens. The formation of these complexes transfers information to the cell and results in the release of histamine and other factors.

Basophils and mast cells also release *heparin, eosinophil chemotactic factor of anaphylaxis* (ECF-A), *kinin-generating enzyme*, and leukotrienes comprising *slow-reacting substance of anaphylaxis* (SRS-A).[234] Histamine and eosinophil chemotactic factor are preformed and are stored in the cell, whereas SRS-A and platelet-activating substance are generated following stimulation by IgE. Degranulation of mast cells in vitro occurs not only with antigen, but also with corresponding divalent anti-IgE or antilight chains.[235]

The release of mediators results in a nonlytic phase in which mast cell lysosomal membranes fuse with each other and cause degranulation.[236]

Asthma. Abnormalities in the airways during an asthmatic attack include smooth muscle spasm, plugging with mucus, mucosal edema, and infiltration by chronic inflammatory cells.[237] Serum levels of IgE are elevated. When

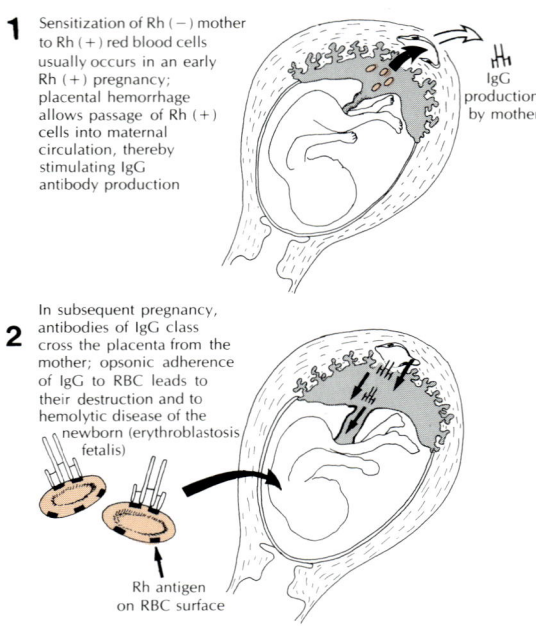

1 Sensitization of Rh (−) mother to Rh (+) red blood cells usually occurs in an early Rh (+) pregnancy; placental hemorrhage allows passage of Rh (+) cells into maternal circulation, thereby stimulating IgG antibody production

IgG production by mother

2 In subsequent pregnancy, antibodies of IgG class cross the placenta from the mother; opsonic adherence of IgG to RBC leads to their destruction and to hemolytic disease of the newborn (erythroblastosis fetalis)

Rh antigen on RBC surface

Figure 3–67. Type II immune response: antibody-dependent cytotoxic injury. Rh disease is a prototype of this form of immune injury.

patients are challenged with an allergen such as pollen, cross-linking of the IgE occurs at the membrane surfaces of mast cells and basophils, and the sequence of events generating histamine, SRS-A, and other factors is activated.

Eosinophils and neutrophils are prominent in the skin and in bronchial mucosa in asthma. In vitro studies suggest that migration of these granulocytes is determined by chemotactic factors produced by target cells in immediate hypersensitivity reactions, complement components, fibrinogen degradation products, plasminogen activators, and kallikrein. Eventually, following repair processes, much of the bronchial wall is replaced by fibrous tissue.

Type II: Cytotoxic Injury

In general, cytotoxic injury activates the complement cascade, with eventual lysis of cells of the immunohematologic organ system (Table 3–57), particularly red blood cells (hemolytic anemias),[238] white blood cells (agranulocytosis), platelets (thrombocytopenic purpura),[239] and vascular endothelia (vascular purpura) (Fig. 3–67). The initial interaction involves cell-surface-bound complement C3b with subsequent generation of the complement cascade. IgM or IgG may both activate complement.[240] In other instances, antibody may bind with target cell membranes as an opsonin promoting cell destruction by phagocytosis in the lymphoreticular system. Other cytotoxic reactions involving killer T, macrophage, or null cells are discussed under "Type V: Delayed (Cell-Mediated) Hypersensitivity."

Table 3–57. *Examples of Cytotoxic Injury*

Hemolytic anemias (red blood cells)
    ABO hemolytic disease of newborn
    Erythroblastosis fetalis
    Transfusion reactions (ABO system)
    Acquired autoallergic hemolytic disease to infectious
      agents, drugs, or neoplasia

Agranulocytosis (white blood cells)
    Neonatal leukopenia
    Acute or chronic agranulocytosis (acquired)

Thrombocytopenia (platelets)
    Post-transfusional thrombocytopenia purpura
    Neonatal thrombocytopenia purpura
    Acute or chronic idiopathic thrombocytopenia

Endothelial vascular purpura (endothelial cells)

The classic example of *cytotoxic injury* is that seen in transfusion reactions in which IgM antibodies are formed against *ABO antigens.* This type of injury is also seen in *Rh* (rhesus) *incompatibility* disease (erythroblastosis fetalis) (Fig. 3–67). In this disease, fetal red blood cells possessing Rh-positive antigens inherited from the father cross the placental barrier into the maternal circulation. This sensitizing process may occur during childbirth or during induced or spontaneous abortion. In the Rh-negative mother, the production of antibodies directed against Rh-positive fetal red blood cells may be induced. Such maternal antibodies may adversely affect subsequent pregnancies with an Rh-positive fetus. Maternal IgG antibodies, formed after previous sensitization, cross the placenta and coat fetal red blood cells, which are then lysed or are subject to phagocytosis in the spleen.

Drugs and toxins may be metabolized to form intermediary products that bind to proteins as *haptens,* thereby becoming antigenic. These antigens stimulate the synthesis of antibodies that adsorb to, or cross-react with, normal cells and bring about lysis with or without complement (Table 3–58). The *acquired hemolytic anemias* associated with certain drugs result from agglutination of red blood cells by antibodies. These agglutinated cells may become sequestered in the spleen or liver and are subject to osmotic lysis and the action of proteases present in leukocytes.

Table 3–58.   *Red Blood Cell Hemolysis Due to Antibodies*

Warm-antibody immunohemolytic anemia
Idiopathic
Systemic lupus erythematosus
Chronic lymphocytic leukemia, lymphocytic lymphoma
Systemic Hodgkin's disease and other rare tumors
Drug-related immune hemolysis
α-methyldopa type
Penicillin type (hapten)
Cold-antibody agglutinin disease
Acute: Mycoplasma infection, infectious mononucleosis
Chronic: Idiopathic, lymphoma
Paroxysmal cold hemoglobinuria

(Adapted from Thorn, G.W., et al. (Eds.): Harrison's Principles of Internal Medicine. 8th Ed. New York, McGraw-Hill, 1977. Used with the permission of McGraw-Hill Book Company.)

Autoimmune Hemolytic Anemia. This disorder is based upon the active binding to membrane receptors on phagocytic cells by antigenic foreign or damaged particles derived from red blood cell membranes.[241]

Type III: Toxic Complex Injury

When antibodies bind to antigen with or without complement, immune complexes may be formed extracellularly or in vascular spaces. These immune complexes may later be deposited in specific tissues and may produce subsequent damage.[242] The addition of complement, if not already present, aggravates a local inflammatory response.

Table 3–59. *Toxic Complex Injury States*

Arthus reaction

Glomerulonephritis
    Serum sickness
    Experimental allergic
    Nephrotoxic
    Poststreptococcal
    Antimembrane
    Hypocomplementemic
    IgA

Infectious disease
    Schistosomiasis
    Syphilis
    Typhoid fever
    Endocarditis
    Thyroiditis
    Hepatitis
    Lymphocytic choriomeningitis

Collagen disease
    Polyarteritis
    Systemic lupus erythematosus
    Systemic sclerosis

Skin diseases
    Erythema nodosa marginatum
    Pemphigus
    Psoriasis
    Dermatitis herpetiformis

Table 3–59 indicates the host of diseases associated with *immune complex formation. Large complexes* are cleared by phagocytosis in the lymphoreticular system. *Small complexes* are excreted in urine, whereas *medium-sized complexes* are deposited in vessels or other tissues.

Sell has grouped together all *toxic complexes* present in tissues, both antibody initially complexed to foreign or altered basement-membrane antigen and true antigen-antibody-precipitated immune complexes formed elsewhere that deposit on the basement membrane. Both reactions bind complement and produce an inflammatory response with infiltration of polymorphonuclear leukocytes (PMN) and subsequent release of lysosomal enzymes.[235]

Arthus Reaction and Serum Sickness. These disorders are experimental models of immune complex disease. The Arthus phenomenon, which is generally studied in the skin but may occur in any organ, is an allergic reaction induced in the presence of *antibody excess* to antigens that have been previously injected. The deposited immune complexes activate C3 and cause migration of PMN with subsequent inflammation and hemorrhage (Fig. 3–68).

Serum sickness, on the other hand, results from deposition of soluble antigen-antibody complexes that have been formed in *antigen excess*. This phenomenon may occur with therapeutic injections of foreign serum, such as horse antidiphtheria globulin, and results in the clinical picture of fever, lymphadenopathy, generalized urticaria, and painful, swollen joints.

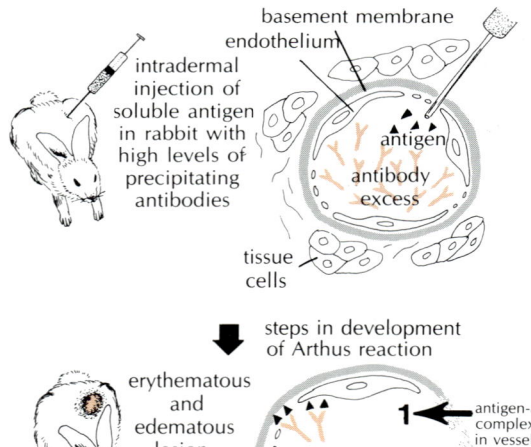

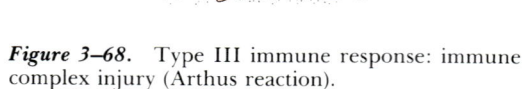

Figure 3–68. Type III immune response: immune complex injury (Arthus reaction).

220   *Agents of Disease*

In both *experimental arthritis* and *nephritis*, researchers have noted the presence of immune complexes attracting PMN and monocytes, which induce selective damage by release of lysosomal hydrolases. The enzymes may arise either from cell death or from the release of the lysosomal granules from viable cells. In vitro, both granulocytes and mac-

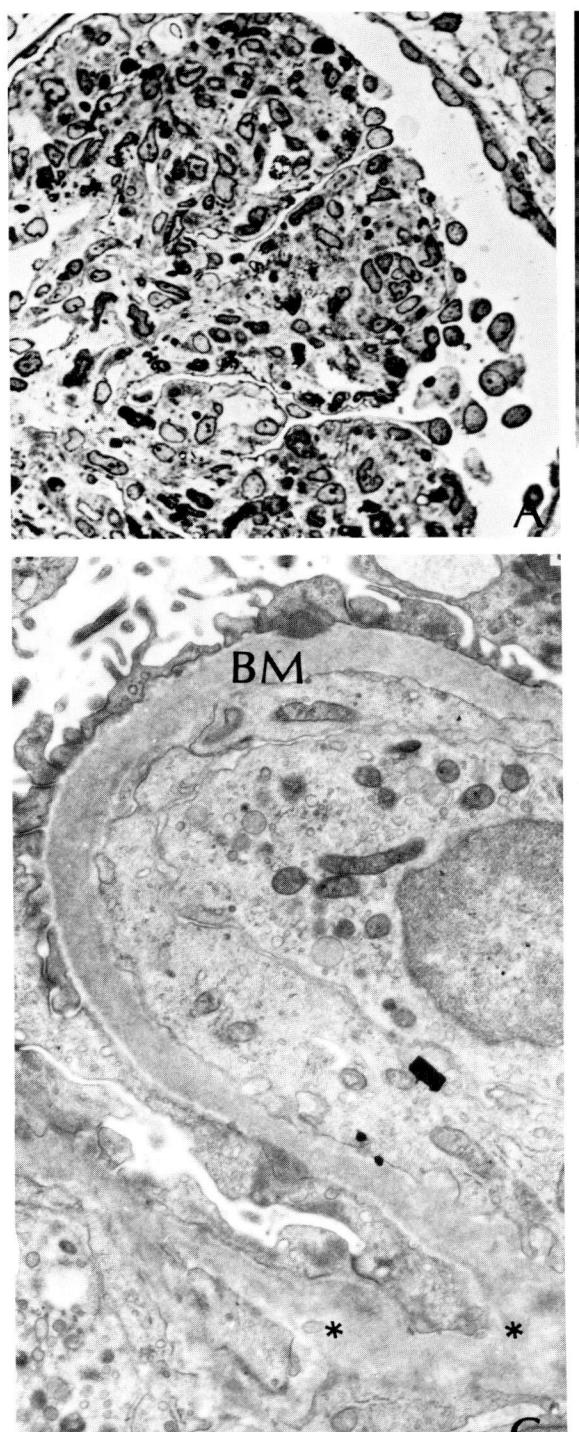

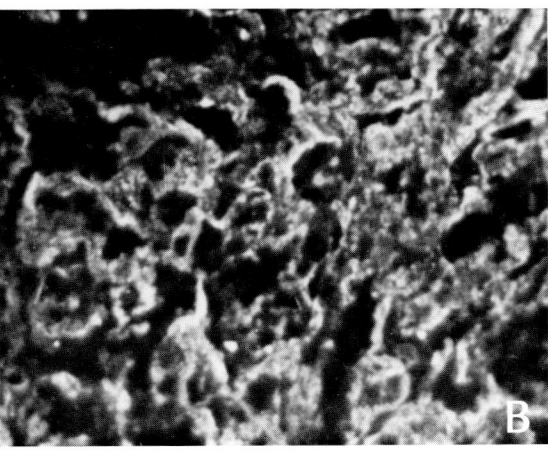

Figure 3–69. Poststreptococcal glomerulonephritis. *A*, Light micrograph shows mild hypercellularity of the glomerular loops. *B*, Immunofluorescence demonstrates immune complexes in the glomerulus. *C*, Electron micrograph shows immune complex deposits (*) in the basement membrane (BM).

rophages, in association with acute and chronic inflammation, can selectively release lysosomal hydrolases with no detectable loss of viability.

Several renal lesions serve as prototypes of immune complex disease. *Poststreptococcal glomerulonephritis* and *systemic lupus erythematosus* are examples of human diseases in which antigen-antibody complexes are deposited within glomeruli (Fig. 3–69).

Velosa et al. noted that immune complexes and components of the classic and alternate complement pathways are regularly present in all hyalinized, senescent, end-stage glomeruli, regardless of the origin of the renal damage.[243] Complement receptors have also been found on mesangial cells.[244] When complement is fixed, the generation of the anaphylatoxins C3a and C5a may release histamine, with consequent vasodilation and chemotaxis of white blood cells. Among the many factors that accentuate glomerular injury are extracellular release of neutral proesterase from PMN, the action of collagenase on collagen with resulting stimulation of kinin production, and the release of polycationic proteins and cathepsins D and E. The consequent damage to walls of blood vessels and the increased vascular permeability also accentuate the injury.

Bayer et al.[245] have reported circulating immune complexes in infective endocarditis. It remains to be proved whether the Osler's nodes and Janeway lesions of infective endocarditis are due to deposition of immune complexes with an inflammatory reaction and whether the antigens present are of host tissue or bacterial membrane origin.

Type IV: Stimulatory and Neutralizing Activity

Stimulatory Antibodies. In one form of immune response, antibodies to a membrane antigen may stimulate hormonal action by virtue of their interaction either with hormone-receptor molecules or antigens closely linked to them on the target-cell membrane (Fig. 3–70 and Table 3–60).

Table 3–60. *Stimulatory and Neutralizing Antibodies*

| Disease | Effect of Immunoglobulin (IgG) | |
	In Vivo	In Vitro
Acanthosis nigricans	Inhibits action of insulin	Inhibits binding of insulin
Myasthenia gravis	Inhibits neuromuscular transmission	Binds to acetylcholine receptor and inhibits binding of bungarotoxin or con-A
Graves' hyperthyroidism	Stimulates thyroid activity	TSI (LATS) inhibits binding of TSH and stimulates thyroid activity

(LATS, long-acting thyroid stimulator; TSH, thyroid-stimulating hormone (thyrotropin); con-A, concanavalin A; TSI, thyroid-stimulatory immunoglobulin.)

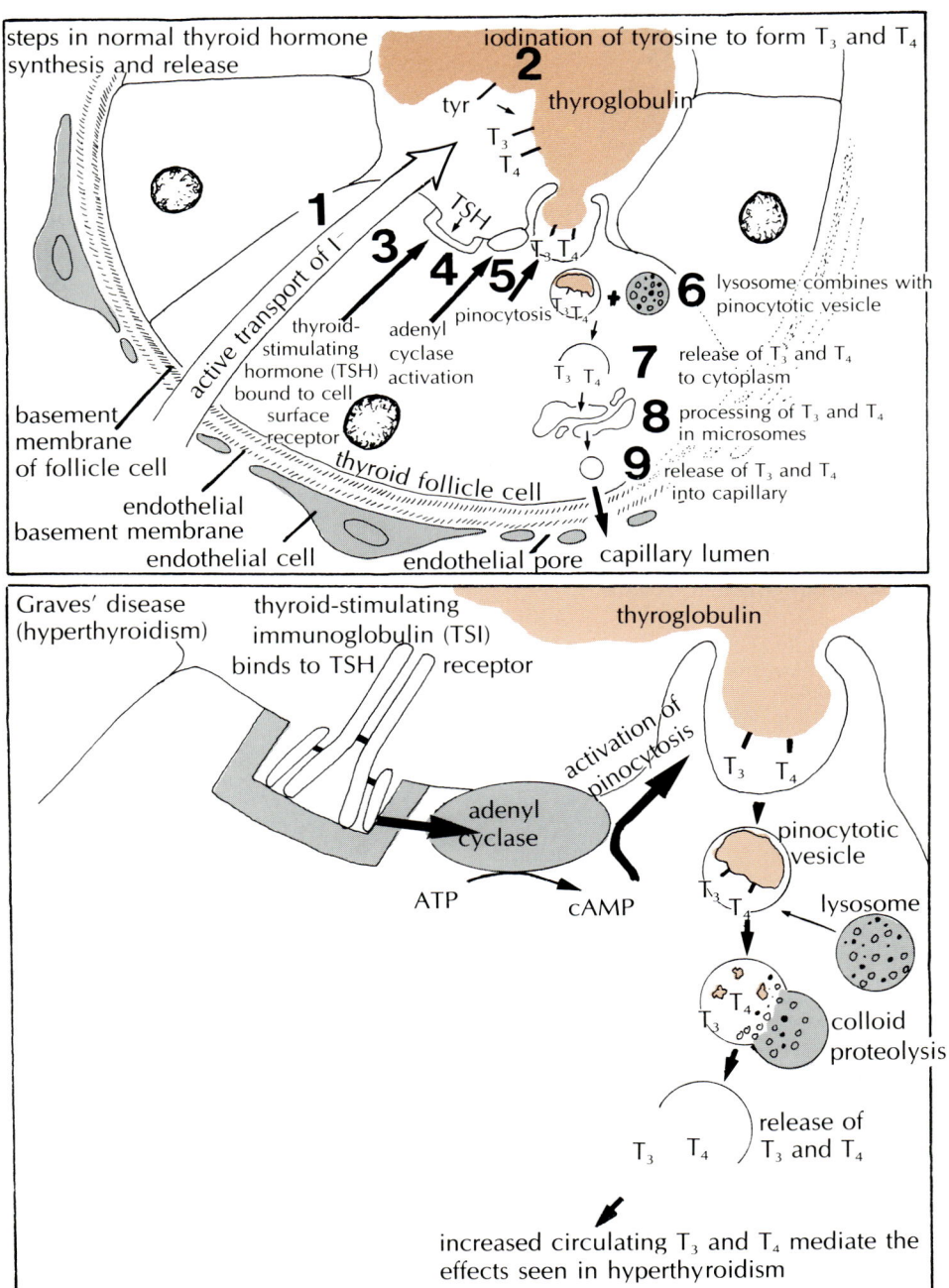

Figure 3–70. Type IV immune response: stimulatory hypersensitivity (Graves' disease). In hyperthyroidism (see lower box), binding of thyroid-stimulating immunoglobulin (TSI) to the TSH receptor mimics TSH action and stimulates (via cAMP) T_3 and T_4 release.

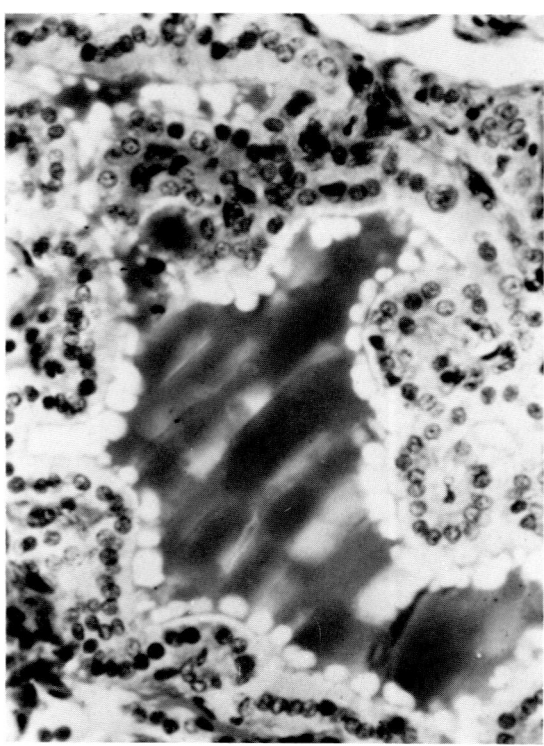

Figure 3–71. Light micrograph of thyroid from a patient with Graves' disease showing prominent scalloping of the intrafollicular colloid.

The *hyperthyroidism* of *Graves' disease* is caused by thyroid-stimulatory immunoglobulin *(TSI)*, previously known as *LATS* (long-acting thyroid stimulator). TSI is an antibody to the thyroid-stimulating hormone *(TSH)* receptor on the thyroid follicular cell surface. The antibody binds to the receptor and thereby mimics the action of TSH. This process stimulates adenyl cyclase, with increased liberation of thyroxine and triiodothyronine; hyperthyroidism results (Fig. 3–71).

Neutralizing Antibodies. These antibodies may bind and inhibit hormones, toxins, enzymes, and clotting or growth factors and may react with cell-surface components including receptors. Autoimmune antibodies have been found to acetylcholine (ACh) receptors, β-adrenergic receptors, and insulin receptors. Antibodies effective in aggravating diabetes have been produced against insulin, islet-cell cytoplasm, and target-cell insulin receptors.

Type V: Delayed (Cell-Mediated) Hypersensitivity

Delayed hypersensitivity reactions (Table 3–61) are usually associated with certain infections such as tuberculosis and viral, fungal, and parasitic diseases, systemic disorders such as thyroiditis and polymyositis, localized "allergic" injurious processes such as contact hypersensitivity, and graft and tumor rejections.[230,246]

Table 3–61. *Delayed (Cell-Mediated) Hypersensitivity*

Infections
Tuberculosis or leprosy
Viral diseases
Fungal diseases
Parasitic diseases
Systemic disorders
Thyroiditis
Polymyositis
Localized "allergic" injurious processes
Contact hypersensitivity
Graft rejection
Tumor rejection

Role of the T Cell. This type of hypersensitivity is not transferable by antibody, but resides in T cells previously exposed to an antigen. Memory T lymphocytes are derived from cells sensitized to a specific antigen. When a person is re-exposed to the antigen, it combines with receptors on these memory T cells and induces blast transformation in them that leads to their mitosis and proliferation.[247] As a result of this activation, the T cells both participate in direct cellular interactions and produce soluble lymphokines.

The ancillary function of macrophages, helper T cells (T_H), and suppressor T cells (T_S) with the B cell in antibody synthesis has been previously discussed. Subsets of both types of these cells remain as memory cells.[248] A third group of T cells (T_D) is involved in delayed hypersensitivity reactions associated with the previously mentioned disease states and is particularly important in the production of lymphotoxins, macrophage-inhibition factor (MIF), chemotactic factors, skin reaction factor, interferon, and macrophage-cytotoxic factor (MCF), sometimes called macrophage-arming factor (MAF). This last factor is especially important in activating macrophages to be capable of killing foreign cells by direct action or with the aid of antibody-dependent cellular cytotoxicity (ADCC).[249] Cytotoxic T lymphocytes (CTL), also known as killer T cells (T_K), are capable of killing cells by direct cell-cell interaction. T cells may possibly destroy cells with the aid of antibody (ADCC).[250]

Although the literature remains confusing, there appear to be three classes of null cells, which are lymphoid cells without consistent cell-surface markers; these cells are capable of reacting with foreign antigens on grafts, tumors, or altered membranes[251] of the host cell and of producing cell destruction[252] (Table 3–62). These include *null cells reacting with ADCC, cytotoxic null cells (N_C)*, which appear to be naturally cytotoxic without antibody against *leukemias*, and *natural killer (N_K)* null cells, which also require no antibody and are particularly effective against *solid tumor antigens*.[253] Table 3–63 lists the similarities and differences between N_C and N_K cells.

Table 3–62. *Nomenclature of Immune Cells (B, T, Null (N) and Macrophages (M))*

T_H	Helper T cell
T_S	Suppressor T cell
T_D	Delayed hypersensitivity T cell producing lymphokines
CTL (T_K)	Cytotoxic or killer T lymphocyte (direct cell interaction)
T (ADCC) ?	Antibody-dependent cellular cytotoxicity (T cell)
N_C	Natural cytotoxic null cell
N_K	Natural killer null cell
B (ADCC)	Antibody-dependent cellular cytotoxicity (B cell)
M (ADCC)	Antibody-dependent cellular cytotoxicity (macrophage)

Table 3–63. *Comparison of Natural Cytotoxic (N_C) and Natural Killer (N_K) Cells*

Similarities	Differences
No H-2 restriction	Strain distribution (beige mouse—
No MuLv specificity	normal N_C, low N_K)
Present in nude mice	Age of appearance
Increased by bacille Calmette	Effect of incubation
Guérin (BCG) vaccine	Fc receptors
Nonphagocytic	Surface Ag (Thy-H-2)
Effects of irradiation	Effects of estrogen

(From a personal communication from Dr. Osias Stutman at the Cancer Biology I Seminar, Given Institute of Pathobiology, Aspen, Colorado, July 7 to 11, 1980.)

Graft Rejection. *Corneal transplants* and properly matched blood transfusions rarely provoke an immune response and are thus not rejected. In contrast, *renal,*[254] heart, and *bone marrow transplants* are fraught with rejection problems. The reactions of the host tissue *(host versus graft)* to the foreign cellular antigens in kidney donor transplants are usually divided into three stages[255] (Fig. 3–72), as described in the following paragraphs.

An immediate *(hyperacute)* rejection may take place on the operating table or within hours following transplantation in which *preformed antibody* in the host reacts with donor tissue antigens on the endothelium of the glomerular capillaries to induce coagulation, clot formation, thrombosis, and infarct with widespread renal cortical necrosis.[256] (*Acute fulminant rejection* is an irreversible, primary episode

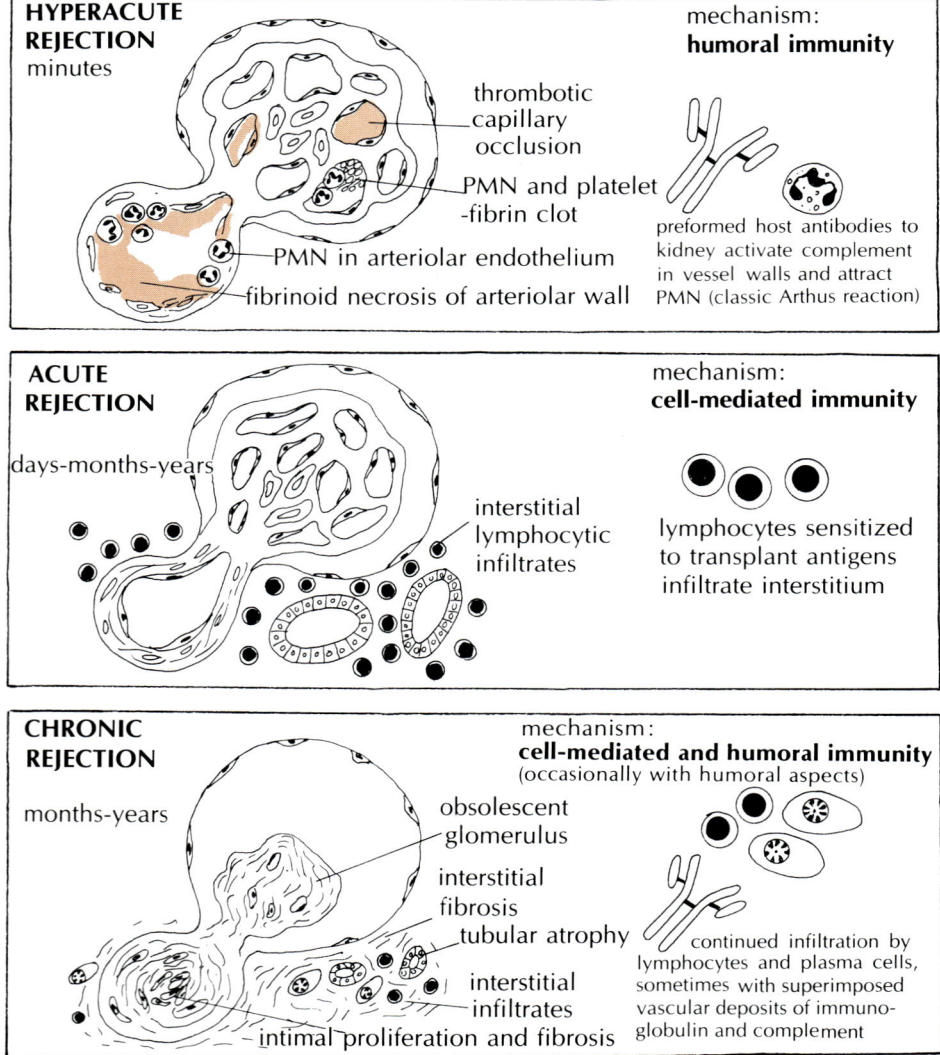

Figure 3–72. Mechanisms of renal transplant rejection.

of rejection that is consistent with *both* acute cellular rejection and hyperacute rejection.)

Acute rejections, which usually occur within weeks, result from the presence of prominent, perivascular, T-lymphoid cell infiltrates and donor cell necrosis. Generally speaking, only this predominantly cellular type of rejection (acute rejection) can be reversed by immunosuppressive therapy.

The third type of rejection, or *chronic stage*, may occur several months or years later. It has characteristics of both *cellular* and humoral antibody responses with an obliterative vascular intimal proliferation.[257] In addition, toxic *glomerulonephritis*, antiglomerular basement membrane nephritis, or pyelonephritis may occur in the later stages.

A rare complication, particularly seen in bone marrow transplants, is *graft versus host* disease.[258] The transfer of a donor cell population of immune-competent lymphocytes may lead to their colonization and proliferation and to the rejection of the antigens of the host, which are perceived as foreign by the donor lymphocytes.

In most human transplants, the immune response is suppressed with a variety of *immunosuppressive drugs* including prednisone and azathioprine. These drugs increase the susceptibility of the patient to infection, particularly with herpes, hepatitis B, and cytomegalic inclusion viruses.

Although the significant increase in lymphoreticular tumors reported in renal transplant patients was previously attributed to depression of the *immune surveillance mechanism* or the *mutagenic carcinogenic* action of immunosuppressive drugs, others believe that the drugs increase susceptibility to mutagens. Frizzera et al. have proposed, from morphologic histochemical analysis, that two types of tumors arise following transplant. They are "polymorphic diffuse B cell hyperplasias" and "polymorphic B cell lymphomas."[259]

Different Types of Delayed Hypersensitivity. Some investigators believe that the delayed hypersensitivity reactions associated with viral disease and graft and tumor rejection can be separated from a second group of hypersensitivity diseases including tuberculosis, leprosy, berylliosis, sarcoidosis, and fungal diseases. The last-mentioned group of diseases is associated with a much more extensive and progressive *epithelioid* and *giant cell* granulomatous reaction (Fig. 3–73), different from that seen with graft and tumor rejection.[230] This granulomatous response is discussed in the chapter on inflammation.

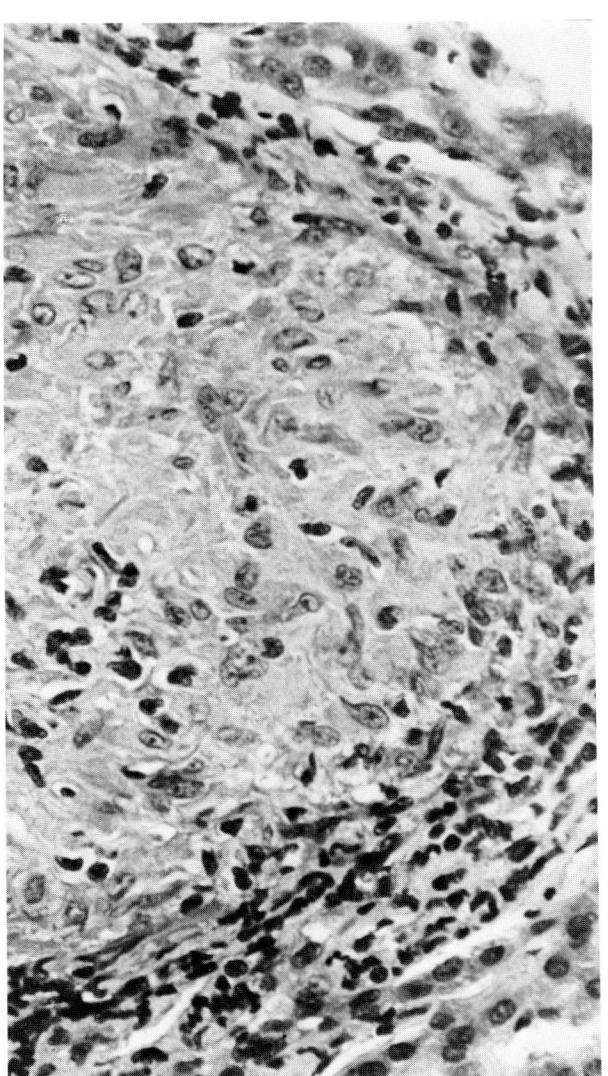

Figure 3–73. Light micrograph of a noncaseating granuloma in a patient with sarcoidosis is composed of a large collection of epithelioid histiocytes.

Autoimmune Disease

The spectrum of diseases attributed partially to autoimmune injury runs from *organ-specific* to generalized *systemic diseases* (Table 3–64). Among the organ-specific diseases are Hashimoto's thyroiditis and thyrotoxicosis (thyroid), pernicious anemia and gastritis (stomach),[260] Goodpasture's disease (lung, kidney), pemphigus (skin), myasthenia gravis (muscle), and primary biliary cirrhosis and chronic active hepatitis (liver). Generalized autoimmune diseases affecting many systems include systemic lupus erythematosus, scleroderma, and rheumatoid arthritis. Cellular destruction may result primarily from humoral antibodies (Hashimoto's thyroiditis), immune complex deposition (systemic lupus erythematosus), cell-mediated delayed hypersensitivity (rheumatoid arthritis), or stimulatory hypersensitivity (thyrotoxicosis).

Table 3–64.   *Genetic Autoimmune Syndromes*

Alopecia areata
Hashimoto's thyroiditis
Pernicious anemia
Thyroid autoantibodies
Hypoadrenocorticism with its hypoparathyroidism and superficial moniliasis
Schmidt's syndrome (diabetes mellitus, Addison's disease, myxedema)
Turner's syndrome
Down's syndrome

(Modified from Martin, G.M.: Genetic syndromes in man with potential relevance to the pathobiology of aging. *In* Genetic Effects of Aging. Edited by D. Bergsma and D.E. Harrison. New York, Alan R. Liss for the National Foundation—March of Dimes, BD:OAS XIV(1), 1978.)

Rheumatoid Arthritis (RA)

Rheumatoid arthritis is an autoimmune disease of unclear etiology that appears in middle age, particularly in women. The disease affects smaller joints bilaterally and is characterized by a *granulomatous pannus* reaction in the joint that is initially painful and later debilitating (Fig. 3–74).

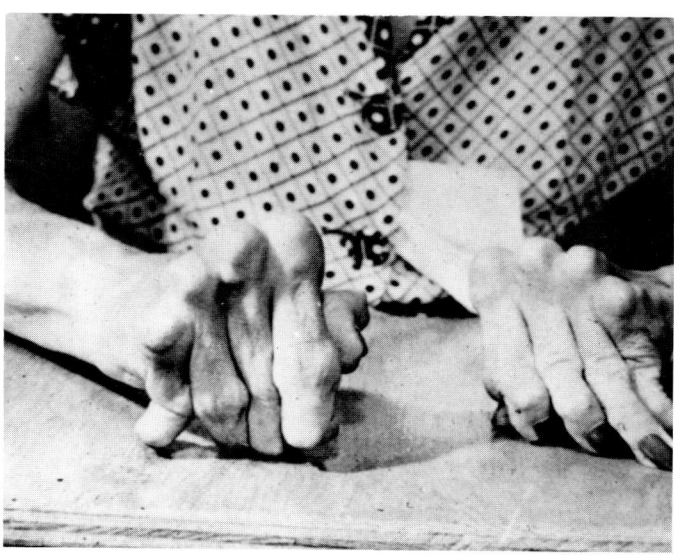

Figure 3–74. Patient with rheumatoid arthritis; note the deformity of the hands with prominent knuckles and deviation of the fingers. (Courtesy of Dr. A. Johnston, Department of Pathology, College of Physicians & Surgeons, Columbia University, New York.)

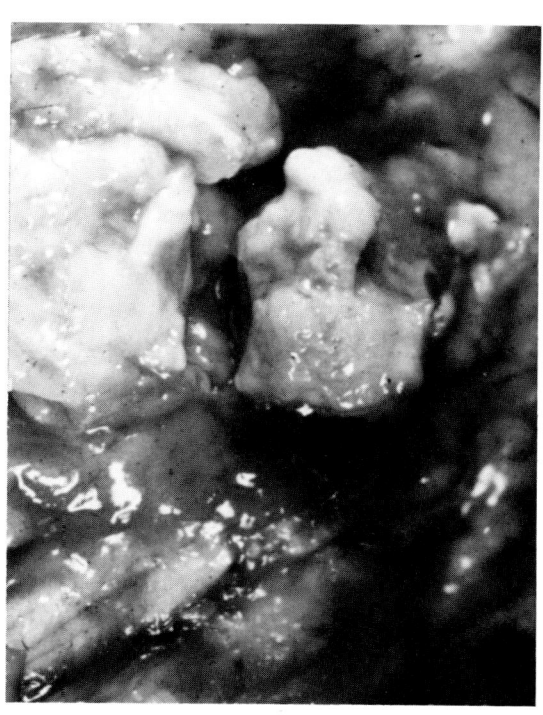

Figure 3–75. Gross picture of a joint surface from a patient with rheumatoid arthritis demonstrating irregular pannus formation. (Courtesy of Dr. A. Johnston, Department of Pathology, College of Physicians & Surgeons, Columbia University, New York.)

The crippling features of RA occur as the joint-bearing surfaces are destroyed and bone alignment is secondarily distorted. The articular cartilage, ligaments, tendons, and bones are destroyed by an invasive, proliferative *pannus* of granulation tissue and collagen (Fig. 3–75). The principal structural proteins of normal joints are destroyed by the activation of latent collagenase in the joint, which degrades Type II collagen from cartilage and Type I collagen from tendons and bone.[261]

Some investigators believe that the primary derangement is in the synovial cell, perhaps initially owing to viral injury.[262] Examination of lymphoid infiltrates in RA shows that whereas 9 to 35% of the cells are B cells and bear surface IgG, the majority of the cells in the infiltrate (70% to 85%) form spontaneous sheep red blood cell rosettes and are therefore T cells.[263]

The nature of the autoantigen in this disorder is still debated. It has been hypothesized that collagen is the culprit. Although vasculitis usually complicates the disease, the major tissue injury is confined to the joint cavity. Complement-derived chemotactic factors attract PMN, which then burst and release their lysosomal enzymes. These enzymes further injure the articular cartilage and enhance pannus formation.[263]

Several immune complexes have been demonstrated in the joints, but the most important is IgM–anti-IgG. A prominent aid in diagnosis is the presence in the serum of *rheumatoid factor*, which represents a 19S IgM macroglobulin synthesized against IgG antibody.[264]

Systemic Lupus Erythematosus (SLE)

SLE is a chronic inflammatory disease of unknown etiology. Its features are attributed to injury by autoimmune reactions following initial injury to the synovial cells, possibly by an infectious, drug, chemical, or other agent (Fig. 3–76). This disease shows a strong predilection for women and displays diverse manifestations. These include fever, a characteristic erythematous malar rash, polyarthralgia and arthritis, polyserositis, and anemia and thrombocytopenia, as well as renal,[265] neurologic, and cardiac abnormalities.

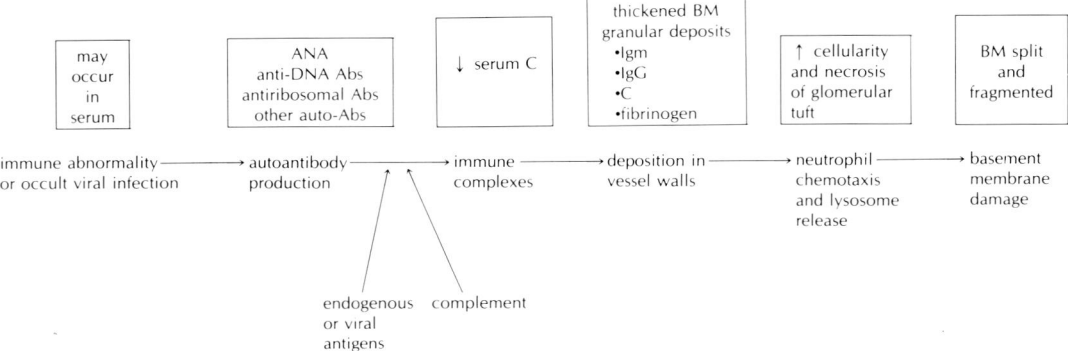

Figure 3–76. Pathogenetic considerations in systemic lupus erythematosus (SLE). C, complement; BM, basement membrane; ANA, antinuclear antibody; Ab, antibody.

The clinical manifestations stem from vascular and tissue inflammation, which follows deposition of immune complexes that form between the patient's antinuclear antibodies and his own nuclear material.[266] A comparison of the autoantibodies seen in SLE and RA is shown in Table 3–65. These autoantibodies may arise because of a defect in suppressor T cells.[267]

Table 3–65. *Comparison of SLE and Rheumatoid Arthritis*

Studies	SLE	Rheumatoid Arthritis
Total white blood cell count	Frequently decreased	Frequently increased
Coombs' test	Frequently positive	Rarely positive
LE preparation	Frequently positive	Negative
Autoantibody		
Antinuclear antibody (ANA)	Positive (high titer)	Rarely positive (low titer)
Anti-DNA antibody	Frequently positive (high titer)	Positive (low titer)
Anti-smooth-muscle antibody	Negative	Negative

(Modified from Rudolph, A.M. (Ed.): Pediatrics. 16th Ed. New York, Appleton-Century-Crofts, 1977.)

On electron-microscopic examination of the renal lesion of SLE, one can see amorphous, electron-dense deposits containing IgG, IgM, complement, and sometimes fibrinogen within and about the basement membrane (Fig. 3–77). Indirect immunofluorescence has often demonstrated properdin in glomeruli and in the dermal-epidermal junction of patients with SLE, indicating involvement of both classic and alternate complement pathways. Autoantibodies to double-stranded DNA and ribosomes have been demonstrated and serve as serologic criteria of disease activity.[268] Interaction of autoantibodies and nuclear material results in the formation of the characteristic *hematoxylin bodies*, bluish purple globular inclusions found within phagocytic cells *(LE cells)*.

The disease has been observed in an animal model. When Schwartz[269] diagnosed SLE in a dalmatian dog, the disease was transferred with ultrafiltrates to seven puppies that later produced antinuclear antibodies. Serologic evidence of a *C-type RNA virus* was also present. Virus-like particles have been noted for years in human kidneys studied by electron microscopists. Independent evidence has also shown that antigen related to C-type RNA virus is present

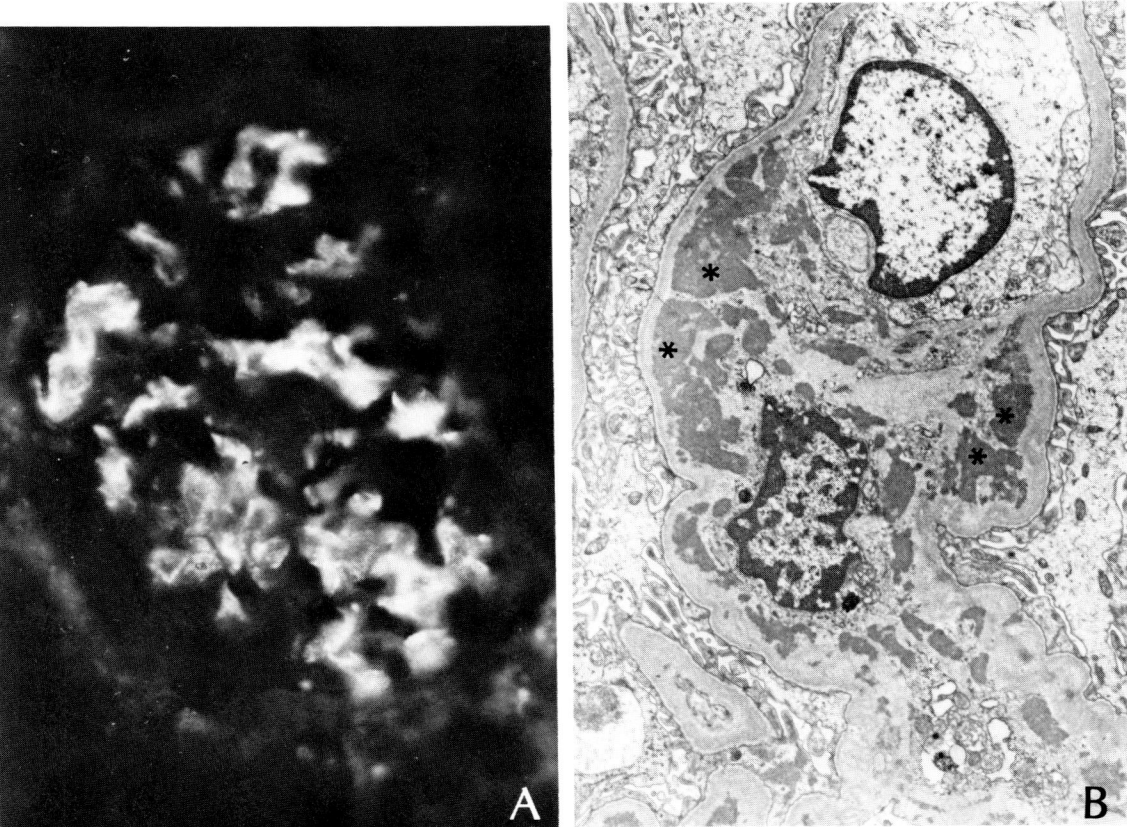

Figure 3–77. The kidney glomerulus in systemic lupus erythematosus. *A,* Immunofluorescence demonstrates the irregular deposition of immune complexes. *B,* Electron micrograph shows deposition of immune complexes (*). (Courtesy of Dr. C. Pirani, Department of Pathology, College of Physicians & Surgeons, Columbia University, New York).

in cells of some patients with SLE.[270] Although viral infection may be a cause of the disease, genetic or familial factors must also be of great importance. HLA-B8 and other major histocompatibility complex (MHC)-related antigens show weak associations.[271]

The *NZB/NZW* hybrid mouse is a naturally occurring experimental model of SLE. Such mice spontaneously develop glomerulonephritis as well as immunopathologic electron-microscopic and serologic findings similar to those found in human SLE. Viral antigens and antibodies, as well as viral reverse transcriptase, have been demonstrated in these animals.

Different *antinuclear antibodies* have also been found in *Sjögren's syndrome, scleroderma* (progressive systemic sclerosis), and *mixed connective tissue disease,*[272] as well as in other diseases (Table 3–66). Antibodies to a special ribonuclear protein (RNP) component called *Sm* fraction were found in 85% of patients with typical SLE, whereas nonspecific anti-RNP antibody was characteristically found in patients with mixed connective tissue disease.

Table 3–66.   *Immunologic Specificity of Antibodies to Nuclear Antigens*

Types of Antibodies	Diseases in Which Antibodies are Seen
Antibodies to native DNA (N-DNA)	
React only with double-stranded DNA (DS-DNA)	Characteristic of SLE; few cases reported
React with both double- (DS-DNA) and single-stranded DNA (SS-DNA)	High levels in SLE; lower levels in other rheumatic diseases
React only with single-stranded DNA	Present in rheumatic and nonrheumatic diseases
Deoxyribonucleoprotein	Found in LE cell antibody in SLE
Histone	Infrequent, present in low titer in SLE
Sm protein (ribonuclease resistant)	Highly diagnostic of SLE
RNP (ribonucleoprotein (ribonuclease sensitive)	High levels in mixed connective tissue disease (MCTD); lower levels in other rheumatic diseases
Scl-1 protein	Highly diagnostic of scleroderma
SS-A protein	High prevalence in Sjögren's syndrome and sicca complex
SS-B protein	High prevalence in Sjögren's syndrome and sicca complex

(Modified from Sharp, G.C., et al.: Association of antibodies to ribonucleoprotein and Sm antigens with mixed connective-tissue disease, systemic lupus erythematosus and other rheumatic diseases. N. Engl. J. Med., 295:1149, 1976.)

Vasculitis

Necrotizing vasculitis, a process characterized by inflammation and necrosis of blood vessels (Fig. 3–78), can exist as the primary manifestation of a disease such as *polyarteritis nodosa,* or it may be a complicating minor component of immune complex deposition in other disorders (Table 3–67). Disseminated vasculitides comprise a broad spectrum of disorders that involve different vessels of different types, sizes, and locations. In general, however, they are either caused directly by, or are closely associated with, immunopathogenic mechanisms involving immune complexes or cell-mediated immune reactions. Antibody may react with antigenic components, such as drugs or virus, it may be present in the wall of the vessel, or it may be a part of antigen-antibody complexes formed elsewhere. Systemic lupus erythematosus and rheumatoid arthritis have vasculitic components.[273]

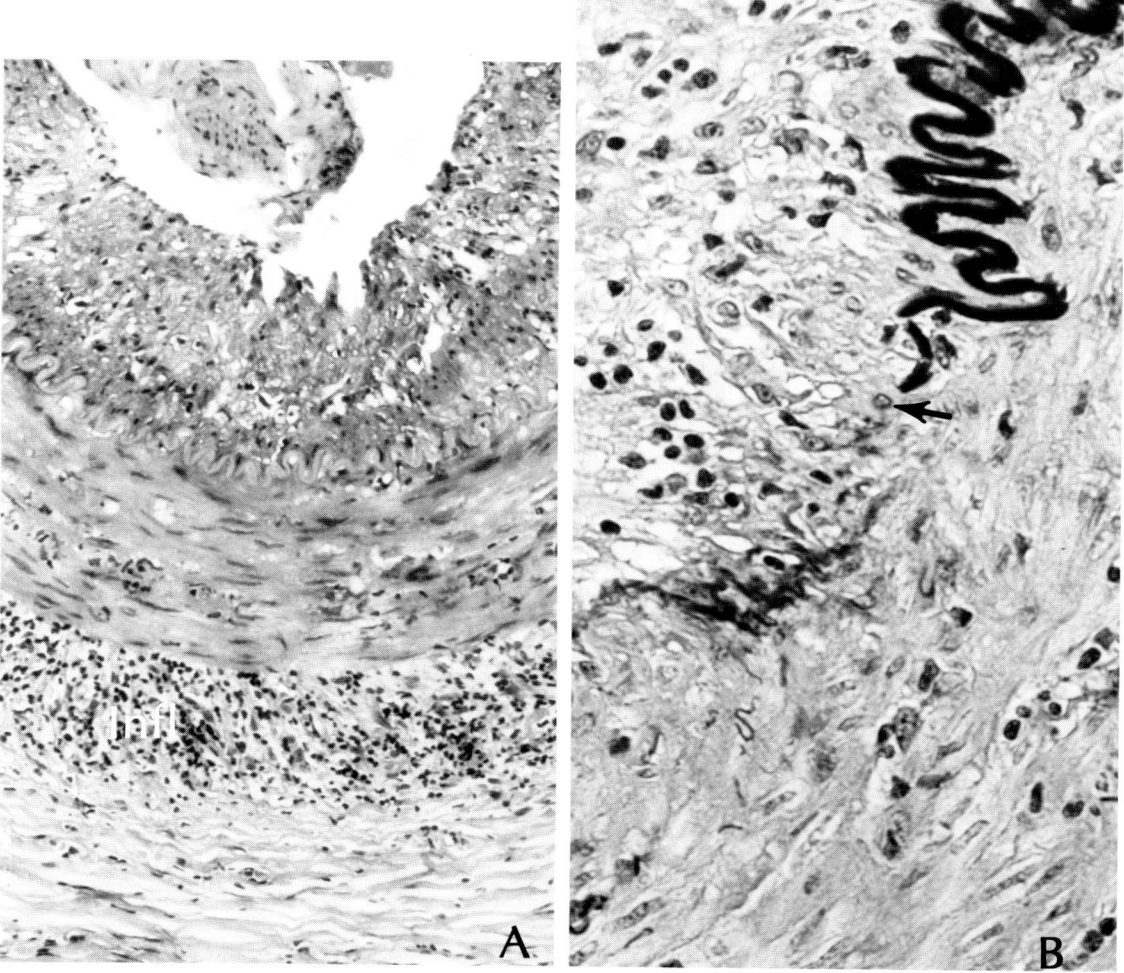

Figure 3–78. Arteritis. *A,* Note the presence of the inflammatory infiltrate (Infl) in the wall of the artery. *B,* When the vessel is stained with an elastic tissue stain, destruction of the elastica is demonstrated (arrow).

Table 3–67. *Spectrum of Vasculitides—Autopsy Study*

	No. of Cases
Polyarteritis nodosa	120
Allergic granulomatosis	20
Hypersensitivity vasculitis	
Rheumatoid arthritis	3
Systemic lupus erythematosus	24
Lymphoma	14
Wegener's granulomatosis	3
Lymphomatoid granulomatosis	2
Giant cell arteritis	4
Takayasu's disease	2
Buerger's disease	63
Miscellaneous vasculitis	9

(Adapted from Branwood, A.W.: The enigma of vasculitis. *In* Progress in Surgical Pathology. Edited by C.M. Fenoglio and M. Wolff. New York, Masson Publishing USA, Inc., 1981.)

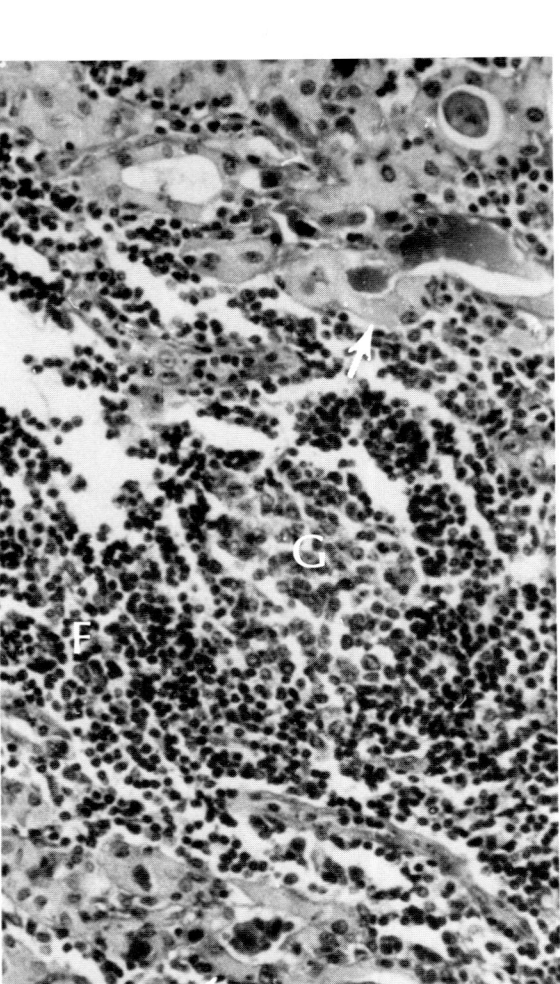

Figure 3–79. Hashimoto's thyroiditis with lymphoid follicle (F) complete with a germinal center (G). The thyroid epithelium has undergone typical oxyphilic change (arrows).

Hashimoto's Thyroiditis

This disease of unknown etiology is first seen either as *acute thyroiditis* with an enlarged, inflamed gland or as *chronic thyroiditis* with atrophy of thyroid follicles and fibrosis (Fig. 3–79). Characteristic of the disease is infiltration by mononuclear cells and lymphoid follicles with germinal centers.[274] Antibodies to thyroglobulin, microsomal antigens and to lipoproteins (organ-specific) are present. T_H lymphocytes may be required to help B lymphocytes bind autoantigens such as thyroglobulin. Antibody is believed to collaborate with N_K or T_K cells in killing acinar cells. *Experimental autoimmune thyroiditis* has been induced in mice with thyroglobulin antigen,[275] and spontaneous autoimmune thyroiditis is found in 90% of the OS strain of chickens.[276]

Endocrine Autoimmune Disorders

Several endocrine deficiencies are clearly mediated by immunologic mechanisms. These include *Graves' disease, Hashimoto's thyroiditis,* and some forms of *diabetes. Graves' disease,* an immunologically mediated, hyperfunctional endocrine disease has previously been discussed. In all these immunologically mediated endocrinopathies, a defect in suppressor cells as well as other possible malfunctions of immune regulation have been suggested. If one postulates the existence of "*forbidden clones*" of lymphocytes, one need not postulate alterations of "self" cellular antigens as the mechanism of disease. A *deficiency* of *suppressor T cells* could allow helper T cells to stimulate B cells to produce autoantibodies.[277]

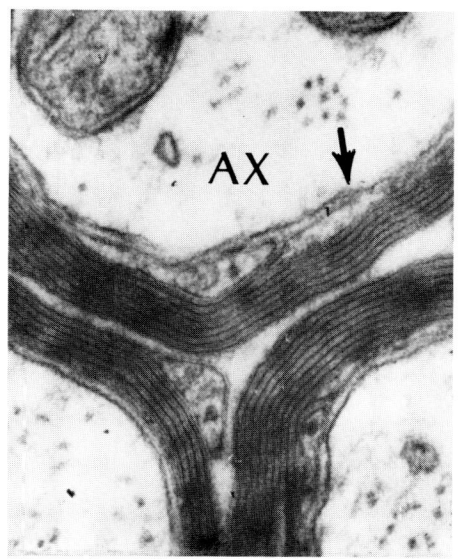

Figure 3–80. The myelin surrounding axons (Ax) is degenerating (arrow) in a case of allergic encephalomyelitis.

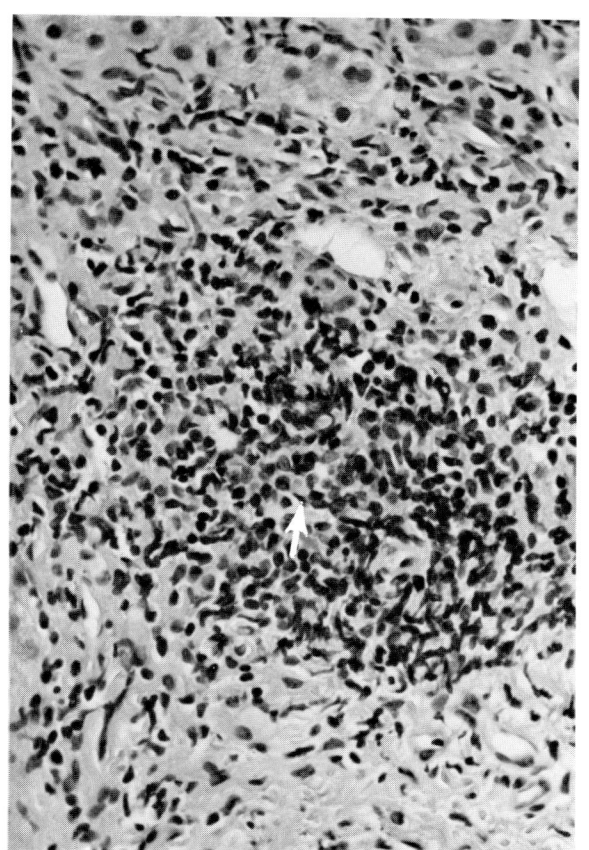

Figure 3–81. The portal tract is inflamed by lymphocytes and plasma cells that surround bile duct epithelium (arrow) undergoing destruction in this "florid bile duct lesion" of primary biliary cirrhosis.

Allergic Encephalomyelitis

Allergic encephalomyelitis is a well-known experimental autoimmune disease. Animals can be induced to react to a component of the myelin sheath called *myelin basic protein (BP)*. To induce this disease experimentally, animals must be injected both with BP and Freund's adjuvant. Lampert[278] showed that demyelination and allergic neuritis occurred concurrently with infiltration of mononuclear cells that attach on the myelin sheath (Fig. 3–80). The experimental model closely resembles other naturally occurring idiopathic forms of human demyelinating diseases.

Chronic Liver Diseases

Chronic active hepatitis, primary biliary cirrhosis (Fig. 3–81), and certain forms of liver disease are believed to be perpetuated by immunologic mechanisms. Circulating immune complexes are important in many of the hepatic and extrahepatic manifestations of these diseases,[279] but this concept is controversial.

Myasthenia Gravis

Myasthenia gravis (MG) is a disease characterized by episodic skeletal muscle weakness secondary to abnormalities of neuromuscular impulse tranmission. This disease most frequently affects the facial, oculomotor, pharyngeal, and respiratory muscles; respiratory insufficiency may be fatal.

The similarity of this disease to curare poisoning and its response to anticholinesterase drugs indicate that the primary site of injury is probably the neuromuscular junction.[280,281]

Clinical Features

Young women are affected twice as often as men, and when men have the disease, they tend to be older.

Myasthenia becomes manifest over several weeks, and partial or complete remissions occur in about 50% of patients. Weakness of ocular muscles with drooping of the eyelids is seen in 90% of patients and is often insidious in onset. Generalized skeletal muscle weakness may also be seen in more advanced cases.

Classically, the affected muscles fatigue easily with partial recovery following rest. In some patients, the weakness is confined to the extraocular muscles and does not become generalized. Testing repetitive or sustained movements of the eyes may bring out inherent eyelid fatigability. Administration of a cholinergic drug (neostigmine) usually also aids in the diagnosis, by improving muscle strength.[282,283]

Normal Neuromuscular Transmission

The neurotransmitter acetylcholine (ACh) is produced in the motor nerve axon terminals and is stored in vesicles for subsequent release into the synaptic junction. Exocytosis, with release of ACh from presynaptic membranes, occurs at specialized release sites situated directly opposite the highest concentration of ACh receptors on postsynaptic membranes. When ACh combines with its receptor, electrolyte permeability is altered, and electrical depolarization takes place. The effect is terminated by diffusion of ACh away from the neuromuscular junction, reuptake by the presynaptic membrane, or by degradation by *acetylcholinesterase* (Fig. 3–82).

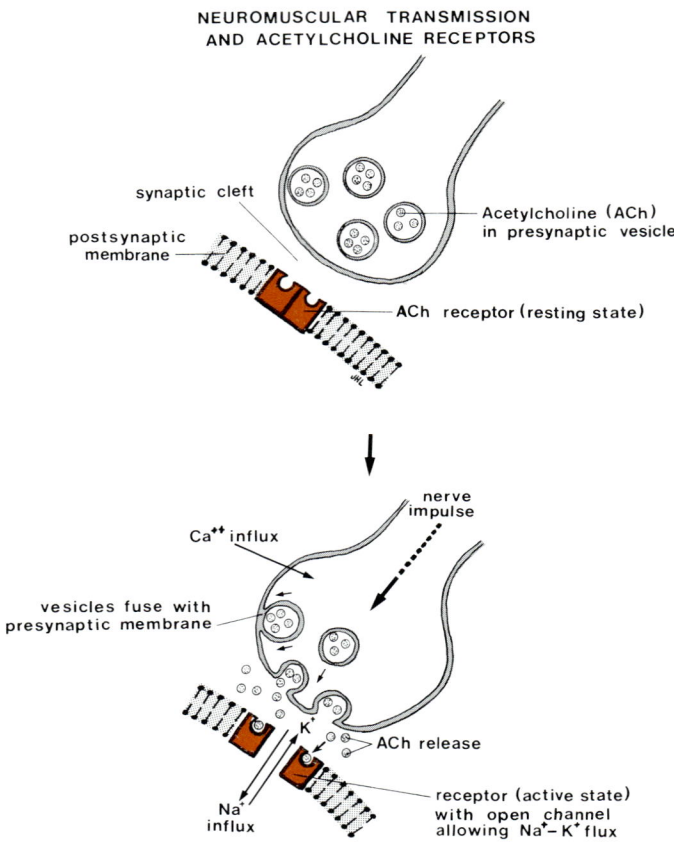

NEUROMUSCULAR TRANSMISSION
AND ACETYLCHOLINE RECEPTORS

Figure 3–82. Diagrammatic representation of normal synaptic transmission.

The specific receptor sites for ACh have been studied with toxins derived from snake venoms, the most common of which is *bungarotoxin*.[284] This substance binds specifically and irreversibly to the active sites of ACh receptors and is used to quantitate and study the number of ACh receptor sites.

The *receptor* is a 300,000-molecular-weight glycoprotein composed of subunits: 2 α subunits contain the active site with monomers of 50,000 and 1 β, 1 γ, and 1 δ subunit. Each receptor molecule has 1 or 2 ACh binding sites. The receptor molecule is believed to have its own ion pore that allows the movement of ions.[285] It is represented in electron microscopy by a negative staining pit 100 × 150 Å.

Pathogenesis

Early studies indicated that the amplitude of the *neuromuscular end plate potential* was reduced in muscles of myasthenic patients. It was suggested that this change was secondary to a reduced synthesis, secretion, or availability of ACh, a reduction of *ACh receptor (AChR)* molecules, a blockade of AChR, or to the synthesis of a false transmitter.[286] Experimental evidence favors an immune pathogenesis related to production of antibodies against AChR[287] (Fig. 3–83).

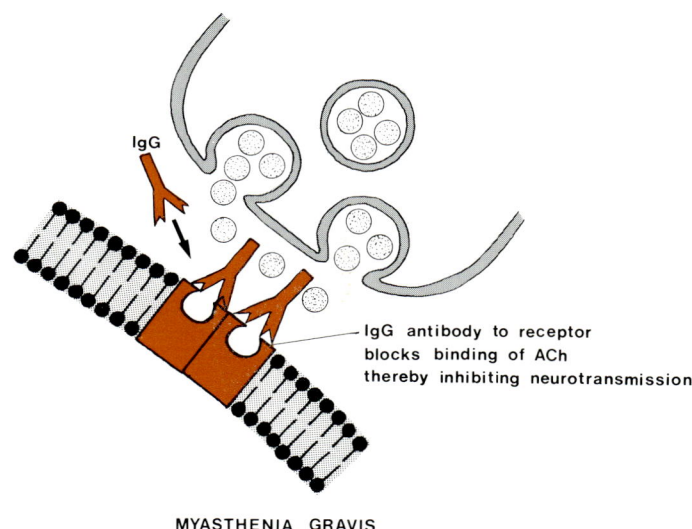

IgG

IgG antibody to receptor blocks binding of ACh thereby inhibiting neurotransmission

MYASTHENIA GRAVIS

Figure 3–83. This diagrammatic representation showing a defect in synaptic transmission in myasthenia gravis.

The technique of immunoperoxidase staining of α-bungarotoxin has allowed visualization of AChR on skeletal muscle. Muscle biopsies from MG patients demonstrate reduced immunoperoxidase bungarotoxin staining at the postsynaptic sarcolemma, a finding consistent with earlier autoradiographic data. This technique led to isolation of *circulating antibodies* that were bound to the AChR (thereby blocking toxin binding) and appeared to play a role in the pathogenesis of MG.[288] More recently, a receptor-specific antibody has proved to be a much better probe than the bungarotoxin, which cross-reacts with other receptors in the brain and hypothalamus.[289]

Ultrastructural studies in experimental and human MG have shown degenerated postsynaptic membrane folds, especially at their tips where the AChR are concentrated, and widened synaptic spaces containing dense globular residues.[290] Both C3 and C4 complement fractions are seen in the synaptic space.

Because many myasthenics have associated thymic abnormalities, it has been suggested that the disease has an autoimmune basis. Indeed, evidence in humans favors the idea that AChR may act as an autoantigen in the pathogenesis of myasthenia. Almon et al. found immunoglobulins in the serum of myasthenics that partially blocked AChR.[288] The ability to induce remission of symptoms in myasthenics with plasmapheresis is consistent with the presence of humoral factors blocking the AChR. Other studies have since confirmed the existence of such antireceptor antibodies. The antibody appears to be an IgG molecule, the effect of which is enhanced by the "early" components of complement.

Antireceptor antibody against the cytoplasmic portion may interfere with receptor function in a variety of ways. It may block the active site of the ACh molecule, or it may mediate increased AChR degradation or decreased synthesis of AChR. Experimental evidence suggests that accelerated AChR degradation occurs with an actual decrease in the number of receptors.[291]

Some of the effects of the disease have been produced in experimental animals immunized with purified AChR protein from the electric eel. These animals developed progressive muscular weakness related to receptor-blocking antibodies. The immunization of rats with purified AChR in Freund's adjuvant has also resulted in the isolation of circulating antibody (IgG) to receptors.[292]

Several lines of evidence suggest that cell-mediated immune responses are also important in the pathogenesis of myasthenia gravis.[293] When lymphocytes from myasthenic patients were cultured in vitro with AChR from the eel, Electrophorus electricus, the lymphocytes underwent blast transformation.

No prominent macrophage invasion takes place in humans, as it does in rats. The lymphorrhagia seen in skeletal muscle biopsies of myasthenic patients may not be at the neuromuscular junctions and may represent a response to other, nonspecific antibodies (Fig. 3–84).[294]

In some patients, general abnormalities in T-cell functions are noted, as well as a decrease in number and abnormal autoreactivity, associated with increased numbers of B cells. It is conceivable that the immunoregulatory function of T cells is sufficiently altered to lead to abnormal humoral autoimmune responses in this disease.

In addition to the role of antibody and cells of the immune system, other substances have been postulated as important in the pathogenesis of the muscle weakness. These include *complement, interferon,* and *thymosin (thymopoietin).* Serial studies of serum complement levels in myas-

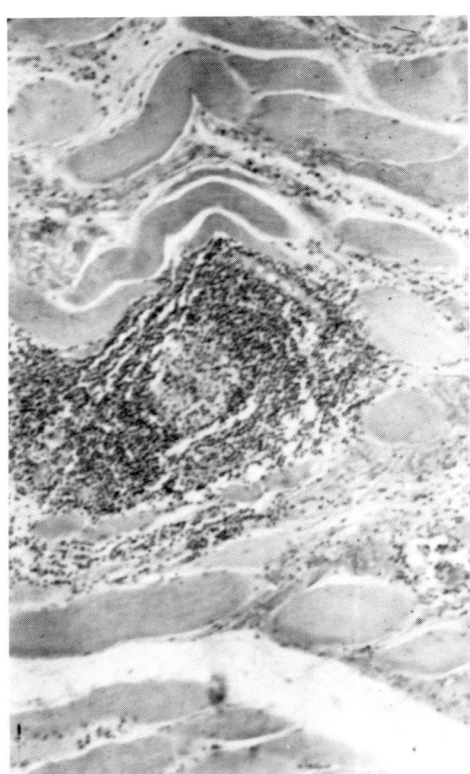

Figure 3–84. Lymphorrhagia in skeletal muscle of a patient with myasthenia gravis.

thenic patients have shown that these levels were lower during active disease, but rose to normal or supernormal levels during remission. It was therefore suggested that a hypersensitivity state exists during exacerbations, whereby complement binds to AChR-Ab complexes and induces lysis of the motor end plate. That thymopoietin, a hormone that regulates some T-cell functions, may also be abnormal accounts for some of the T-cell abnormalities and thymic disorders that are features of myasthenia gravis.

What is the origin of the autoimmune response directed against the AChR? The thymus is believed to be involved, because thymic abnormalities are common, and thymectomy often alleviates some of the symptoms (Table 3–68). Patients with MG have a high proportion of thymic abnormalities. These are 9% thymoma, 66% hyperplasia, and 25% normal, involuted thymus.[295] The thymus normally contains *myoid cells* that can be grown out in tissue culture in addition to its lymphoid cells.[296]

Table 3–68. *Clinicopathologic Correlations in Myasthenia Gravis*

Organ	Lesion
Thymus	Thymoma
	Lymphoid T-cell hyperplasia
Skeletal muscle (ocular, bulbar, neck, limb, respiratory)	Lymphorrhagia
	Muscle fiber atrophy (Type I or Type II fibers)
	Muscle necrosis with infiltrative inflammatory cells

An antibody directed against striated muscle has been identified and has been found to cross-react with the myoid cells of the thymus.[297] If antigenic material similar to AChR were located on the surface of these myoid cells, it might be released following certain thymic inflammatory or neoplastic processes. Subsequent formation of antibodies directed against myoid cell AChR could then cross-react with peripheral skeletal muscle AChR (Fig. 3–85).

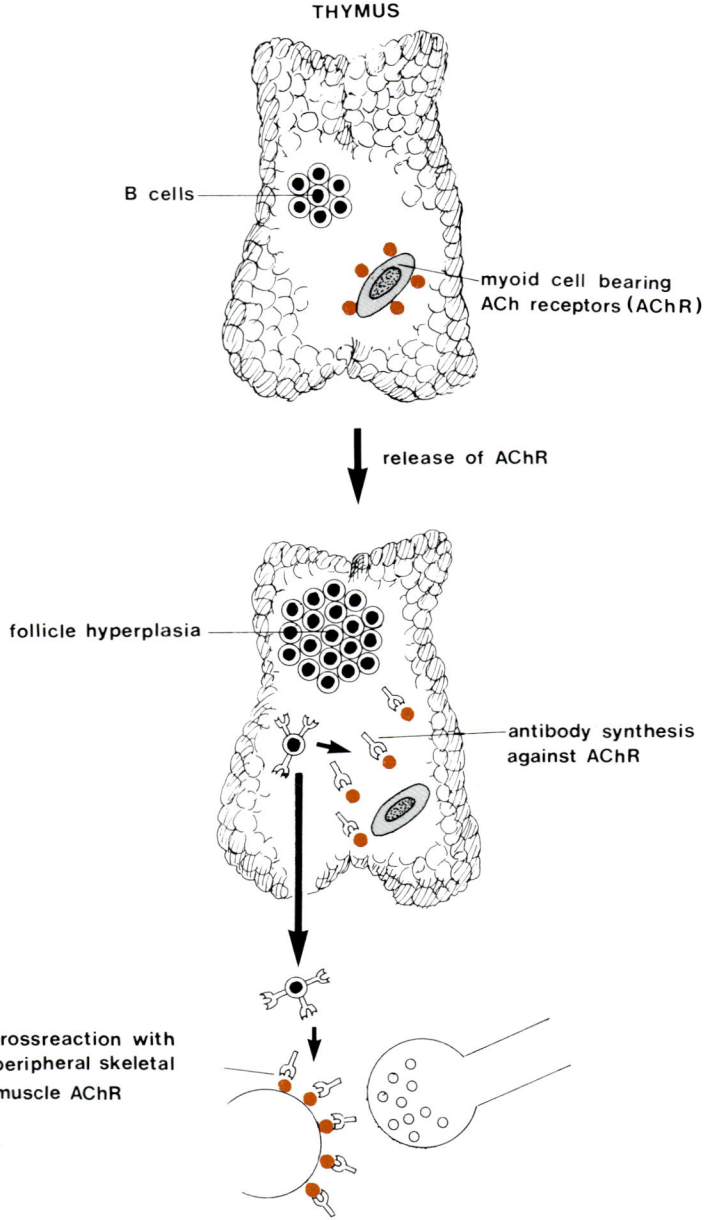

THYMUS

B cells

myoid cell bearing
ACh receptors (AChR)

release of AChR

follicle hyperplasia

antibody synthesis
against AChR

crossreaction with
peripheral skeletal
muscle AChR

Figure 3–85. Postulated interaction of antibodies to thymic myoid cells and skeletal muscle acetylcholine (ACh) receptors.

Young MG patients who have not undergone thymectomy have decreased T-cell reactivity to *alloantigens* in mixed lymphocyte cultures. After thymectomy, a rapid loss of a small population of T cells is associated with prompt reversal of the decreased reactivity to alloantigens.[298] The presence of a population of these suppressor T cells (short-lived lymphocytes with decreased reactivity) might alter the humoral immune response to self antigen and might prevent the appearance of *"blocking"* antibodies. This sequence of events might then allow the appearance of other humoral or cellular immune responses to AChR antigens and might cause an autoimmune disorder manifested as *myasthenia gravis*. This hypothesis is provocative in light of the higher-than-expected frequency of other autoimmune phenomena such as *antinuclear* and *antithyroid* antibodies in myasthenic patients. Alternately, the primary effector role of T cells, lymphokines, and macrophages may initiate the damage seen in myasthenia gravis (Fig. 3–86).

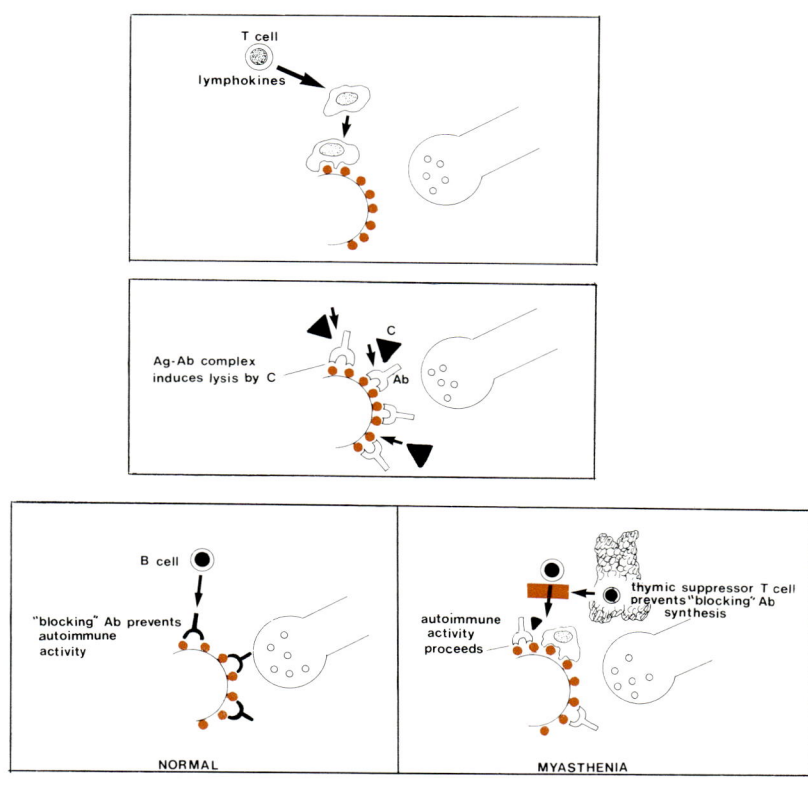

Figure 3–86. Immune attack against motor end plates in myasthenia gravis is postulated.

It has been proposed that a breakdown of immunologic tolerance, probably genetically determined, may be manifested as myasthenia gravis.[299] Immunogenetic studies of myasthenic patients have supported this proposal. These studies have enabled us to divide myasthenic patients into two groups: (1) MG with early onset (under 40 years), predominance of females, increased HLA-B8 frequency, and low incidence of antimuscle antibodies; and (2) MG with late onset (over 40 years), predominance of males, increased HLA-B2 frequency, and relatively high incidence of thymomas and antimuscle antibodies.

In summary, the pathogenesis of myasthenia gravis remains controversial, although current investigation indicates a primary role for antibodies against acetylcholine receptors at the neuromuscular junction. The inciting cause of the antigenic stimulation is also unclear. Considerations of *autoimmune* phenomena demand an examination of the role of B and T lymphocytes, the thymus, thymosin, macrophages, complement, and other implicated factors.

The intricate roles of components of immune cells such as C3 and Fc receptors are being evaluated in clinical and experimental trials.

The use of anticholinesterases,[300] corticosteroids,[301] immunosuppression,[302] and plasmapheresis[303] in managing myasthenic patients is also helpful in theorizing possible mechanisms of this disease.

MULTIFACTORIAL DISORDERS—DIABETES MELLITUS

Diabetes mellitus (DM) serves as a prototype for a large group of diseases in which we find a group of etiologic factors rather than a single agent. Juvenile diabetes mellitus has a genetic susceptibility, probably a relationship to a viral infection, and certainly an autoimmune component.

Diabetes mellitus affects about 4.5 million adults and children in the United States. It occurs in two forms: *Juvenile (acute-onset) diabetes* and *adult (maturity-onset) diabetes.* Juvenile diabetes is the more serious disease and occurs in 0.1% of people. These individuals tend to be thin, are prone to ketosis, and require exogenous insulin. This type of diabetes is strongly associated with histocompatibility antigens *HLA-B8* and *HLA-BW15.* Although this form is typical of children, it can occur at any age.[304]

Maturity-onset diabetics are usually obese, non-insulin-dependent individuals who do not demonstrate any known HLA associations, are less prone to ketotic episodes, and are often treated by diet alone. This form of diabetes may also occur in young individuals who may have a strong family history of the disease.

The hallmarks of insulin deficiency in diabetes are *hyperglycemia* and *glycosuria.* Uncontrolled diabetes with *ketosis* and *metabolic acidosis* may result in coma and death.[305] Diabetics also have an increased incidence of obesity, vascular disease, and susceptibility to infection.

Diabetes antedating pregnancy is an important cause of maternal morbidity, birth defects, intrauterine fetal death, and neonatal morbidity and death. Thirty-six percent of neonates born to these women are macrosomic (greater than ninetieth percentile of birth weight for the gestational age), and 9% have associated major congenital anomalies.[306]

Biochemistry of Diabetes

Diabetes is a disease in which metabolism of carbohydrates is impaired, whereas that of fats and proteins is increased (Fig. 3–87). Ingested glucose, or glucose mobilized from body stores, cannot be assimilated into fat or muscle cells and therefore builds up in the blood (*hyperglycemia*) or is excreted in the urine *(glycosuria)*. Proteins are degraded for energy, and this process leads to an increased blood urea nitrogen level. Increased breakdown of fats leads to the formation of *ketone bodies.*

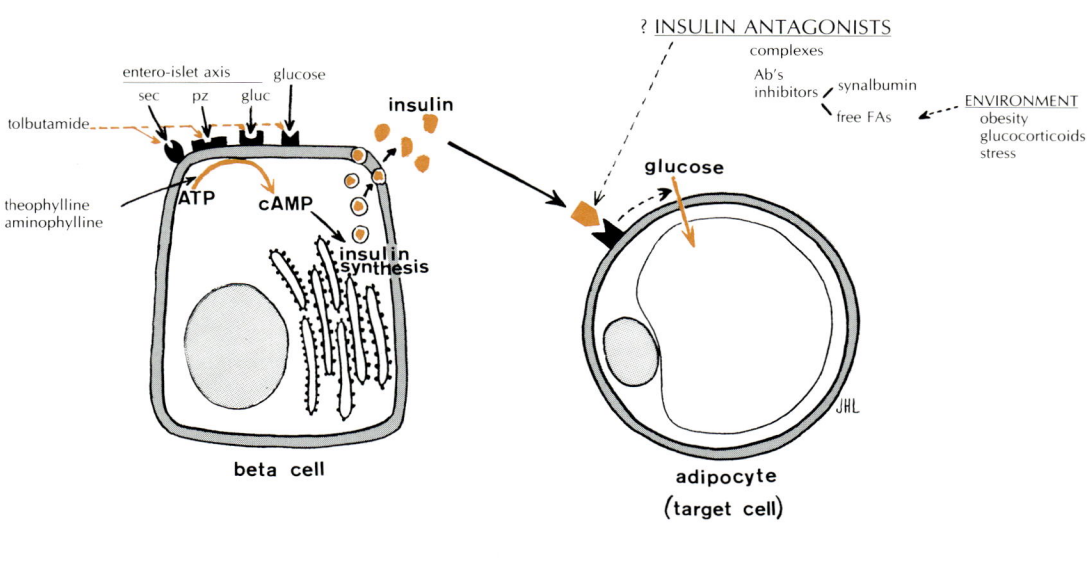

DIABETES: ONE OR MORE ABNORMALITIES AT HORMONE OR GLUCOSE RECEPTOR SITES IN β CELL CAUSES HYPERGLYCEMIA & RELATIVE OR ABSOLUTE INSULIN DEFICIENCY

Figure 3–87. The pathogenesis of diabetes mellitus involves abnormalities of hormone-producing cells and target cells.

The excretion of glucose and ketones results in loss of water and electrolytes and causes dehydration and thirst. If ketone bodies increase, then *ketoacidosis, coma,* and *death* may result. In some cells, much of the glucose is converted to sorbitol, which accumulates and damages tissue (cataracts, nerve damage).[307]

Marked insulin deficiency results in a metabolic state similar to starvation because important substrates cannot be stored effectively for later use. This metabolic state brings about a decreased synthesis of proteins, lipids, and glycogen, an inhibited peripheral glucose uptake, a reversal of the glycolytic pathway and the production of glucose from amino acids in the liver, the mobilization of fat from adipose tissue that leads to marked increases in plasma lipids, cholesterol, triglycerides, and free fatty acids, and finally, ketoacidosis. Insulin-deficient diabetics are in a catabolic state, and despite huge food intakes, such patients lose weight. The clinical triad of *polyphagia, polydipsia,* and *polyuria* is well known.[308]

Insulin itself regulates other substances besides blood glucose. Diabetics have impaired K^+ tolerance that is corrected by insulin administration. Other factors such as metabolic acidosis contribute to *hyperkalemia* in diabetics.[309]

Hemoglobin A$_{1C}$ (HbA$_{1C}$)

Diabetics have increased levels of an abnormal hemoglobin (*HbA$_{1C}$*), which appears to be a manifestation of the severe metabolic abnormalities present in diabetes. Normally, about 5% of hemoglobin in the red blood cell is covalently linked to glucose to form HbA$_{1C}$. This linkage is the result of a nonenzymatic glycosylation of the molecule at its β-chain amino terminal valine[310] (Fig. 3–88).

HbA$_{1C}$ comprises 3 to 6% of total hemoglobin in normal people and is increased to 6 to 12% of total hemoglobin in both juvenile and maturity-onset diabetics. HbA$_{1C}$ can be used to monitor glucose control in diabetic mothers; this process allows optimal maternal and fetal care. The HbA$_{1C}$ variant has a decreased affinity for oxygen, and therefore, red blood cells containing it are less efficient in carrying O_2 to tissues. This phenomenon predisposes diabetics to local tissue hypoxia and can result in a functional microangiopathy that progresses to true vascular injury with endothelial damage and proliferation.[311]

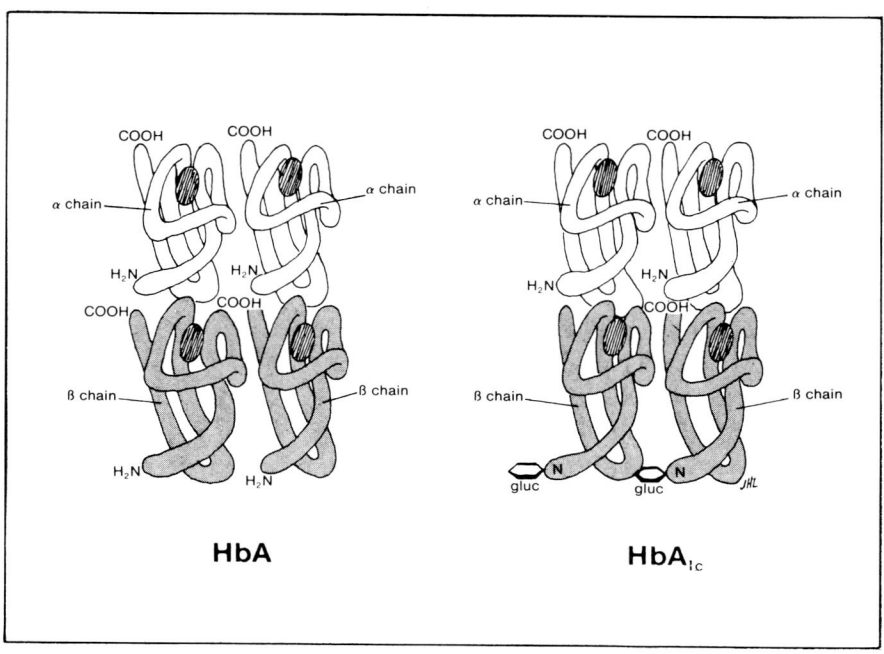

Schematic comparison of HbA and HbA$_{1c}$. HbA$_{1c}$ is produced by the addition of a glucose molecule to the terminus of the β chains of normal adult hemoglobin.

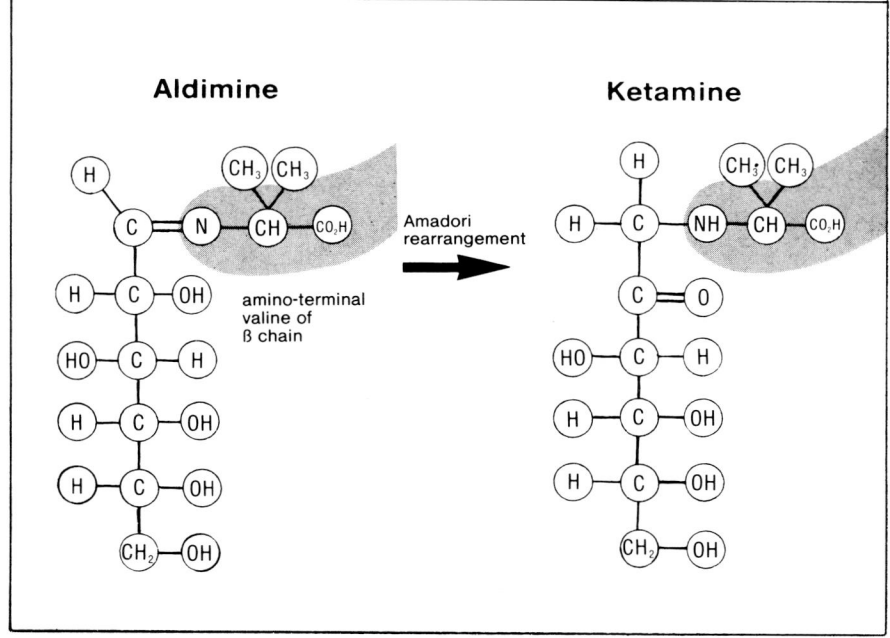

The nonenzymatic production of HbA$_{1c}$ requires the formation of a Schiff base between the aldehyde of the glucose and the amino-terminal valine of the β chain, followed by an Amadori rearrangement to the relatively more stable ketamine.

Figure 3–88. The formation of hemoglobin A$_{1c}$ in diabetes.

Insulin (Structure, Synthesis, Secretion, and Action)

Insulin consists of 2 peptide chains, an *A-chain* with 21 amino acids, and a *B-chain* with 30 amino acids. The molecule contains 3 disulfide bridges that confer its configuration. Two of these bridges connect the A- and B-chains, and one binds the number 6 and number 11 amino acids of the A-chain.

Preproinsulin is a large molecule that is not readily detectable because it is cleaved to *proinsulin* almost immediately following its synthesis. This cleavage results in a loss of 24 amino acids from the preproinsulin molecule. Proinsulin consists of a single, long chain of amino acids, of which 51 are destined to become the A- and B-chains, linked by an extra connecting peptide of 31 amino acids known as the *C-peptide*. Proinsulin is transported to the Golgi apparatus, where it is cleaved by proinsulin cleavage enzymes into insulin plus the C-peptide. This enzyme cleaves the

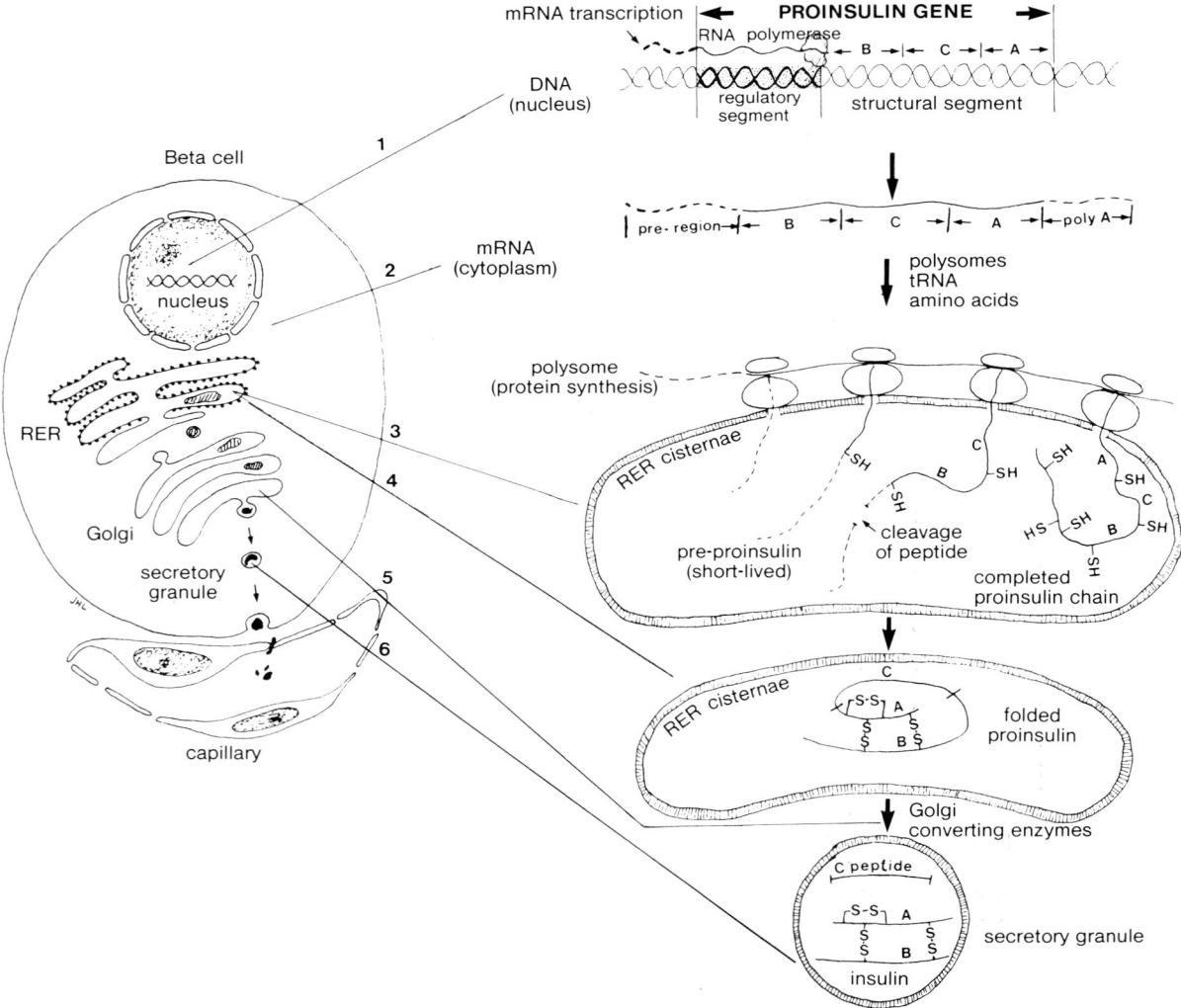

Figure 3-89. Diagrammatic representation of insulin synthesis.

molecule at the C-peptide-A and -B chain linkage. The C-peptide remains intact. This reaction normally produces equal amounts of insulin and C-peptide, in addition to a little circulating proinsulin[312] (Fig. 3–89).

Errors in insulin synthesis and structure do occur. Gabbay et al. described a kindred in which there is a genetic defect such that proinsulin becomes the major part of the insulin immunoreactive material. The defect may represent either a deficiency in the proinsulin cleaving enzyme(s) or an abnormal species of proinsulin.[313]

Given et al.[314] described an abnormal species of insulin in a patient with adult-onset diabetes. This study defined a mutation in the receptor-binding region of the insulin molecule in which a leucine molecule was substituted for one of two adjacent phenylalanine residues in the B-chain. This patient's insulin had low biologic activity and reduced ability to bind insulin receptors so that diabetes resulted.

The insulin molecule is transported to the Golgi apparatus from the ER and is transmitted to the cell surface in the form of a granule within a vesicle. This transport is probably aided by the microtubular system. The transformation of proinsulin begins in the Golgi apparatus. Granules are released in an ordered manner along the membrane by the process of emiocytosis.[315,316]

The release of insulin from the cell is controlled by a variety of factors, including nutrients in the intestine[317] such as fatty acids, protein, and glucose; enzymes such as secretin, gastrin, and pancreatic enzymes; and the CNS, including cholinergic and β-adrenergic hormones of the autonomic nervous system. Calcium is also absolutely required.[318] Once released from the cell, insulin travels with the α and β globulin fractions of the serum, but a specific carrier protein has not been identified. The three principal target tissues of insulin are liver, muscle, and fat.

Although one of its principal effects is accelerated transport of glucose into the cell, insulin also influences ion transport mechanisms of the cell membrane. While depressing *glycogenolysis* and *gluconeogenesis* in muscle, in addition to having an indirect effect of regulating the concentration of free fatty acids in the serum, insulin stimulates glycogen synthesis and perhaps affects a uridine diphosphoglucose (UDPG) transferase enzyme. It also accelerates glucose transport through the membrane and increases protein synthesis. In adipose tissue, insulin stimulates transport of glucose across the cell membrane and promotes the phosphorylation of glucose.[319]

Target Cell Insulin Receptors

The binding of insulin to its target tissue involves a specific receptor(s) on the outer cell membrane as well as on the membranes of specific organelles, such as the Golgi apparatus. The receptors at these two sites appear to be identical; however, the regulation of insulin binding to them

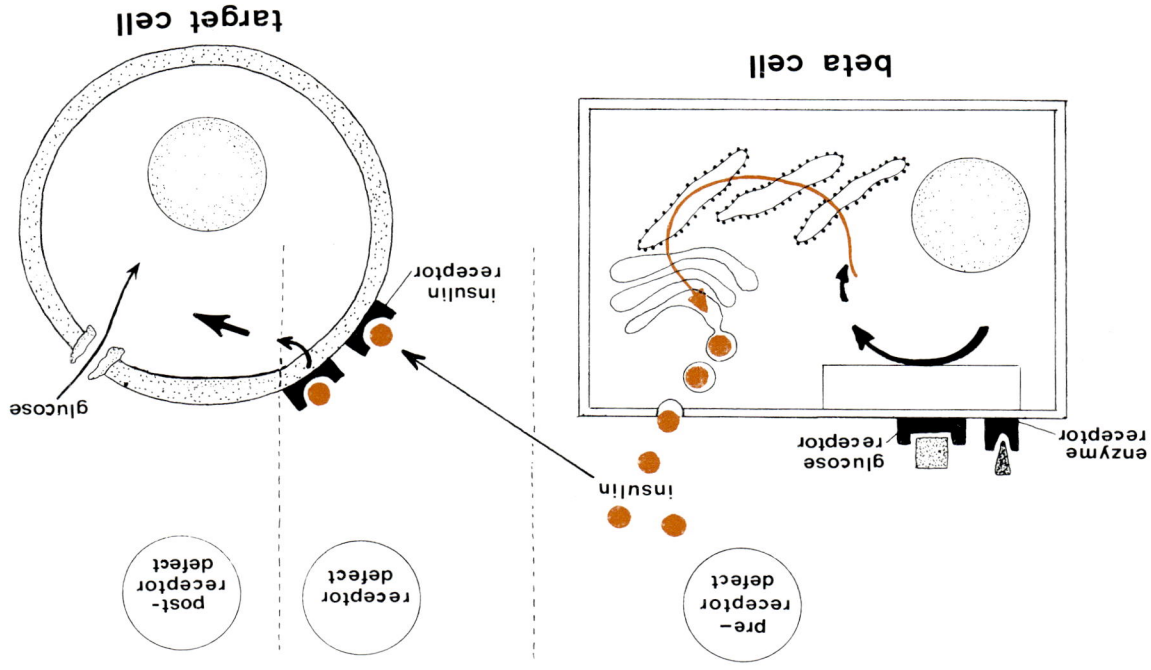

Figure 3–90. Defects in diabetes are postulated at several sites.

appears to differ. These receptors are found on the plasma membrane of traditional insulin target cells such as fat, liver, skeletal, muscle, as well as on other cells such as lymphocytes and kidney.[320]

Olefsky and Chang[321] showed that insulin receptors are clustered rather than diffusely distributed over cell membranes. The number of receptors for each cell type is finite, and the binding of the hormone to its receptor is saturable, reversible, and specific. Inhibition of lipolysis, protein synthesis, glucose oxidation, lipogenesis, and glucose, potassium, and amino acid transport can all be controlled by insulin molecules occupying the receptor in the fat cell.[322] The affinity of the receptor for insulin seems to be controlled by factors such as fasting or feeding.[323] Because receptor number and affinity are also increased in fetal life, perhaps a correlation exists with the active prenatal growth process.[324] Conversely, fewer receptors have been found in diabetes.[325]

The interaction of insulin with its receptor is not sufficient to trigger hormone action because enzymes that degrade insulin have been localized in the plasma membrane. Rather, hormone binding triggers a chain of cellular events mediating hormonal action. The receptor-bound insulin undergoes rapid compartmentalization in the cell. The receptor sites and degradation sites have differing affinities for insulin and operate at different pH, ionic strengths, and temperatures.[326,327]

It has become clear that the concentration of insulin receptors on cells is controlled by and rapidly adapts to insulin

levels; that is, insulin regulates its own receptor concentration.

Abnormalities of insulin-receptor interaction may be classified as *preceptor, receptor,* or *postreceptor defects* (Fig. 3–90). Theoretically, prereceptor defects involve abnormal insulin molecules or errors in synthesis, assembly, or secretion. Receptor defects involve loss of receptor sites, changes in receptor sensitivity, or attachment of insulin antibodies to the receptor. Postreceptor defects involve lack of an effect on the target cells once insulin binds to the receptor.

Insulin Resistance

Circulating antibodies to the insulin receptor have been identified in patients with extreme insulin resistance. These antibodies are predominantly IgG, but some IgM activity is also present. Different autoantibodies bind to different determinants on the insulin receptor molecule.[328] Such antibodies may have a real role in the pathogenesis of diabetes in a manner analogous to the antibodies to AChR in myasthenia gravis. In fact, one patient with insulin receptor antibodies, manifested clinically by severe insulin resistance, underwent spontaneous remission of her diabetes; during remission, the antibodies to the insulin receptor disappeared.[329]

Diseases in which severe insulin resistance exists include obesity, *acanthosis nigricans,*[330] *nonketotic diabetes,* and *ataxia telangiectasia.*[331] *Obesity* is associated with increased insulin secretion; however, fat cells may be insulin resistant, probably secondary to an abnormal insulin receptor.[332] *Nonketotic diabetics* also have decreased insulin receptors without abnormal insulin or circulating antagonists.

In one form of diabetes with severe insulin resistance and *acanthosis nigricans,* an antireceptor antibody was found in the IgG fraction that bound to adipocytes in vitro, where the antibody exhibited insulin-like effects. *Ataxia telangiectasia* also probably has circulating inhibitors of insulin binding.

Other Hormones and Diabetes

Other hormones that also appear to have key roles in diabetes include glucagon, prolactin, somatostatin, prostaglandins, and growth hormone (somatotropin)[333] (Table 3–69). Glucagon is released from alpha cells of pancreatic islets and is generally elevated when insulin is deficient. Orci[316] cites three lines of evidence supporting a role for glucagon in diabetes: (1) an increased concentration of glucagon is always seen with hyperglycemia; (2) when both glucagon and insulin secretion are depressed, hyperglycemia is not seen unless the glucagon level is raised; and (3) the suppression of glucagon release induced by somatostatin in diabetics restores blood sugar levels to normal.[334]

Table 3–69. Interrelationship of Insulin and Other Hormones

Glucagon	Increases in concentration with hyperglycemia
	Regulates liver-mediated mobilization of stored glucose
	Regulates oxidation of fatty acids in liver
Prolactin	Stimulates lipid metabolism
	Decreases sensitivity to insulin
Somatostatin	Inhibits release of growth hormone from pituitary and may have glucagon-like activity
	Suppresses glucagon release in diabetics, restores blood sugar levels to normal
	Inhibits release of insulin and glucagon
Growth Hormone	Alters tissue responsiveness to insulin by interfering with insulin binding to cell surfaces
Prostaglandins	Play a role in abnormal beta cell function
Insulin	Regulates transfer of glucose from blood to storage sites in liver, fat and muscle

Prolactin stimulates lipid metabolism and decreases the sensitivity to insulin.[335] *Somatostatin* (somatotropin release-inhibiting factor) inhibits the release of *growth hormone from the pituitary* and may have glucagon-like activity.[336] The site of action of somatostatin is the pancreas, where it inhibits the release of both insulin and glucagon. *Growth hormone* is known to alter tissue responsiveness to insulin by interfering with insulin binding to cell surfaces. The "glucoreceptor" hypothesis of diabetes postulates that diabetic patients' beta cells fail to respond normally to glucose signals. Certain endogenous, and perhaps pancreatic, *prostaglandins* may have a role in abnormal beta cell function in this disease.[337]

The major role of *insulin* is to regulate the transfer of glucose from the blood to storage sites in the liver, fat, and muscle. *Glucagon*, on the other hand, regulates the liver-mediated mobilization of stored glucose. It also regulates the oxidation of fatty acids in the liver. The suppression of glucagon secretion by somatostatin prevents ketoacidosis in man.

Morphologic Changes in Diabetes

Pancreatic Islets

The earliest morphologic changes in diabetes are demonstrable in pancreatic islets, with *degranulation* of *beta cells*, which indicates a lack of cellular insulin synthesis. Juvenile-onset diabetics may have an extensive inflammatory infiltration of the islets (*insulitis*) with islet cell necrosis. This reaction is most common in patients under ten years old[338] and leads to progressive *fibrosis, atrophy,* and *amyloid deposition.* This amyloid may represent crystallized insulin or insulin precursors (Fig. 3-91).

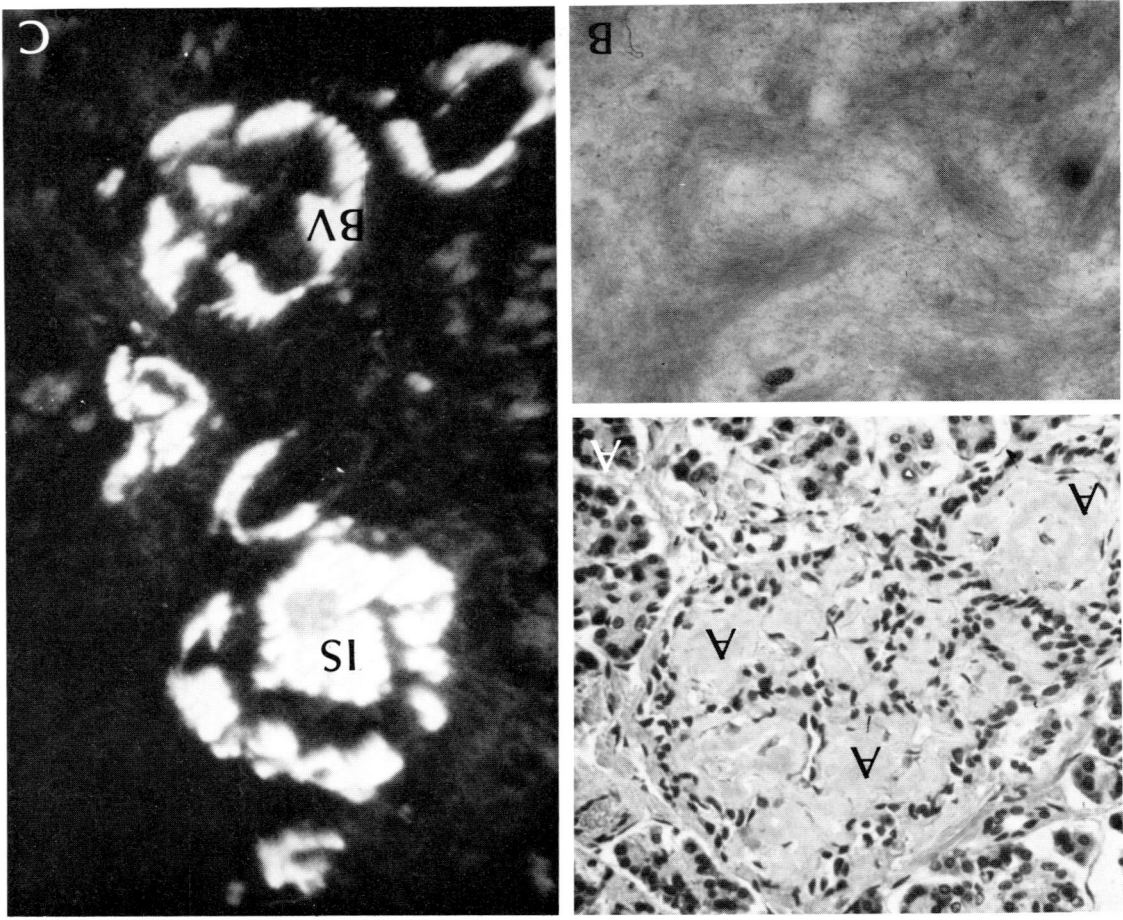

Figure 3-91. The pancreas in diabetes. A. The islets contain large amounts of eosinophilic material compatible with amyloid (A). B. Electron microscopy of these deposits demonstrates the characteristic fibrils of amyloid. C. When the section of pancreas is stained with thioflavin T, amyloid is identified in the islets (IS) and in the blood vessels (BV).

Basement Membranes

The indirect effects of insulin deficiency in diabetes are seen in several organ systems including *blood vessels, nerves, retina,* and *kidney;* these effects are primarily the result of angiopathies and basement membrane abnormalities.[339] Indeed, many of the complications in diabetes are caused by diffuse basement membrane thickening thought to be due to the increased deposition of glycoproteins.[340]

Serious retinal and glomerular abnormalities appear to be absent at the onset of juvenile diabetes, but their frequency increases with the duration of the disease. Basement membrane thickening probably is not the primary lesion in patients with carbohydrate intolerance, but rather is secondary to it. Abnormal glycosylation reactions character-istic of diabetics are responsible for the development of cataracts, peripheral neuropathy, and cerebral edema.[341,342] A collagen-like molecule that contains more hydroxylysine and hydroxyproline than usual collagen has been found in the glomerular basement membrane. An isolated lysyl-hydroxylase elevation is also present. Insulin administration restores this enzyme to normal levels and also increases glucosyltransferase.[343]

Microangiopathy—Small-Vessel Disease

Disease of small and large blood vessels occurs commonly in diabetes, and although *microangiopathic* disease is an in-herent part of the diabetic state, large-vessel disease differs from normal aging only by its prematurity in diabetics. There is heterogeneity in the vascular expression of dia-betes: up to 25% of patients with insulin-dependent dia-betes never develop vascular disease. Controversy still exists as to whether the vascular abnormalities are primary lesions or are secondary to disordered metabolism.[344] *Microangiopathy* may begin as a functional disorder with variations in blood-vessel caliber secondary to changes in oxygen tension. In diabetic acidosis, pH levels drop, and intracellular glycolysis is inhibited. This process leads to frequent variations in oxygen consumption. Another factor is the inherent abnormality in the red blood cell membrane in diabetes; that is, *reduced deformability* as in sickle cell dis-ease. Sludged red blood cells and decreases in local oxygen tension may contribute to small-vessel disease. Basement membrane thickening, with deposits of glycoprotein, is a significant lesion.[345]

Another aspect of the vascular disease in diabetics may involve *platelets;* it has been shown that diabetic patients have an increased sensitivity to platelet aggregation by ADP, epinephrine, and collagen. Indeed, small-vessel *thrombosis* is a common finding.[346]

Macroangiopathy—Large-Vessel Disease

Progressive macrovascular disease, including *atherosclē-rosis,* is a recognized complication of diabetes, and the re-

lationship of abnormal lipid metabolism to this progression is under investigation. Persistent *hyperglycemia* and *hypoinsulinemia* are associated with *elevated blood lipid levels,* the inability to clear neutral lipids or triglycerides, and elevated cholesterol levels. The Framingham study has shown an association among diabetes, obesity, decreased high-density lipoprotein levels, and a high incidence of *coronary artery* disease in women. This finding reinforces the concept of the *protection* from vascular disease offered by high levels of *high-density lipoproteins.*[347]

Retinopathy

Diabetic retinopathy is also a characteristic lesion in diabetic patients. This retinal vascular disorder is the most serious encountered by the internist because of its prevalence and because it often also reflects the state of renal microangiopathy. *Retinopathy* may be *intra-* or *extraretinal.* The latter involves a *proliferative vascular response.*[348] The retina in this disorder is characterized by vascular attenuation, optic nerve pallor, pigment dispersion, and replacement of neovascularization by avascular glial tissue.[349]

Heart Disease

Accelerated vascular changes often lead to concurrent cardiac disease. It has recently been postulated that cardiac involvement may not be only on the basis of *obliterative coronary artery disease,* but also on the basis of a *cardiomyopathy.* Most normotensive diabetics with long-standing disease do not have clinically evident heart disease, yet functional studies indicate a presymptomatic *left ventricular abnormality.* It appears that the ventricle has an increased stiffness that may be related to altered interstitial glycoprotein and collagen accumulation diffusely throughout the ventricle. This stiffness could lead to progressively abnormal cardiac function.[350]

Kidney Disease

One of the major organs injured in diabetes is the kidney, especially the glomerulus. Mesangial proliferation and collagen synthesis result in both nodular and diffuse forms of glomerulosclerosis. The nodular form of the disease is classically known as *Kimmelstiel-Wilson disease.* IgG, IgM, HbA$_{1c}$, and albumin have all been demonstrated in a linear pattern in the glomerular basement membrane. It has been suggested that insulin-anti-insulin antigen-antibody complexes are deposited in the manner of other immune complex diseases. This deposition may merely reflect increased leakiness of abnormal basement membranes.[351] The formation of crescents in diabetic glomeruli correlates with the degree of vascular and glomerular damage

and with renal function and proteinuria. Crescent formation may result from the leakage of fibrin through the
abnormal basement membrane into the urinary space; this
leakage stimulates proliferation of parietal cells, which then
produce collagen. The lesion becomes progressive.[352]

Another lesion frequently found in diabetics is the presence of glycogen vacuoles in renal tubular epithelium (Armanni-
Ebstein lesion), as well as in nuclei of hepatocytes of the liver.
The glycogen is deposited singly, as rosettes, or as reticular
threads and is believed to diffuse through the nuclear
pores.[353]

Polyneuropathy

Polyneuropathies, especially symmetrical distal polyneuropathies, are common, but their pathogenesis is unclear.
Occlusive arterial diseases or microangiopathies are not always responsible, and some investigators feel that the neurologic disease reflects chronic metabolic disturbances.[354]
Insulin deficiency and hyperglycemia, as well as alterations
in inositol metabolism, appear to be important factors in the
pathogenesis of the neuropathy. Levels of myoinositol, a normal constituent of cells, are reduced in the diabetic state,
especially within tissues such as nerves and the lens.

Histologically, the most prominent changes involve the
distal parts of peripheral nerves, with loss of myelinated
and unmyelinated nerve fibers, proliferation of Schwann
cells, and increased amounts of connective tissue.[355]

The muscle cells may also be abnormal and may show a
depletion of glycogen and the presence of lipid vacuoles.[356]

Wound Healing and Infection

Diabetics characteristically have poor wound healing and a
high incidence of wound infections.[357] It has been suggested
that this phenomenon is secondary to microvascular disease. Other factors such as decreased collagen production
may also play a role, however. In vitro systems have shown
that fibroblasts respond to insulin by an increase in DNA
and RNA synthesis and by cellular proliferation. Therefore, in insulin deficiency states, fibroblastic responses may be
poor.[358] Furthermore, impairment of phagocytosis may result in ineffective elimination of organisms. Healing may
be delayed.

Etiology

The pathogenesis of diabetes is an enigma. Most investigators in this area today consider juvenile diabetes to result from multiple factors, including genetic inheritance,
cell injury by viral infection, and resultant autoimmune
states involving disorders of the beta cells and target organs.
Adult-onset maturity diabetes is even more complex and
may relate to the aging process.[359]

Experimental Diabetes

Several experimental models of diabetes include genetic strains of mice and production of the disease by viruses, drugs, and chemicals.

Strains of *ob/ob* and *db/db* mice are single-gene mutants that are obese and spontaneously develop diabetes with different clinical features, depending on their genetic backgrounds. Both strains of animals are associated with an early islet cell proliferation followed by extensive necrosis. The ob/ob mouse manifests myriad disease signs, with reduced oxygen consumption, decreased body temperature, and excess body fat.[360]

A major defect in these animals is the hyposecretion of insulin. Both strains have significant alterations in somatostatin functions, which thereby alter glucagon and blood glucose levels. Insulin receptors have also been found to be lacking.[361]

Encephalomyocarditis virus (M variant) and *Coxsackie virus* characteristically produce pancreatic islet necrosis and diabetes.[362]

Experimental diabetes may also be produced by administering *alloxan* or *streptozotocin*. Both these drugs degranulate pancreatic beta cells and cause insulin deficiency.[363]

Human Disease

Genetic Inheritance. The inheritance of diabetes mellitus is still uncertain, but it is evident that diabetic patients represent a genetically heterogenous group and that the expression of their disease is modified by other factors such as diet and obesity. Although a familial tendency to insulin-dependent diabetes has been noted, fewer than 20% of patients have first-degree relatives with a history of diabetes. In studies of identical twins, no clear-cut evidence has been seen for increased numbers of viral infections in a twin with diabetes, when compared to a nondiabetic twin. The etiology of this disease is believed to be multifactorial, and its inheritance may differ in juvenile and maturity-onset forms.

HLA Antigens

The association of particular HLA types with juvenile diabetes has been the subject of several reports. Rubenstein et al.[364] described at least two different genetic groups for the susceptibility to juvenile diabetes mellitus. One form had a strong immune response to insulin and appeared to be associated with HLA-BW15. The other form had no humoral immunoreactivity to insulin and was associated with the presence of HLA-B8 and the absence of HLA-B7. What do these HLA-type disease associations mean? They may be related to ethnic stratification, disease causation, or disease association. Ethnic stratification implies that a dis-

ease happens to be more common in an ethnic group in which the HLA type is also common. Causation implies that the HLA type is in the direct chain of events leading to the disease. Association is the situation in which the HLA alleles are linked to one or more alleles that are responsible for the predisposition to a disease.[365]

Role of Viral Infection

An interesting aspect of the etiology of diabetes concerns the role of viruses. It is certainly possible that they account for some cases of this disease, which is probably multifactorial in origin.

Craighead et al. showed that by administering the *encephalomyocarditis (EMC) virus* one can induce a form of diabetes in mice that resembles juvenile diabetes.[366] When the myocardiotrophic variant (M variant) is used, isolated pancreatic islet cell necrosis occurs, with edema and an inflammatory infiltrate of macrophages, lymphocytes, and neutrophils. Eventually, the islet cells are totally destroyed. Vascular changes are also present. This virus is interesting because it has five antigenically related variants that have different tissue tropisms. *Reoviruses* type 3 also produce an insulitis when inoculated into mice. Reovirus antigens are demonstrable in the pancreatic beta cells.

Despite the murine model, a viral etiology has never been definitely proved in man. Recently, however, at the National Institutes of Health, the death of a diabetic patient led to the isolation of a *Coxsackie virus* from the pancreas that, when injected into mice, produced diabetes.[367] Viruses may well play some role in the initiation of juvenile-onset diabetes. *Mumps, rubella,* and *Coxsackie B1* and *6* are the viruses most associated with human diabetes, and attempts to infect cells with these viruses in vitro have been successful. The link with rubella is strongest in patients with prenatal rubella infections. It is also possible that the HLA-B8 or HLA-BW15 genes are related to membrane attachment of virus, and infection may be followed by an immune-mediated destruction of islet cells.[368]

Autoimmune Reactions

A variety of autoantibodies have been identified in the juvenile form of diabetes and may be associated with HLA-B8 and *HLA-BW15 haplotypes.* These HLA antigens are also present with increased frequency in *Graves' disease, Addison's disease,* and *pernicious anemia.*[369] Juvenile diabetics have an increased incidence of *thyroid* and *gastric cross-reacting autoantibodies* directed against beta cells as well as against glucagon- and somatostatin-secreting cells. Twenty-four percent of patients with diabetes have pancreatic islet cell antibodies at the onset of their disease, and 59% develop them within a year of diagnosis.[370] In addition to being directed against specific tissue, an-

tibodies may be directed against the receptor molecule or against insulin.[371] Autoantibodies against the insulin receptor have been described in the serum of insulin-resistant diabetics. These autoantibodies bind to and block the cell membrane receptor sites and thereby alter the receptor-insulin interaction by reducing the receptor affinity or number.

Antibodies to insulin belong to IgG and IgE classes. IgE specific to insulin has been found in diabetics with a generalized insulin allergy. This antibody is also found in low titers in all diabetics treated with insulin.[372]

Histologically, the pancreatic islets manifest a lymphocytic infiltrate similar to that present in experimental EMC virus-induced diabetes or in the lesion produced by injecting complete Freund's adjuvant in addition to insulin. This same pattern is seen in other delayed hypersensitivity reactions. Cytotoxicity to islet cells may rest with these lymphocytes.[373]

In addition to specific, abnormal cellular responses directed against certain target tissues, generalized abnormalities of cell-mediated responses are also seen and possibly account for increased susceptibility to infection. Some patients appear to have defects in phagocytosis, but have intact neutrophil chemotaxis. Abnormal cell-mediated responses may be modulated through the action of insulin because many cells of the immune system have receptors for insulin on their surfaces. Such cells include monocytes, macrophages, granulocytes, and T cells. It is known that insulin inhibits antibody-dependent cytotoxicity.[374]

Treatment

Because diabetes is associated with insulin deficiency, it is not surprising that the first agent used to treat the disorder was insulin. Its administration to insulin-dependent diabetics remains a major mode of therapy, and insulin pumps have recently been implanted in the abdomen to give regulated dosages. The use of parenteral bovine and bovine-porcine insulin preparations may be associated with the induction of anti-insulin antibodies.

Oral antidiabetic agents taken by mouth once or twice a day are often more acceptable to the patient than insulin, which must be injected. Two of these drugs, tolbutamide and phentolamine, partially restore acute insulin responses to glucose in diabetics. However, these agents have been associated with increased risk of coronary thrombosis.

Human insulin genes isolated with recombinant DNA techniques allow one to introduce the gene into plasmids, and in vitro production of insulin has been accomplished. The administration of human insulin should diminish the risk of inducing anti-insulin antibodies.

Dietary management often permits control of adult-onset diabetes. Restoration of electrolyte and fluid balance along with control of infection continue to be crucial therapy in the decompensated patient. Recent experience with experimental transplantation in mice of fetal pancreas cultured in vitro may hold added dividends for the treatment of the human disease in the future.[375]

REFERENCES

1. Robinson, A.: Genetic counseling. Adv. Pathobiol., 3:95, 1976.
2. Stanbury, J.B., Wyngaarden, J.B., and Fredrickson, D.S.: The Metabolic Basis of Inherited Diseases. 4th Ed. New York, McGraw-Hill, 1978.
3. Miller, O.J., and Erlanger, B.T.: Immunochemical probes of chromosome organization. Adv. Pathobiol., 3:55, 1976.
4. Ricciuti, F.C., and Ruddle, F.H.: Assignment of three gene loci (PGK, HGPRT, G8PD) to the long arm of the human X chromosome by somatic cell genetics. Genetics, 74:661, 1973.
5. Bach, F.: The variable condition of euchromatin and heterochromatin. Int. Rev. Cytol., 45:25, 1976.
6. Milunsky, A.: Prenatal diagnosis of genetic disorders. N. Engl. J. Med., 295:378, 1976.
7. Hirschhorn, D.: Prenatal diagnosis of genetic disease. Adv. Pathobiol., 3:87, 1976.
8. Garrod, A.E.: Inborn errors of metabolism (Croonian Lectures). Lancet, 2:1, 73, 142, 214, 1908.
9. Erbee, R.W.: Principles of medical genetics (second of two parts). N. Engl. J. Med., 294:480, 1976.
10. Kalckar, H.M., Kinoshita, J.H., and Donnell, G.N.: Galactosemia: biochemistry, genetics, pathophysiology and developmental aspects. In Biology of Brain Dysfunction. Vol. 1. Edited by G.E. Gaull. New York, Plenum Press, 1972.
11. Van der Ploeg, L.H.T., et al.: α-β-thalassaemia studies showing that deletion of the α- and δ-genes influences β-globin gene expression in man. Nature, 283:637, 1980.
12. Straja, D., Steiner, G., and Kwiterovich, P.O.: Plasma high-density lipoproteins and ischemic heart disease. Studies in a larger kindred with familial hypercholesterolemia. Ann. Intern. Med., 89:871, 1978.
13. Cartwright, G.E.: Diagnosis of treatable Wilson's disease. N. Engl. J. Med., 298:1347, 1978.
14. Cartwright, G.E., et al.: Hereditary hemochromatosis. Phenotypic expression of the disease. N. Engl. J. Med., 301:175, 1979.
15. Kidd, K.K.: Genetic linkage and hemochromatosis. N. Engl. J. Med., 301:209, 1979.
16. Pyeritz, R.E., and McKusick, V.A.: The Marfan syndrome: diagnosis and management. N. Engl. J. Med., 300:772, 1979.
17. German, J.: Chromosomes and Cancer. New York, John Wiley & Sons, 1974.
18. Lewandowski, R.C., and Yunis, J.J.: Phenotypic mapping in man. In Chromosomes in Biology and Medicine. New Chromosomal Syndromes. Edited by J.J. Yunis. New York, Academic Press, 1977.
19. Oakley, G.P.: Natural selection, selection bias and the prevalence of Down's syndrome. N. Engl. J. Med., 299:1068, 1978.
20. Davidson, W.M., and Smith, D.R.: Human Chromosomal Abnormalities. Springfield, IL, Charles C Thomas, 1961.
21. Goldis, D.W., et al.: The Philadelphia chromosome in human macrophages. Blood, 49:367, 1977.
22. Holmes, L.B.: Inborn errors of morphogenesis. A review of localized hereditary malformations. N. Engl. J. Med., 291:763, 1974.
23. Legator, M.S.: Teratogenesis, Carcinogenesis and Mutagenesis. Vol. 1. New York, Alan R. Liss, 1980.
24. Marx, J.L.: Cytomegalovirus: a major cause of birth defects. Science, 190:1184, 1975.
25. Lux, S.E., John, K.M., and Karnovsky, M.J.: Irreversible deformation of the spectrin-actin lattice in irreversibly sickled cells. J. Clin. Invest., 58:955, 1976.
26. Lessin, L.S., Jensen, W.N., and Klug, P.: Ultrastructure of the normal and hemoglobinopathic red blood cell membrane. Arch. Intern. Med., 129:306, 1972.
27. Korpman, R.A., et al.: The red cell shape as an indicator of membrane structure: Ponder's rule reexamined. Blood Cells, 3:315, 1977.

28. Patel, V.P., and Fairbanks, G.: Spectrin phosphorylation and shape change of human erythrocyte ghosts. J. Cell Biol., *88*:430, 1981.
29. Nienhuis, A.W., and Benz, E.J.: Regulation of hemoglobin synthesis during the development of the red cell. N. Engl. J. Med., *297*:1318, 1371, 1430, 1977.
30. Kazazian, H.H., and Woodhead, A.P.: Hemoglobin A synthesis in the developing fetus. N. Engl. J. Med., *289*:58, 1973.
31. Bookchin, R.R., et al.: Polymerisation of haemoglobin SA hybrid tetramers. Nature, *269*:526, 1977.
32. Palek, J.: Red cell membrane injury in sickle cell anaemia. Br. J. Haematol., *35*:1, 1977.
33. Snyder, L.M., et al.: Partition of catalase and its peroxidase activities in human red cell membrane: effect of ATP depletion. Biochim. Biophys. Acta, *470*:290, 1977.
34. Grasso, J.A., Sullivan, A.L., and Sullivan, L.W.: Ultrastructural studies of the bone marrow in sickle cell anaemia. I. The structure of sickled erythrocytes and reticulocytes and their phagocytic destruction. Br. J. Haematol., *31*:135, 1975.
35. Grasso, J.A., Sullivan, A.L., and Sullivan, L.W.: Ultrastructural studies of the bone marrow in sickle cell anaemia. II. The morphology of erythropoietic cells and their response to deoxygenation *in vitro*. Br. J. Haematol., *31*:381, 1975.
36. Orkin, S.H., et al.: Improved detection of the sickle mutation by DNA analysis. Application to prenatal diagnosis. N. Engl. J. Med., *307*:32, 1982.
37. Rosenblate, H.J., Eisenstein, R., and Holmes, A.W.: The liver in sickle cell anemia. Arch. Pathol., *90*:235, 1970.
38. Walker, B.R., et al.: Glomerular lesions in sickle cell nephropathy. JAMA, *215*:437, 1971.
39. Friedman, M.J., and Trager, W.: The biochemistry of resistance to malaria. Sci. Am., *244*:184, 1981.
40. Dean, J., and Schechter, A.N.: Sickle-cell anemia: molecular and cellular bases of therapeutic approaches. N. Engl. J. Med., *299*:752, 804, 863, 1978.
41. Benesch, R., and Benesch, R.: Antisickling drugs and water structure. Nature, *289*:637, 1981.
42. Scriver, C.R.: Diets and genes: euphenic nutrition. N. Engl. J. Med., *297*:202, 1977.
43. Andres, R.: Influence of obesity on longevity in the aged. Adv. Pathobiol., *7*:238, 1980.
44. Van Itallie, T.B., and Yang, M-U.: Current concepts in nutrition. Diet and weight loss. N. Engl. J. Med., *297*:1158, 1977.
45. Ambrus, C.M., et al.: Phenylalanine depletion for the management of phenylketonuria: use of enzyme reactors with immobilized enzymes. Science, *201*:817, 1978.
46. Law, D.H.: Current concepts in nutrition. Total parenteral nutrition. N. Engl. J. Med., *297*:1104, 1977.
47. Cohen, S.S.: On biochemical variability and innovation. Science, *139*:1017, 1963.
48. Haussler, M.R., and McCain, T.A.: Basic and clinical concepts related to vitamin D metabolism and action. N. Engl. J. Med., *297*:974, 1041, 1977.
49. Adams, J.S., et al.: Vitamin-D synthesis and metabolism after ultraviolet irradiation of normal and vitamin-D-deficient subjects. N. Engl. J. Med., *306*:722, 1982.
50. Broadus, A.E., et al.: The importance of circulating 1,25-dihydroxy-vitamin D in the pathogenesis of hypercalciuria and renal-stone formation in primary hyperparathyroidism. N. Engl. J. Med., *302*:421, 1980.
51. Ulmer, D.D.: Current concepts. Trace elements. N. Engl. J. Med., *297*:318, 1977.
52. Crosby, W.H.: Current concepts in nutrition. Who needs iron? N. Engl. J. Med., *297*:543, 1977.
53. Mendeloff, A.I.: Current concepts. Dietary fiber and human health. N. Engl. J. Med., *297*:811, 1977.
54. Trier, J.S., et al.: Celiac sprue and refractory sprue. Gastroenterology, *75*:307, 1978.
55. Sleisenger, M.H.: Malabsorption syndrome. N. Engl. J. Med., *281*:1111, 1969.
56. David, T.J., Ajdukiewicz, A.B., Read, A.E.: Dermal and epidermal atrophy in celiac sprue. Gastroenterology, *64*:539, 1973.

57. Reunala, T., et al.: Gluten-free diet in dermatitis herpetiformis. Br. J. Dermatol., 97:473, 1977.
58. Seah, P.P., et al.: A comparison of histocompatibility antigens in dermatitis herpetiformis and adult coeliac disease. Br. J. Dermatol., 94:131, 1976.
59. Strober, W., et al.: The pathogenesis of gluten-sensitive enteropathy. Ann. Intern. Med., 83:242, 1975.
60. Katz, J., and Kantor, F.: Intestinal antibodies to wheat fractions in celiac disease. Ann. Intern. Med., 69:1149, 1968.
61. Eterman, K.P., and Feltkamp, T.E.W.: Antibodies to gluten and reticulin in gastrointestinal diseases. Clin. Exp. Immunol., 31:92, 1978.
62. Holmes, G.K.T., Asquith, P., and Cooke, W.T.: Cell-mediated immunity to gluten fraction III in adult coeliac disease. Clin. Exp. Immunol., 24:259, 1976.
63. Ferguson, A., et al.: Cell mediated immunity to gliadin within the small intestinal mucosa in coeliac disease. Lancet, 1:895, 1975.
64. Halter, S.A., Greene, H.L., and Helinek, G.: Gluten-sensitive enteopathy: Sequence of villous regrowth as viewed by scanning electron microscopy. Hum. Pathol., 13:811, 1982.
65. Challacombe, D.N., and Robertson, K.: Enterochromaffin cells in the duodenal mucosa of children with coeliac disease. Gut, 18:373, 1977.
66. Granditsh, G., and Wick, G.: Immunologische studies an kindern mit coeliakie. Klin. Paediatr., 188:408, 1976.
67. Baklien, K., Brandtzaeg, P., and Fausa, O.: Immunoglobulins in jejunal mucosa and serum from patients with adult coeliac disease. Scand. J. Gastroenterol., 12:149, 1977.
68. Trier, J.S.: Organ culture methods in the study of gastrointestinal-mucosal function and development. N. Engl. J. Med., 295:150, 1976.
69. Trump, B.F., Jesudason, M.L., and Jones, R.T.: Ultrastructural features of diseased cells. In Diagnostic Electron Microscopy. Vol. I. New York, John Wiley & Sons, 1978.
70. Garcia, J.H., et al.: Cerebral ischemia: the early structural changes and correlation of these with known metabolic and dynamic abnormalities. In Cerebral Vascular Diseases. Edited by J.P. Whisnant and B.A. Sandok. New York, Grune & Stratton, 1975.
71. Rennie, D.: Give me air! But not much. N. Engl. J. Med., 297:1285, 1977.
72. Halliwell, B.: Biochemical mechanisms accounting for the toxic action of oxygen on living organisms. The key role of superoxide dismutase. Cell Biol. Int. Rep., 2:113, 1978.
73. Balin, A.K., et al.: Oxygen sensitive stages of the cell cycle of human diploid cells. J. Cell Biol., 78:390, 1978.
74. Hittner, H.M., et al.: Retrolental fibroplasia: efficacy of vitamin E in a double-blind clinical study of preterm infants. N. Engl. J. Med., 305:1365, 1981.
75. Cohen, J.J.: Disorders of potassium balance. Hosp. Pract., 14:119, 1979.
76. Means, A.R., and Chafouleas, J.G.: Calmodulin in endocrine cells. Ann. Rev. Physiol., 44:667, 1982.
77. Parving, H-H., et al.: Mechanisms of edema formation in myxedema-increased protein extravasation and relatively slow lymphatic drainage. N. Engl. J. Med., 301:460, 1979.
78. Falop, M.: Current concepts. Serum potassium in lactic acidosis and ketoacidosis. N. Engl. J. Med., 300:1087, 1979.
79. Narins, R.G., Rudnick, M.R., and Bastl, C.P.: Lactic acidosis and the elevated anion gap (II). Hosp. Pract., 15:91, 1980.
80. Gralnick, H.R.: Intravascular coagulation. I. Differential diagnosis and conditioning mechanisms. Postgrad. Med., 62:68, 1977.
81. Heller, H.G., Crenshaw, L.I., and Hammel, H.T.: The thermostat of vertebrate animals. Sci. Am., 239:102, 1978.
82. Jeske, A.H., Fonteles, M.C., and Karow, J.R.: Functional preservation of the mammalian kidney. III. Ultrastructural effects of perfusion with DMSO. Cryobiology, 11:170, 1974.
83. Marx, J.L.: Low-level radiation: just how bad is it? Science, 204:160, 1979.
84. Cerutti, P.A.: Base damage induced by ionizing radiation. In Photochemistry and Photobiology of Nucleic Acids. Edited by S.Y. Wang. New York, Academic Press, 1976.
85. Committee on the Biological Effects of Ionizing Radiation: The

Effects on Populations of Exposure to Low Levels of Ionizing Radiation: 1980. Washington, National Academy Press, 1980.

86. Anderson, R.E., Standefer, J.C., and Scaletti, J.V.: Radiosensitivity of defined populations of lymphocytes. VI. Functional, structural, and biochemical consequences of *in vitro* irradiation. Cell. Immunol., *33*:45, 1977.

87. Hillis, L.D., and Braunwald, E.: Myocardial ischemia. N. Engl. J. Med., *296*:971, 1977.

88. Streja, D., Steiner, G., and Kwiterovich, P.O.: Plasma high-density lipoproteins and ischemic heart disease. Ann. Intern. Med., *89*:871, 1978.

89. Slone, D., et al.: Relation of cigarette smoking to myocardial infarction in young women. N. Engl. J. Med., *298*:1273, 1978.

90. Shine, K.I., et al.: Pathophysiology of myocardial infarction. Ann. Intern. Med., *87*:75, 1977.

91. Erhardt, L.R., Lundman, T., and Millstedt, H.: Incorporation of I^{125}-labelled fibrinogen into coronary arterial thrombi in acute myocardial infarction in man. Lancet, *1*:387, 1973.

92. Maseri, A., et al.: Coronary vasospasm as a possible cause of myocardial infarction. N. Engl. J. Med., *299*:1271, 1978.

93. Braunwald, E.: Coronary spasm and acute myocardial infarction—new possibility for treatment and prevention. N. Engl. J. Med., *299*:1301, 1978.

94. Prizel, K.R., Hutchins, G.M., and Bulkley, B.U.: Coronary artery embolism and myocardial infarction. Ann. Intern. Med., *88*:155, 1978.

95. Ross, R., and Glomset, J.A.: The pathogenesis of atherosclerosis. N. Engl. J. Med., *295*:420, 1976.

96. Benditt, E.P., and Benditt, J.M.: Evidence for a monoclonal origin of human atherosclerotic plaques. Proc. Natl. Acad. Sci. USA, *70*:1753, 1973.

97. Thomas, W.A., et al.: Alterations in population dynamics of arterial smooth muscle cells during atherogenesis. Exp. Mol. Pathol., *24*:244, 1976.

98. Anderson, R.G.W., Goldstein, J.S., and Brown, M.S.: A mutation that impairs the ability of lipoprotein receptors to localize in coated pits on the cell surface of human fibroblasts. Nature, *270*:695, 1977.

99. Rosenberg, L.E., et al.: Cystinuria: biochemical evidence for three genetically distinct diseases. J. Clin. Invest., *45*:365, 1966.

100. Siseher-Dzoga, K., Sraser, R., and Wissler, R.W.: Stimulation of proliferation in stationary primary cultures of monkey and rabbit. I. Effects of lipoprotein fraction of hyperlipemic serum and lymph. Exp. Mol. Pathol., *24*:346, 1976.

101. De Duve, C.: General properties of lysosomes: the lysosome concept. *In* Ciba Foundation Symposium on Lysosomes. Edited by A.V.S. de Reuck and M.P. Cameron. Boston, Little, Brown, 1963.

102. Kritchevsky, D., and Story, J.: Atherosclerosis: dietary factors other than the usual lipids. Fed. Proc., *41*:2790, 1982.

103. Bierman, E.L., and Ross, R.: Aging and atherosclerosis. *In* Atherosclerosis Reviews. Vol. 2. Edited by R. Paoletti and A.M. Gotto. New York, Raven Press, 1977.

104. Minick, C.R., Alonzo, D.R., and Rankin, L.: Role of immunological arterial injury in atherosclerosis. Thromb. Haemost., *39*:304, 1978.

105. Longley, W.: A new crystalline form of tropomyosin. J. Mol. Biol., *115*:381, 1977.

106. Rose, A.G., Opie, L.H., and Bricknell, O.L.: Early experimental myocardial infarction. Evaluation of histologic criteria and comparison with biochemical and electrocardiographic measurement. Arch. Pathol. Lab. Med., *100*:516, 1976.

107. Jones, C.E., et al.: Acute changes in high-energy phosphates, nucleotide derivatives and contractile force in ischemic and non-ischemic canine myocardium following coronary occlusion. Cardiovasc. Res., *10*:275, 1976.

108. Boor, P.J., and Reynolds, E.S.: Myocardial infarct size: clinicopathologic agreement and discordance. Hum. Pathol., *8*:685, 1977.

109. Mallory, G.K., Kite, P.D., and Salcedo-Salger, J.: The speed of healing of myocardial infarction: a study of the pathologic anatomy in 72 cases. Am. Heart J., *18*:647, 1939.

110. Lodge-Patch, I.: The ageing of cardiac infarcts and its influence on cardiac rupture. Br. Heart J., *13*:37, 1951.

111. Fishbein, M.D., et al.: The histopathologic evolution of myocardial infarction. Chest, *73*:843, 1978.

112. Bouchardy, B., and Majno, G.: Histopathology of early myocardial infarcts. Am. J. Pathol., 74:301, 1974.
113. Trump, B.F., et al.: Recent studies on the pathophysiology of ischemic cell injury. Beitr. Pathol., 158:363, 1976.
114. Neely, J.R., et al.: Effects of ischemia on function and metabolism of the isolated working rat heart. Am. J. Physiol., 225:651, 1973.
115. Jennings, R.B., and Ganote, C.E.: Structural change in the myocardium during acute ischemia. Circ. Res., 35:156, 1974.
116. Yeter, W., et al.: Comparison of clinical and pathologic aspects of coronary artery disease in men of various ages. Ann. Intern. Med., 34:352, 1951.
117. DeMaria, A.N., et al.: Left ventricular thrombi identified by cross-sectional echocardiography. Ann. Intern. Med., 90:14, 1979.
118. Eaton, L.W., et al.: Regional cardiac dilatation after acute myocardial infarction. N. Engl. J. Med., 300:57, 1979.
119. Galen, R.: Isoenzymes of CPK and LDH in myocardial infarction and certain other diseases. *In* Clin. Enzyme Symp. Edited by A. Berlina and L. Galzigna. Padua, Piccin Medical Books, 1979.
120. Kloster, F.E., et al.: Coronary bypass for stable angina. N. Engl. J. Med., 300:149, 1979.
121. Mackowiak, P.A.: Microbial synergism in human infections. N. Engl. J. Med., 298:24, 1978.
122. Mims, C.A.: Aspects of the pathogenesis of virus diseases. Bacteriol. Rev., 28:30, 1964.
123. Morrison, D.C., and Ulevitch, R.J.: The effects of endotoxins on host mediation systems. A review. Am. J. Pathol., 93:528, 1978.
124. Wadstrom, T., and Jeljaszewicz, J.: Bacterial Toxins and Cell Membranes. London, Academic Press, 1978.
125. Kaslow, H.R., et al.: Cholera toxin can catalyze ADP-ribosylation of cytoskeletal proteins. J. Cell Biol., 91:410, 1981.
126. Boquet, P., and Pappenheimer, A.M. Jr.: Interaction of diphtheria toxin with mammalian cell membranes. J. Biol. Chem., 251:5770, 1976.
127. Sanford, J.P.: Current concepts. Legionnaire's disease—the first thousand days. N. Engl. J. Med., 300:654, 1979.
128. Fraser, D.W.: Legionnaire's disease: four summers' harvest. Am. J. Med., 68:1, 1980.
129. Schulman, J.L.: Epidemiology of influenza. J. Am. Clin. Pathol., 70:141, 1978.
130. Krizanova, O.: Interaction of plasma membranes with influenza virus. IV. Changes in adenosine triphosphatase and uridine triphosphatase activities. Acta Virol., 18:97, 1974.
131. Craighead, J.E.: Chronic and persistent viral infections. Introduction. Fed. Proc., 38:2659, 1979.
132. Roizman, B., and Buchman, T.: The molecular epidemiology of Herpes simplex viruses. Hosp. Pract., 14:95, 1979.
133. Roizman, B.: Molecular organization and expression of Herpes simplex DNA. Adv. Pathobiol., 5:54, 1976.
134. Galloway, D.A., et al.: Detection of Herpes simplex RNA in human sensory ganglia. Virology, 95:265, 1979.
135. Albrecht, T., et al.: Cytomegalovirus. Development and progression of cytopathic effects in human cell culture. Lab. Invest., 42:1, 1980.
136. Lee, F.K., Nahmias, A.J., and Stagno, S.: Rapid diagnosis of cytomegalovirus infection in infant by electron microscopy. N. Engl. J. Med., 299:1266, 1978.
137. Joseph, B.S., and Oldstone, M.B.A.: Immunologic injury in measles virus infection. II. Suppression of immune injury through antigenic modulation. J. Exp. Med., 142:864, 1975.
138. Tyrrell, D.A.: Immunologic methods in virology. *In* Handbook of Experimental Immunology. Applications of Immunologic Methods. Vol. 3. Edited by D.M. Weir. Oxford, Blackwell Scientific Publications, 1978.
139. Drutz, D.J.: Urban coccidiodomycosis and histoplasmosis. N. Engl. J. Med., 301:381, 1979.
140. Bloom, B.R.: Games parasites play: how parasites evade immune surveillance. Nature, 279:21, 1979.
141. Godfrey, O.G.: Identification of economically important parasites. Nature, 273:600, 1978.
142. Binford, C.H., and Connor, D.H.: Pathology of Tropical and Extraordinary Diseases. Washington, D.C., Armed Forces Institute of Pathology, 1976.

143. Krogstad, D.J., Spencer, H.C., and Healy, G.R.: Current concepts in parasitology. Amebiasis. N. Engl. J. Med., *298*:262, 1978.
144. Jordan, A.M.: Principles of the eradication or control of tsetse flies. Nature, *273*:607, 1978.
145. Masur, H., et al.: An outbreak of community-acquired Pneumocystic carinii pneumonia. Initial manifestation of cellular immune dysfunction. N. Engl. J. Med., *305*:1431, 1981.
146. Marsden, P.O.: Current concepts in parasitology. Leishmaniasis. N. Engl. J. Med., *300*:350, 1979.
147. Lainson, R., and Shaw, J.J.: Epidemiology and ecology of leishmaniasis in Latin America. Nature, *273*:595, 1978.
148. Miller, L.H., et al.: Influence of erythrocyte membrane components on malaria merozoite invasion. J. Exp. Med., *138*:1597, 1973.
149. Miller, L.H., Aikawa, M., and Dvorak, J.A.: Malaria *(Plasmodium knowlesi) merozoites:* immunity and the surface coat. J. Immunol., *114*:1237, 1975.
150. Aikawa, M., Miller, L.H., and Rabbege, J.: Caveola-vesicle complexes in the plasmalemma of erythrocytes infected by *Plasmodium vivax* and *P. cynomolgi.* Unique structure related to Schuffner's dots. Am. J. Pathol., *79*:285, 1975.
151. Levy, M.R., and Chou, S.C.: Activity and some properties of an acid proteinase from normal and *Plasmodium berghei*-infected red cells. J. Parasitol., *59*:1064, 1973.
152. Maskrey, P., et al.: Cytotoxic substances in sera from *P. knowlesi*-infected rhesus monkeys. Trans. R. Soc. Trop. Med. Hyg., *67*:15, 1973.
153. Soni, J.L., and Cox, H.W.: Pathogenesis of acute avian malaria. I. Immunologic reactions associated with anemia, splenomegaly, and nephritis of acute *Plasmodium gallinaceum* infections in chickens. Am. J. Trop. Med. Hyg., *23*:577, 1974.
154. Gould, S.E.: Trichinosis in man and animals. Springfield, IL, Charles C Thomas, 1970.
155. Warren, K.S.: The pathology, pathobiology and pathogenesis of schistosomiasis. Nature, *273*:609, 1978.
156. Schater, J.: Chlamydial infections. N. Engl. J. Med., *298*:540, 1978.
157. Walker, D.H., and Cain, B.G.: The rickettsial plaque. Evidence for direct cytopathic effect of *Rickettsia rickettsii.* Lab. Invest., *43*:388, 1980.
158. Blumberg, B.S., et al.: Current concepts. Australia antigen and hepatitis. N. Engl. J. Med., *283*:349, 1970.
159. Bianchi, L., et al.: Viral hepatitis. *In* Pathology of the Liver. Edited by R.N.M. MacSween, P.P. Anthony, and P.J. Scheuer. Edinburgh, Churchill Livingstone, 1979.
160. Krugman, S., Friedman, H., and Lattimer, C.: Viral hepatitis type A: identification by specific complement fixation and immune adherence tests. N. Engl. J. Med., *292*:1141, 1975.
161. Gerin, J.L., Shih, J.W-K., and Hoyer, B.H.: Biology and characterization of hepatitis B virus. *In* Viral Hepatitis. 1981 International Symposium. Edited by W. Szmuness, H.J. Alter, and J.E. Maynard. Philadelphia, Franklin Institute Press, 1982.
162. Yamada, G., et al.: Electron and immunoelectron microscopic study of Dane particle formation in chronic hepatitis B virus infection. Gastroenterology, *83*:348, 1982.
163. Rimland, D., et al.: Hepatitis B outbreak traced to an oral surgeon. N. Engl. J. Med., *296*:953, 1977.
164. Dienstag, J.L., and Purcell, R.H.: Recent advances in the identification of hepatitis viruses. Postgrad. Med. J., *53*:364, 1977.
165. Parker, H.W., et al.: Venereal transmission of hepatitis B virus; the possible role of vaginal secretions. Obstet. Gynecol., *48*:410, 1976.
166. Rappaport, A.M.: The microcirculatory acinar concept of normal and pathological hepatic structure. Beitr. Pathol., *157*:215, 1976.
167. Bianci, L., et al.: Acute and chronic hepatitis revisited. Lancet, *2*:914, 1977.
168. U.S. Government Printing Office: Diseases of the Liver and Biliary Tract. Standardization Nomenclature, Diagnostic Criteria, and Diagnostic Methodology. Washington, D.C., Fogerty International Center Proceedings No. 22. DHEW Publication No. (NIH) 76-725, 1976.
169. Dehoratius, R.J., Henderson, C., and Strickland, R.G.: Lymphocytotoxins in acute and chronic hepatitis. Clin. Exp. Immunol., *26*:21, 1976.

170. Baker, A.L., et al.: Polyarteritis associated with Australia antigen-positive hepatitis. Gastroenterology, 62:105, 1972.
171. Nowoslawski, A., et al.: Tissue localization of Australia antigen immune complexes in acute and chronic hepatitis and liver cirrhosis. Am. J. Pathol., 68:31, 1972.
172. Johnson, P.J., et al.: Hepatocellular carcinoma in Great Britain: influence of age, sex, HB$_S$Ag status and aetiology of underlying cirrhosis. Gut, 19:1022, 1978.
173. Shafritz, D.A., et al.: Integration of hepatitis B virus DNA into the genome of liver cells in chronic liver disease and hepatocellular carcinoma. N. Engl. J. Med., 305:1067, 1981.
174. Bréchot, C., et al.: Evidence that hepatitis B virus has a role in liver-cell carcinoma in alcoholic liver disease. N. Engl. J. Med., 306:1384, 1982.
175. Szmuness, W., et al.: Hepatitis B vaccine. Demonstration of efficacy in a controlled clinical trial in a high-risk population in the United States. N. Engl. J. Med., 303:833, 1980.
176. Purcell, R.H., et al.: Modification of chronic hepatitis B-virus infection in chimpanzees. Administration of an interferon inducer. Lancet, 2:757, 1976.
177. Chadwick, R.G., et al.: Inhibition of hepatitis B virus DNA polymerase activity by adenine arabinoside. Ital. J. Gastroenterol., 10:165, 1978.
178. Garry, V.F., and Weston, J.T.: Environmental pathology: new directions. Hum. Pathol., 10:1, 1979.
179. Kolbye, A.: Personal communication. Chronic Toxicity Testing and the Food Industry Seminar. Aspen, CO, Given Institute of Pathobiology, August 22, 1976.
180. Mahaffey, K.R., et al.: National estimates of blood lead levels: United States, 1976–1980. Association with selected demographic and socioeconomic factors. N. Engl. J. Med., 307:573, 1982.
181. Cleveland, W.S., and Graedel, T.E.: Photochemical air pollution in the northeast United States. Science, 204:1273, 1979.
182. U.S. Department of Health, Education and Welfare: The Changing Cigarette. Supplementary Report of the Surgeon General. Washington, D.C., Government Printing Office, 1981.
183. Auerbach, O., Hammond, E.C., and Garfinkel, L.: Changes in bronchial epithelium in relation to cigarette smoking. 1955–1960 vs. 1970–1977. N. Engl. J. Med., 300:381, 1979.
184. Bhagauan, B.S., and Koss, L.G.: Secular trends in prevalence and concentration of pulmonary asbestos bodies 1940–1972. Arch. Pathol. Lab. Med., 100:539, 1976.
185. Pintar, K., Funahashi, A., and Siegesmund, K.A.: A diffuse form of pulmonary silicosis in foundry workers. Arch. Pathol. Lab. Med., 100:535, 1976.
186. Bekesi, J.G., et al.: Lymphocyte function of Michigan dairy farmers exposed to polybrominated biphenyls. Science, 199:1207, 1978.
187. Collins, W.T., et al.: Effect of polychlorinated biphenyl (PCB) on the thyroid gland of rats. Am. J. Pathol., 89:119, 1977.
188. Bahn, A.K., et al.: Hyperthyroidism in workers exposed to polybrominated biphenyls. N. Engl. J. Med., 302:31, 1980.
189. Martin, J.F., et al.: Vinyl-chloride associated liver disease. Ann. Intern. Med., 84:717, 1976.
190. Study Group of Minamata Disease: Minamata Disease. Kumamoto, University of Japan, 1968.
191. Physicians' Desk Reference. 36th Ed. Oradell, NJ, Medical Economics, 1982.
192. Koblin, D.O., and Egen, E.I.: Current concepts. Theories of narcosis. N. Engl. J. Med., 301:1222, 1979.
193. Hruban, Z., et al.: Ultrastructural changes during cholestatis induced by chlorpromazine in the isolated perfused rat liver. Virchows Arch. (Cell Pathol.), 26:289, 1978.
194. Herbst, A.L., Cole, P., and Nohusis, M.J.: Epidemiologic aspects and factors to survival in 384 registry cases of clear cell adenocarcinoma of the vagina and cervix. Am. J. Obstet. Gynecol., 135:876, 1979.
195. Richardson, G.S., and MacLaughlin, D.T. (Eds.): Hormonal Biology of Endometrial Cancer. Vol. 42. Geneva, VICC Technical Report Series, 1978.
196. Hammond, C.B.: Effect of long-term estrogen replacement therapy. Am. J. Obstet. Gynecol., 133:525, 1979.
197. Christopherson, W.M., Mays, E.T., and Barrows, G.H.: Liver tumors in young women: a clinical pathologic study of 201 cases in the

Louisville registry. *In* Progress in Surgical Pathology. Vol. II. Edited by C.M. Fenoglio, and M. Wolff. New York, Masson Publishing USA, 1980.

198. Bagheri, S.A., and Boyer, J.L.: Peliosis hepatitis associated with androgenic-anabolic steroid therapy. Ann. Intern. Med., *81*:610, 1974.

199. Sterling, K.: Thyroid hormone action at the cell level. N. Engl. J. Med., *300*:117, 1979.

200. Mauer, A.M.: Cell kinetics and practical consequences for therapy of acute leukemia. N. Engl. J. Med., *293*:389, 1975.

201. Smuckler, E.A.: Alcoholic drink, its production and effects. Fed. Proc., *34*:2038, 1975.

202. Lieber, C.S.: Pathogenesis and early diagnosis of alcoholic liver injury. N. Engl. J. Med., *298*:888, 1978.

203. Rutstein, D.D., and Veech, R.L.: Genetics and addiction to alcohol. N. Engl. J. Med., *298*:1140, 1978.

204. Blass, J.P., and Gibson, G.E.: Abnormality of a thiamine-requiring enzyme in patients with Wernicke-Korsakoff syndrome. N. Engl. J. Med., *297*:1367, 1977.

205. Lieber, C.S., et al.: Differences in hepatic and metabolic changes after acute and chronic alcohol consumption. Fed. Proc., *34*:2060, 1975.

206. Review by an International Group: Alcoholic liver disease: Morphological manifestations. Lancet, *1*:707, 1981.

207. Gregory, D.H., and Levi, D.F.: The clinical-pathologic spectrum of alcoholic hepatitis. Am. J. Dig. Dis., *17*:479, 1977.

208. Popper, H.: Alcoholic hepatitis—an experimental approach to a conceptual and clinical problem. N. Engl. J. Med., *290*:159, 1974.

209. Rubin, E., and Lieber, C.S.: Fatty liver, alcoholic hepatitis and cirrhosis produced by alcohol in primates. N. Engl. J. Med., *290*:128, 1974.

210. Chen, T.S.N., and Leevy, C.M.: Collagen biosynthesis in liver disease of the alcoholic. J. Lab. Clin. Med., *85*:103, 1975.

211. Powell, W.J. Jr., and Klatskin, G.: Duration of survival in patients with Laennec's cirrhosis. Am. J. Med., *44*:406, 1968.

212. Popper, H., and Schaffner, F.: Structural studies in alcohol and drug induced liver injury. *In* Skandia International Symposia on Alcoholic Cirrhosis and Other Toxic Hepatopathies. Stockholm, Nordiska Bokhandelns Forlag, 1970.

213. Tinberg, H.M., et al.: Mallory bodies. Isolation of hepatocellular hyalin and electrophoretic resolution of polypeptide components. Lab. Invest., *39*:483, 1978.

214. Ma, M.H.: Ultrastructural pathologic findings of the human hepatocyte. Arch. Pathol., *94*:554, 1972.

215. Iseri, O.A., and Gottlieb, L.S.: Alcoholic hyalin and megamitochondria as separate and distinct entities in liver disease associated with alcoholism. Gastroenterology, *60*:1027, 1971.

216. Koch, O.R., et al.: Biochemical lesions of liver mitochondria from rats after chronic alcohol consumption. Exp. Mol. Pathol., *27*:213, 1977.

217. Cederbaum, A.I., and Rubin, E.: Molecular injury to mitochondria produced by ethanol and acetaldehyde. Fed. Proc., *34*:2045, 1975.

218. Rubin, E.: Alcoholic myopathy in heart and skeletal muscle. N. Engl. J. Med., *301*:28, 1979.

219. Perkoff, G.T., Hardy, P., and Velez-Garcia, E.: Reversible acute muscular syndrome in chronic alcoholism. N. Engl. J. Med., *274*:1278, 1966.

220. Worden, R.D.: Pattern of muscle-nerve pathology in alcoholism. Ann. N.Y. Acad. Sci., *273*:351, 1979.

221. Deitrich, R.A.: Neurochemistry of ethanol. Fed. Proc., *34*:1929, 1975.

222. Squires, K.C., Chu, N-S., and Starr, A.: Acute effects of alcohol on auditory brainstem potentials in humans. Science, *201*:174, 1978.

223. Centerwall, B.S., and Criqui, M.H.: Prevention of the Wernicke-Korsakoff syndrome. A cost-benefit analysis. N. Engl. J. Med., *299*:285, 1978.

224. Gordon, J.J., et al.: Effect of alcohol (ethanol) administration on sex-hormones metabolism in normal men. N. Engl. J. Med., *295*:794, 1976.

225. Raskin, N.H., Sligar, K.P., and Steinberg, R.H.: A pathophysiologic role for alcohol dehydrogenase: is retinol its "natural" substitute? Ann. N.Y. Acad. Sci., *273*:317, 1976.

226. Zetterman, R.K., Luisada-Opper, A., and Leevy, C.M.: Cell-me-

diated immunological response to alcoholic hyalin. Gastroenterology, *63*:1020, 1972.

227. Leevy, C.M., Chen, T., and Zetterman, R.: Alcoholic hepatitis, cirrhosis, and immunologic reactivity. Ann. N.Y. Acad. Sci., *252*:106, 1975.

228. Gell, P.G.H., Coombs, R.R.A., and Lachmann, P.J.: Clinical Aspects of Immunology. 3rd Ed. Oxford, Blackwell Scientific Publications, 1975.

229. Roitt, I.M.: Essential Immunology. 2nd Ed. Oxford, Blackwell Scientific Publications, 1975.

230. Sell, S.: Immunology, Immunopathology and Immunity. 3rd Ed. New York, Harper & Row, 1980.

231. Paterson, R., Zeiss, C.R., and Kelly, J.F.: Classification of hypersensitivity reactions. N. Engl. J. Med., *295*:277, 1976.

232. Soter, N.A., et al.: Release of mast-cell mediators and alterations in lung function in patients with cholinergic urticaria. N. Engl. J. Med., *302*:604, 1980.

233. Newman, S.A., Rossi, G., and Metzger, H.: Molecular weight and volume of the cell-surface receptor for immunoglobulin E. Proc. Natl. Acad. Sci. USA, *74*:869, 1977.

234. Atkins, P.C., et al.: Release of neutrophil chemotactic activity during immediate hypersensitivity reactions in humans. Ann. Intern. Med., *86*:415, 1977.

235. Sullivan, T.J., and Parker, C.W.: Pharmacologic modulation of inflammatory mediator release by rat mast cells. Am. J. Pathol., *85*:437, 1976.

236. Dvorak, A.M., et al.: Degranulation mechanisms in human leukemic basophils. Clin. Immunol. Immunopathol., *5*:235, 1976.

237. Schatz, M., Patterson, R., and Fink, J.: Immunologic lung disease. N. Engl. J. Med., *300*:1310, 1979.

238. Frank, M.M., et al.: Pathophysiology of immune hemolytic anemia. Ann. Intern. Med., *87*:210, 1977.

239. Aster, R.H.: TTP: New clues to the etiology of an enigmatic disease. N. Engl. J. Med., *297*:1400, 1977.

240. Parrillo, J.E., and Fanci, A.S.: Apparent direct cellular cytotoxicity mediated via cytophilic antibody. Immunology, *33*:839, 1977.

241. Shohet, S.B., and Ness, P.M.: Hemolytic anemias. Med. Clin. North Am., *60*:913, 1976.

242. McCluskey, R.T., Hall, C.L., and Colvin, R.B.: Immune complex mediated diseases. Hum. Pathol., *9*:71, 1978.

243. Velosa, J., Miller, K., and Michael, A.F.: Immunopathology of end-stage kidney. Immunoglobulin and complement component deposition in nonimmune disease. Am. J. Pathol., *84*:149, 1976.

244. Gelfand, M.C., Frank, M.M., and Green, I.: A receptor for the third component of complement in the human renal glomerulus. J. Exp. Med., *142*:1024, 1975.

245. Bayer, A.S., et al.: Circulating immune complexes in infective endocarditis. N. Engl. J. Med., *295*:1500, 1976.

246. Zinkernagel, R.M.: Major transplantation antigens in host responses to infection. Hosp. Pract., *13*:83, 1978.

247. Shiftan, T.A., and Mendelsohn, J.: The circulating "atypical" lymphocyte. Hum. Pathol., *9*:51, 1978.

248. Teh, H-S., Phillips, R.A., and Miller, R.G.: Quantitative studies on the precursors of cytotoxic lymphocytes. III. The lineage of memory cells. J. Exp. Med., *146*:1280, 1977.

249. Pearson, G.R.: *In vitro* and *in vivo* investigations on antibody-dependent cellular cytotoxicity. Microbiol. Immunol., *80*:65, 1978.

250. Nelson, D.L., Sachs, D.H., and Dickler, H.B.: Antibody-dependent cellular cytotoxicity effector cells lack Ia antigens. J. Immunol., *119*:1034, 1977.

251. Riethmuller, G., Wernet, P., and Cudkowicz, G. (Eds.): Natural and Induced Cell-Mediated Cytotoxicity. Effector and Regulatory Mechanisms. New York, Academic Press, 1979.

252. Kall, M.A., and Koren, H.S.: Heterogeneity of human natural killer cell populations. Cell. Immunol., *40*:58, 1978.

253. Beverly, P., and Knight, D.: Killing comes naturally. Nature, *278*:119, 1979.

254. Guttman, R.D.: Renal transplantation. N. Engl. J. Med., *301*:975, 1038, 1979.

255. Suciu–Foca, N., Godfrey, M.M., and Khan, R.: HLA–D–DR relationships: PLT studies of HLA-D specificities associated with DR1, DR2 and DR4. Hum. Immunol., *2*:295, 1981.

256. Paul, L.C., et al.: Accelerated rejection on a renal allograft associated with pretransplantation antibodies directed against donor antigens on endothelium and monocytes. N. Engl. J. Med., *300*:1258, 1979.
257. Ettenger, R.B.: Anti-B lymphocytotoxins in renal-allograft rejection. N. Engl. J. Med., *295*:305, 1976.
258. Reinherz, E.L., et al.: Aberrations of suppressor T cells in human graft-versus-host disease. N. Engl. J. Med., *300*:1061, 1979.
259. Frizzera, G., et al.: Lymphoproliferative disorders (LPD) in renal transplant recipients: a morphologic and biologic spectrum. Lab. Invest., *44*:21A, 1981.
260. Vandelli, C., et al.: Autoantibodies to gastrin-producing cells in antral (type B) chronic gastritis. N. Engl. J. Med., *300*:1406, 1979.
261. Woolley, D.E., et al.: Collagenase immunolocalization in cultures of rheumatoid synovial cells. Science, *200*:773, 1978.
262. Hirschhorn, R.: The blind men and the rheumatoid elephant. N. Engl. J. Med., *293*:554, 1975.
263. Zvaifler, N.J., and Greenberg, P.O.: Immunopathology of rheumatoid arthritis. *In* Mechanism of Immunopathology. Edited by P.A. Ward and R.T. McClusky. New York, John Wiley & Sons, 1979.
264. Zvaifler, N.J.: Immunopathogenesis of Rheumatoid Arthritis and Systemic Lupus Erythematosus. Kalamazoo, MI, Upjohn, 1974.
265. Appel, G.B., et al.: Renal involvement in systemic lupus erythematosus (SLE): a study of 56 patients emphasizing histologic classification. Medicine, *57*:371, 1978.
266. Frank, M.M., et al.: Defective reticuloendothelial system Fc-receptor function in systemic lupus erythematosus. N. Engl. J. Med., *300*:518, 1979.
267. Tatal, N., et al.: Biological significance of IgM and IgG antibodies to DNA and RNA in autoimmune disease. Am. J. Clin. Pathol., *68*:643, 1977.
268. Fretzler, M.J., and Taan, E.M.: Antibodies to histones in drug-induced and idiopathic lupus erythematosus. J. Clin. Invest., *62*:560, 1978.
269. Schwartz, R.S.: Viruses and systemic lupus erythematosus. N. Engl. J. Med., *293*:132, 1973.
270. Panem, S., et al.: Viral immune complexes in systemic lupus erythematosus. Specificity of C-type viral complexes. Lab. Invest., *39*:413, 1978.
271. Reinertsen, J.L., et al.: B-lymphocyte alloantigen associated with systemic lupus erythematosus. N. Engl. J. Med., *299*:515, 1978.
272. Nakamura, R.M., and Tan, E.M.: Recent progress in the study of autoantibodies to nuclear antigens. Hum. Pathol., *9*:85, 1978.
273. Fauci, A.S., Haynes, B.F., and Katz, P.: The spectrum of vasculitis: clinical pathologic, immunologic and therapeutic considerations. Ann. Intern. Med., *89*:660, 1978.
274. Rose, N.R.: Autoimmunity revisited. Nature, *275*:88, 1978.
275. Esquivel, P.S., Kong, Y.M., and Rose, N.R.: Evidence for thyroglobulin-reactive T cells in good responder mice. Cell. Immunol., *37*:14, 1978.
276. Rose, N.R., Bacon, C.D., and Sundick, R.S.: Genetic determinants to thyroiditis in the OS chicken. Transplant. Rev., *31*:264, 1976.
277. Volpe, R.: The role of autoimmunity in hypoendocrine and hyperendocrine function. Ann. Intern. Med., *87*:86, 1977.
278. Lampert, P.W.: Autoimmune and virus-induced demyelinating diseases. A review. Am. J. Pathol., *91*:176, 1978.
279. Goldberg, M.J., et al.: Evidence against an immune complex pathogenesis of primary biliary cirrhosis. Gastroenterology, *83*:677, 1982.
280. Engel, A.G.: Myasthenia gravis. *In* Handbook of Clinical Neurology. Edited by P.J. Vinken and G.W. Bruyn. Amsterdam, North-Holland, 1979.
281. Drachman, D.B.: Medical progress. Myasthenia gravis. N. Engl. J. Med., *298*:136, 298, 1978.
282. Koell, G.B.: Anticholinesterase agents. *In* The Pharmacological Basis of Therapeutics. 5th Ed. Edited by L.S. Goodman and A. Gilman. New York, Macmillan, 1975.
283. Grob, D.: Introduction: myasthenia gravis in perspective. Ann. N.Y. Acad. Sci., *274*:1, 1976.
284. Fertuck, H.C., and Salpeter, M.M.: Localization of acetylcholine receptor by ^{125}I-labeled α-bungarotoxin binding at mouse motor endplates. Proc. Natl. Acad. Sci. USA, *71*:1376, 1974.
285. Eldefrawi, M.E., Eldefrawi, A.T., and Shamoo, A.E.: Molecular and

functional properties of the acetylcholine-receptor. Ann. N.Y. Acad. Sci., *264*:183, 1975.

286. Rash, J.E., et al.: Studies on human myasthenia gravis: Electrophysiological and ultrastructural evidence compatible with antibody attachment to acetylcholine receptor complex. Proc. Natl. Acad. Sci. USA, *73*:4584, 1976.

287. Satyamurti, S., Drachman, D.B., and Slone, F.: Blockade of acetylcholine receptors: a model of myasthenia gravis. Science, *187*:955, 1975.

288. Almon, R.R., Andrew, C.G., and Appel, S.H.: Serum globulin in myasthenia gravis: inhibition of α-bungarotoxin binding to acetylcholine receptors. Science, *186*:55, 1974.

289. Grob, D.: Myasthenia gravis. Ann. N.Y. Acad. Sci., *377*, 1981.

290. Engel, A.G., et al.: Experimental autoimmune myasthenia gravis: a sequential and quantitative study of the neuromuscular junction ultrastructure and electrophysiologic correlation. J. Neuropathol. Exp. Neurol., *35*:569, 1976.

291. Drachman, D.B., Angus, C.W., and Adams, R.N.: Myasthenia antibodies cross-link acetylcholine receptors to accelerate degradation. N. Engl. J. Med., *298*:1116, 1978.

292. Lennon, V.A., Lindstrom, J.M., and Seybold, M.E.: Experimental autoimmune myasthenia: a model of myasthenia gravis in rats and guinea pigs. J. Exp. Med., *141*:1365, 1975.

293. Richman, D.P., et al.: Cellular immunity to acetylcholine receptor in myasthenia gravis: relationship to histocompatibility type and antigenic site. Neurology, *29*:291, 1979.

294. Abransky, O., et al.: Cellular immune response to acetylcholine receptor-rich fraction in patients with myasthenia gravis. Clin. Exp. Immunol., *19*:11, 1975.

295. Castleman, B.: The pathology of the thymus gland in myasthenia gravis. Ann. N.Y. Acad. Sci., *135*:496, 1966.

296. Van de Velde, R.I., and Friedman, N.B.: Thymic myoid cells and myasthenia gravis. Am. J. Pathol., *59*:347, 1970.

297. Kao, I., and Drachman, D.B.: Thymic muscle cells bear acetylcholine receptors: Possible relation to myasthenia gravis. Science, *195*:74, 1977.

298. Abdou, N.I., et al.: The thymus in myasthenia gravis: evidence for altered cell populations. N. Engl. J. Med., *291*:1271, 1974.

299. Pirskanen, R.: On the significance of HL-A and LD antigens in myasthenia gravis. Ann. N.Y. Acad. Sci., *274*:451, 1976.

300. Mulder, D.G., Herrmann, C., and Buckberg, G.D.: Effect of thymectomy in patients with myasthenia gravis: a sixteen year experience. Am. J. Surg., *128*:202, 1974.

301. Brunner, N.G., et al.: Corticotropin and corticosteroids in generalized myasthenia gravis: comparative studies and role in management. Ann. N.Y. Acad. Sci., *274*:577, 1976.

302. Matell, G., et al.: Effects of some immunosuppressive procedure on myasthenia gravis. Ann. N.Y. Acad. Sci., *274*:659, 1976.

303. Vincent, A., et al.: Circulating anti-acetylcholine receptor antibody in myasthenia gravis treated by plasma exchange. Neurology, *27*:364, 1977.

304. Barta, L., and Simon, S.: Role of HLA-B8 and BW 15 antigens in diabetic children. N. Engl. J. Med., *296*:397, 1977.

305. Felts, P.W.: Current concepts. Coma in the Diabetic. Kalamazoo, MI, Upjohn, 1974.

306. Kitzmiller, J.L., et al.: Diabetic pregnancy and perinatal morbidity. Am. J. Obstet. Gynecol., *131*:550, 1978.

307. Winegrad, A.I., and Greene, D.A.: Diabetic polyneuropathy: the importance of insulin deficiency hyperglycemia and alterations in myoinositol metabolism in its pathogenesis. N. Engl. J. Med., *295*:1416, 1976.

308. Kreisbert, R.A.: Diabetic ketoacidosis: new concepts and trends in pathogenesis and treatment. Ann. Intern. Med., *88*:681, 1978.

309. Cox, M., Sterno, R.H., and Singer, I.: The defense against hyperkalemia: the roles of insulin and aldosterone. N. Engl. J. Med., *299*:525, 1978.

310. Bunn, H.F.: Nonenzymatic glycosylation of protein: relevance to diabetes. Am. J. Med., *70*:325, 1981.

311. Ditzel, J., and Standl, E.: The problem of tissue oxygenation in diabetes mellitus. I. Its relation to the early functional changes in the microcirculation of diabetic subjects. Acta Med. Scand. (Suppl.), *578*:49, 1975.

312. Horowitz, D.L., Kuzuya, H., and Rubenstein, A.H.: Circulating serum C-peptide. A brief review of diagnostic implications. N. Engl. J. Med., 295:207, 1976.
313. Gabbay, K.H., et al.: Familial hyperproinsulinoma. An autosomal dominant defect. N. Engl. J. Med., 294:911, 1976.
314. Given, B.D., et al.: Diabetes due to secretion of abnormal insulin. N. Engl. J. Med., 302:129, 1980.
315. Lacy, P.E.: Endocrine secretory mechanisms. A review. Am. J. Pathol., 79:170, 1975.
316. Orci, L.: A portrait of the pancreatic B-cell. Diabetologia, 10:163, 1974.
317. Gabbay, K.H., Korff, J., and Schneiberger, E.E.: Vesicular binesis: glucose effect on insulin secretory vesicles. Science, 187:177, 1975.
318. Yasuda, K., et al.: Glucose tolerance and insulin secretion in patients with parathyroid disorders. Effect of serum calcium on insulin release. N. Engl. J. Med., 292:501, 1975.
319. Czech, M.P.: Molecular basis of insulin action. Annu. Rev. Biochem., 46:359, 1977.
320. Posner, B.I., et al.: Different regulation of insulin receptors in intracellular (Golgi) and plasma membranes from livers of obese and lean mice. Proc. Natl. Acad. Sci. USA, 75:3302, 1978.
321. Olefsky, J.M., and Chang, H.: Insulin binding to adipocytes: evidence for functionally distinct receptors. Diabetes, 27:946, 1978.
322. Kahn, C.R., and Baird, K.: The fate of insulin bound to adipocytes: Evidence for compartmentalization and processing. J. Biol. Chem., 253:4900, 1978.
323. Olefsky, J.M.: Effects of fasting on insulin binding glucose transport and glucose oxidation in isolated rat adipocytes. J. Clin. Invest., 58:1450, 1976.
324. Thorsson, A.V., and Hintz, R.L.: Insulin receptors in the newborn. N. Engl. J. Med., 297:908, 1977.
325. Roth, J., et al.: Receptors for insulin, NSILA-s and growth hormones: application to disease states in man. Recent Prog. Horm. Res., 31:95, 1975.
326. Hepp, K.D.: Studies on the mechanism of insulin action: basic concepts and clinical implications. Diabetologia, 13:177, 1977.
327. Zeleznik, A.J., and Roth, J.: Demonstration of the insulin receptor in vivo in rabbits and its possible role as a reservoir for the plasma hormone. J. Clin. Invest., 61:1363, 1978.
328. Flier, J.S., et al.: Characterization of antibodies to the insulin receptor. J. Clin. Invest., 58:1442, 1976.
329. Blackard, W.G., Anderson, J.H., and Mullinax, F.: Anti-insulin receptor antibodies and diabetes. Ann. Intern. Med., 86:584, 1976.
330. Pulini, M., et al.: Insulin resistance and acanthosis nigricans. Ann. Intern. Med., 85:749, 1976.
331. Bar, R.S., et al.: Extreme insulin resistance in ataxia-telangiectasia. N. Engl. J. Med., 298:1164, 1978.
332. Kasuga, M., et al.: Effects of anti-insulin receptor. Autoantibodies on the metabolism of human adipocytes. Diabetes, 27:938, 1978.
333. Soman, V., et al.: Insulin binding and insulin sensitivity in isolated growth hormone deficiency. N. Engl. J. Med., 299:1026, 1978.
334. Unger, R.H.: Glucagon, pancreatectomy and ketoacidosis. N. Engl. J. Med., 297:559, 1977.
335. Landgraf, R., et al.: Prolactin: a diabetogenic hormone. Diabetologia, 13:99, 1977.
336. Gerich, J.E., et al.: Prevention of human diabetic ketoacidosis by somatostatin. N. Engl. J. Med., 292:985, 1975.
337. Maugh, T.H.: New hormones promise more effective therapy. Science, 188:920, 1975.
338. Junker, K., et al.: An autopsy study of the islets of Langerhans in acute-onset juvenile diabetes mellitus. Acta Pathol. Microbiol. Scand. [A], 85:699, 1977.
339. Winegrad, A.I., and Greene, D.A.: The complications of diabetes mellitus. N. Engl. J. Med., 298:1250, 1978.
340. Koenig, R.J., and Cerami, A.: Synthesis of hemoglobin$_{A1C}$ in normal and diabetic mice. Potential model of basement membrane thickening. Proc. Natl. Acad. Sci. USA, 72:3687, 1975.
341. Stevens, V.J., et al.: Diabetic cataract formation: potential role of glycosylation of lens crystallins. Proc. Natl. Acad. Sci. USA, 75:2918, 1978.
342. Gabbay, K.H.: The sorbitol pathway and the complications of diabetes. N. Engl. J. Med., 288:831, 1973.

343. Cohen, M.P., and Khalifa, A.: Effect of diabetes and insulin on rat renal glomerular protocollagen hydroxylase activities. Biochem. Biophys. Acta, *496*:88, 1977.
344. Wautier, J.-L., et al.: Increased adhesion of erythrocytes to endothelial cells in diabetes mellitus and its relation to vascular complications. N. Engl. J. Med., *305*:237, 1981.
345. Jackson, R.L., and Guthrie, R.A.: Current Concepts. The Child with Diabetes Mellitus. A Scope Monograph. Kalamazoo, MI, Upjohn, 1975.
346. Mustard, J.F., and Packham, M.A.: Platelets and diabetes mellitus. N. Engl. J. Med., *297*:1345, 1977.
347. Gordon, R., et al.: Diabetes, blood lipids and the role of obesity in coronary heart disease risk for women. The Framingham Study. Ann. Intern. Med., *87*:393, 1977.
348. Patz, A.: Current concepts in ophthalmology. Retinal vascular diseases. N. Engl. J. Med., *298*:1451, 1978.
349. Ramsay, W.J., et al.: Involutional diabetic retinopathy. Am. J. Ophthalmol., *84*:851, 1977.
350. Regan, T.J., and Weisse, A.B.: The question of cardiomyopathy in diabetes mellitus. Ann. Intern. Med., *89*:1000, 1978.
351. Westberg, N.: Biochemical alterations of the human glomerular basement membrane in diabetes. Diabetes, *25 (Suppl. 2)*:920, 1976.
352. Elfenbein, S.B., and Reyes, J.W.: Crescents in diabetic glomerulopathy. Incidence and clinical significance. Lab. Invest., *33*:687, 1975.
353. Schulz, H., and Hahnel, E.: Die ultrastruktor des glykogens in lochkernen der menschlichen leberepithelzellen bei diabetes mellitus. Virchows Arch. (Cell Pathol.), *3*:282, 1969.
354. Wingrad, A.I., and Greene, D.A.: Diabetic polyneuropathy: the importance of insulin deficiency, hyperglycemia and alterations in myoinositol metabolism in its pathogenesis. N. Engl. J. Med., *295*:1416, 1976.
355. Jakobsen, J.: Axonal dwindling in early experimental diabetes. Diabetologia, *12*:539, 1976.
356. Naccarato, R., et al.: The muscle in diabetes mellitus. Virchows Arch. (Cell Pathol.), *4*:283, 1970.
357. Goodson, W.H., and Hunt, R.K.: Studies of wound healing in experimental diabetes mellitus. J. Surg. Res., *22*:221, 1977.
358. Teng, M.H., Bartholomew, J.C., and Bissell, M.J.: Insulin effect on the cell cycle: analysis of the kinetics of growth parameters in confluent chick cells. Proc. Natl. Acad. Sci. USA, *73*:3173, 1976.
359. Craighead, J.E.: Current views on the etiology of insulin-dependent diabetes mellitus. N. Engl. J. Med., *299*:1439, 1978.
360. York, D.C., Bray, G.A., and Yukimura, Y.: An enzymatic defect in the obese (ob/ob) mouse: Loss of thyroid-induced sodium and potassium dependent adenosinotriphosphatase. Proc. Natl. Acad. Sci. USA, *75*:477, 1978.
361. Birglund, O., Frankel, B.J., and Hellman, B.: Development of the insulin secretory defect in genetically diabetic (db/db) mouse. Acta Endocrinol., *87*:543, 1978.
362. Woon, J.W., et al.: Antibody to encephalomyocarditis virus in juvenile diabetes. N. Engl. J. Med., *297*:1235, 1977.
363. Craighead, J.E.: Animal model of disease. Am. J. Pathol., *78*:538, 1975.
364. Rubinstein, P., Suciu-Foca, N., and Nicholson, J.F.: Genetics of juvenile diabetes mellitus. N. Engl. J. Med., *297*:1036, 1977.
365. Neel, J.V.: The genetics of juvenile-onset diabetes mellitus. N. Engl. J. Med., *297*:1062, 1977.
366. Craighead, J.E., Kanish, R.E., and Kessler, J.B.: Lesions of the islets of Langerhans in encephalomyocarditis virus infected mice with diabetes mellitus-like disease. Am. J. Pathol., *74*:287, 1974.
367. Ross, M.E., et al.: Virus-induced diabetes mellitus. V. Biological differences between the M variant and other strains of encephalomyocarditis virus. Infec. Immun., *12*:1224, 1975.
368. Yoon, J.W., et al.: Virus-induced diabetes mellitus. Diabetes, *27*:778, 1978.
369. Vanthiel, D.H., et al.: A syndrome of IgA deficiency, diabetes mellitus, malabsorption and a common haplotype. Ann. Intern. Med., *86*:10, 1977.
370. Little, J.A., et al.: Insulin antibodies and clinical complications in diabetics treated for five years with Lente or sulfated insulin. Diabetes, *26*:980, 1977.

371. Flier, J.S., et al.: Auto-antibodies to the insulin receptor. J. Clin. Invest., *60*:784, 1977.
372. Kumar, D.: Anti-insulin IgE in diabetes. J. Clin. Endocrinol. Metab., *45*:1159, 1977.
373. Fialkow, P.G., Zavala, C., and Nielsen, R.: Thyroid autoimmunity: increased frequency in relatives of insulin-dependent diabetes mellitus. Ann. Intern. Med., *83*:170, 1975.
374. Bar, R.S., Kahn, C.R., and Koren, H.S.: Insulin inhibition of antibody-dependent cytotoxicity and insulin receptors in macrophages. Nature, *265*:632, 1977.
375. Lacy, P.E.: Prolongation of islet allograft survival following *in vitro* culture (24° C) and a single injection of ALS. Science, *204*:312, 1980.

Chapter 4

NEOPLASIA

The canker galls the infants of the spring.

—Hamlet I, iii

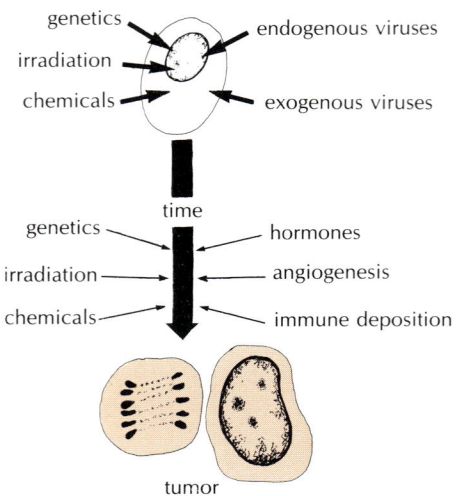

Figure 4–1. Some of the multiple factors involved in the development of cancer.

GENERAL FEATURES OF NEOPLASIA

Cancer is a complex disease.[1] Our understanding of it is plagued by myriad controversies concerning its etiology, diagnosis, and therapy. The burgeoning literature makes it even more difficult to understand. Like heart disease, hypertension, and atherosclerosis, cancer probably has a multifactorial origin (Fig. 4–1), although a specific etiologic agent may be recognized in certain instances. For example, polyvinyl chloride exposure may result in angiosarcomas of the liver, Epstein-Barr virus has been associated with Burkitt's lymphoma, some forms of radiation cause leukemia, diethylstilbestrol therapy has been linked with carcinoma of the vagina, and cigarette smoking has been associated with carcinoma of the lung. It has proved valuable to concentrate on these examples to learn more about the host's reaction to carcinogenic agents and the pathogenesis of cancer.

Environment

The majority of tumors occur in an atmosphere that contains a sea of known and unknown carcinogens; we cannot underestimate the effect of the environment.[2] This effect is apparent when we study the incidence of certain cancers in populations that migrate from one country to another. For example, cancer of the stomach is more common in Japan than in the United States. Conversely, colon, breast, and prostate cancers are much rarer in Japanese than in Americans. When Japanese emigrate to the United States, however, these differences are lost within a generation or two.

The evidence for an environmental origin for human cancers can be considered at two levels. At one level are those cancers in which strong evidence suggests that a specific stimulus is involved. This group includes cancers related to personal habits, such as smoking, which causes cancer of the lung or lip, and to certain occupations, such as construction (mesothelioma). The second group includes those cancers in which a specific etiologic agent is not yet identified, but in which the most rational interpretation of the available data implicates the environment.[3]

The prevention of environmental contamination by carcinogens is a difficult task for regulatory agencies, which can only concentrate on obvious, prominent violators; therefore, the early detection of tumors is emphasized. This approach has proved successful for carcinoma of the cervix and breast;[4] however, efforts at early detection of most cancers depend on extensive monitoring, continuing research, and the development of educational programs.

The critical factors that determine whether or not malignant disease occurs in most patients are related to genetic susceptibility and resistance of the individual.[5] These factors have been documented with other diseases such as viral

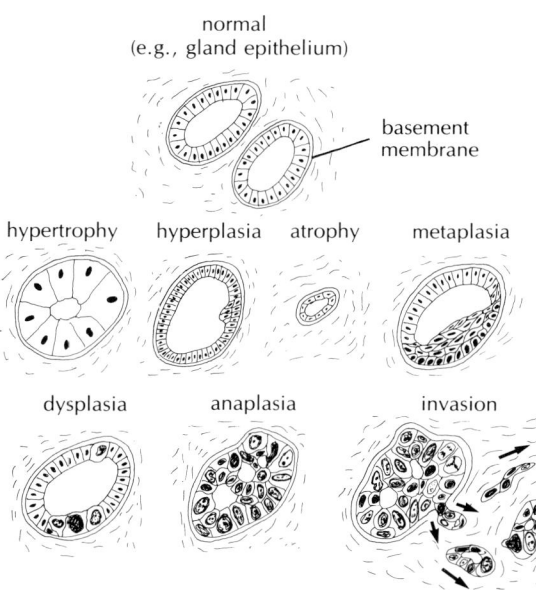

normal
(e.g., gland epithelium)

basement
membrane

hypertrophy hyperplasia atrophy metaplasia

dysplasia anaplasia invasion

Figure 4–2. Schematic depiction of the terminology used in neoplasia.

hepatitis, infectious mononucleosis, tuberculosis, and poliomyelitis, and it appears logical that cancer will prove to be similar in this regard.

Nomenclature

We have previously defined the terms (Table 4–1) *hyperplasia* (increase in number of cells), *hypertrophy* (increase in size of cells), *atrophy* (decrease in number or size of cells), *metaplasia* (replacement of one adult cell type by another adult cell type), and *neoplasia* (change in cytologic features and organization in tissues) (Fig. 4–2).

Table 4–1. *Nomenclature of Growth Phenomena*

Atrophy	Decrease in number or size of cells
Hypertrophy	Increase in size of cells
Hyperplasia	Increase in number of cells
Metaplasia	Replacement of one adult cell type by another
Dysplasia	Loss of cellular differentiation and tissue organization
Neoplasia	Change in cytologic features and organization in tissues often associated with invasion and metastasis

Hyperplasia may be physiologic or neoplastic. The former is due to an extracellular stimulus and usually subsides when the stimulus is removed. Neoplastic cell proliferation, however, is due in part to a heritable abnormality within the cell[6] and continues even if the initial stimulus is removed.

Dysplasia refers to abnormal cells that show atypical cytologic features and tissue architecture with proliferation. Dysplasia often precedes frank malignancy. Malignant cells are capable of *invasion,* which is infiltration of tumor cells into surrounding tissue, and *metastasis,* which means the growth of tumor cells at distant sites. Tumors may have all degrees of differentiation; the least differentiated are called *anaplastic.* Generally, when we speak of tumors, we mean benign or malignant growths. The word "tumor," however, literally means "swelling" and may therefore also refer to an inflammatory mass, a pregnancy, or a cyst, as well as a true neoplastic growth.

The term cancer refers to a malignant process, which is classified according to its histogenesis into three broad groups (Table 4–2): *carcinomas* arising in epithelium, *sar-*

Table 4–2. *Nomenclature of Malignant Tumors*

Carcinomas	Tumors arising in epithelium
Sarcomas	Tumors arising in mesenchymal tissues
Leukemias, lymphomas	Tumors arising in mesenchymal stem cells of bone marrow and lymphoid tissues
Carcinosarcomas	Tumors containing both malignant epithelial and mesenchymal elements
Teratocarcinomas	Malignant tumors containing tissue from the three primitive germ layers

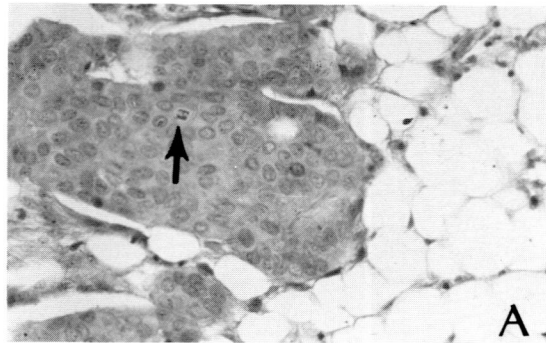

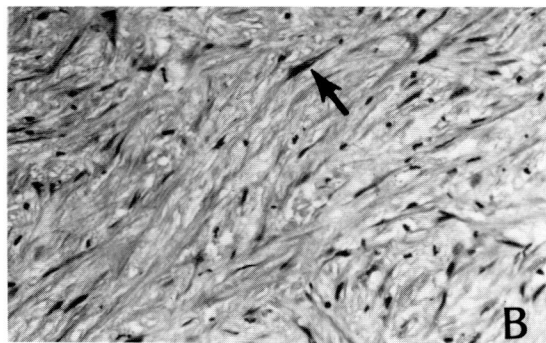

Figure 4–3. Epithelial versus mesenchymal neoplasms. *A*, Carcinoma is composed of a nest of epithelial cells with prominent mitosis (arrow) invading fatty tissue. *B*, Low-grade sarcoma is composed of spindle-shaped cells demonstrating nuclear pleomorphism (arrow).

Table 4–3. *Nomenclature of Leukemias and Lymphomas*

Cell Involved	Disease
Stem cell	Undifferentiated stem cell leukemia
Monomyeloblast	Monomyeloblastic leukemia
Monocyte	Monocytic leukemia
Granulocyte	
Myelocyte	Myelocytic leukemia
Eosinophil	Eosinophilic leukemia
Basophil	Basophilic leukemia
Lymphocyte (B, N, T)	Lympho(blastic)cytic leukemia
Plasma cell	Plasma(blastic)cytic leukemia
Lymphocytes or lymphoblasts	Lympho(blastic)cytic lymphoma
Monocyte	Mono(blastic)cytic lymphoma
Histiocytes and lymphocytes	Mixed type lymphoma
Plasma cell (or plasmablast)	Multiple myeloma

comas arising in mesenchymal tissues, and *leukemias* and *lymphomas* (Table 4–3) arising in the blood-forming cells of the bone marrow and lymph nodes (Fig. 4–3).

Cancers may also be classified according to their site of origin, for example, cancers of the lung or prostate. Tumors occasionally contain both malignant epithelial and mesenchymal elements; these are referred to as *carcinosarcomas*. Tumors that contain tissue from each of the three primitive germ layers (ectoderm, mesoderm, and endoderm) are called *teratomas* when benign or *teratocarcinomas* when malignant.

A term that describes benign proliferations of squamous epithelial tissue is *papilloma* (Table 4–4). Malignant squamous cell epithelial tumors are called epidermoid or *squamous cell carcinomas*. Benign tumors of glandular tissue are called *adenomas;* their malignant counterparts are called *adenocarcinomas*. Mesodermal tumors take their name from their cell of origin. Finally, a few tumors retain eponyms in honor of their discoverers (Table 4–5), for example,

Table 4–4. *Nomenclature of Tumors*

	Cell Type of Origin	Benign	Malignant
Epithelial	Squamous cell	Papilloma	Epidermal (squamous cell) carcinoma
	Glandular cell	Adenoma	Adenocarcinoma
Mesenchymal	Fibroblast	Fibroma	Fibrosarcoma
	Fat cell	Lipoma	Liposarcoma
	Endothelial cell	Angioma	Angiosarcoma
	Cartilage cell	Chondroma	Chondrosarcoma
	Bone cell	Osteoma	Osteosarcoma

Table 4–5. *Eponyms of Common Tumors*

Brenner	Epithelial ovarian tumor
Burkitt's	Lymphoma
Ewing's	Sarcoma of bone
Grawitz's	Carcinoma of the kidney
Kaposi's	Hemangiosarcoma
Krukenberg's	Carcinoma of ovary (usually metastatic from stomach)
Pancoast's	Carcinoma of pulmonary sulcus
Rathke's	Craniopharyngioma of pituitary
Warthin's	Tumor of salivary gland
Wilms'	Adenomyosarcoma of kidney

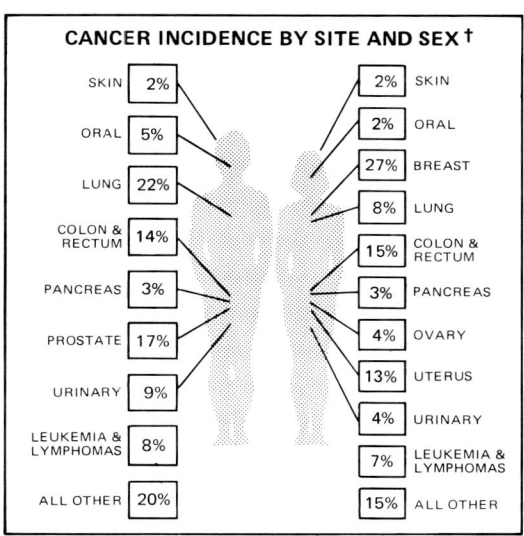

CANCER INCIDENCE BY SITE AND SEX †

SKIN	2%		2%	SKIN
ORAL	5%		2%	ORAL
LUNG	22%		27%	BREAST
COLON & RECTUM	14%		8%	LUNG
PANCREAS	3%		15%	COLON & RECTUM
PROSTATE	17%		3%	PANCREAS
URINARY	9%		4%	OVARY
LEUKEMIA & LYMPHOMAS	8%		13%	UTERUS
ALL OTHER	20%		4%	URINARY
			7%	LEUKEMIA & LYMPHOMAS
			15%	ALL OTHER

A † Excluding non-melanoma skin cancer and carcinoma in situ.

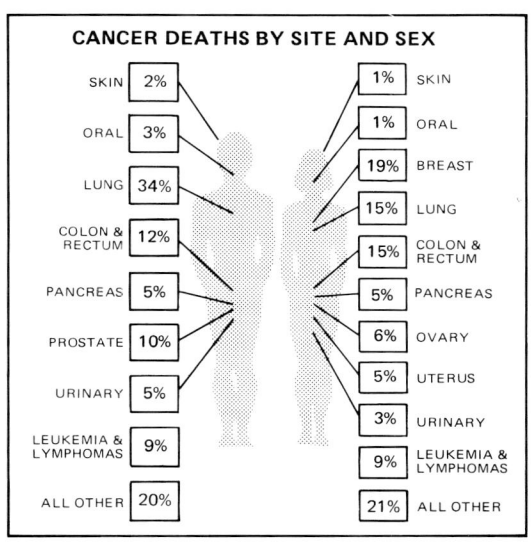

CANCER DEATHS BY SITE AND SEX

SKIN	2%		1%	SKIN
ORAL	3%		1%	ORAL
LUNG	34%		19%	BREAST
COLON & RECTUM	12%		15%	LUNG
PANCREAS	5%		15%	COLON & RECTUM
PROSTATE	10%		5%	PANCREAS
URINARY	5%		6%	OVARY
LEUKEMIA & LYMPHOMAS	9%		5%	UTERUS
ALL OTHER	20%		3%	URINARY
			9%	LEUKEMIA & LYMPHOMAS
			21%	ALL OTHER

B

Figure 4–4. 1981 American Cancer Society's estimates of cancer incidence *(A)* and cancer deaths *(B)* by site and sex. (From Cancer 1981. Facts and Figures. New York, American Cancer Society.)

Wilms' tumor of the kidney, *Ewing's* sarcoma of bone, and *Warthin's* tumor of the salivary gland.

Because a continuum of growth patterns frequently exists among benign and malignant tumors, it is occasionally difficult to distinguish between the two categories on the basis of histology, expected behavior of the lesion, or both. Generally speaking, benign tumors are well-encapsulated lesions, whereas malignant tumors are usually nonencapsulated and have infiltrative growth patterns. A hallmark of a malignant neoplasm is its tendency to metastasize. Even this tendency is not an exclusive property of malignant cells, however, because certain benign proliferations can appear at sites distant from their tissue of origin. An example is benign endometrial tissue appearing in the abdomen or fallopian tubes in the phenomenon known as *"endometriosis."*

Incidence

The incidence of human cancers increases with age. Because a large proportion of the United States population is over age 65 (23 million), we may expect the number of cancer patients to increase above the current figure of 25% of the population. Nevertheless, it should be kept in mind that prevention or cure of all cancers, although of great benefit to the young and middle-aged, would probably not change the ultimate life span of humans by more than 2 to 3 years (see Chap. 5).

Statistically, the most common malignant tumors are carcinomas of the skin.[7] These tumors are usually diagnosed early, are readily treatable, and therefore are not generally fatal. Of the fatal tumors in males, carcinoma of the lung and colon predominate. In females, carcinoma of the breast, uterus, colon, and lung are predominant. Carcinomas of the gastrointestinal tract are the most common fatal tumor in both sexes (Fig. 4–4).

Some tumors are associated with specific age groups. The significant incidence of cancer at birth increases through adolescence.[8] The cancers of infancy and childhood are largely leukemias, but occasionally, congenital tumors such as Wilms' tumors, neuroblastomas, and brain tumors are seen. In late adolescence, lymphomas, particularly Hodgkin's disease, predominate. Following adolescence, the incidence of cancer declines, then increases again in the forties and reaches a peak during the sixties and seventies.

Of course, one should not forget that a given tumor may take 10 to 20 years to develop, and many of the tissues forming tumors after middle age may have shown preneoplastic changes in the patient's thirties and forties.

The incidence of tumors may be altered by many factors (Table 4–6). Evidence suggests that the incidence of cancer in those who are exposed to certain types of air pollutants or who ingest certain carcinogens in the diet is high. Tumors develop concurrently with changes in hormone synthesis, secretion, and activity as individuals approach age 50. At this age, carcinoma of the prostate, ovary, thyroid, cervix, and breast commonly occur.

Table 4–6. *Estimated Cancer Risks*

	Risk/year
Cosmic and Other Radiation Risks	
Being an airline pilot flying 30 hrs/mo at 35,000 feet	5×10^{-5}
Being a frequent airline passenger	1.5×10^{-5}
Living in Denver as compared to New York	10^{-5}
Undergoing average United States diagnostic medical x-ray studies	10^{-5}
Food and Alcohol	
Eating 4 tablespoons peanut butter/day (aflatoxin)	4×10^{-5}
Eating $1/_2$-lb. charcoal broiled steak once a week (cancer risk only; heart attack, etc. additional)	4×10^{-7}
Drinking alcohol (averaged over smokers and nonsmokers)	5×10^{-5}
Tobacco	
Smoking, cancer only	1.2×10^{-3}
Smoking, all effects (including heart disease)	3×10^{-3}
Being in room with smoker	10^{-5}
Miscellaneous	
Taking contraceptive pills regularly	2×10^{-5}

(Conference on Chronic Toxicity Testing and the Food Industry. Given Institute of Pathobiology, Aspen, Colorado, August 22, 1976.)

Course

Human cancers have different morphologic characteristics from their benign counterparts and have capacities to invade and metastasize. Osteogenic sarcoma and acute myelogenous leukemia in young adults have a high fatality rate, whereas chronic lymphocytic leukemia in the elderly may persist for a long time. Over 30% of men over 60 have *occult carcinoma* of the prostate, which remains undetected. Melanoma characteristically may have long latent periods of 10 to 20 years before metastases become evident.

Tumors of the gastrointestinal tract and reproductive organs often metastasize to the liver and lung. Breast, lung, thyroid, kidney, and prostate tumors commonly go to bone and sometimes to brain.

Relation to Occupation and Life Style

Although many exceptions exist, certain tumors have been associated with particular life styles, occupations, and geographic regions (Table 4–7). Examples include the following: carcinoma of the cervix, associated with early sexual relations and many partners; carcinoma of the vagina, related to estrogen therapy to the mother during pregnancy; carcinoma of the breast and endometrium, associated with nulliparity and late pregnancies; carcinoma of the skin, often seen in sailors, farmers, and persons exposed to the sun; carcinoma of the lung, associated with smokers and miners; mesothelioma, seen in construction workers; carcinoma of the liver, seen in Africa, where aflatoxin ingestion is common; gastric carcinoma in Japan, where it is attributed to high consumption of smoked fish; carcinoma of the oral cavity, common in smokers and drinkers; carcinoma of the bladder, found in smokers and in workers in chemical plants; and leukemia, seen in radiation workers, following poor shielding from x-ray and nuclear radiation.

Table 4–7. *Relation of Tumors to Environment*

Tumor	Occupation, Activity, or Geographic Region
Carcinoma of cervix	Early sexual relations and many partners
Carcinoma of vagina	Estrogen therapy to mother during pregnancy
Carcinoma of breast and endometrium	Nulliparity and late pregnancies
Carcinoma of skin	Sailors, farmers, and outdoorsmen
Carcinoma of lung	Smokers and miners
Mesothelioma of pleura	Construction workers
Carcinoma of liver	Africa, from aflatoxin ingestion, HBV infection
Carcinoma of stomach	Japan, from high consumption of smoked fish
Carcinoma of oral cavity	Smokers and drinkers
Carcinoma of bladder	Smokers and chemical plant workers
Leukemia	Radiation workers following poor shielding from x-ray and nuclear radiation

Mechanism of Death

The mechanism of death as a result of cancer (Table 4–8) is often unknown. Unfortunately, except for tumors readily detected on easily examined sites such as skin, cervix, mouth, and breast, the first signs of cancer are often insidious and nonspecific. Weight loss may be followed by anorexia, cachexia, and, too late, the appearance of a mass.

Table 4–8. *Immediate Causes of Death Associated with Tumors*

Destruction of tissue	Interference with vital synthetic functions (e.g., hepatocellular carcinoma)
Hemorrhage	Major: Erosion of blood vessels (e.g., gastric carcinoma)
	Minor: Continual bleeding (e.g., bowel carcinoma) resulting in anemia
Obstruction	Obstruction of important passageways (e.g., sigmoid carcinoma)
Infection	Abscess surrounding tumor (e.g., empyema of lung)
	Susceptibility to intercurrent bacterial, viral, or fungal infection
Metastasis	Spread to vital areas and interference with essential regulatory functions (e.g., cerebral metastasis)
Cardiac failure	Increased stress on cardiovascular system

Tumors occasionally replace large quantities of tissue and thus interfere with vital synthetic functions, as in hepatocellular carcinoma. Carcinomas may erode blood vessels and may cause death by hemorrhage, as in gastric carcinoma. They may obstruct important passageways or may cause death by rupture, as in colonic carcinoma with peritonitis, or they may metastasize to vital areas and may thereby interfere with essential regulatory functions, as in cerebral metastasis. Infection becomes a predominant feature in many cancer patients. In the older literature, frequent references were made to tumor "toxic factors," none of which have been identified.

The psychologic and emotional factors erupting prior to a definitive diagnosis of cancer and during the course of malignant disease cannot be underestimated. The role these factors play, in conjunction with better-defined immune, genetic, and chemical mechanisms, has barely been studied. Unfortunately, these emotional factors are commonly the ones with which the practicing physician comes into contact in the day-to-day care of the cancer patient. Enlightened supportive care and concern for the individual patient are perhaps the most important forms of therapy.

ETIOLOGY OF CANCER

The etiology of most specific cancers remains obscure in humans. Many have attempted to identify a single initiating etiologic agent, even though it appears obvious that several promoting and inhibiting agents, as well as host factors, are of major significance in most cancers. With our refined technologies, it is likely that we will find that the neoplastic cell is an altered phenotype that may result from the cell's interaction with many agents. Any of these agents may serve to activate unexpressed latent information in the cell that eventually leads to its uncontrolled growth. Thus, it may be a mistake to look for "the cause" of cancer. Nevertheless, we can identify certain agents that have been associated with the induction of cancer. These are discussed later.

The ability of a few specific malignant tumors to differentiate to benign forms, specifically the change in children of a malignant neuroblastoma to a benign ganglioneuroma, has suggested that some tumors represent not dedifferentiation, but rather a delay or failure to differentiate fully.

Sachs has isolated a maturation factor which, in vitro in tissue culture and in vivo in mice, is apparently able to produce maturation of myeloblastic leukemic cells into mature granulocytes.[9] This finding implies that viruses, chemicals, and other oncogenic agents stimulate division and growth of stem cells, prevent normal maturation and differentiation, and thus establish neoplasia.

In discussing the etiology and pathogenesis of neoplasia, we attempt to divide carcinogenic factors into major etiologic groups. As we shall see, these divisions are often purely arbitrary because factors such as genetics, viruses, chemicals, and hormones are closely linked in their effects (see Fig. 4–1). Both animal experiments and studies on human cancers are discussed with respect to each of these potential causes.

Genetic Oncogenic Factors

Experimental Tumors

It has been recognized for many years that certain inbred strains of mammals, particularly mice, rats, and hamsters, have definite incidences of spontaneous tumors. The Paris R3 mouse strain has a 100% incidence of mammary tumors and the C3H strain has a 75 to 80% incidence of mammary cancer and a 90% incidence of leukemia.[10] It must be kept in mind, however, that these strains of animals carry oncogenic viruses. It is difficult to determine whether the virus itself or the genetic susceptibility plays the greater role.

The genetic membrane markers that have been identified appear to be of great importance in the susceptibility for the development of cancers. In particular, some H-2 transplantation markers in mice, analogous to HLA antigens in humans, have shown particular propensities for tumorigenesis.[11] The portions of the MHC that code for immune responses may alter the host's immune response to the antigenically foreign cells, thereby leading to increased incidence of cancer.

Human Tumors

Just as certain strains of mice have a predilection for developing certain tumors, certain human genomes are associated with a marked tendency to develop tumors (Tables 4–9, 4–10, and 4-11). A striking example of this tendency is one type of retinoblastoma, which is inherited as an autosomal dominant. In some cases of familial retinoblastoma there is an association with a constitutional deletion of chromosome 13q14, suggesting that the predisposition to retinoblastoma may be attributed to the loss of specific genetic material.[12] In this genetically predisposed group of patients, the incidence of osteogenic sarcoma is also increased. The risk of developing a sarcoma

Table 4–9. *Dominantly Inherited Autosomal Tumors and Neoplastic Syndromes*

Hereditary multiple endocrine adenomatosis syndrome (multiple endocrine neoplasia type I)
Testicular feminization syndrome (sex cord tumors)
Carcinoma of breast in association with other malignant neoplasms
Retinoblastomas
Neurofibromatosis
Multiple nevoid basal cell carcinoma syndrome

(Modified from Lynch, H.T., et al.: Familial cancer syndromes: a survey. Cancer, *39*:1867, 1977.)

Table 4–10. *Recessively Inherited Autosomal Tumor Syndromes*

Xeroderma pigmentosum
Werner's syndrome
Ataxia-telangiectasia
Bloom's syndrome
Chédiak-Higashi syndrome
Fanconi's aplastic anemia
Down's syndrome
D chromosome deletion syndrome
Trisomy D and Klinefelter's and alpha-1-antitrypsin syndrome

(Modified from Lynch, H.T., et al.: Familial cancer syndromes. a survey. Cancer, *39*:1867, 1977.)

Table 4–11. *Sex-linked Cancers*

Disorder	Predominant Cancers
Aldrich's syndrome (Wiskott-Aldrich syndrome)	Leukemia, lymphoma
Bruton's agammaglobulinemia	Acute leukemia
Dyskeratosis congenita	Squamous cell carcinoma of skin and mucous membranes
Reticuloendothelial syndrome with hyperglobulinemia	Reticuloendothelial cancer
Duncan's syndrome (X-linked lymphoproliferative syndrome)	Lymphoma

(Adapted from Martin, G.M.: Genetic syndromes in man with potential relevance to the pathobiology of aging. *In* Birth Defects. Vol. 14. Genetic Effects of Aging. Edited by D. Bergsma and D.E. Harrison. New York, Alan R. Liss, 1978.)

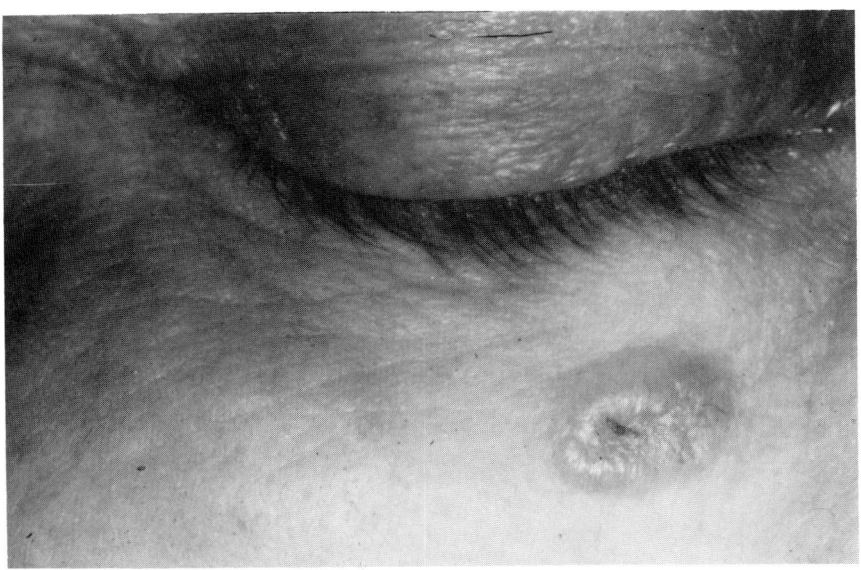

Figure 4–5. Basal cell carcinoma.

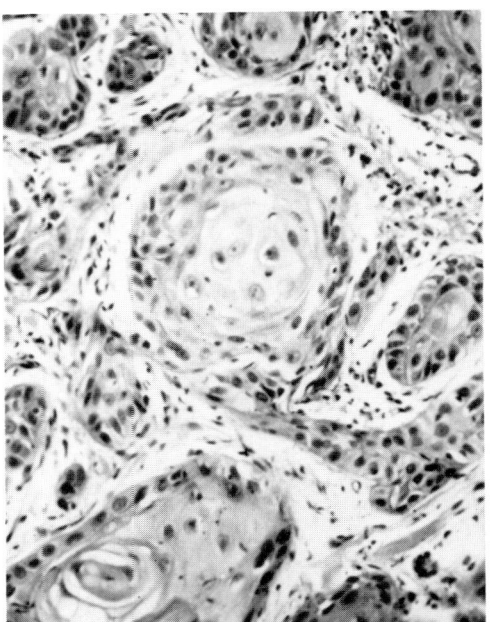

Figure 4–6. Well-differentiated squamous cell carcinoma containing areas of keratinization.

rapidly increases in individuals who receive intensive radiation therapy for their retinoblastoma.[13] A form of kidney cancer has been shown to be inherited, associated with a defect on chromosome 3–8, different from the Wilms' tumor deletion in chromosome 11.[14]

Four genetically unstable conditions associated with a genetic predisposition to cancer are *xeroderma pigmentosum, Bloom's syndrome, Fanconi's syndrome,* and *ataxia-telangiectasia.*[15] All these patients have abnormal DNA repair mechanisms, as well as frequent sister chromatid exchanges. The frequency of tumors in these conditions may be increased by exposure to chemical mutagens, x-rays, and UV light.

Xeroderma Pigmentosum (XP). In this rare autosomal recessive disease that progressively affects multiple organ systems, one of seven different enzyme defects may occur. The skin is the major target organ; the most common cancers that occur are *basal cell* and *squamous cell carcinomas* (Figs. 4–5 and 4–6). The most important change following ultraviolet (UV) radiation is the formation of chemical linkages between adjacent pyrimidine bases on the nucleic acid chain that produce dimers. This change distorts the DNA molecule and, if not repaired, interferes with normal synthesis of daughter DNA molecules.[16] The biochemical defect is due to failure of the DNA excision-repair mechanism in skin cells. The defect is associated with lack of a specific endonuclease, which normally initiates excision of the damaged DNA.[17]

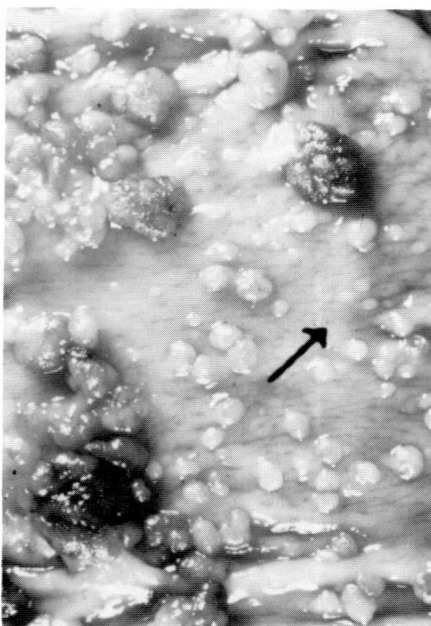

Figure 4–7. In the colon of patient with familial polyposis, numerous adenomas of varying size are present. Even the small smooth elevations (arrow) represent adenomatous polyps.

Bloom's Syndrome. This is another rare genetic disorder characterized by retarded growth, sun-sensitive eruptions on the face, disturbed immune function, and a predisposition to *skin cancer*. The dividing cells from such patients display increased numbers of chromatid breaks and rearrangements. A characteristic feature of this genetic instability is increased exchanges between homologous chromatid sites.[18]

Colon Cancer. Several premalignant diseases are also known to have a genetic origin. In *familial polyposis* of the colon (Fig. 4–7), 100% of patients develop colonic adenocarcinoma by age 50, and only prophylactic colectomy is preventive.[19] Other colon cancers occur in excess in one group of patients on a site-specific basis in the absence of familial polyposis. Patients with this disorder have an autosomal mode of inheritance, early onset of cancer, and a predisposition to multiple tumors in the right side of the colon.

Other Familial Cancers. Many tumors have been classified according to autosomal, recessive or dominant, and to sex chromosomal, recessive or dominant, inheritance. Familial origins have also been suggested for sarcomas, leukemias, and brain tumors. Von Recklinghausen's disease, an autosomal dominant disorder, is associated with benign neurofibromata. Sipple's syndrome (multiple endocrine neoplasia type IIa) is an autosomal dominant disorder associated with medullary carcinoma of the thyroid, pheochromocytoma, and parathyroid adenomas or hyperplasia. Each of these autosomal dominant neoplasms may have a varying degree of penetrance.

Gonadal tumors may also have a genetic background.[20] Dysgenetic gonads are frequently associated with ovarian neoplasms. Klinefelter's syndrome is associated with ovarian, breast, and testicular neoplasms. The Peutz-Jeghers (multiple polyposis) syndrome is often associated with ovarian tumors.

Physical Oncogenic Factors

Experimental Animal Tumors

Radiation is associated with the experimental production of tumors in animals. Low doses of radiation over a long period or high doses in short periods produce tumors in almost every organ in the mouse and rat with a high dose/effect correlation. If a single large dose of radiation is given, severe necrosis, ulceration, scarring, and later, development of tumors may result.[21]

In the initial stages of radiation-induced injury, destruction of lipid membranes is initiated by a series of chain reactions and the generation of free radicals. This process results in extensive membrane lipid peroxidation of various organelles. Once the tumor is established, the host fails to reject the antigenic tumors that are produced. This response indicates the initial failure of the immune surveillance mechanisms and the subsequent failure to respond immunologically to the established tumor.[22]

Tumors have also been produced in experimental animals following implantation of plastics, injury by heat, and other forms of physical trauma.

Human Tumors

In many well recognized situations, carcinomas result from continued exposure to physical agents, especially various forms of radiation.

Basal cell and squamous cell carcinomas are especially well known in sailors, farmers, and sportsmen who are continually exposed to solar UV radiation. A high incidence of leukemia and carcinoma of the hand in radiologists was formerly commonplace before proper shielding. Radiation therapy of tonsils, adenoids, and thymuses in childhood has led to a high incidence of carcinoma of the thyroid years later.[23] In fact, there was a 50% increase in this tumor from 1947 to 1971.

The incidence of neoplasms of the skin and salivary glands that were previously exposed in the radiation fields has increased.[24] Radiation therapy for squamous carcinoma of the lip is often followed by sarcomatous changes in the underlying scar tissue. The nuclear explosion at Hiroshima produced a marked increase in leukemia in individuals exposed to radiation doses insufficient for immediate death. Later, increases in carcinoma in the thyroid and lung were significant[25] (Fig. 4–8).

In the past 2 decades, we have seen the emergence of tumors related to the injection of a radioactive contrast solution, *Thorotrast*, used in roentgenographic studies between 1929 and 1956. This radioactive drug provides a more detailed model for oncogenesis than other forms of radiation. Tissue effects of this agent have been essentially twofold: physicochemical damage resulting in progressive fibrosis, and local irradiation damage linked to the induction of neoplasia. Over 120 cases of malignant liver tumors, following administration of a 25% colloidal solution of *thorium dioxide* (ThO_2), have been documented, and estimates indicate there are currently 50,000 to 100,000 Thorotrast injected patients in whom neoplasia may yet occur.[26]

Thorium, a radioactive element with a half-life of 400 or more years, emits approximately 90% α, 9% β, and 1% γ rays. When thorium decays it produces radium and thoron. The 5 separated sources of radiation dosage from Thorotrast (all α-emitters) are ^{232}Th, ^{228}Th, ^{224}Ra, the pair ^{220}Rn-^{216}Po, and ^{212}Bi. Approximately 70% of administered ThO_2 is deposited in the liver; spleen, regional lymph nodes, and bone receive smaller percentages. Thorotrast granules, amorphous, singly refractile, 10- to 50-μ light brown granules, are phagocytosed by lymphoreticular cells in *liver,*

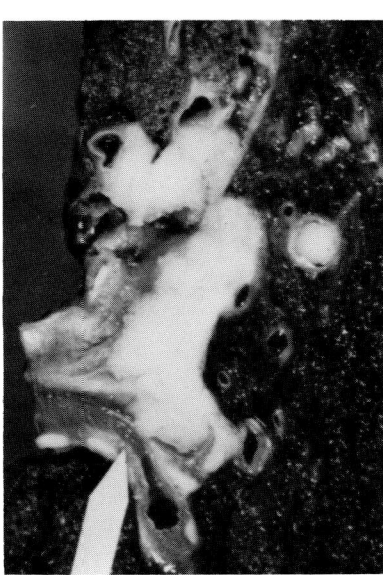

Figure 4–8. This carcinoma of the lung has arisen in a bronchus (arrow). The solid white neoplastic tissue is invading the underlying lung parenchyma.

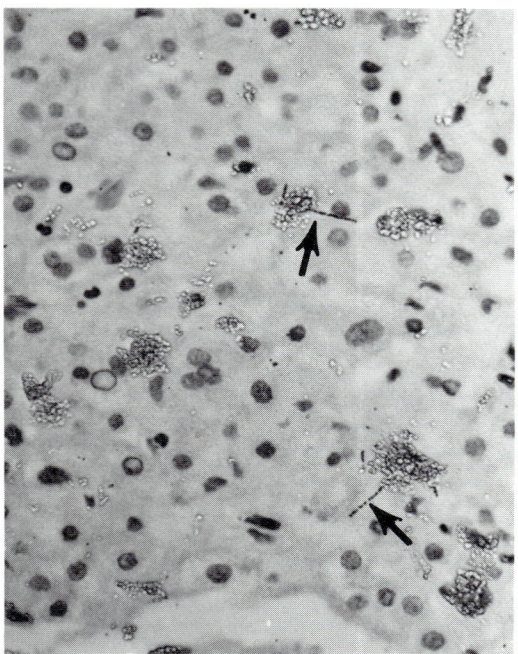

Figure 4–9. Thorotrast in liver is seen as refractile granules. When radioautographs are done on tissues containing this material, characteristic alpha-tracks (arrows) are produced.

PRODUCTIVE INFECTION

virus   permissive cell

viral uncoating

viral transcription and translation

cell lysis with release of viral progeny

NONPRODUCTIVE INFECTION

nonpermissive cell

virus

integration of viral genome into host genome

synthesis of viral transformation antigens

transformed cells

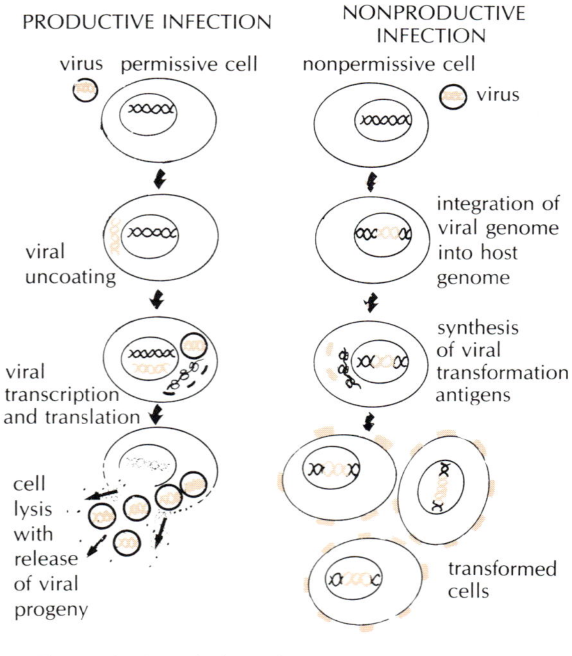

Figure 4–10. Viral productive and nonproductive infections.

spleen, bone, and *lymph nodes.* Degradation of phagocytes elicits progressive fibrosis and, subsequently, extracellular Thorotrast extravasation.

The sequence of liver damage by Thorotrast appears to be as follows: at one month or less, Kupffer cells are filled with the granules, and liver cell vacuolation, foci of necrosis, and some inflammation are present. Lymphocytic infiltrates predominate at 2 to 3 months. At 15 months to 7 years, fibrosis, especially in portal areas, becomes progressively more severe and is associated with extracellular extravasates of Thorotrast. This late, irregular distribution generates a lacy, reticular pattern in the liver on abdominal x-ray studies. Many years later, Thorotrast becomes irregularly located in Kupffer cells, with greater extracellular deposits and strong association with connective tissue septa and the periphery of lobules (Fig. 4–9). This extensive portal fibrosis results in a clinical picture of biliary obstruction, and along with the marked subcapsular fibrosis, leads to coarsely nodular gross appearances of the liver. Electron microscopy has demonstrated Thorotrast in Kupffer-cell and liver-cell cytoplasm and lysosomes and in the space of Disse.[27] The spleen and regional lymph nodes, to which Thorotrast-bearing phagocytes may have migrated, also undergo fibrotic changes.

In 1947 MacMahon reported the first *Thorotrast-associated malignant* tumor, an *angiosarcoma* developing 12 years after parenteral administration. Since then, the association between angiosarcomas of the liver and Thorotrast has been strong. Other neoplasms reported to occur include primary *hepatocellular carcinoma,*[28] *bile duct carcinomas,* and *leukemias.*

Infectious Oncogenic Agents

With the exception of the parasite Schistosoma haematobium, associated with bladder cancer, viruses are the major class of oncogenic infectious agents.[29] Bacteria, spirochetes, fungi, and rickettsiae have never been convincingly shown to play significant roles in the induction of neoplasia.

RNA and DNA Viruses

The two major types of viruses contain either RNA or DNA. We are mainly concerned here with their ability to transform cells into the neoplastic state. Their ability to infect cells depends upon the cell type, species, susceptibility, and resistance. These factors determine the ultimate outcome: cell lysis, latent or abortive infection, or proliferation with or without the induction of cancer.

When a virus enters a cell that is normally its host, it replicates, and cytolysis may occur, with the release of thousands of new viral particles. Such cells are said to be *"permissive,"* and the infection is *"productive"* (Fig. 4–10). When a virus enters a cell that is not its natural host *(nonpermissive cells),* viral particles are often not produced (a *nonproductive infection),* and *malignant transformation* may or may not occur. Successful tumor induction by oncogenic viruses depends on many factors: genetic susceptibility, age of the host, dose, route of infection, specific membrane receptors, and previous exposure to viruses.[30]

Cell Transformation

Examination of early biochemical events during viral transformation, either by RNA or DNA viruses, discloses that the induction of several enzymes is necessary for DNA synthesis. The viral genome enters the host cell and usually persists in cells transformed by the oncogenic viruses, although viral particles may not be detectable. The viral genome may be present and may be transmitted in an integrated form in the chromosomes or in a nonintegrated form in the cell. The presence of the viral genome is demonstrated by the appearance of virus-specific antigens in the nucleus, cytoplasm, or on cell membranes,[31] by the presence of structural proteins of the virus on the membranes of neoplastic cells,[32] by molecular hybridization studies for demonstrating genetic sequences complementary to the viral genome in the host cell and by the presence of virus-specific mRNA.[33] This presence is also demonstrated by complex changes in the type, concentration, and properties of a number of cellular polypeptides.[34]

Experimental Tumor Viruses

Most work on virally induced tumors has involved studies in animal models. Oncornaviruses *(oncogenic RNA viruses),* now called *retroviruses,* are divided into two main classes, B and C (Fig. 4–11). (Type A RNA viruses are not oncogenic.)

Most type C oncogenic RNA viruses produce mesenchymal tumors such as leukemias, lymphomas, and sarcomas. These viruses contain a compact, almost spherical central nucleoid surrounded by an electron-lucent lipid layer that

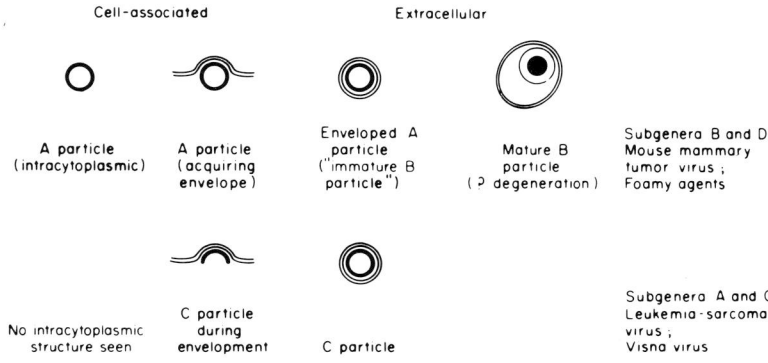

Figure 4–11. Morphogenesis of leukoviruses and the differences among A, B, and C type particles.

makes the virus look like a target. The membrane has small, irregularly spaced surface glycoprotein spikes.

Fewer type B RNA viruses are known; they have been associated primarily with murine breast cancers. These viruses have a more irregular, eccentric nucleoid, and the surface spikes are larger and are more regularly spaced than those of type C particles.[35]

The most important characteristic of this group of viruses is their possession of an RNA-directed DNA polymerase *(reverse transcriptase)*, discovered independently by Baltimore and by Temin.[36] This group of viruses also shares a common density of 1.15 to 1.19 in sucrose gradients and a viral genome that is always a 70S RNA[37] (Table 4–12).

Table 4–12. *Retroviruses Containing RNA*

C-type oncorna retroviruses (central nucleoid)
   Mammalian leukemia-sarcoma viruses
      Murine: murine leukemia virus (MLV), murine sarcoma virus (MSV)
         (e.g., Friend, Moloney, and Rauscher)
      Feline: feline leukemia virus (FLV) and feline sarcoma virus (FSV)
      Primate: simian sarcoma (woolly monkey) and gibbon ape viruses
   Avian leukemia-sarcoma viruses (e.g., Rous sarcoma virus (RSV), avian
      myeloblastosis virus (AMV)
   Adult T cell leukemia virus
   Leukemia retrovirus (ATLV)

B-type retrovirus (eccentric nucleoid)
   Murine mammary tumor virus (MMTV)
   Human milk particle
   Mason-Pfizer monkey virus

(Modified from Green, M.: DNA and RNA tumor viruses—molecular events of virus replication and T cell transformation and role in human cancer. Adv. Pathobiol., 2:13, 1976.)

When the retrovirus enters the cell and sheds its protein coat, a DNA copy of the viral RNA genome is produced by the reverse transcriptase enzyme. This intermediate form is called a *provirus*.[38] Once the DNA provirus is formed, it is believed to be integrated into the host cell's genome to produce a *virogene,* which is a gene template for production of virus. The virus contains all the enzymes necessary for cleaving host DNA (endonuclease, exonuclease), inserting the provirus, and healing the break (ligase). If the virogene is present in germ cells, it will be vertically transmitted to offspring of the infected animal.

The infected cell has three possible fates: (1) replication of the cell containing the virogene without the production of viral particles and without transformation of the cell; (2) activation of the virogene by unknown stimuli with the production of new viruses that can infect neighboring cells or may cause individual horizontal transmission: and (3) activation of the virogene resulting in host cell transformation.

It has been suggested by Temin that many, if not all, oncornaviruses evolved from normal cellular components;

at some point, endogenous viruses mutated so that they were freed from the cell's genetic control.[38] Gallo further postulated that evolutionary pressures then allowed these viruses to cross species lines.[39] An analysis of the virogenes (gene sequences related to the RNA of a virus) show that Old World monkeys, apes, and man have a baboon virus virogene in common.[40]

The "oncogene" theory of carcinogenesis, first proposed by Heubner and Todaro,[41] suggests that viral genetic material introduced hundreds of thousands of years ago, but now completely endogenous in the genome, produces malignant cells after appropriate derepression by chemicals, radiation, or other carcinogenic agents. A wide range of oncogenic nucleotide sequences of cellular origin have been identified. The prototype of the oncogene is the retroviral Onc gene of the Rous sarcoma virus (the Src gene). A large part of the Src gene is derived from the virus; a smaller part derives from the normal chicken cell genome. It is unclear how this combined genome of the Src gene occurs, but it is clear that once the chicken genome undergoes activation and transduction with a component retrovirus, it exhibits strong transforming capabilities.[42]

Other cellular genes are capable of inducing transformation upon mobilization by a transducing retrovirus. These genes are highly conserved in nature, suggesting that they may have a normal cellular differentiation function. Only rarely do they interact with a retroviral genome, thereby allowing them to assume a malignant role.

The cellular precursor of the transforming gene is termed C-Onc or retro-oncogene. The active transforming retroviral gene is referred to as V-onc.

A different class of oncogene has been identified in gene transfer (transfection) experiments. DNA fragments obtained with restriction enzymes of several tumors are able to transform 3T3 cells in vitro. These tumors include human bladder,[43] breast, lung, and colon.[44] These tumors are not known to have an association with retroviruses.

Thus, the two classes of oncogenes are the onc genes affiliated with the retroviruses and the oncogenes defined by transfection experiments. Both groups have in common a block in normal cellular DNA synthesis. The genes defined by the transfection experiments are potentially activatable by viruses as well as by other agents such as chemicals and irradiation.

RNA Viral Tumors in Experimental Animals. Studies in animals relating RNA viruses to cancer may be summed up as follows: (1) in several species of animals, such as chickens, mice, rats, and cats, leukemias and lymphomas can be transmitted by viruses; (2) certain strains of animals with low incidences of leukemia can be induced to produce leukemia by exposure to x irradiation; a virus can be isolated from the leukemic tissue and may be passed into new animals in which it also induces leukemia; (3) characteristic viral particles have been found in organs of many animals with leukemias, lymphomas, mammary tumors, kidney cancer, and sarcomas; these particles are usually found in the intercellular spaces; (4) some viruses are only oncogenic in certain species; in other species, they merely produce an inflammatory reaction; and (5) the presence of viral proteins, for example, gp 52 of murine mammary tumor virus, in an animal's plasma is correlated with the presence of a tumor; these proteins are, therefore, potentially useful indicators of malignant disease.

DNA Viral Tumors in Experimental Animals. As with RNA viruses, many DNA viruses (Table 4–13) have produced tumors in experimental animals. These include papilloma-, polyoma-, and herpesviruses. Marek's disease, an infectious neoplastic condition of chickens caused by a herpesvirus, has recently been shown to be preventable by a variety of methods. These include the development of a genetically resistant strain of chickens, strict isolation procedures to prevent spread of the virus, treatment with a benzimidasole derivative, and vaccination with turkey herpesvirus vaccine. Induction of tumor with a DNA virus usually does not require reverse transcriptase and may not need actual integration.

Table 4–13. *Oncogenic DNA Viruses*

Papillomaviruses (warts in man, dog, cow, rabbit, and other species)
Polyomaviruses: SV40-related viruses (human: BK, JC, and PML-viruses); SV40 (monkey); polyoma virus (mouse)
Adenoviruses: > 50 human strains are oncogenic in other species
Herpesviruses: Epstein-Barr virus (? Burkitt's lymphoma, nasopharyngeal carcinoma); HSV2 (? cervix), CMV (? Kaposi's), HBV (? hepatoma)
Marek's disease virus (chicken leukosis)
Lucké's carcinoma virus (frog carcinoma)

(Modified from Green, M.: DNA and RNA tumor viruses—molecular events of virus replication and T cell transformation and role in human cancer. Adv. Pathobiol., 2;13, 1976.)

RNA Human Tumor Viruses

Leukemias, Lymphomas, and Sarcomas. Some evidence suggests that viral agents are present in association with human leukemias, lymphomas, and sarcomas, but no definite proof is available.[45] Many of these tumors possess viral reverse transcriptase. If a suitable DNA probe is available, RNA-DNA hybridization techniques can detect virus-specific RNA (70S RNA) in human tumors. Spiegelman and his associates have used a simultaneous detection assay for the 70S RNA and the reverse transcriptase of virus in human leukemias.[46] These agents are found in morphologically abnormal leukemic cells as well as in some normal-appearing leukocytes from patients in remission.

Other studies that link *C-type RNA* viruses to human leukemia include the detection of subviral components in

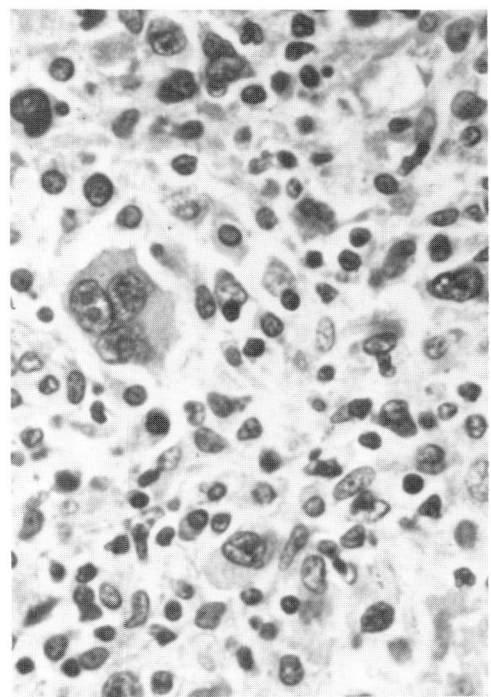

Figure 4–12. In Hodgkin's disease, the neoplasm is composed of a heterogeneous cell population. A characteristic multinucleated Reed-Sternberg cell is seen.

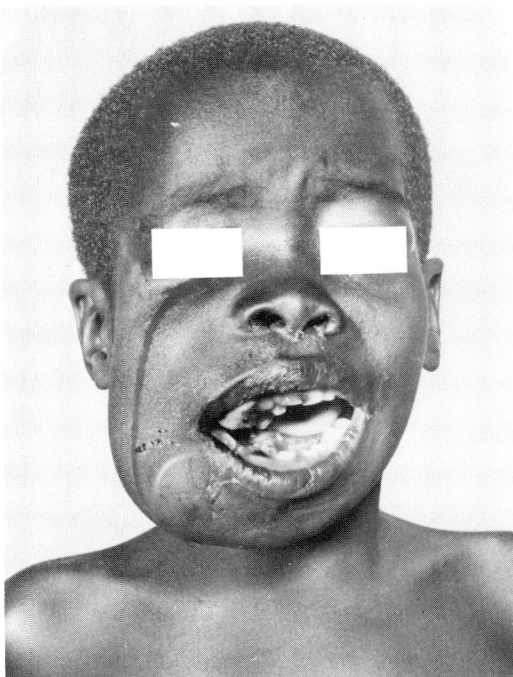

Figure 4–13. Burkitt's lymphoma in African child. (From Ziegler, Z.L., and Magrath, I.T.: Burkitt's lymphoma. Pathobiol. Annu., *4*:129, 1974.)

leukocytes,[147] transient release of virus-like particles from short-term culture of these cells, and the rare isolation of infectious virus from cultured leukemic cells.

A primate C-type virus p30 antigen has been found in human white blood cells from leukemic patients.[48] These viral structures have generally been found to be contaminating strains of murine virus, however. Most recently, the laboratories of Gallo[49] and Hinuma[50] have isolated a new retro-C-type virus from T cells cultured from a patient with a T-cell leukemia. This virus has been seen by electron microscopy, contains a reverse transcriptase, stimulates antibody in the patient's serum, and appears different from all murine viruses.

When cells from patients with *genetic diseases (Fanconi's anemia, Down's syndrome)* that predispose them to leukemia are grown in culture and are exposed to viruses, these cells are 35 to 50 times more susceptible to transformation than normal cells. Thus, the higher incidence of leukemia in patients with genetic instability may be due to their increased susceptibility to environmental carcinogens, including viruses.[51]

Breast Cancer. Some evidence associates RNA viruses with human breast cancer. Particles similar to oncogenic RNA tumor virus have occasionally been seen in human milk and in breast tumor tissue. The serum of breast cancer patients enhances the neutralization of infective *mouse mammary tumor virus (MMTV)*. Simultaneous detection assays for reverse transcriptase and 70S RNA have demonstrated the presence of both in human breast tumors.[37] More recently, immunohistologic localization techniques have demonstrated a mouse mammary tumor virus-like antigen (gp 52) in a number of human breast tumors.[52]

Hodgkin's Disease. An important epidemiologic question concerns the transmissibility of oncogenic viruses in man. It has been convincingly demonstrated that feline leukemia is horizontally transmissible among cats within a household.[53] Of interest are a number of suggestions that *Hodgkin's disease* (Fig. 4–12) is also a transmissible viral disease, since cases of this lymphoma sometimes appear in clusters among school classmates. The evidence remains weak, however, because of poor controls.[54]

DNA Human Tumor Viruses

At the present time, the only documented human tumor caused by a DNA virus (a *papovavirus*) is the common *wart*.

Burkitt's Lymphoma. Over the past decade, the evidence that *Epstein-Barr virus (EBV)* produces Burkitt's lymphoma (BL) (Figs. 4–13 and 4–14) and nasopharyngeal carcinoma

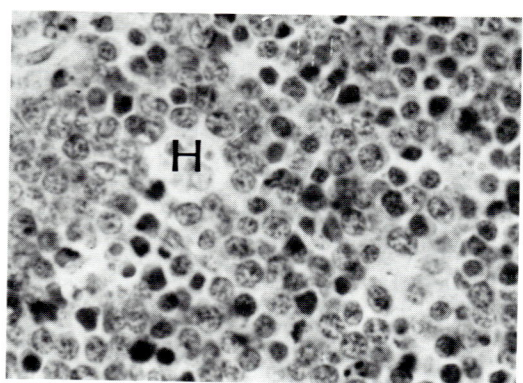

Figure 4–14. Burkitt's lymphoma is composed of malignant lymphocytes and reactive histiocytes (H) producing a typical "starry sky" pattern.

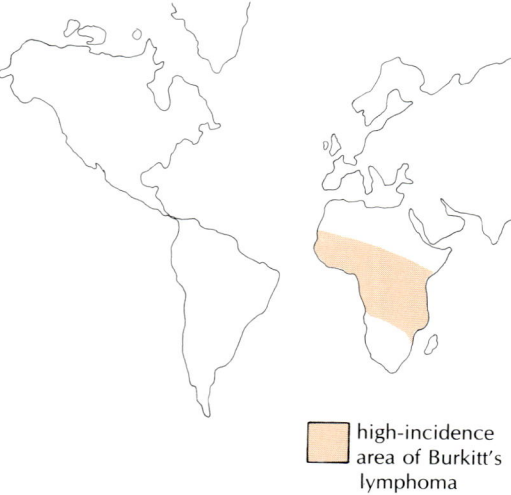

high-incidence area of Burkitt's lymphoma

Figure 4–15. The geographic distribution of Burkitt's lymphoma.

has become strong.[55] EBV is found in adults of all countries, but only in Africa and other scattered areas does it appear to produce malignant tumors[56] (Fig. 4–15). In Africa, the virus infects over 80% of children under the age of 5. The virus selectively infects B cells by binding to a specific receptor.

The virus is generally transmitted horizontally, and EBV shedding has been demonstrated in the saliva and oropharynx. In the United States, EBV infects lower socioeconomic groups in childhood, and clinical disease may not be detected. When teenagers of higher socioeconomic groups in the United States are infected, the manifestations of infectious mononucleosis and positive heterophil antibody tests are more commonly found probably because these persons visit physicians more often.[57]

It is interesting that the atypical cells present in the blood of patients with infectious mononucleosis are T lymphocytes, despite the predilection of EBV for B cells. The atypical T lymphocytes may be a manifestation of cellular immune response to the virus. In normal individuals, it is believed that T_s lymphocytes control the B cell proliferation that ensues following infection; and as a result, neoplasia does not occur.[58]

One interesting aspect of the patient with BL is the evidence that suggests that coinfection with EBV and malaria is necessary for malignant transformation to occur. The geographic distribution of both BL and malaria are similar, but the interaction of these two diseases is unclear.[59]

Various *EBV-determined antigens* that may be detected on BL cells include early antigen (EA), viral capsid antigens (VCA), nuclear antigen (NA), true membrane-determined antigens (MA), and lymphocyte membrane-determined antigen (LMDA).[60] The lymph nodes have a classic "starry sky" appearance (Fig. 4–14).

EBV is detected in most cells cultured from BL by hybridization studies. Between 80 and 90% of the tumors contain multiple copies of the EBV DNA genome.[55]

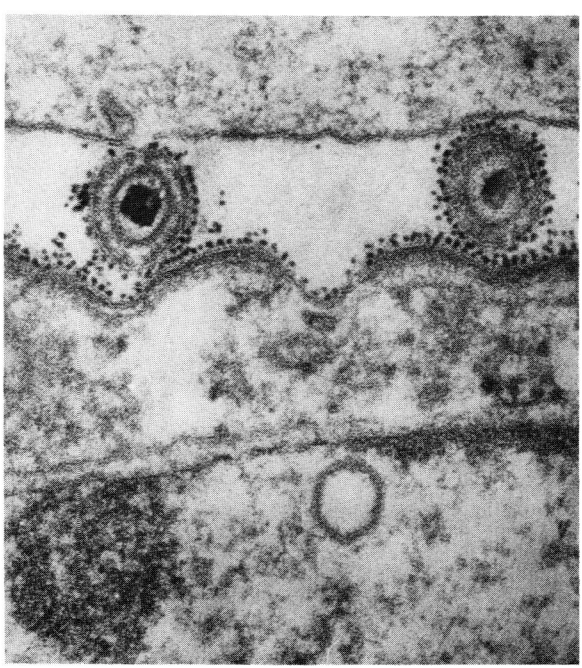

Figure 4–16. Two herpesvirus particles are seen outside virus-infected cells grown in tissue culture. (Courtesy of Dr. Councilman Morgan, National Research Center, Washington, D.C.)

Cervical Carcinoma. Another herpesvirus suspected of being oncogenic in man is *Herpesvirus genitalis (herpes simplex virus 2) (HSV-2)* (Fig. 4–16). Epidemiologic surveys and the increased incidence of herpesvirus antigen and antibody in the serum of patients with cervical cancer and its precursors link HSV and cervical cancer. More recently HSV-specific mRNA has been detected in neoplastic cervical cells by in situ hybridization techniques.[61] Three possible explanations for the association of cervical neoplasia and HSV are as follows: (1) neoplastic cells are more readily infected with HSV; (2) cervical cancer and HSV occur in similar epidemiologic situations, but HSV is not oncogenic; and (3) HSV acts as a carcinogen either alone or in combination with other cocarcinogens and promoters to produce cervical cancer.

Recent evidence suggests that human papilloma virus (HPV) type 6 may also have a role in the genesis of cervical cancer.[62] In some patients, the intraepithelial phase of the disease may be preceded by the presence of a flat condyloma. The latter lesion is known to be caused by HPV. Areas of direct transition between the flat condyloma and cervical neoplasia have been observed. Furthermore, genetic material for HPV has been demonstrated in neoplastic cervical cells by molecular hybridization studies.

Nutritional Oncogenic Factors

Burkitt[63] suggested that carcinoma of the bowel may result from the accumulation of toxic metabolites, some of which may be produced by bacterial metabolism. He compared the African population, which has a low incidence of colon carcinoma, a low-sugar and high-fiber diet, and a short transit time, with Western populations, which have a high incidence of colon carcinoma, a high-sugar and low-fiber diet, and a long transit time. From this comparison, he reasoned that in patients with a slow transit time of fecal contents, possible carcinogenic bacterial metabolites or ingested carcinogenic agents would have a longer time to interact with the colonic epithelial tissue.

A relationship between gastric cancer and diet has been postulated in patients with a high intake of hydrocarbons found in smoked foods.[64] Experimentally, high doses of vitamin C have prevented the formation of nitrosamines believed to be implicated in the genesis of stomach and liver cancers.[65,66]

A high-fat diet in rodents yielded a higher number of experimentally induced colon cancers. Fatty diets have also been associated with an increased incidence of colon cancer in man. This finding has been linked to lipid peroxidation, increased bacterial metabolites, and increased susceptibility of the fully dilated bowel.

Liver cancer is found in patients in Africa following the ingestion of grains contaminated with *aflatoxins* produced by the fungus, Aspergillus flavus.[67]

The cycad nut contains *cycasin*, which, although harmless itself, gives rise to a carcinogen when exposed to the normal intestinal tract flora. This discovery has led to the theory that people with large numbers of anaerobic bacteria in their gastrointestinal tracts dehydrogenate bile acids, which may then act as local carcinogens in the colon. Thus, *bile acids* may play a role in the pathogenesis of large bowel carcinoma.[68] Moreover, it has been suggested that a high level of vitamin K is required to act as a hydrogen acceptor before carcinogens can be formed.

Some anticarcinogens are naturally occurring antioxidants and therefore inhibit the formation of free radicals. *Vitamin E* (α-tocopherol), one such natural antioxidant, prevents the formation of free radicals and inhibits lipid peroxidation and perhaps precarcinogen activation.[69] Further, it has been reported that diets high in vitamin E inhibit experimental tumor induction by *methylcholanthrene*. Vitamin E therapy has had no demonstrable effect in humans.

Chemical Oncogenic Agents

The largest group of oncogenic agents are chemicals, both those that occur naturally in the environment as well as those that are man–made. We encounter these in the air, where we work, in the home, in what we eat, and, unfortunately, in our current medical therapeutic techniques. Treatment of cells in tissue culture with chemical agents can result in cell transformation and malignant disease[70] (Tables 4–14 and 4–15). Cells with a regular pattern of growth and a limited in vitro life span that are not tumorigenic in vivo are converted into cells with a random pattern of cell growth and the ability to grow continuously in culture and to form tumors in vivo.

Table 4–14. *Basic Biologic and Biochemical Facts on Chemical Carcinogenesis*

1. Carcinogenesis is dose dependent.
2. A long lag exists between exposure and the appearance of tumors. In humans, this is from about 5 to 30 years.
3. Conversion of a normal tissue to a malignant neoplasm is a multistep process.
4. The action of certain types of carcinogens, so-called initiating agents, is enhanced by promoting agents, hormonal agents, and various cofactors.
5. Cellular proliferation enhances carcinogenesis (e.g., polyps).
6. Carcinogens are subject to both metabolic activation and detoxification in vivo.
7. The metabolically activated forms are reactive electrophiles that bind covalently to nucleophilic residues in cellular proteins and nucleic acids.
8. The binding to nuclear and cytophilic protein is quantitatively greater than binding to nucleic acids and has a specific activity of about 1 residue of carcinogen/10^3 to 10^4 amino acid residues.
9. Both RNA and DNA are targets, and the specific activity is about 1 residue of carcinogen/10^4 to 10^5 nucleoside residues. Most carcinogens bind preferentially to guanine, but adenine and cytosine are also targets.

(Modified from Weinstein, I.B.: Molecular events in chemical carcinogenesis. Adv. Pathobiol., 4:106, 1976.)

Table 4–15. *Chemical Carcinogens—Early Effects on Macromolecular Synthesis*

1. *Replication.* The binding to DNA induces unscheduled DNA synthesis (excision repair) and single- and double-stranded DNA breakage. Most, but not all, carcinogens are mutagens. They can induce base pairing errors, frame shift errors, deletions, and chromosomal breakage.
2. *Transcription.* An early inhibition of RNA synthesis is preferential for the 45S ribosomal RNA precursor.
3. *Translation.* An early inhibition of protein synthesis is often associated with release of ribosomes bound to the endoplasmic reticulum and disaggregation of polysomes.
4. *Regulation.* Enzyme induction (tyrosine aminotransferase) may be blocked. The pattern of transcription is altered.

(Modified from Weinstein, I.B.: Molecular events in chemical carcinogenesis. Adv. Pathobiol., 4:106, 1976.)

The classes of chemical carcinogens (Table 4–16) are largely divisible into two major groups: (1) those with no apparent need for metabolic conversion *(proximate carcinogens)* and (2) those that are inactive until converted to metabolically active derivatives *("ultimate" carcinogens).*

Carcinogens are converted to ultimate carcinogens by *mixed-function oxidases,* which are inducible by their substrates. This inducibility is under genetic control in mice. Ironically, the mixed-function oxidases are also the major detoxifying enzymes of the body.[71,72]

The liver is a potent metabolizer of potential carcinogens. Tissues that generate ultimate carcinogens appear to do so by producing either an alkylated or an arylated derivative, which then interacts with many of the host's cellular macromolecules (DNA, RNA, protein) to alter their regulatory control or metabolic properties.[73]

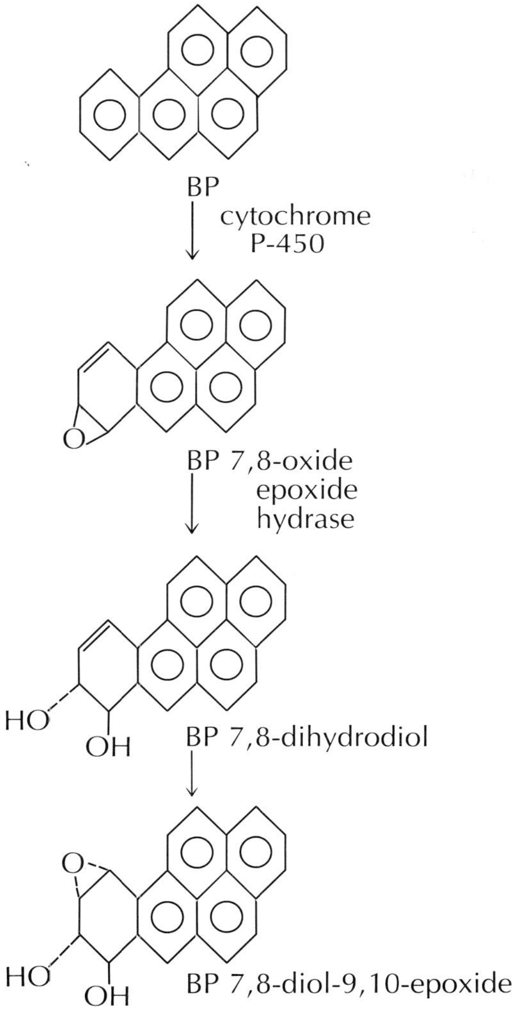

Figure 4–17. The metabolism of benzpyrene (BP) to ultimate carcinogenic species.

Table 4–16. *Major Classes of Chemical Carcinogens*

Polycyclic hydrocarbons (benzo(a)pyrene)
Azo- dyes
Aromatic amines (acetylaminofluorene or AAF)
Mycotoxin (aflatoxin)
Inorganic compounds (arsenic, chromium)
Nitroso- compounds (nitrates, nitrites)
Aliphatic compounds (benzidine)

Experimental Chemical Carcinogens

Polycyclic Hydrocarbons. *Benzo(a)pyrene* (BP), the prototype of the polycyclic hydrocarbons (Fig. 4–17), is converted in the liver by a microsomal enzyme, *aryl hydrocarbon hydroxylase* (AHH) to an *epoxide.*[74] The epoxide may act as the ultimate carcinogen and may interact with DNA to produce cytotoxicity, mutation, and malignant transformation.[75] It may also be converted enzymatically to a *phenol,* or it may be metabolized to nontoxic 7- or 8-dihydrodiols by the enzyme epoxide hydrase (Fig. 4–17). The conversion appears to take place in the endoplasmic reticulum and on the nuclear membrane.

The major enzyme systems that metabolize BP are aryl hydrocarbon hydroxylase, the microsomal nicotinamide-adenine dinucleotide phosphate (NADPH)-dependent mixed function oxidases (containing cytochromes P448 or P450), and BP epoxide hydratase.[76]

Nitrosamines. Although capable of producing mutation and being carcinogenic after a single dose, the nitrosamines require microsomal activation before reacting with nucleic acids and protein macromolecules. The activation of aromatic amines proceeds by N-hydroxylation followed by sulfate ester formation.[77] It appears that the most important reaction is oxidative dealkylation, which generates unstable nitrosamines. These are potentially potent alkylating or arylating agents capable of interacting with many of the cell's nucleophilic groups.

Nitrosamides. These substances require no metabolic activation before acting, and some have a propensity for particular organs. Ethylnitrosourea (ENU) produces tumors, particularly affecting the central nervous system (CNS) and peripheral nerves.

N-methyl-N-nitrosourea is a potent organotropic carcinogen that alkylates (methylates) cellular macromolecules, especially the guanine moieties of nucleic acids.[78] This class of drugs is often cytotoxic as well as carcinogenic, and it has been shown that the cyanate ion generated during the metabolism of these compounds is responsible for their cytotoxicity.

Aflatoxins. Metabolites of a mold (Aspergillus flavus), aflatoxins are both toxic and hepatocarcinogenic in that they cause both hepatitis and hepatocellular carcinoma.[79] They are activated by mixed function oxidases and are then capable of binding to DNA and RNA. Aflatoxin B_1, the most potent known hepatocarcinogen, is activated to an epoxide (Fig. 4–18).

Following exposure to aflatoxins, the liver cells progress through a defined series of events during the genesis of a primary liver cell tumor. The earliest changes involve cytopathic effects of the carcinogenic chemical that result in liver cell necrosis.[80] This necrosis is followed by the production of hyperplastic liver cell foci and nodules. Both these alterations are considered to be preneoplastic. Finally, frankly malignant foci appear. The characteristic morphologic and biochemical alterations discernible during each of the stages in the progression are discussed in the following paragraphs; these changes are similar to those seen with *acetoaminofluorene* (AAF) administration (Fig. 4–19).

Aromatic Amines. The propensity of the aromatic amine carcinogens to induce tumors only at sites distant from the point of entry supports the suggestion that these compounds require metabolic conversion for their oncogenicity.[81] *AAF,* an example of an aromatic amine, undergoes N-hydroxylation by a microsomal enzyme to a *"proximate"*

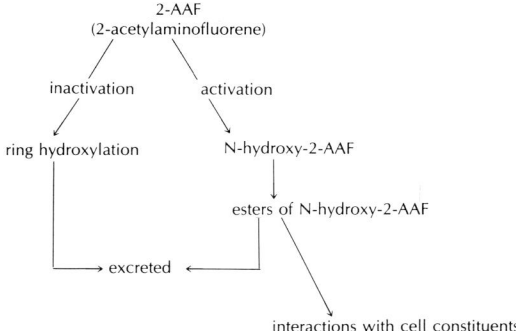

Figure 4–19. Aromatic amino acids such as 2-AAF may undergo detoxification (inactivation) pathways or alternate (activation) pathways that produce ultimate carcinogens. (Adapted from Farber, E.: On the pathogenesis of experimental hepatocellular carcinoma. *In* Hepatocellular Carcinoma. Edited by K. Okuda and R.L. Peters. New York, John Wiley & Sons, 1976.)

carcinogen form (Fig. 4–19). These proximate carcinogens are sulfate, phosphate, glucuronidate, and acetate esters.

Because the enzymatic compositions of cells differ, it is probable that the tissue and species specificity for tumor induction by the aromatic amines is a reflection of their hydroxylating and esterifying enzymes.

Experimental Liver Tumors

With both aromatic amine and aflatoxin carcinogenesis, a malignant cell population appears as a progressive sequence of discontinuous steps, each of which is associated with a new population of cells.

Some of the characteristics of the hyperplastic nodules produced by chemical carcinogens have been summarized.[82]

Small islands or foci of cells are first detected by changes in their histochemical enzyme pattern and not by their morphologic appearance. Adenosine triphosphatase (ATPase), glucose-6-phosphatase, β-glucuronidase, alkaline phosphatase, serine dehydrase, and iron uptake are decreased. Later, early discrete nodules containing two or more cell-thick hyperplastic liver cell plates with attempts at maturation, differentiation, and remodeling of normal architecture become apparent. Finally, one sees nodules that show less success at remodeling and differentiation and more distortion of the normal liver architecture. This distortion is accompanied by ductal proliferation, piecemeal necrosis of liver cells, and hyperbasophilia of the hepatic cytoplasm. Foci of frank carcinoma may be identified in the separate nodules.[83]

Alterations in the carbohydrate metabolism of these cells are reflected by altered glycogen phosphorylase activity and glycogen structure. The changes related to the proliferative activity include a high labeling index (with tritiated thymidine) and the presence of annulate lamellae in nuclei. The DNA shows changes in spectrographic absorption, buoyant density, ultrastructural morphology, and melting point.[84]

It has recently been shown that AAF binds in a nonrandom fashion to the DNA in the nucleosomes of the chromatin fiber. The most prominent ultrastructural changes during cancer induction with AAF are hypertrophy and dilatation of the rough endoplasmic reticulum (RER) and the presence of abundant smooth endoplasmic reticulum (SER).[85]

Human Tumors Produced by Chemicals

The initial clue that chemical agents could cause human cancer was noted in 1775 by *Sir Percival Pott,* who called attention to the high incidence of scrotal cancer among the chimney sweeps of London and who attributed the cause of the disease to continual exposure to coal methyl tars.

Current examples of environmental carcinogens include benzo(a)pyrene and other polycyclic aromatic hydrocarbons, as in cigarette smoke, polluted city air, and charcoal-broiled meat; aflatoxins, as in moldy grains and peanuts; and possibly nitrates from preserved meats (Table 4–17). Nitrates interact with amino acids in the stomach to form nitrosamines, which are believed to be important in the development of gastrointestinal cancer.

A survey of United States cancer mortality rates from 1950 to 1969 was conducted in counties where the petroleum industry was most heavily concentrated. Males living in these areas had significantly higher incidence rates of cancer of the lung, nasal cavity, sinus, and skin than males from counties with otherwise similar demographic characteristics.[86]

If one excludes skin cancer, believed to be caused by exposure to UV light, it has been broadly stated that be-

Table 4–17. *Agents Recognized as Carcinogenic in Man*

Agent	Site of Cancers
Chemical mixtures	
Soots, tars, oils	Skin, lungs
Cigarette smoke	Lungs
Hematite (mining)	Lungs
Industrial chemicals	
2-Naphthylamine	Urinary bladder
Benzidine, benzene	Urinary bladder
4-Aminobiphenyl	Urinary bladder
Chloromethyl methyl ether	Lungs
Nickel compounds	Lungs, nasal sinuses
Chromium compounds	Lungs
Cadmium oxide	Lungs
Asbestos	Lungs
Arsenic compounds	Skin, lungs
Phenytoin	Urinary bladder
Vinyl chloride	Liver, brain, lung
Oxymetholone	Lung
Drugs	
N, N-bis (2-chloroethyl)-2-naphthylamine	Urinary bladder
Bis (2-chloroethyl) sulfide (mustard gas)	Lungs
Diethylstilbestrol	Vagina
Phenacetin (acetophenetidin)	Renal pelvis
Oral contraceptives	Adenoma (benign liver tumor)
Chloramphenicol	Leukemia, bone marrow
Cyclophosphamide (Cytoxan)	Leukemia, bone marrow
Melphalan	Bone marrow
Chlornaphazine	Bladder
Estrogen (postmenopausal)	Endometrium
Naturally occurring compounds	
Betel nuts	Buccal mucosa
Aflatoxins	Liver
Radiation including isotopes	
Phosphorus	Acute leukemia (blood)
Radium	Osteosarcoma and carcinoma (bone and sinus)
Thorotrast	Angiosarcoma (liver)
Ultraviolet light	Skin

(Modified from Weinstein, I.B.: Molecular events in chemical carcinogenesis. Adv. Pathobiol., 4:106, 1976.)

tween 70 and 90% of the remaining cancers are caused by chemicals in the environment. At least 24 chemicals in our environment have definitely been found to be carcinogenic in man.[87]

Individual differences in rates of carcinogen metabolism might determine an agent's carcinogenic potential. "Rapid metabolizers" might have a different susceptibility to carcinogens than "slow metabolizers." It has in fact been demonstrated that basal activities and inducibility of enzymes, important in the conversion of carcinogens to active forms, vary among individuals. The inducibility of these enzymes can be measured in vitro in cultured lymphocytes and macrophages.[88]

Levels of aryl hydrocarbon hydroxylase (AHH), one of these enzymes, are different in patients with lung cancer than in those without cancer. The lung cancer patient group was seen to contain a higher percentage of persons with high levels of AHH than an age-matched group of noncancer patients.[88] Using techniques such as this, one could possibly screen the population to determine which individuals are uniquely sensitive to the carcinogens in cigarette smoke.

Hormonal Oncogenic Factors

Experimental Hormonal Factors

A common denominator in neoplasia is the failure of homeostatic mechanisms, especially of the endocrine system, to control cell growth. If cells fail to recognize the usual restraining influence of hormones, they are called hormone-independent or autonomous. If, on the other hand, the homeostatic control is incomplete, the neoplastic cells may be stimulated or inhibited and are said to be hormone-responsive. Few examples of complete hormone dependence in human tumors have been reported.[89,90]

Estrogens. Early experiments of Biskind and Biskind in 1944[91] showed that ovaries, after bilateral removal and transplantation into the spleen, developed tumors. This development was attributed to the *inactivation* of *estrogen* by the liver following passage of the hormone through the portal circulation. The lack of estrogen feedback increased the production of gonadotropin by the pituitary, with the subsequent stimulation of *ovarian tumors* (Fig. 4–20). Huggins et al. showed that mice were more sensitive to the initiation of tumors by chemical carcinogens at an age that corresponded to the period of greatest estrogen release.[92]

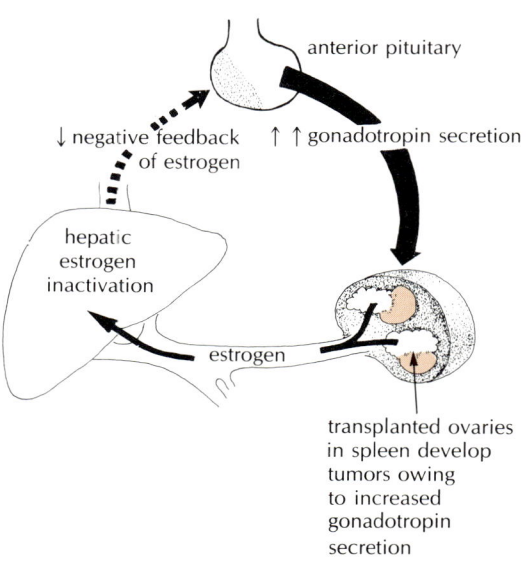

anterior pituitary

↓ negative feedback of estrogen   ↑ ↑ gonadotropin secretion

hepatic estrogen inactivation

estrogen

transplanted ovaries in spleen develop tumors owing to increased gonadotropin secretion

Figure 4–20. The Biskind experiments demonstrated the importance of the estrogen-pituitary axis in tumorigenesis.

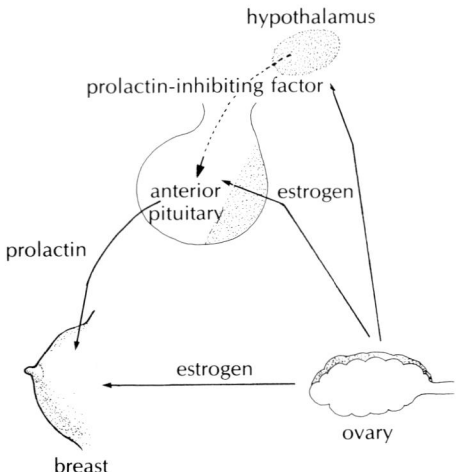

Figure 4–21. Interaction of the hypothalamic-pituitary axis with estrogens and prolactin control breast secretory activity and influence the growth of breast tumors.

Prolactin. This polypeptide hormone is believed to be influential in the growth of breast tumors. Prolactin is produced by the pituitary and is under the control of hypothalamic neurohormones that act as releasing and inhibiting factors. The role of prolactin is not isolated, in that it may be regulated by other hormones (Fig. 4–21). Estrogens reduce prolactin-inhibiting factor and directly cause prolactin release in rodents.[93]

A precursor lesion to mouse mammary carcinoma (hyperplastic alveolar nodules) has also been shown to be pituitary hormone dependent, the principal hormone being prolactin.[94] Conversely, mice that are chronically prolactin deficient are relatively refractory to tumor development, have hypoplastic breast epithelium, and are refractory to carcinogenic agents such as viruses.

Furth[95] demonstrated that injection of mammary tumor hormone, presumably prolactin, produced tumors in 58% of radiated mice, in 85% of methylcholanthrene-treated rats, and in 40% of virus-treated mice. That none of these agents alone produced tumors in the doses used thus demonstrates the cocarcinogen or promoter role of the hormone.

Human Hormonal Factors

Estrogens. The human tumors in which hormones are believed to play an important etiologic role include *clear cell vaginal carcinomas* in young women exposed to diethylstibestrol in utero,[96] *endometrial cancer* in postmenopausal women,[97,98] *breast cancers*,[99] and *liver cancers*.[100] Ironically, estrogen is also used in palliative treatment, as an inhibitor rather than a stimulator, in carcinoma of the prostate.

The endocrine-dependent nature of some human breast tumors was noted by Bateson over 75 years ago, and since that time, a number of ablative endocrine procedures have been used to palliate metastatic disease.[92] Another fact that points to the underlying endocrine abnormality in breast cancer is the known risk factors for its development. They include an early age at menarche, a delayed age of first pregnancy, and a delayed age of the menopause.[101,102]

One aspect of hormonal regulation and the development of cancer that currently engages our attention is that of the estrogen receptor. Jensen investigated the affinity of estrogens for human breast and endometrial tumor cells. He found that the *primary estrogen receptor* resides in the cytoplasm. Once the receptor-estrogen complex is formed, it translocates to the nucleus and interacts with DNA.[103]

Bresciani et al. modified this theory in the following way: Estrogen enters the cytoplasm and forms a complex with the native form of the receptor. A Ca^{++}-activated receptor-transforming factor, a proteolytic enzyme, splits an estrogen-binding fragment from the native receptor. The resulting mobile complex enters the nucleus and binds to a basic acceptor protein, which is part of chromatin. This process results in stimulation of DNA, RNA, and protein synthesis.[104,105]

Assaying for estrogen receptors can help to predict which patients will be responsive to endocrine therapy[106] because the absence of estrogen receptors is associated with a poor response to oophorectomy (Table 4–18). The presence of such receptors does not guarantee a positive response, however.

Table 4–18. *Breast Tumor Regressions In Patients with Hormone Therapy*

Therapy	Estrogen Receptor +	Estrogen Receptor −
Adrenalectomy	40/76	4/41
Castration	28/43	2/74
Hypophysectomy	9/14	0/12
TOTAL	77/133 = 58%	6/127 = 5%
Androgen	10/28	2/22
Estrogen	38/60	2/49
Glucocorticoid	15/32	0/19
TOTAL	63/120 = 52%	4/90 = 4%
Antiestrogens	9/21	5/29
Other	13/24	4/36
TOTAL	22/45 = 49%	9/65 = 14%

(Modified from McGuire, W.L.: Current status of estrogen receptors in human breast cancer. Cancer, 36:638, 1975.)

About two-thirds of primary breast cancers are estrogen-receptor-positive. Of these, about 50 to 70% respond to endocrine therapy.[107] A possible explanation for the failure to respond may relate to abnormalities in recognizing the hormone receptor complex in the nucleus. This failure may also reflect tumor heterogeneity.

The relationship between peptide and steroid hormones in the hormonal control of mammary carcinogenesis is complicated and involves many hormones. One human breast cancer cell line has been found to possess high-affinity receptors for estrogens, progesterone, androgens,[108] and corticosteroids. This finding provides a potential mechanism for interaction of various hormones in the growth regulation of breast epithelial tumors.[109]

Antiestrogens may also affect some tumors. The binding of estrogens to tumor cells normally leads to cellular proliferation. When supplied to these cells in vitro, antiestrogens compete for the 17 B-estradiol binding sites and inhibit cell growth.[110]

Prolactin. The role of prolactin in human breast cancer is far less conclusively known in man than in rodents, although evidence appears to indicate that it may be important in some cases [111,112]

Androgens. These hormones may also be carcinogenic in man. Liver cell cancers have been reported following the administration of androgenic hormones. Even the liver tumors associated with oral estrogen contraceptives may be androgen related because the progestational agents used are generally 17-substituted testosterone derivatives.[113] The liver tumors produced by oral contraceptives are usually benign *(adenomas)*, and their major morbidity is secondary to hemorrhage.[114] Androgens may also have a role in the pathogenesis of certain breast tumors.[115]

Immunologic Oncogenic and Protective Factors

Originally, it was thought that neoplastic cells arose from previously suppressed forbidden clones that escaped inhibition in later life. It was later postulated that neoplastic cells with altered surface antigens were formed constantly as a result of environmental carcinogenic agents such as chemicals or viruses.

In 1909, Paul Ehrlich postulated the theory of *"immune surveillance,"* later popularized by Thomas and Burnett. This theory suggested that both humoral antibody (IgG, IgM) and cellular immune responses, such as null cells (NC or NK) and killer T cells and killer macrophages, were able to remove malignant cells (Fig. 4–22) that were being constantly formed throughout life.[116,117,118]

The protective role of the thymus against oncogenesis was demonstrated experimentally by the observation that neonatal thymectomy increased the incidence of virally induced tumors.[119] Normally, immune surveillance mechanisms appear to deal efficiently with ubiquitous viruses in their natural hosts, but they are less able to cope with chemical carcinogens.

Experimental Animal Studies

The reasons for undisturbed growth of a new tumor at a given site are complex. Several theories have been advanced to explain why antigenic differences on the surfaces of neoplastic cells often fail to induce tumor rejection.[120] Indeed, previous investigators showed *enhancement of Ehrlich cell tumor growth* when tumor membranes were injected before whole tumor cells. It was suggested that when tumor membranes were injected, antibodies were formed to membrane antigens. These antibodies later served to block certain cellular receptor sites that would have been stimulated by whole tumor cell antigens and thereby enabled tumor cells to proliferate without inhibition. A number of host *immune deficiencies* may exist, or the antigen expression may be modified so as not to be recognized as foreign.[121] Cell-mediated and hormonal functions may also be abrogated.

The *"sneaking through" hypothesis* theorized that a nascent tumor does not provide a sufficient antigenic stimulus to induce an immune response until the tumor has reached

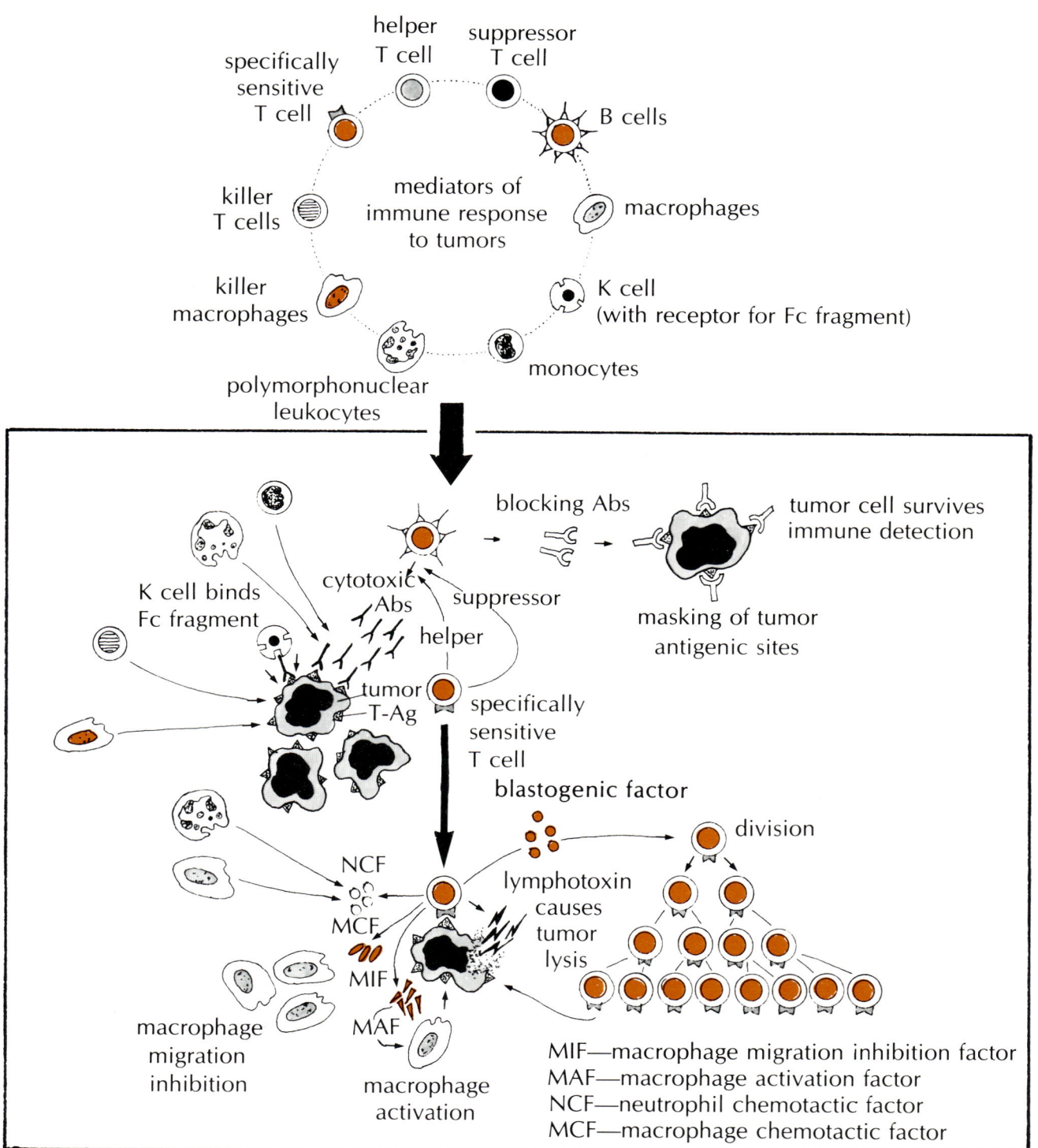

Figure 4–22. Immune responses to tumors (immune surveillance).

a size beyond host control.[122] Snyderman and others have described the release of *factors* by neoplasms that *inhibit* the *migratory function* of inflammatory cells and thereby protect the neoplasms from the destructive influences of macrophages during the early phases of tumor growth.[123,124]

The *major histocompatibility complex (MHC)* is involved in the immunologic control of neoplasia. *Immune response (Ir)* genes are a part of this complex, and influence all types of immune responses that have a genetic component. These immune responses include antigen recognition by T cells, T cell-B cell cooperations, and antibody formation by B cells. Paul and Benacerraf suggest that the Ia antigen on macrophages and B cells is the essential site for T-cell recognition.[125]

The H-2 antigens displayed on the surfaces of murine cells are incorporated into viral envelope structures as the virus buds from the host cell membrane. Killing by T cells requires recognition of the H-2 antigens as well as specific tumor antigens.[126]

Human Lymphoreticular Tumors

It is well known that the incidence of cancer increases with age. This increase may be secondary to the failure of normal control mechanisms or to dose-related phenomena because the longer one lives, the longer one is exposed to environmental carcinogens. The body's regulatory devices suffer progressive impairment after age 40. These regulatory homeostatic mechanisms, for example, control of temperature, electrolytes, and glucose, along with an altered immune surveillance mechanism, fail to eliminate metabolically altered cells. Furthermore, genetic instability and the incidence of chromosomal breaks increase with age. Only rarely do cells bearing breaks become neoplastic, but when they do, the altered metabolic and immune functions may allow unrestricted proliferation and resultant neoplasia.

The concept of immune surveillance in human tumors is presently in disfavor. Several investigators demonstrated that the incidence of tumors was not increased in nude mice. Prehn and Prehn[127] have shown that T-cell deficient animals and man have no increase in nonlymphomatous neoplasms. On the other hand, children born with immune deficiencies of B- and T-cell origin, but predominantly thymic aplasia, do have an increased incidence of lymphoreticular tumors.

Leukemia and Lymphoma. The use of *immunosuppressive drug therapy* results in lack of synthesis of immunoglobulins, in lack of proliferation of immunocytes, and in direct lymphocyte toxicity by the drug. That an increased incidence of *tumors*, predominantly of the *lymphoreticular type*, has been noted in such immunosuppressed patients seems to support the immune surveillance theory. Others suggest that immunosuppressive drugs such as azathioprine (Imuran) are directly mutagenic and carcinogenic.[128] A widely favored hypothesis suggests that cytotoxic-suppressive drugs increase the susceptibility of lymphoid cells to oncogenic viruses or to chemical carcinogens. Recently, retroviruses have been found in association with some leukemias.[129]

A *new immunodeficiency disease* associated with unusual susceptibility to EBV has been described by Purtilo.[130] Two phenotypes were found in the boys affected by this X-linked recessive lymphoproliferative syndrome: (1) In the proliferative phenotypes involving B cells, boys developed *American Burkitt's lymphoma,* immunoblastic sarcoma of B cells, fatal infectious mononucleosis, and plasmacytosis; and (2) in the nonproliferative phenotypes, these patients developed agammaglobulinemia, agranulocytosis, or aplastic anemia. The tentative designation of a "lymphoproliferative control virus" on the X chromosome is a provocative speculation as regards the immune and genetic control of neoplasia.

Thymic Tumors. Thymic abnormalities have been demonstrated in a variety of autoimmune disorders, for example, myasthenia gravis, that are associated with an increased cancer risk.[131] Patients with *myasthenia gravis* also have abnormal concentrations of immunoglobulins, most notably IgA, which may contribute to altered immune responses. The incidence of *mammary tumors, lymphomas,* and *leukemias* is increased in patients with *thymic hyperplasia* or *thymic tumors.*

Assays of Mutagenesis and Carcinogenesis

We have seen that a variety of agents, either alone or in combination, have the capacity to alter *DNA* in a way that is heritable. In some instances, this is due to the *insertion* of foreign genetic material (viruses). In others, the DNA is *altered* by the carcinogenic agent (chemicals and x rays). One would ideally like to be able to test the carcinogenic capabilities of different substances. This type of testing classically has been done in tissue culture in which morphologic and functional criteria, including contact inhibition, growth in agarose, and sister chromatid exchange, are assayed. Bioassays in animals have been done for many years, although direct applicability to man is difficult because of differences in genetic susceptibility, life span, route of administration, and dosage.

Recently, Ames and others[132,133,134] proposed in vitro bioassays for chemically caused mutagenesis (Fig. 4–23). The assays assume that mutation is synonymous with carcinogenic activity. Although mutation does have a high correlation with known carcinogenicity, it remains that certain mutagens are not carcinogenic, and certain carcinogens, such as hormones, are not mutagenic. The mutagenic dose necessary for carcinogenesis is presumably related to individual susceptibility, resistance, and cellular repair processes of individual host cells. A new approach has been

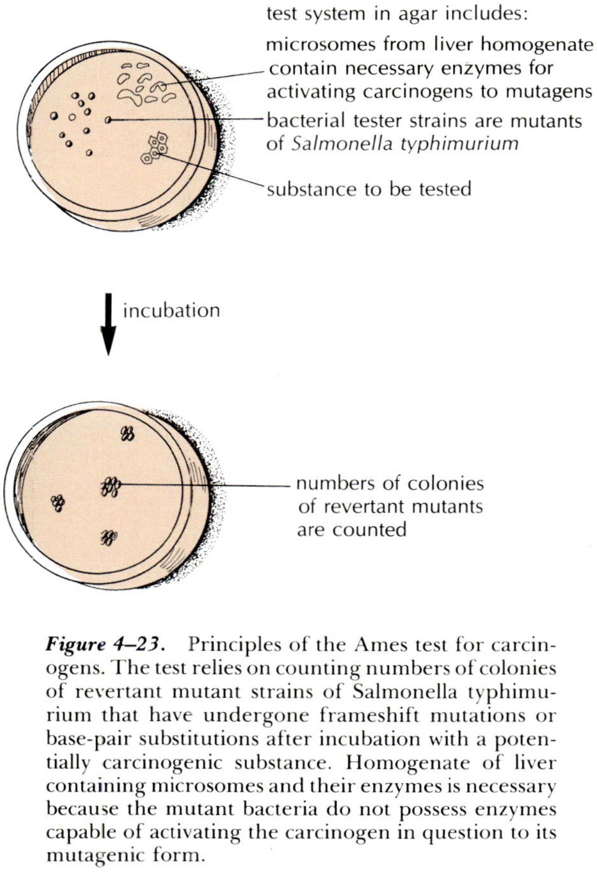

test system in agar includes:

microsomes from liver homogenate contain necessary enzymes for activating carcinogens to mutagens

bacterial tester strains are mutants of *Salmonella typhimurium*

substance to be tested

incubation

numbers of colonies of revertant mutants are counted

Figure 4–23. Principles of the Ames test for carcinogens. The test relies on counting numbers of colonies of revertant mutant strains of Salmonella typhimurium that have undergone frameshift mutations or base-pair substitutions after incubation with a potentially carcinogenic substance. Homogenate of liver containing microsomes and their enzymes is necessary because the mutant bacteria do not possess enzymes capable of activating the carcinogen in question to its mutagenic form.

proposed to assay for mutagenesis and carcinogenesis, called the "decision point approach." It involves four stages: (1) definition of chemical structure; (2) short-term tests in vitro; (3) limited bioassays in vivo; and (4) long-term bioassay.[134]

MORPHOLOGY, PHYSIOLOGY, AND BIOCHEMISTRY OF CANCER CELLS

Although no new cellular organelles, metabolic pathways, or physiologic responses are seen in cancer cells, they may display quantitative changes as a group when compared with normal cells. The criteria for neoplastic transformation are indicated in Table 4–19.

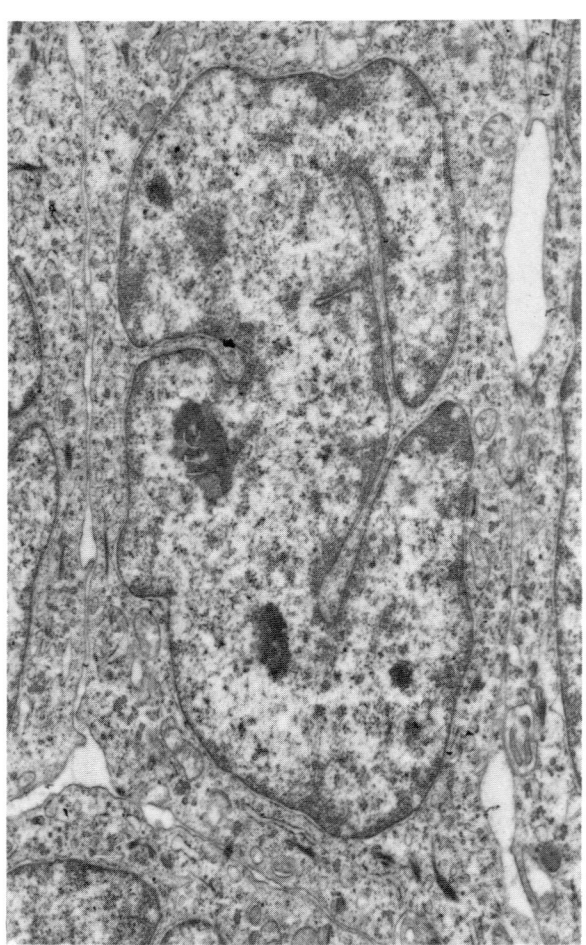

Figure 4–24. Transmission electron micrograph of squamous cell carcinoma of the cervix demonstrating an irregular nucleus and a paucity of cellular organelles.

Table 4–19. *Criteria for Neoplastic Transformation*

Production of biologically malignant neoplasms
Immortality of transformed cells in culture
Growth of transformed cells in soft agar
   Growth on glass independent of serum concentrations
Difference in morphologic and growth characteristics
   Surface microvilli increased
   cAMP decreased
   Microtubules and microfilaments disorganized
Loss of contact inhibition of cell replication
Increase in saturation density
Agglutination of transformed cells by plant lectins
Demonstration in culture of antigenic alterations in cells transformed by chemicals or viruses
Demonstration of karyotypic changes in transformed cells
Demonstration in transformed cells of cloning efficiency greater than in nontransformed cells

(Modified from Pitot, H.C.: Cell-carcinogen interaction in tissue culture. Am. J. Pathol., *85*:707, 1976.)

Nucleus

The nucleus of a malignant cell is often enlarged, pleomorphic, and hyperchromatic, and the nuclear/cytoplasmic ratio is increased[135] (Fig. 4–24). Nuclear pleomorphism correlates with an abnormal chromosomal number, tetraploidy, aneuploidy, and abnormal DNA content. The mechanism for the shift from the diploid to the tetraploid state has been studied in a number of systems including myeloma cells. The loss of cytokinesis, with subsequent formation of binucleate cells, appears to be one of the mechanisms for the formation of tetraploid states.[136]

Chromatin

The chromatin may be dispersed along the periphery of the nucleus, and this dispersal produces prominent peripheral clumping.[137] When the chromatin becomes condensed into chromosomes, normal or abnormal mitotic figures may form. The number of mitoses is generally increased in neoplastic tissues, and this criterion is used in some types of tumors to make the diagnosis of cancer.

Histones

Novikoff hepatocellular carcinoma ascites cells have been found to have a unique nonhistone protein that stimulates nucleolar RNA polymerase activity.[138] In cancer cells, the histones may also possess biochemical modifications. The major modification is the extent to which the histones are phosphorylated. This change, in turn, appears to be related to the proliferative rate and the cyclic nucleotide concentration.[139]

Chromosomes

If chromosome preparations are made from tumor cells, grossly abnormal chromosomal morphologic features may be detectable (Table 4–20). These changes include breaks, deletions, ring forms, and abnormal chromosomal karyotypes. Considerable evidence now suggests that chromosomal variation is a nonrandom event and that certain genotypes are more favorable for the development of malignant disease than others.

Table 4–20. *Abnormal Karyotypes in Neoplasms*

Disorder	Chromosomal Abnormality
Chronic myelogenous leukemia	Philadelphia chromosome (22–9 translocation)
Meningioma	22 missing in 50% of cases
Benign parotid tumor	3–8 translocation
Papillary serous cystadenocarcinoma	6–14 translocation
Retinoblastoma	Deletion of 13 in somatic cells
Wilms' tumor	Deletion of 11
Renal cell carcinoma	3–8 translocation
Burkitt's lymphoma	8–14 translocation, 8–22 translocation

Of particular interest are the consistent changes seen in chromosomes 1 and 17 in a variety of hematologic disorders. Rowley[140] has shown that patients with hematologic abnormalities, including acute leukemia, polycythemia vera, and myelofibrosis, showed trisomy for bands 1q25 to 1q32. Chromosome 17 showed either a duplication of the entire long arm or a translocation of part of the long arm to chromosome 15.

The best example of a specific chromosomal abnormality associated with cancer is the well-known *Philadelphia chromosome* (chromosome 22), whose long arm is translocated to chromosome 9 and is seen in chronic myelogenous leukemia[141] (Fig. 4–25). Many *Burkitt's lymphoma* patients have an 8- to 14-chromosome translocation, and chromosomal abnormalities are associated with many solid tumors, including meningiomas and colon cancers.[142]

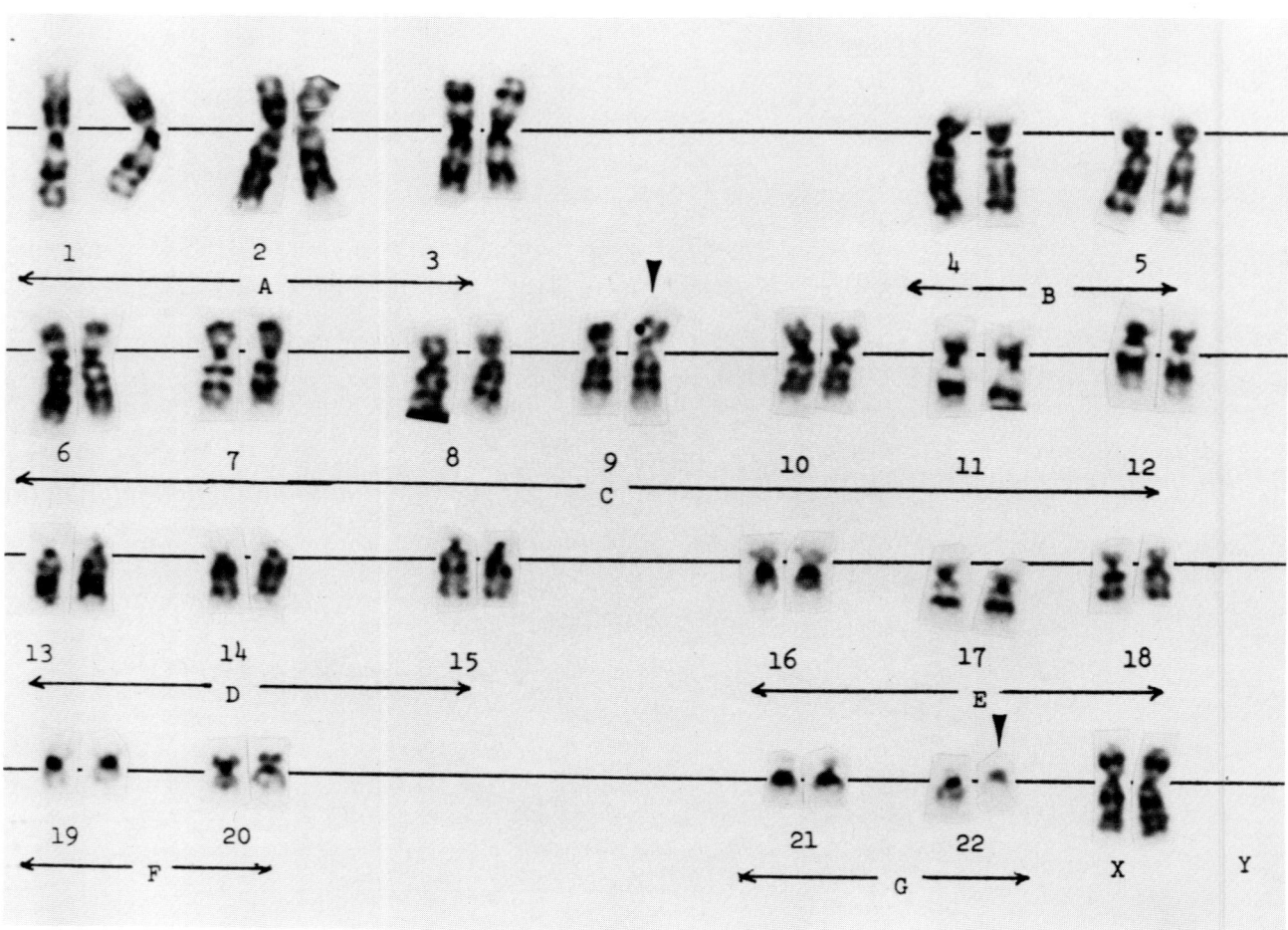

Figure 4–25. A karyotype of a cell containing the Philadelphia chromosome (arrow). (Courtesy of Dr. T.T. Puck, University of Colorado, Denver.)

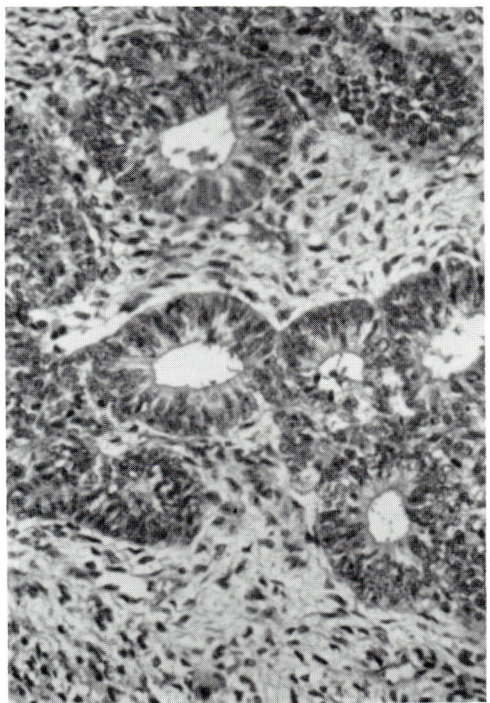

Figure 4–26. Wilms' tumor composed of primitive tubules surrounded by a cellular stroma.

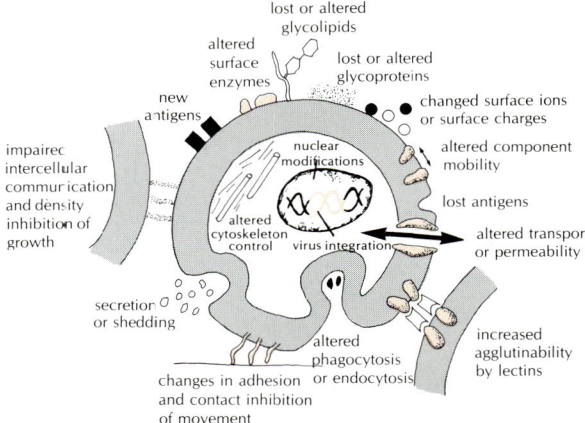

Figure 4–27. Cell surface changes occurring after neoplastic transformation. (Modified from Nicolson, G.L., and Poste, G.: N. Engl. J. Med., *295*:253, 1976.)

One inherited renal carcinoma, *Wilms' tumor* (Fig. 4–26) shows a deletion in chromosome 11, and another renal carcinoma shows a translocation of chromosomes 3 to 8.[143] Patients who bear a deletion in the long arm of chromosome 13 in all their somatic cells are genetically predisposed to develop *retinoblastomas*.[144] Other common abnormalities include 1p−, +17, and −22.[145] It is of interest that the prognosis is better in patients who initially have normal karyotypes.[146]

Nucleolus, Nuclear Membrane, and Pores

Other nuclear changes occur in neoplastic cells. Altered nucleolar morphologic features may contribute to *nuclear hyperchromatism*. These nucleolar changes are thought to reflect altered RNA metabolism. The nuclear membrane and chromatin organization may contribute to the nuclear changes in malignant disease.[135] The nuclear membrane may show blebbing, pockets, and projections as, for example, in some lymphoma cells. These changes are associated with diminished numbers of nuclear pores. The nuclear pore has been associated with DNA replication sites.

Other Nuclear Structures

Structures that are not usually found in the nucleus may be present in neoplastic cells. These structures include *viral particles, inclusions, crystalloid structures, filaments, annulate lamellae,* or prominent *fibrous lamina.*[147] The annulate lamellae may also be seen in the cytoplasm of actively proliferating neoplastic cells.[148] None of these nuclear structures are specific for malignant disease, however.

Cytoplasm

Plasma Membrane

The *plasma membrane*, which has been extensively studied in neoplasia, has a number of structural and functional differences from the normal plasma membrane (Fig. 4–27). Generally, neoplastic cells have a more complex surface architecture,[149] less complex glycolipids, altered membrane fluidity, decreased amounts of the glycoprotein known as the "large external transformation substance" (*LETS*),[150] now called *fibronectin*, altered membrane enzymes, decreased amounts of actin-like membrane-associated proteins, and *loss* of *contact inhibition*.[151] Differences in intrinsic membrane function are inferred from transport studies.[152] Reports demonstrate differences in the distribution of intramembranous particles between normal and transformed cells and increased *lectin agglutinability*.

The changes listed in the previous paragraph may also be present in the precancerous states, although not as ob-

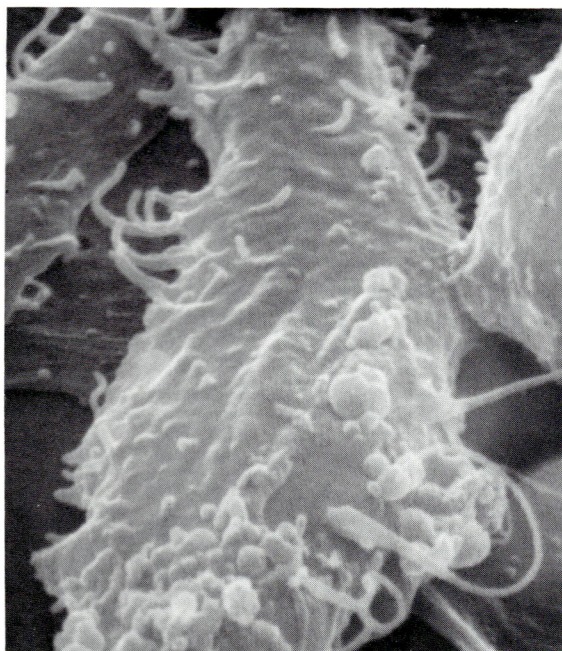

Figure 4–28. Scanning electron micrograph of a cell transformed by radiation demonstrating a complex surface feature with irregular filopodia and membrane knobs.

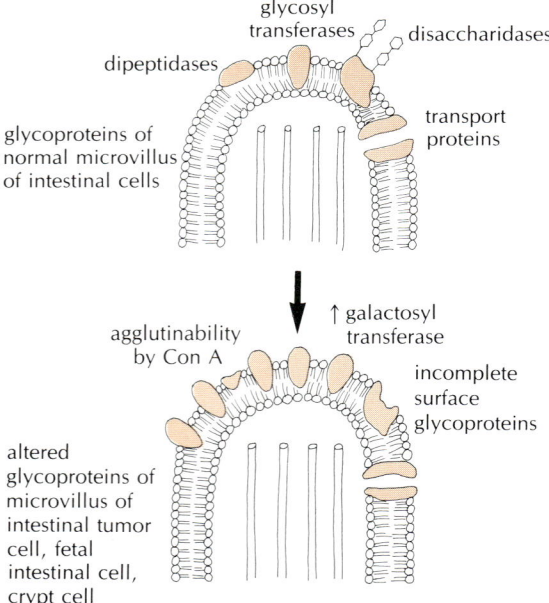

Figure 4–29. The tip of a microvillus of intestinal cells is represented schematically to show the normal glycoprotein components (above). With malignant transformation to cells that are undifferentiated (below), changes in glycoproteins with agglutinability by Con A occur.

viously or dramatically as in the full-blown cancers. Furcht et al. showed that independent alterations in cell shape and *intramembranous particle* distribution also occurred following cytochalasin and colchicine treatment of both normal and neoplastic cells.[153]

The normal anatomic and physiologic organization of multicellular organisms dictates that cell division be limited by the number of a particular cell type needed for functioning of the organism. This restriction of cell division and development of cellular maturation is abnormal in neoplastic cells and is believed to reflect changes in the genome. For example, malignant cells are no longer responsive to the density-dependent inhibition of growth; they continue to proliferate in an uncontrolled fashion. Because the plasma membrane is the structure through which cells communicate and interact, the membrane changes outlined in the following paragraphs appear to result in decreased cellular cohesion and in lost growth control.

Membrane structure has been investigated using lectin proteins that bind to specific sites on the cell surface. Some neoplastic cells have an increased agglutinability by these proteins through the exposure of cryptic sites, through the concentration of exposed sites, by a decreased cellular size, or by rearrangement of the exposed sites without a decrease in cell size.[154]

One hypothesis links the low cyclic adenosine monophosphate (cAMP) concentration and complex microvillous surfaces of neoplastic cells to their increased agglutinability by lectins through microvillous extensions. Willingham and Pastan[155] found that by increasing intracellular cAMP levels in neoplastic cells, the number of microvilli on cell surfaces decreased and thus led to poor agglutination by lectins (Fig. 4–28).

That *increased agglutinability* and alterations in transport are not necessarily confined to neoplastic cells was well demonstrated by Isselbacher, who studied the *intestinal crypt* and found that it contained a mixed population of differentiated and undifferentiated cells.[156] The epithelial generative zone in the bottom of the crypt contains undifferentiated, mitotically active cells that migrate up the villus and become differentiated and mitotically inactive.

The brush-border membranes of fetal small-intestinal cells, crypt cells, and neoplastic cells have similar enzymatic properties.[156] Furthermore, mitotically active nonmalignant cells of other types also have increased concanavalin A (Con A) agglutinability (Fig. 4–29), altered surface features, and transport properties in common with malignant cells.

Transformed cells have profound surface alterations and increased sugar transport. Some believe that this change partially accounts for the high anaerobic and aerobic glycolysis seen in tumors.

Cellular Adhesiveness and Invasion. Alterations in membrane structure and biochemical composition may be

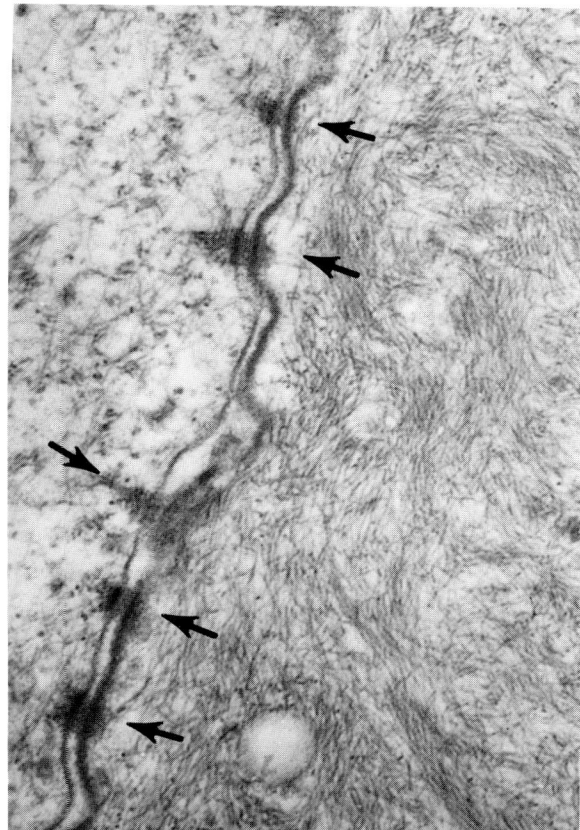

Figure 4–30. Endometrioid carcinoma of the ovary demonstrating numerous junctions between two adjacent cells (arrows).

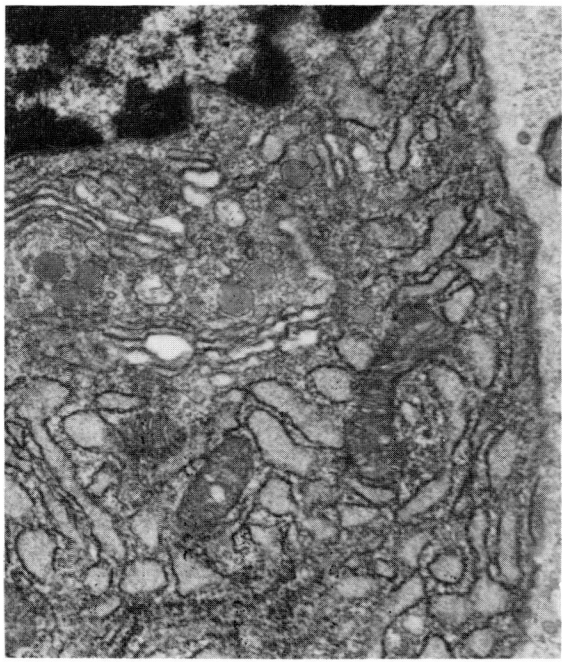

Figure 4–31. In this plasma cell in multiple myeloma with prominent endoplasmic reticulum, the nucleus is present in the upper left-hand corner.

important in the expression of the neoplastic state.[157] That changes in glycoproteins decrease cellular adhesiveness may be an important factor in invasion and subsequent metastasis. The loss or distortion of membrane surface receptors may allow the escape of neoplastic cells from neuroendocrine regulatory influences, with resultant increased transport of nutrients that stimulate growth.[158]

Intracellular Junctions. Plasma membranes of many cells have specialized regions that function in intercellular recognition, adhesions, electrical coupling, and communication. These regions possess a number of characteristic morphologic appearances and are known as intercellular junctions. Just as with other parts of the plasma membrane, these too may be altered in the neoplastic cell.

Poorly developed tight junctions and *desmosomes* have been described in a number of tumors[159] and have been repeatedly related to the decreased cellular cohesion and the ability to invade and metastasize (Fig. 4–30).

The junction currently receiving great attention is the *gap junction* or *nexus*. It consists of two closely apposed plasma membranes, each of which contains aggregates of intramembranous particles. The junctional particles appear to bridge the extracellular space and associate with complementary areas on the opposite plasma membrane. Studies of neoplastic cells have demonstrated decreased electrical coupling, and ultrastructural studies have reported reduced numbers of gap junctions in epithelial tumors when compared to the corresponding normal epithelial cells. This work remains controversial, however.[160]

Cell Communication. Malignant change may be associated with a loss not only of the ability to communicate, but also of the specificity of the communication. A change in the pattern of communication may have selective advantages for metastasizing tumor cells that enable them to ignore inhibitory signals from surrounding epithelial cells while still receiving stimulatory signals from nearby cells such as fibroblasts.[161]

Alterations at the cell surface reflect, in some ways, intracellular events. Some believe that the cyclic nucleotides are mediating signals transmitted from the membrane to the nucleus and vice versa, thereby regulating growth. Low levels of cAMP and high levels of guanosine monophosphate (cGMP) are usually associated with stimulation of cell division. The cyclic nucleotides are believed to interact with microtubules, microfilaments, and lysosomes in the transmission of certain signals.[162]

Endoplasmic Reticulum and Golgi Apparatus

The structure of the endoplasmic reticulum reflects the synthetic capabilities of the neoplastic cell. A differentiated tumor that continues to produce exported cellular products, for example, plasma cell myeloma or mucin-producing carcinoma, may have a well-developed RER (Fig. 4–31) and may be stimulated to become hyperplastic, with

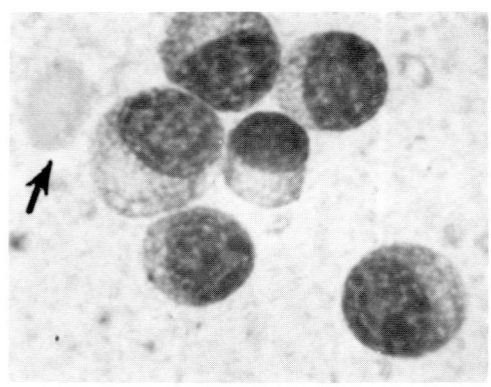

Figure 4–32. Six plasma cells and Russell body in surrounding area (arrow).

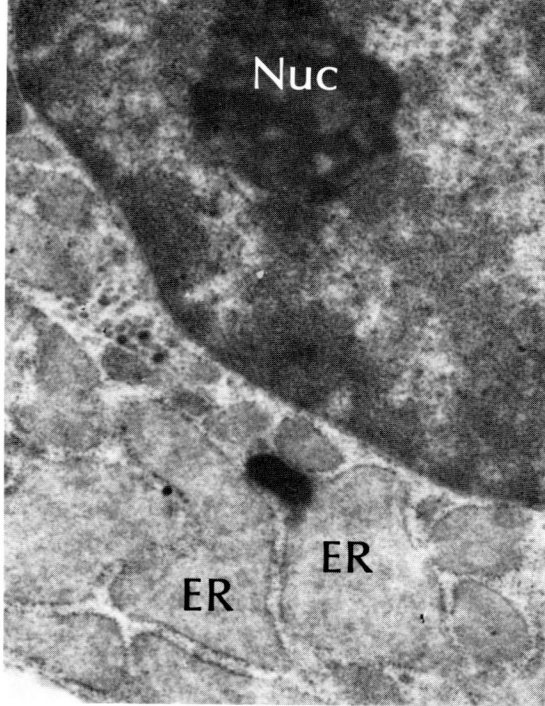

Figure 4–33. In this electron micrograph of a plasma cell in multiple myeloma, the endoplasmic reticulum (ER) is distended with immunoglobulin. A prominent nucleolus (Nuc) is present within the nucleus.

increased production of several metabolic enzymes, particularly of the mixed-function oxidase type.

Those enzymes associated with the microsomal fraction of cells have an important role in chemical carcinogenesis. For example, hypertrophy of the SER is seen in early stages of experimental nodular hyperplasia of the liver following the administration of a carcinogen. In other tumors, the prominent feature of undifferentiated tumor cells is increased number of free ribosomes.

Special Structures of the Endoplasmic Reticulum. Abnormal ER morphologic features may be present in some types of tumors. For example, certain tumors contain whorled arrangements of SER known as *"nebenkern,"*[163] and neoplastic lymphocytes and meningiomas may contain ER crystalline-like structures known as ribosomal-lamellar complexes.

Immunoglobulin (Ig) Synthesis in Multiple Myeloma. Perhaps one of the more intriguing facets of ER and Golgi function in neoplastic states has come to light through investigations of immunoglobulin production in multiple myeloma. The synthesis of the Ig molecules is well understood, and different mutant myeloma cell lines show varying blocks in assembly, glycosylation, or secretion of these immune molecules. For example, the mutant M3.11 has an H chain with a molecular weight of 40,000 for which known blocks in both assembly and glycosylation[164] exist. Intracytoplasmic inclusions *(Russell bodies)* found in cells of multiple myelomas are localized within the cisternae of the ER and represent synthesized but unreleased immunoglobulins[165] (Figs. 4–32 and 4–33).

Lysosomes

The malignant cell contains variable numbers of lysosomes. In general, the number of lysosomes and autophagic vacuoles is increased, especially in actively growing tumors and in those with a compromised blood flow. In at least two instances, the presence of increased levels of a lysosomal enzyme presages the presence of an underlying tumor. It has been noted that increased serum and urinary *lysozyme (muramidase)* is found in *monocytic leukemia* and in some hairy cell leukemias.[166] Increased *serum acid phosphatase* is found with carcinoma of the prostate, particularly with bony metastases.

Mitochondria

Mitochondria in tumor cells may be normal or abnormal in number or structure. The structural abnormalities include swelling, decreased numbers of cristae, intramitochondrial dense bodies, intercristal fusion, and intramitochondrial rodlets.[167] *Giant mitochondria* are noted in some leukemias. Mitochondrial DNA synthesis may also be abnormal.[168]

The most striking change presently seen in the number of mitochondria is in *"oncocytomas,"* in which neoplastic cells become packed with excessive numbers of mitochondria. Such mitochondrion-rich cells have been seen in salivary (Fig. 4–34), parathyroid, thyroid, and renal tumors.

The major function of mitochondria is cellular respiration; it is therefore not surprising that oxidative phosphorylation in neoplastic cells is frequently abnormal. In some instances, activity of the aceto-acetate-hydroxybutyrate "shuttle" of the membrane is impaired. That poorly differentiated tumors have increased glycolysis and fewer mitochondria may partially account for decreased cellular respiration. This was a major hypothesis of Warburg.[169]

Mitochondria of some tumors, which may also have abnormal fatty acid biosynthesis, are associated[170] with alterations in acetylcoenzyme A (acetyl-CoA)-carboxylase activity.

Microtubules and Microfilaments

Microtubules and microfilaments are often altered in tumor cells, the alteration depending on the cell type. Microtubules help to maintain surface structure and membrane fluidity. Some authors have stated that these organelles are decreased in number, are shorter, and are arranged at random in neoplastic cells.

Others report that microtubular cytoskeletons are clearly visualized in both normal and transformed cells (see Fig. 4–30).

In some autochthonous and chemically induced skin cancers, cytoplasmic microfilaments that resemble actin filaments are increased.[171] These microfilaments are disorganized. Others have reported an increased amount of smooth-muscle-associated antigen, presumably actin, in other tumors.[172] This finding has led to the hypothesis that microfilaments are involved in tumor cell movement and invasiveness. These changes may also account for the reduced ability of neoplastic B cells to "cap" various surface markers.[173]

Cytoplasmic Matrix

The term *"structuredness* of the *cytoplasmic matrix"* is used to describe the physical state of organization of the cytoplasmic matrix at the molecular level. It reflects the interactions among water, ions, macromolecules, and substances such as cAMP and is measurable by fluorescence polarization and other techniques. Neoplastic cells can be differentiated from their non-neoplastic counterparts on the basis of changes in this matrix following incubation with lectins or tumor-specific antigens.[174]

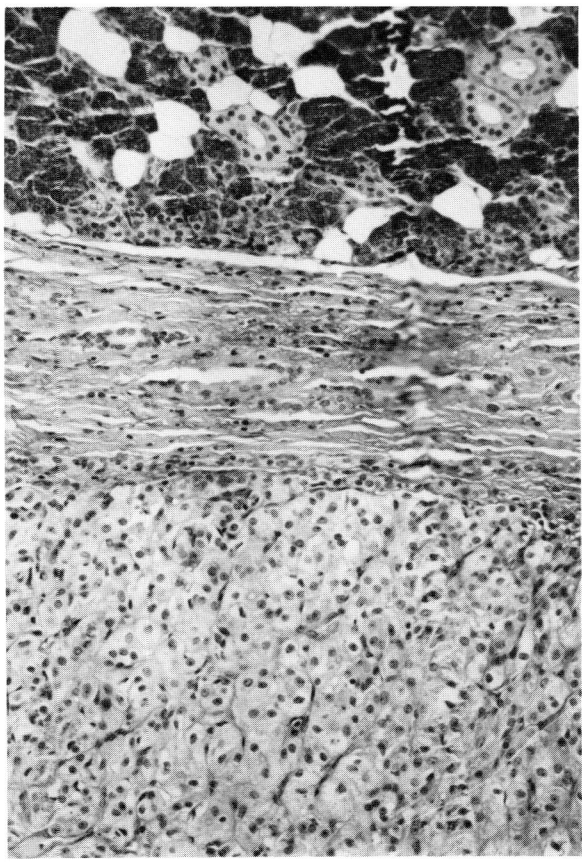

Figure 4–34. Oncocytoma of parotid gland (bottom) shows granular cells rich in mitochondria.

Tumor Markers (Hormones, Enzymes, Antigens)

A tumor marker may be defined as a substance produced by neoplastic cells that can be found on tumor cells or in the blood, spinal fluid, or urine[175,176] (Table 4–21).

When considering tumor-cell markers, one should recall that the expression of any of these markers varies from cell to cell and site to site in a given neoplasm during a patient's clinical course. Tumor cell products naturally vary with the progression of the tumor. Heterogeneous cell populations may arise as the tumor progresses from a preneoplastic state to early neoplasia and finally to far-advanced metastatic disease.[177] All these markers, whether hormones, antigens, or enzymes, represent products of the genome that have been activated during carcinogenesis.[178] Similarly, the appearance of hormonal receptors on the surfaces of neoplastic cells may represent retrogenic expression.

Table 4–21. *Tumor-Cell Markers*

Marker	Tumor
Cytology	Aspirates, exudates, urine, brushings
Antigens	
Carcinoembryonic antigen	Many solid tumors
Alpha-fetoprotein	Liver, ovary, testis
Tumor-specific cell mediated reactions	
Cytotoxicity tests	Many solid tumors
Delayed hypersensitivity reaction to tumor extracts	Many solid tumors
Ectopic hormones	
Human chorionic gonadotropin	Many tumors
Parathormone	Kidney, lung
Adrenocorticotropic hormone	Lung
Antidiuretic hormone	Lung
Melanin-stimulating hormone	Lung
Thyroid-stimulating hormone)	Placenta (choriocarcinoma)
Insulin	Lung
Isoenzymes	
Acid phosphatase	Metastatic prostate cancer
Lactic-dehydrogenase	Many tumors
Lysozyme (muramidase)	Leukemia
Elevated normal substances	
Immunoglobulins	Multiple myeloma
Insulin	Islet cell tumors
Serotonin	Carcinoid tumors
Parathormone	Parathyroid tumors
Prolactin	Pituitary tumors
Gastrin	Islet cell tumors
Human chorionic gonadotropin	Choriocarcinoma
Calcium	Medullary carcinoma (thyroid), parathyroid tumors

Hormones

One biochemical characteristic of some tumors is *inappropriate hormone synthesis*[179] (Table 4–21). Examples include the many tumors that produce adrenocorticotropic hormone (ACTH), insulin, human chorionic gonadotropin

(HCG), parathormone,[180] and erythropoietin in the so-called "paraneoplastic" syndromes.

One of the best clinical markers for tumors is HCG. A high serum level is useful in diagnosing and monitoring a lesion that is rare in the United States, trophoblastic disease—choriocarcinoma. Elevated HCG levels are not specific for trophoblastic neoplasia, however, and may be increased to a lesser degree in other malignant diseases as well.[181]

A tumor may also be detected by the presence of abnormally high serum levels of normal substances. These substances may be associated with signs and symptoms that herald the presence of underlying lesions. Examples include the presence of flushing and watery diarrhea secondary to 5-hydroxytryptamine (serotonin) release from carcinoid tumors, hirsutism from increased androgen production seen in some ovarian tumors, and increased calcitonin levels in medullary carcinoma of thyroid.[182]

Enzymes

Weber[183] suggests that key enzymes regulate gene control. He divides enzymes seen in neoplasia into *"transformation-linked" enzymes*, which are present in all tumors, and *"progression-linked" enzymes*, which are positively or negatively correlated with the expression of malignant disease. Cancer cells have an imbalance in pyrimidine and DNA metabolism that is linked to both transformation and progression. Weber believes that the ratio of the rate of incorporation of thymine into DNA to the rate of degradation of thymine to CO_2 provides the best correlation with tumor growth rate and degree of malignancy of all the biochemical markers.[183]

The enzyme *"convergence"* phenomenon, whereby the enzyme pattern of many tumors resembles that of other tumors more strongly than the enzyme pattern of the tissue of origin, was defined by Greenstein.[184]

A decrease in substances normally present within a given cell type may also mark the neoplastic state. *Decreased* leukocyte *alkaline phosphatase* levels have been described in *monocytic leukemia,* and blood-group antigens are lost in many malignant diseases.

We have mentioned that the urine may be assayed for *lysozyme (muramidase)* in patients with *monocytic leukemia.* Terminal deoxynucleotidyl transferase is present in the neoplastic cells of patients with leukemia and lymphoblastic lymphoma, as well as on the surfaces of normal thymocytes.[185] Deficiencies of *adenosine deaminase* with *leukemia*[186] and β-glucuronidase with *lymphomas* have recently been associated.[187]

In certain instances, an enzyme elevation signifies that a malignant tumor is no longer confined to its original anatomic site; for example, *serum acid phosphatase* becomes elevated in *metastatic prostatic carcinoma.*[188]

anti-LETS protein (fibronectin) antiserum shows prominent staining in the area of contact between two cells (arrow). (Courtesy of Dr. J.K. McDougall, Fred Hutchinson Cancer Center, Seattle.)

latter is a protein also known as *fibronectin* (MW 230,000), which is lost when fibroblasts and other cells become transformed, and especially when metastasis occurs[150] (Fig. 4–36)

Isoenzymes. From the previous discussion, it is clear that enzyme alterations are characteristic of certain neoplastic states. Weinhouse[189] has shown that well-differentiated hepatocellular carcinomas usually contain the adult form of the enzyme aldolase, whereas moderately well differentiated tumors contain approximately equal amounts

The modulation of expression of membrane antigens may result in changes that are especially significant in metastatic lesions.

GROWTH OF TUMORS

Initiation and Promotion

Regardless of their etiology, cancers develop from cells that have become transformed and are no longer under the normal intrinsic or extracellular control mechanisms. The tumor, which may grow at a fast or a slow pace, becomes a true cancer when it invades normal tissue and eventually metastasizes. This progression varies with the tumor, the site, the age, and numerous other factors in the host. We now appreciate that many cancers take years to develop. Often new cell populations appear that represent the progressive steps in a continuum from normal, initiated, and preneoplastic to malignant neoplasia.[72] How the cellular properties of these different cell populations relate to the subsequent development of a fully malignant neoplasm remains unknown.

When two agents play a role in carcinogenesis, they are considered to be *cocarcinogens*. Carcinogenesis, which occurs in two distinct stages, that is, *initiation* and *promotion*, has been demonstrated in a number of experimental systems[195,196] (Fig. 4–37).

In 1941, Rous and Kidd first suggested a two-stage mechanism for the development of cancer: an *initiation step* followed by a *promotion stage* by another agent.[197] This hypothesis was extended by the studies of Berenblum and Shubik in the late 1940's.[198] Investigators of murine skin carcinomas used methylcholanthrene as the initiating carcinogen and croton oil as the promoting agent.[199] Neither agent produced tumors when given separately.

Heidelberger has made the interesting observation that when a *promoting phorbol ester* is added to cells grown in tissue culture immediately following the removal of the initiating hydrocarbon, DNA synthesis is inhibited and prevents the cell division necessary to "fix" the *transformed state*.[200]

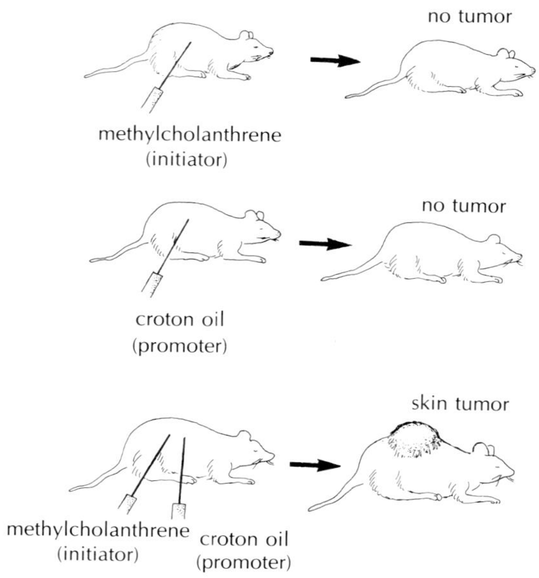

Figure 4–37. Experimental conditions of carcinogenesis demonstrate the roles of cocarcinogens in initiation and promotion of tumors.

Table 4–22. *Comparison of Initiator and Promoter Substances*

Initiator Substances	Promoter Substances
Single exposure sufficient for initiation	Given after initiation
Rapid, irreversible process	Requires prolonged exposure and is reversible during early stages
Initiators usually metabolically converted to electrophilic reactants that bind covalently to DNA and other macromolecules	No metabolic conversion or covalent binding necessary
Administration of two initiators is additive	Only weakly carcinogenic when given without prior treatment with initiator
Carcinogenic alone at high doses	Number of cancers formed increases when given after low doses of initiating agent

(Modified from Weinstein, I.B.: Molecular events in chemical carcinogenesis. Adv. Pathobiol., 4:106, 1976.)

Initiation is an irreversible step, but promotion is reversible if exposure to promoters is stopped before the cells gain the ability to multiply independently (Table 4–22). *Initiation* implies that cancer can develop after the brief exposure to the initiating agent (a few hours or days)[72] to the carcinogen and this agent never need be present again; however, this brief exposure does not induce a neoplastic event, but rather gives rise to a cell or cell populations that can be differentially stimulated to produce a focal proliferation. Because the initiated cells do not grow autonomously, they may not be considered to be neoplastic, and the effect of the initiator is only demonstrable once a promoting agent acts on these cells to produce an altered phenotype that is now manifest by relatively autonomous growth processes. The term *promotion* is used to designate the process by which these initiated cells are encouraged or accelerated to become neoplastic. The concept of initiation and promotion is most useful in discussing chemical agents. Radiation, viruses, and hormones may be both initiators and promoters; in these situations, the initiation and promotion phases are not clearly defined as in chemical carcinogenesis.

Single-Cell Clone Origin Versus Field Theory

Considerable thought has been given to whether a cancer arises from a single cell, which then proliferates widely, or from several cells in multiple foci that proliferate approximately simultaneously (field theory).

These theories have been tested on women who are heterozygous for the enzyme marker glucose-6-phosphate dehydrogenase (G6PD). This enzyme has two isoenzymes showing either a fast (A) or a slow (B) electrophoretic mobility, and each is located on a separate X chromosome. During the blastula stage, one of the X chromosomes is inactivated in each cell randomly. If a tumor arises from a single cell, only one chromosome will be expressed, and only one enzyme will be synthesized. If the tumor arises from a mosaic of several cells, the tumor will contain both isoenzymes on the electrophoretic pattern.[201]

It has been found that tissue culture cells from benign warts, leiomyomas, and carcinoma of the cervix all have only one isoenzyme and thus arise from one cell. Hepatocellular carcinomas formed experimentally with chemical carcinogens (AAF) arise in a multifocal pattern, and in humans, multiple bladder papillomas (carcinomas) also appear to arise simultaneously. This multiple pattern could represent either simultaneous cell transformation within several foci or, conceivably, horizontal transmission of an infectious agent.

Progression

"Neoplastic progression" of a tumor means worsening of the abnormal biologic potential, but not necessarily an increase in the tumor's size or extent. After a certain period of time, some tumors become more malignant and have a higher histologic grade. This finding appears to involve a simple selection advantage of the more malignant over the less malignant cells.[202]

The morphologic features of a cancer reflect its degree of differentiation (Table 4–23). The more a cancer resembles its tissue of origin, the better differentiated it is said to be. Conversely, the less it resembles normal tissues, the more undifferentiated it is. One may consider differentiation to be the process whereby cells develop specialized functions at the expense of other functions, such as proliferation; however, many metastatic tumors may appear to be highly differentiated, yet retain both functional and proliferative capacities.

Table 4–23. *Histologic Grading of Malignant Tumors: General Principles*

Grade I (Well differentiated)	Tumor tissue closely resembles tissue of origin (e.g., gland formation in adenocarcinoma, keratinization and epithelial pearls in squamous cell carcinoma) Few mitoses Little variation in size and shape of tumor cells
Grade II (Moderately differentiated)	Tumor tissue resembles tissue of origin less well Increased mitoses Increased variation in size and shape of tumor cells
Grades III, IV (Poorly differentiated)	Tumor tissue does not closely resemble tissue of origin Many mitoses Large variation in size and shape of tumor cells

The state of cytologic differentiation and tissue organization are used to estimate a cancer's histologic *"grade"* (Table 4–23), a concept introduced by *Broders*. He found that the histologic grade of a tumor was relevant to the prognosis of the patient.

Similarly, the *"staging"* of a cancer in a patient is related to survival. Staging is determined by an assessment of the degree of invasion or metastasis (Table 4–24). The survival rate is far higher in a patient with an early-stage lesion, that is, confined to the site of origin, than in a patient with late-stage disease with widespread metastasis.[203]

Table 4–24. *Staging of Cancer of the Cervix (International Classification)*

Stage I	Carcinoma confined to cervix
Stage II	Carcinoma extending beyond the cervix, but not onto the pelvic wall; may involve the vagina, but not the lower third
Stage III	Carcinoma extending onto the pelvic wall; may involve lower third of vagina
Stage IV	Carcinoma extending beyond the true pelvis or involving the mucosa of the bladder or rectum

It is unclear how many neoplasms arise as benign growths and then undergo progression and how many are malignant from the start. Clear examples exist in which cancer arises from a preexisting benign lesion, as in the adenomatous polyp that may progress to colon cancer.[204] In the other instances, a premalignant lesion progresses to malignancy, as in cervical intraepithelial neoplasia giving rise to cervical cancer.[205]

In some malignant diseases, neither a benign nor a premalignant phase is clinically recognized; however, it is possible that premalignant cells were present in these cases.

We recognize both morphologic and biochemical attributes of tumor progression. Generally, this progression involves inflexibility of cellular enzyme patterns with a decreased capacity to cope with environmental stresses. This failure eventually leads to invasion and sometimes metastasis.

Another aspect of progression is seen in endocrine-dependent tumors. During their early stages, these tumors retain their ability to respond to hormones; this responsiveness is often lost as neoplastic progression occurs.

Following the early experiments of Pierce[206] and Gurdon and Woodland,[207] Mintz has been able to fuse a *malignant teratoma* cell with an embryonic mouse blastula to produce a normal *chimeric mouse*.[208] The question arises whether the teratoma cell was malignant, as all cells in a malignant teratoma are not truly malignant. Nevertheless, this experiment explores the interesting aspect of the effect of cellular environment on tumorigenesis.

Cell Growth in Vitro

Contact inhibition of growth (density-dependent regulation) is a form of in vitro growth control, the loss of which is directly correlated with tumorigenicity in vivo.[209] This direct correlation is evidenced by the relationship between the loss of contact inhibition, measured by increasing the saturation densities of the cultures, and the ease of transplantability in vivo, particularly into nude mice in which the immune rejection responses are limited.

The loss of contact inhibition can be reversed in some neoplastic cell lines, most notably *melanoma,* by the addition of a diffusible factor produced by contact-inhibited cells. The factor, known as *melanocyte contact-inhibitory factor,* has a MW of 160,000 and is a glycoprotein.[210]

Whereas the foregoing in vitro characteristics are helpful in distinguishing between neoplastic and nonneoplastic phenotypes, they are less useful in certain cell systems. The gross structure of primary cultures of normal and neoplastic mouse mammary epithelial cells is not significantly different, and their growth rates and saturation densities are similar. Differences in surface architecture do exist, however, and are readily detectable by Con A-mediated hemadsorption assays. Malignant cells are readily responsive to this lectin at low doses, whereas normal cells do not react, even at high doses.[211]

Cell Growth Regulators in Vivo

One characteristic feature of tumors is increased division with a high number of mitotic figures, although many tumors do have a low mitotic index. Regulators of growth include inhibitory chalones and stimulatory growth factors associated with epidermal, neural,[212] fibroblastic, and T cells (Table 4–25). It is likely that, in the future, specific inhibitory and stimulatory factors will be isolated for all specialized cells.

Table 4–25. *Growth Factors*

Epidermal growth factor (EGF)
Neural growth factor (NGF)
Mesodermal stimulating factor (MSF)—somatomedin
Fibroblast (endothelial) growth factor (FGF)
Sarcoma growth factor (SGF)
Interleukin II (T-cell factor)
Macrophage colony stimulating factor (M-CSF)
Granulocyte-monocyte colony stimulating factor (GM-CSF)
Granulocyte colony stimulating factor (G-CSF)
Macrophage-granulocyte inducing protein (MGIP)

Following tumor initiation, many factors influence subsequent tumor growth. Chalones are a group of endogenous substances that inhibit the mitotic activity of a given cell type. They are tissue-specific, noncytotoxic glycoproteins and glycopeptides. Chalones appear to act by increasing the intracellular contents of cAMP, and they keep cells in the G_0 stage of division. Cells with decreased intracellular concentration of cAMP pass into the "S" phase. The growth stimulatory activity of phorbol esters (a "promoter" substance) is counteracted by chalones.[213]

Epidermal growth factor (EGF), a cell growth regulator produced by normal cells, can be abnormal in the neoplastic state. EGF acts as a *potent mitogen* for many cells because when it binds to a specific receptor on the target cell surface, cellular DNA synthesis occurs. These EGF receptors may be altered by viral transformation. EGF is a protein of about 6,000 MW. DeLarco and Todaro consider it a possible oncogene product because it is conserved throughout the species. The production of a growth factor by a *sarcoma cell* line has also been described.[214]

Tumor Angiogenesis Factor

An important requirement for growth is a tumor's ability to maintain an adequate blood supply. In some carcinomas, the growth process of the tumor may be aided by the elaboration of a protein known as *tumor angiogenesis factor (TAF)*.

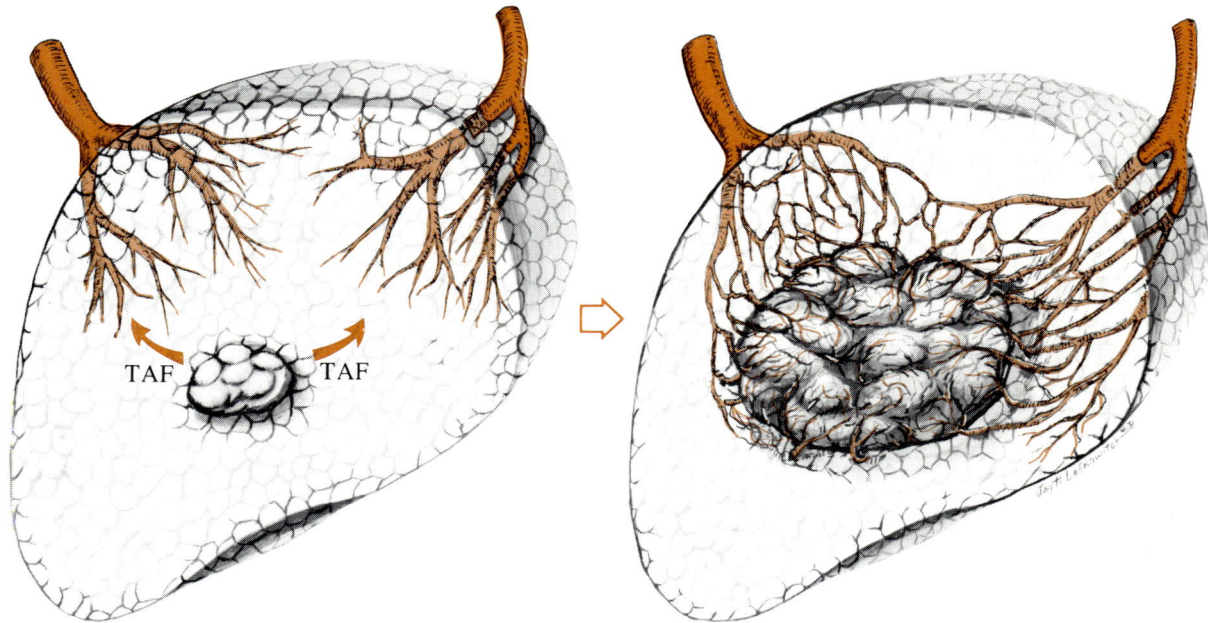

Figure 4–38. Tumor angiogenesis factor (TAF), a molecule with a molecular weight of 100,000 that is synthesized by tumor cells, causes mitogenesis in endothelial cells and thereby stimulates new capillary ingrowth to supply an enlarging tumor mass. (From Young, S.: Determinants of malignant tumor growth. Resident Staff Physician, *4*:89, 1978.)

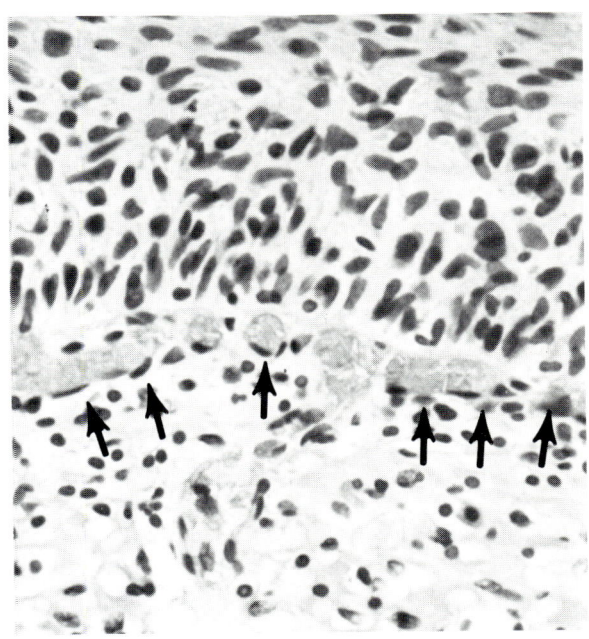

Figure 4–39. Cervical intraepithelial neoplasia Grade 1 (mild dysplasia) with prominent vessels is seen at the epithelial-stromal junction (arrows).

Folkman has postulated that a tumor induces the host to increase its network of blood vessels by releasing diffusible TAF[215] (Figs. 4–38 and 4–39).

TAF stimulates neighboring blood vessels to sprout new capillaries, which grow toward the tumor and finally penetrate it. Endothelial cells undergo a proliferative response with a marked increase in cytoplasmic RER and increased incorporation of H^3 thymidine into their nuclei. TAF is also produced by tumor cells when grown in tissue culture.[216]

TAF appears to be unique to the neoplastic state and has not been found associated with normal or fetal tissues, nor has it been isolated from richly vascularized healing wounds.[217] Angiogenesis may also be evoked by a variety of fetal tissues, by allogenic lymphocytes, and by other mechanisms,[218] however.

In the brain, vessel proliferation is accompanied by a proliferation of histiocytes in the peripheral part of the vacular wall. This proliferation is followed by the deposition of collagen around the vessel wall.[219]

Invasion

Extracellular Hydrolysis and Chemotaxis

The malignant cell develops the ability to invade and to metastasize to other areas of the body. Reich and others

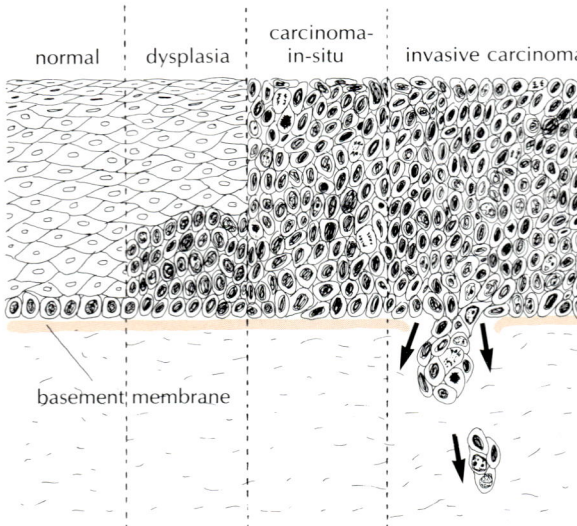

normal | dysplasia | carcinoma-in-situ | invasive carcinoma | basement membrane

Figure 4–40. Cytologic changes occurring in the development of invasive carcinoma.

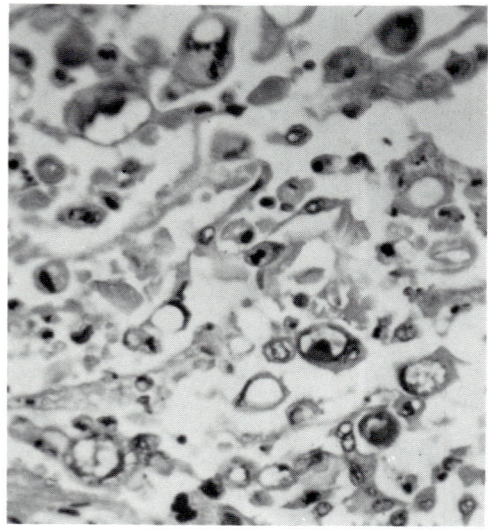

Figure 4–41. Gastric carcinoma composed of numerous signet ring cells.

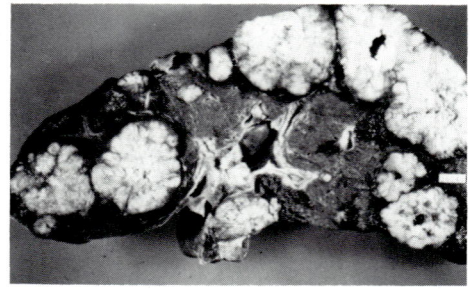

Figure 4–42. Metastatic colon carcinoma in liver.

have isolated a *plasminogen activator* from a variety of tumor cells and a similar factor from 22 other normal cell lines in tissue cultures.[220] Reich's factor is a protease capable of converting plasminogen to plasmin *(fibrinolysin)*.[221]

The hydrolysis of fibrinogen and other extracellular proteins may facilitate the diffusion of nutritive plasma proteins. It may also permit neoplastic cells to migrate more easily through ground substance into capillaries and lymphatic channels.[222] Hyaluronidase production by tumor cells has a similar effect. Several chemotactic factors isolated from tumor tissue increase the mobility of certain neoplastic cells.[223] One of these factors appears to be a neutral protease. Tumor cells may also produce chemotactic inhibitory factors in vivo and in vitro.[224]

Membrane Changes

Membrane abnormalities may also contribute to the capacity for invasion. We have already described alterations in intercellular cohesion. Metastasis is positively correlated with decreased calcium in the membrane and a high negative surface charge.[220] We know that neoplastic cells also have an increased motility and a loss of contact inhibition.

The *basement membrane* (basal lamina) normally separates epithelial cells from their underlying stroma, and capillary basement membranes must be traversed for metastasis to occur. The growth of epithelial neoplastic cells through the basement membrane constitutes an invasive process. The restriction of neoplastic cells to the area above the basement membrane is termed *intraepithelial neoplasia* or *carcinoma-in-situ* (Fig. 4–40).

The *basal lamina* has a variable appearance in malignant disease; it may be intact, reduplicated, or focally disrupted.[225] The destructive consequences of invasion arise from the migration of malignant cells into adjacent tissues and their subsequent growth in their new location (Figs. 4–41 and 4–42). It has been suggested that the presence of an intact basal lamina retards invasive growth, and it is true that an early change in invasive cancer is focal disruption of the basal lamina. This explanation cannot be complete, however, because basal lamina material is also synthesized in a variety of invasive tumors.[226]

Although invasive properties are characteristic of malignant disease, nonmalignant cells also demonstrate limited forms of invasive behavior during inflammation, wound healing, and other nonneoplastic processes.

Metastasis

Once invasion has occurred, metastasis often follows (Table 4–26). In general, *carcinomas metastasize* through the *lymphatic system* and *sarcomas* through the *blood* (Fig. 4–43). In advanced disease, however, hematogenous spread of carcinomas occurs, as well as lymphatic dissemination of sarcomas. These metastatic foci may, in turn, seed cells leading to further satellite metastases.[227] Not all cells shed into the circulation survive and give rise to metastases. Most are destroyed or are dormant at a distant site.

Table 4–26. *Metastatic Tumor Involvement in Autopsy Cases*

Site of Metastatic Involvement	In 1000 Consecutive Autopsies (%)	In 167 Cases of Primary Breast Cancer (%)	In 160 Cases of Primary Lung Cancer (%)	In 118 Cases of Primary Colon Cancer (%)
Abdominal nodes	50	44	29	59
Liver	49	61	40	65
Lungs	47	77	47	37
Mediastinal nodes	42	67	83	14
Pleura	28	65	28	14
Bone	27	73	33	9
Adrenal	27	54	36	14
Gastrointestinal tract	27	15	11	27
Diaphragm	20	25	16	11
Brain (cerebrum)	18	9	43	—

(Adapted from Gwynne, J.F.: Death certification in Dunedin hospitals. N.Z. Med. J., 86:77, 1977.)

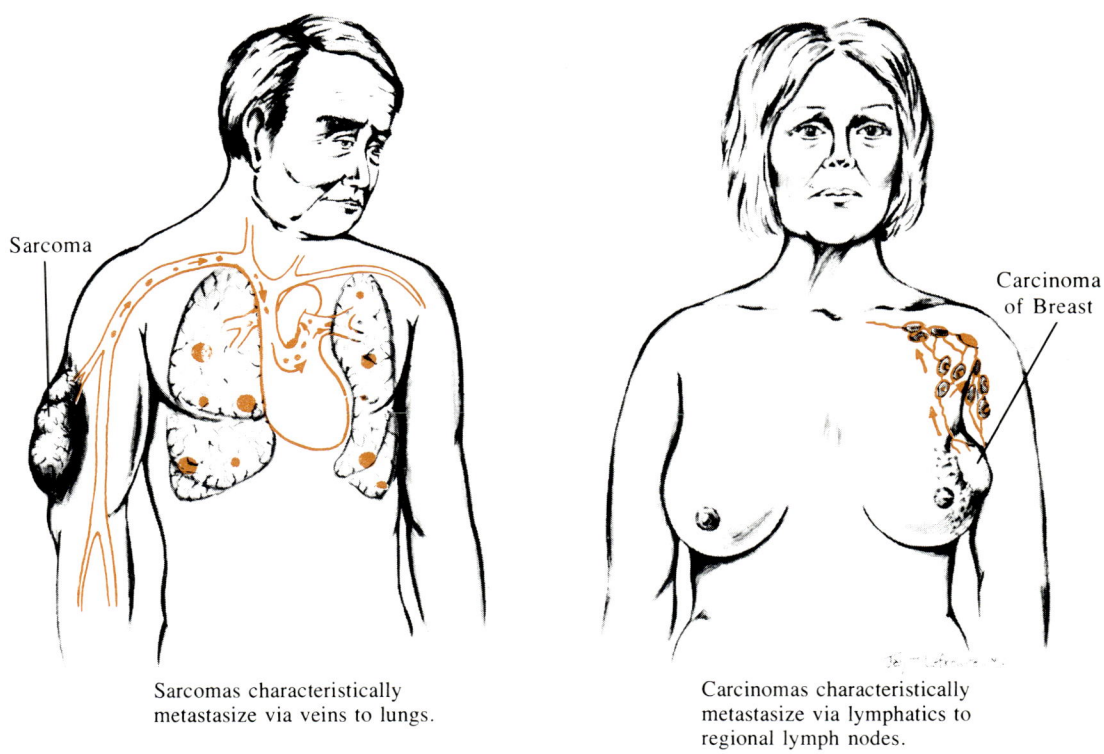

Sarcoma

Carcinoma of Breast

Sarcomas characteristically metastasize via veins to lungs.

Carcinomas characteristically metastasize via lymphatics to regional lymph nodes.

Figure 4–43. Patterns of metastasis of carcinomas and sarcomas. (From Young, S.: Determinants of malignant tumor growth. Resident Staff Physician, 4:89, 1978.)

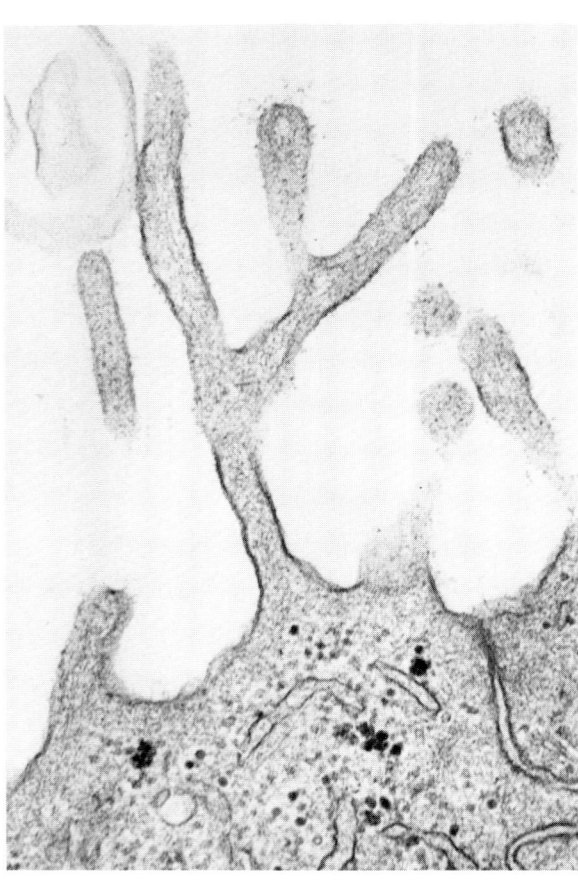

Figure 4–44. The surface of an ovarian cancer cell demonstrates an abnormal, branched microvillus structure.

Sugarbaker has shown a "homing" mechanism in mice whereby malignant cells taken from a metastatic lesion return to a similar organ upon venous reinjection into another animal.[228]

The formation of blood-borne metastases includes the following steps:

1. Growth of the primary tumor with seeding of viable tumor cells into the blood directly through vascular invasion or indirectly through lymphatic channels.
2. Transport of tumor-cell microemboli to distant organs.
3. Arrest of these blood-borne cells in distant vascular beds, often with thrombus formation.
4. Penetration of the blood vessel walls.
5. Continued growth of the metastatic cells in distant sites.

Surface microvilli are important in the attachment of tumor cells (Fig. 4–44) to endothelium; such tumor attachments may also be associated with dense *platelet thrombi.* Indeed, some patients with cancer have been shown to have hypercoagulable states that reflect the role of platelet activation. Once attached to the vessel wall, neoplastic cells may penetrate the capillaries between the junctions of adjacent endothelial cells. These neoplastic cells later undergo mitosis and form nests.[229] It has been suggested that deposits of *tumor* cells in *thrombi* are important in the genesis of metastatic foci. It has also been noted that the administration of coagulation-inhibiting substances such as heparin and dicumarol decreases the risk of metastatic spread.[230]

High levels of fibrinolysin stimulated by plasminogen activator released by the tumor could either retard the formation of tumor cell thrombi or help to release tumor cells from the thrombus at the site of metastasis.

Metastasis to Lymph Nodes

Metastasis to lymph nodes (Fig. 4–45) leads to alterations in the vascularity of the nodal tissues, with a transitory hypervascularity near the metastatic focus.[231] Certain histologic changes in regional nodes of a tumor are associated with a better prognosis, such as the presence of large numbers of lymphocytes and proliferation of sinus histiocytes. In contrast, a poorer prognosis is associated with a fibrotic pattern in lymphocyte- and histiocyte-depleted lymph nodes. The immune response to the tumor may thus play a role in tumor progression or regression.

Skeletal Metastasis

Skeletal metastases are a serious problem in patients with *breast, thyroid, renal, pulmonary,* and *prostatic cancers.* These metastases are often associated with extensive bone destruction, mediated by osteoclasts. Some tumors secrete a diffusible osteoclast-activating factor that causes osteolysis of bone trabeculae. New bone growth, that is, osteoblastic activity, is prominent in some cancers, such as prostatic carcinoma.[232]

Inflammatory and Immune Responses

Inflammatory Cellular Infiltrates

As previously noted, the surface of neoplastic cells may display new antigenic determinants that provoke an immune response in the patient. Invasive cancer cells are often surrounded by a prominent *mononuclear cell infiltrate.* A positive relationship between the prognosis of the patient and the presence of such an infiltrate is documented in *medullary carcinoma* of the *breast* and in *Hodgkin's disease.*[233] This relationship has been challenged by some authors when analyzing other tumors.[234]

The dense tumor and peritumor inflammatory infiltrate, when present, contrasts with its usual absence in surrounding tissues unless necrosis and infection are present. Lymphocytes, plasma cells, and macrophages insinuate themselves among neoplastic cells. Ultrastructurally, complex interdigitations and intimate contacts may exist between the tumor cells and infiltrating lymphocytes and macrophages. Tumor cell necrosis, perhaps due to these interactions or to ischemia, is often seen.[235]

Inflammatory infiltrates are not only seen in invasive tumors. Ioachim[236] noted that prominent lymphocytic and plasmacytic infiltrates are associated with intraepithelial carcinomas in a variety of sites. He concluded that in the early stages of malignant melanoma growth, infiltrates of lymphoid cells are present at the tumor site, and that in some cases, this infiltrate is associated with regression of the tumor. Furthermore, Ioachim[236] found that the amount

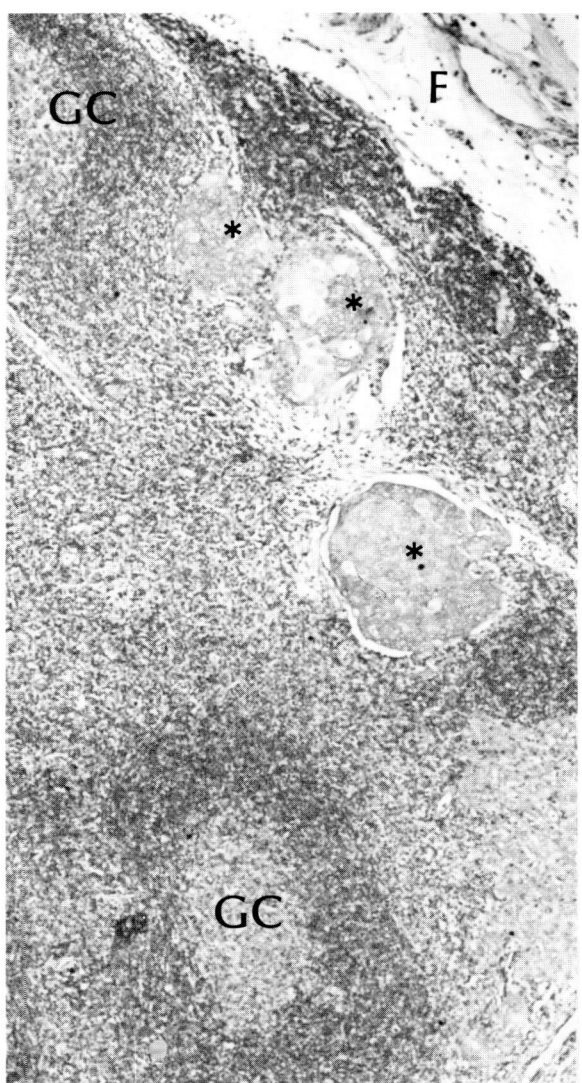

Figure 4–45. Carcinoma of breast metastatic to an axillary lymph node. The perinodal fat (F) is free of tumor. Three nests of malignant cells (asterisks) are identified near the subcapsular sinus. Lymphoid follicles with germinal center (GC) are seen nearby.

of inflammatory infiltrate paralleled the histologic grade of the tumor.

Tumor Cell Cytolysis

New *foreign antigens* in tumor membranes not only provoke cellular immune responses, but also may induce the synthesis of *humoral antibodies* including cytophilic antibody and blocking antibody. *Cytophilic antibody* acts with complement and B cells or macrophages to produce tumor cytolysis. *Blocking antibody* inhibits the cytotoxic T-cell response by masking antigenic sites.

In the absence of blocking antibody, sensitized and unsensitized *null (natural killer) cells* are capable of destroying tumor cells in vitro.[237,238] The susceptibility of target cells to N_K-mediated lysis may be dependent in part on the differentiation of the neoplastic cell.[239] In addition, *sensitized T lymphocytes* elaborate a variety of *lymphokines*, some of which (lymphotoxins) are directly cytotoxic to tumor cells. Other lymphokines may endow macrophages with enhanced cytotoxic capacities. *"Killer" macrophages* or "killer" T cells destroy tumor cells by an unknown mechanism involving cell-cell interaction.[240] In this pattern of response, specifically sensitized cells interact with *membrane antigens* and appropriate *HLA determinants* on the tumor target cell.

Tumor Immunodeficiency

That the tumor-bearing host is frequently immunodeficient has led to an interminable debate on which is the cart and which is the horse. Immunosuppressed individuals and children with immune deficiencies certainly have an increased incidence of certain types of tumors. It is also clear that patients who were not originally immunodeficient may develop deficient immune responses when a cancer occurs.

CANCER THERAPY

The treatment of cancer includes surgery, radiotherapy, chemotherapy, immunotherapy, or a combination thereof (Table 4–27).

Table 4–27. Classic Therapeutic Procedures

Treatment	Site or Type of Cancer
Surgery	Colon
	Breast
	Ovary
	Lung
	Thyroid
	Skin
Chemotherapy	Lymphoma
	Leukemia
	Choriocarcinoma
	Ovary
	Combined with surgery (all above)
Radiation	Seminoma
	Breast
	Uterus or cervix
	Lymphoma
	Lung
	Combined with surgery in many tumors
Hormones	Breast
	Prostate
	Endometrium

Surgery and Radiation

Surgery remains the mainstay of therapy in the patient with a localized solid tumor. Surgical treatment of tumors detected early has proved to be of great value, particularly in *breast, cervix, colon,* and *thyroid*. *Radiation* has proved to be of particular value in *seminoma* and as palliative therapy in many tumors affecting the nervous system and other sites. Perhaps with greater use of computerized axial tomography and ultrasound, heretofore undetected small lesions in lung, stomach, and pancreas may be detected early and more effective therapy instituted.

Chemotherapy

Chemotherapy has been most effective with *Hodgkin's disease, leukemia,* and, in females, *choriocarcinoma.* Many classes of chemotherapeutic agents are often used concurrently in definitive protocols in major cancer centers throughout the world[241,242,243] (Table 4–28).

Table 4–28. *Classes of Chemotherapeutic Drugs*

Hormones	Estrogens
	Androgens
Alkylating agents	Nitrogen mustard
	Cyclophosphamide
	Chlorambucil
Antimetabolites	Methotrexate (choriocarcinoma)
	Cytosine arabinoside (leukemia)
	Aminopterin (pancreas)
	Bromouridyldeoxyriboside (BUDR)
	Fluorouridyldeoxyriboside (FUDR)
Antibiotics	Daunorubicin
	Doxorubicin (Adriamycin)
	Actinomycin D
	Bleomycin
Mitotic inhibitors	Vincristine
	Vinblastine

Steroid Hormones

Charles Huggins used *estrogen* to produce remission in cancer of the prostate.[244] Other hormones now used for remission or palliation include *androgens, progesterone, prednisone,* and *cortisone.* The mechanism of action, often unclear, is believed to relate to the presence of appropriate receptors on the neoplastic cells.

Antiestrogens and Other Hormones

Many of these substances are structurally related to estrogens. Adrenal suppression with aminoglutethimide is useful in some breast cancers.[245] *Tamoxifen* increases the steroid-binding globulins in patients with breast cancer.[246] In rat models, this agent appears to exert its antitumor effects by binding to estrogen receptors.

Alkylating Agents

These agents cross-link cellular DNA and impede its ability to function as a template for RNA synthesis. Examples of agents in this class are nitrogen mustard, nitrosoureas, cyclophosphamide, and chlorambucil.[247,248]

Antimetabolites

These agents interfere with the biosynthesis of nucleic acids by substituting for normal metabolites in certain en-

Table 4–29. Mechanism of Action and Cellular Changes of Common Chemotherapeutic Drugs

Agent	Mechanism of Action	Cellular Change
Actinomycin D	Prevents transcription (polymerase) Inhibits tRNA, mRNA synthesis Inhibits protein synthesis	Nucleolar segregation
Mitomycin C	Damages kinetochore	Chromosomal exchange, nucleolar disruption
Bleomycin	Inactivates DNA template	Pyknosis, swelling, vacuolization of nucleus Single-strand and double-strand breaks
Rifampin	Inhibits transcription	
Cytosine arabinoside	Inhibits initiation of DNA replication units Inhibits DNA polymerase Leads to premature termination of nucleic acid chains	Chromosome breaks in G_2
Doxorubicin (Adriamycin)	Binds to DNA by intercalating between the base pairs (A–T) Uncoils the helix Inhibits DNA-directed RNA polymerase	Isochromatid break Peripheral nuclear clumping Nuclear filaments Nucleolar segregation

zyme reactions (Table 4–29). *Methotrexate*, a folic acid analogue, inhibits the enzyme dihydrofolate reductase and secondarily inhibits purine and subsequently protein synthesis.[249] Methotrexate toxicity may be relieved by administering folinic acid (citrovorum factor) several hours after methotrexate treatment ("citrovorum rescue").

Other members of this drug class include *cytosine arabinoside*, which inhibits DNA polymerase. It only affects cells in the early phase of the cell cycle and is used mainly in tumors with high proliferative rates.[250]

Bromouridyldeoxyriboside (BUDR), fluorouridyldeoxyriboside (FUDR), and aminopterin are all antimetabolites that bring about thymineless death. Thymine deprivation is the basis of action of many chemotherapeutic agents.[251] Although continued RNA and protein synthesis may occur for a period of time with thymine deprivation, cell division eventually stops, and irreparable cellular damage develops.

Antibiotics

These complex, naturally occurring compounds are produced by microbial fermentation. Some, such as doxorubicin *(Adriamycin)* and *actinomycin D*, inhibit transcription. Adriamycin is thought to bind nonspecifically to cellular DNA and thus to interfere with its transcription. *Bleomycin* is an antibiotic that inhibits the progression of cells through the cell "S" cycle by causing fragmentation of the DNA.

Mitotic Inhibitors

Among these drugs are the vinca alkaloids, *vincristine* and *vinblastine*. These agents arrest mitotic cells in metaphase by combining with tubulin. This then halts cell division.[252]

Miscellaneous Agents

Some chemotherapeutic drugs do not fall into any of the previous categories. For example, *L-asparaginase* hydrolyzes asparagine in the blood. A few special types of leukemias require an external source of asparagine, and this enzyme destroys this substrate.

Hydroxyurea, although not strictly an antimetabolite, resembles one by inhibiting the enzyme ribonucleoside diphosphate reductase. This action blocks the conversion of cytidylic acid to deoxycytidylic acid, a component of DNA.

Immunotherapy and Bone Marrow Transplantation

Immunotherapy may be either specific or nonspecific.[253] The former confers immunologic responsiveness to a particular set of antigenic determinants. *"Transfer factor"* is perhaps the best-known specific immunotherapeutic agent, although it is of limited usefulness in cancer. This agent, present in T lymphocytes, converts normal lymphocytes to specific antigen-responsive states in vivo and in vitro. Complete bone marrow transplants following total body radiation has been successful in some 50% of irreversible childhood leukemias. Unsuccessful patients die of graft versus host rejection or intercurrent infection.

Interferon, a heterogeneous protein product of leukocytes and fibroblasts, is an antiviral agent being investigated for potential therapy of certain neoplasms.[255] As of now, it has proved to be of little value in studies with leukemia and myeloma. One may postulate that even if these tumors had a viral etiology, the virus might well be unnecessary once the transformed neoplastic state had occurred, and the interferon would therefore not be useful.

Nonspecific immunotherapy generally serves to augment all aspects of the immune response, particularly the cellular one. This end is sometimes accomplished with agents such as methanol-extracted residues of bacille Calmette-Guérin (BCG) or Corynebacterium parvum. More recently, monoclonal antibodies directed against tumor antigens have been used for the early detection of tumors as well as for the specific delivery of radioisotopes, drugs, and toxins to them.[256]

Tumorigenic Effects

In many patients, therapy, whether chemical, surgical, radiation, or immune, has sometimes been successful in curing, or more frequently inducing remissions in, tumor growth. This development has not been without its drawbacks, however. It is now reported that some patients cured of childhood leukemia or lymphoma by *chemotherapy* developed new tumors many years later as a consequence of their therapy (Table 4–30).

Table 4–30. *Tumors Arising Secondary to Therapy of Hodgkin's Disease*

Treatment	No. Patients	Man Years Observed	Tumors Observed	Tumors Expected	Ratio
Radiotherapy	149	562	4	1.05	3.8
Chemotherapy	110	371	4	0.98	4.9
Combined Therapy	62	265	6	0.43	14.5
None	131	543	2	1.2	1.6

(Modified from Canellos, G.P., et al.: Second malignancies complicating Hodgkin's disease in remission. Lancet, *1*:947, 1975.)

Similarly, decades after receiving *radiotherapy*, especially of the thymus, some patients developed a second tumor in the field of radiation, for example, carcinoma of the thyroid. Finally, because both radiation and chemotherapy induce considerable *toxicity* and further compromise already immunodeficient patients, these persons are rendered more susceptible to infection, and morbidity.

REFERENCES

1. Doll, R.: An epidemiological perspective of the biology of cancer. Cancer Res., *38*:3573, 1978.
2. Comar, C.: Environmental assessment: a pragmatic view. Science, *198*:467, 1977.
3. Higginson, J., and Muir, C.S.: The role of epidemiology in elucidating the importance of environmental factors in human cancer. Cancer Detect. Prevent., *1*:79, 1976.
4. Foster, R.S., et al.: Breast self-examination practices and breast cancer stage. N. Engl. J. Med., *299*:265, 1978.
5. Purtilo, D.T., Paquin, L., and Gindhart, T.: Genetics of neoplasia—impact of ecogenetics on oncogenesis. Am. J. Pathol., *91*:609, 1978.
6. Gelfant, S.: A new concept of tissue and tumor cell proliferation. Cancer Res., *37*:3845, 1977.
7. Cancer Facts and Figures. New York, American Cancer Society, 1978.
8. Ioachim, H.L.: Perinatal viral carcinogenesis: the role of immunity. Natl. Cancer Inst. Mongr., *51*:193, 1979.
9. Sachs, L.: Control of cell differentiation in normal hematopoietic and leukemic cells. Adv. Pathobiol., *6*:124, 1977.
10. Green, E.L. (ed.): Biology of the Laboratory Mouse. 2nd Ed. New York, McGraw-Hill, 1966.
11. Benacerraf, B., and McDevitt, H.O.: Histocompatibility-linked immune response genes. Science, *175*:273, 1972.
12. Strong, L.C., et al.: Familial retinoblastoma and chromosome 13 deletion transmitted via an insertional translocation. Science, *213*:1501, 1981.
13. Knudson, A.G.: Heredity and human cancer. Am. J. Pathol., *77*:77, 1974.
14. Cohen, A.J., et al.: Hereditary renal cell carcinoma associated with chromosomal translocation. N. Engl. J. Med., *301*:592, 1979.
15. Galloway, S.M.: Ataxia telangiectasia. The effect of chemical mutagens and x-rays on interchromatid exchanges in blood lymphocytes. Mutat. Res., *45*:343, 1977.
16. Setlow, R.B.: Repair deficient human disorders and cancer. Nature, *271*:713, 1978.
17. Akiha, H., et al.: Defective DNA repair replication in xeroderma pigmentosum fibroblasts and DNA repair of somatic cell hybrids after UV radiation. Tohuko J. Exp. Med., *117*:1, 1975.
18. Chaganti, R.S.K., Schonberg, S., and German, J.: A manyfold increase in sister chromatid exchanges in Bloom's syndrome lymphocytes. Proc. Natl. Acad. Sci. USA, *71*:4508, 1974.
19. Bussey, H.J.R.: Familial polyposis coli: Family studies, histopathology, differential diagnosis, and results of treatment. Baltimore, Johns Hopkins University Press, 1975.

20. Simpson, J.L., and Photopoulos, G.: Hereditary aspects of ovarian and testicular neoplasia. Birth Defects, *12*:51, 1976.
21. Stenback, F.: Cellular injury in cell proliferation in skin carcinogenesis by UV light. Oncology, *31*:61, 1975.
22. Fisher, M.S., and Kripke, M.L.: Systemic alteration induced in mice by ultraviolet light irradiation and its relationship to ultraviolet carcinogenesis. Proc. Natl. Acad. Sci. USA, *74*:1688, 1977.
23. Division of Cancer Control and Rehabilitation, National Cancer Institute: Irradiation-related thyroid cancer. Bethesda, MD, U.S. Dept. of Health, Education and Welfare, Public Health Service, National Institutes of Health, Publication No. (NIH) 77–1120, 1977.
24. Refetoff, S., et al.: Continuing occurrence of thyroid carcinoma after irradiation to the neck in infancy and childhood. N. Engl. J. Med., *292*:171, 1975.
25. Walfish, P.G., and Volpe, R.: Irradiation-related thyroid cancer. Ann. Intern. Med., *88*:261, 1978.
26. Swarm, R.L. (ed.): Distribution, retention, and late effects of thorium dioxide. Ann. N.Y. Acad. Sci., *145(3)*:523, 1967.
27. Popper, H., et al.: Development of hepatic angiosarcoma in man induced by vinyl chloride, thorotrast, and arsenic. Am. J. Pathol., *92*:349, 1978.
28. Battifora, H.A.: Thorotrast and tumors of the liver. *In* Hepatocellular Carcinoma. Edited by K. Okuda and R.L. Peters. New York, John Wiley and Sons, 1976.
29. Friend, C.: The coming of age of tumor virology: Presidential address. Cancer Res., *37*:1255, 1977.
30. Wold, W.S.M., Green, M., and Mackey, J.K.: Methods and rationale for analysis of human tumors for nucleic acid sequences of oncogenic human DNA viruses. *In* Methods in Cancer Research. Vol. 15. Edited by H. Busch. New York, Academic Press, 1978.
31. Weinberg, R.A.: How does T antigen transform cells? Cell, *11*:243, 1977.
32. Ledbetter, J., Nowinski, R.C., and Emery, S.: Viral proteins expressed on the surface of murine leukemia cells. J. Virol., *22*:65, 1977.
33. Gross, L.: The role of viruses in the etiology of cancer and leukemia. JAMA, *230*:1029, 1974.
34. Strand, M., and August, J.T.: Polypeptides of cells transformed by RNA and DNA tumor viruses. Proc. Natl. Acad. Sci. USA, *74*:2729, 1977.
35. Gross, L.: The role of C-type and other oncogenic virus particles in cancer and leukemia. N. Engl. J. Med., *294*:724, 1976.
36. Temin, H.M.: The role of tumor viruses. Proc. Natl. Acad. Sci. USA, *69*:1016, 1972.
37. Schlom, J., and Spiegelman, S.: Evidence for viral involvement in mouse and human mammary adenocarcinoma. Am. J. Clin. Pathol., *160*:44, 1973.
38. Temin, H.M.: Ribodeoxyviruses and cancer. JAMA, *230*:1043, 1974.
39. Gallo, R.C.: Type-C viruses and leukemia. Adv. Pathobiol., *4*:47, 1976.
40. Todaro, G.J.: Type C virogenes: Genetic transfer and interspecies transfer. Adv. Pathobiol., *4*:38, 1976.
41. Huebner, R., and Todaro, G.J.: Oncogenes of RNA tumor viruses as determinations of cancer. Proc. Natl. Acad. Sci. USA, *64*:1087, 1969.
42. Weinberg, R.A.: Fewer and fewer oncogenes. Cell, *30*:3, 1982.
43. Shih, C., and Weinberg, R.A.: Isolation of a transforming sequence from a human bladder carcinoma cell line. Cell, *29*:161, 1982.
44. Murray, M.J., et al.: Three different human tumor cell lines contain different oncogenes. Cell, *25*:355, 1981.
45. Hehlmann, R., et al.: Molecular evidence for a viral etiology of human leukemias, lymphomas, and sarcoma. Am. J. Clin. Pathol., *60*:65, 1973.
46. Spiegelman, S., et al.: Human cancer and animal viral oncology. Cancer, *34*:1406, 1974.
47. Axel, R., Gulati, S.C., and Spiegelman, S.: Particles containing RNA-instructed DNA polymerase and virus related RNA in human breast. Proc. Natl. Acad. Sci. USA, *69*:3133, 1972.
48. Sherr, D.J., and Todaro, G.J.: Primate type C virus p30 antigen in cells from humans with acute leukemia. Science, *187*:855, 1975.
49. Kalyanaraman, V.A., et al.: Antibodies in human sera reactive against

an internal structural protein of human T-cell lymphoma virus. Nature, *294*:271, 1981.

50. Hinuma, Y.: Adult T-cell leukemia: antigen in an ATL cell line and detection of antibodies to the antigen in human sera. Proc. Natl. Acad. Sci. USA, *78*:6476, 1981.

51. Miller, R.W., and Todaro, G.J.: Viral transformation of cells from persons at high risk of cancer. Lancet, *1*:81, 1969.

52. Mesa-Tejada, R., et al.: Detection in human breast carcinoma of an antigen immunologically related to a group-specific antigen of the mouse mammary tumor virus. Proc. Natl. Acad. Sci. USA, *75*:1529, 1978.

53. Vianna, N.J.: Evidence for infectious component of Hodgkin's disease and related considerations. Cancer Res., *36*:663, 1976.

54. Smith, P.G., and Pike, M.C.: Current epidemiological evidence for transmission of Hodgkin's disease. Cancer Res., *36*:660, 1976.

55. Ziegler, J.L.: Burkitt's lymphoma. N. Engl. J. Med., *305*:735, 1981.

56. Klein, G.: The Epstein-Barr virus and neoplasia. N. Engl. J. Med., *293*:1353, 1976.

57. Niederman, J.C., et al.: Infectious mononucleosis. Epstein-Barr virus shedding in saliva and the oropharynx. N. Engl. J. Med., *294*:1355, 1976.

58. Tosato, G., et al.: Activation of suppressor T cells during Epstein-Barr-virus-induced infectious mononucleosis. N. Engl. J. Med., *301*:1133, 1979.

59. Morrow, R.H., Gutensohn, N., and Smith, P.G.: Epstein-Barr virus-malaria interaction models for Burkitt's lymphoma: implications for preventive trials. Cancer Res., *36*:667, 1976.

60. Courtney, R.J.: Immunologic and biochemical characterization of individual polypeptides induced by herpes simplex virus types 1 and 2. Adv. Pathobiol., *5*:87, 1976.

61. McDougall, J.K., et al.: Herpesvirus-specific RNA and protein in carcinoma of the uterine cervix. Proc. Natl. Acad. Sci. USA, *79*:3853, 1982.

62. Fenoglio, C.M.: Viruses in the pathogenesis of cervical neoplasia: an update. Hum. Pathol., *13*:785, 1982.

63. Goldin, B., and Gorbach, S.L.: Alterations in fecal microflora enzymes related to diet, age, lactobacillus supplements and dimethyl hydrazine. Cancer, *40*:2421, 1977.

64. Lijinsky, W.: Nitrosamines and nitrosamides in the etiology of gastrointestinal cancer. Cancer, *40*:2446, 1977.

65. Swarm, R.: Personal communication.

66. Cameron, E., Pauling, L., and Leibovitz, B.: Ascorbic acid and cancer: a review. Cancer Res., *39*:663, 1979.

67. Peer, F.G., and Linsell, C.A.: Dietary aflatoxin and human liver cancer: a population based study in Kenya. Br. J. Cancer, *27*:473, 1973.

68. Weisburger, J.H., Reddy, B.S., and Wynder, E.L.: Colon cancer: its epidemiology and experimental production. Cancer, *40*:2414, 1977.

69. Hackstra, W.G.: Biochemical function of selenium and its relation to vitamin E. Fed. Proc., *34*:2083, 1975.

70. Harris, C.C., and Saffiotti, U.: Carcinogenesis studies in human cells and tissues. Cancer Res., *38*:474, 1978.

71. Weinstein, I.B.: Molecular events in chemical carcinogenesis. Adv. Pathobiol., *4*:106, 1976.

72. Farber, E.: Chemical carcinogenesis: A biologic perspective. Am. J. Pathol., *106*:271, 1982.

73. Miller, E.C., and Miller, J.A.: Mechanisms of chemical carcinogenesis. Cancer, *47*:1055, 1981.

74. Smith, B.R., et al.: Pulmonary metabolism of epoxides. Fed. Proc., *37*:2480, 1978.

75. Neidle, S.: Carcinogens and DNA. Nature, *283*:135, 1980.

76. Pietropaolo, C., and Weinstein, I.B.: Binding of (3H) benzo(a)pyrene to natural and synthetic nucleic acids in a subcellular microsomal system. Cancer Res., *35*:2191, 1975.

77. Knox, P.: Carcinogenic nitrosamides and cell cultures. Nature, *259*:671, 1976.

78. Murthy, A.S.K., Vewter, G.F., and Bhaktavizian, A.: Neoplasms in Wistar rats after an N-methyl-N-nitrosourea injection. Arch. Pathol., *96*:53, 1973.

79. Kalengayi, M.M.R., and Desmet, V.J.: Sequential histological and histochemical study of the rat liver after single-dose aflatoxin B$_1$ intoxication. Cancer Res., *35*:2836, 1975.

80. Kalengayi, M.M.R., and Desmet, V.J.: Sequential histological and histochemical study of the rat liver during aflatoxin B_1 induced carcinogenesis. Cancer Res. *35*:2845, 1975.

81. Conney,H.A.: Carcinogen metabolism and human cancer. N. Engl. J. Med., *289*:971, 1973.

82. Farber, E.: Hyperplastic liver nodules. Methods Cancer Res., 7:345, 1973.

83. Pitot, H.C.: Carcinogenesis and aging—two related phenomena? Am. J. Pathol., *87*:444, 1977.

84. Metzger, G., Wilhelm, F.X., and Wilhelm, M.L.: Non-random binding of a chemical carcinogen to the DNA in chromatin. Biochem. Biophys. Res. Comm., *75*:703, 1977.

85. Flaks, B.: Permanent changes in the fine structure of rat hepatocytes following prolonged treatment with 2-acetylaminofluorene. Eur. J. Cancer, *4*:297, 1968.

86. Blot, W.J., et al.: Cancer mortality in U.S. counties with petroleum industries. Science, *198*:51, 1977.

87. Report of an IARC Working Group: An evaluation of chemicals and industrial processes associated with cancer in humans based on human and animal data: IARC monographs, Volumes 1 to 20. Cancer Res., *40*:1, 1980.

88. McLemore, T.L., et al.: Reassessment of the relationship between aryl hydrocarbon hydroxylase and lung cancer. Cancer, *48*:1438, 1981.

89. Furth, J.: Hormones as etiological agents in neoplasia. *In* Cancer. Vol. 1. Edited by F.F. Becker. New York, Plenum Publishing, 1950.

90. Miller, A.B.: An overview of hormone-associated cancers. Cancer Res., *38*:3985, 1978.

91. Biskind, M.S., and Biskind. G.R.: Development of tumors in the rat ovary after transplantation into the spleen. Proc. Soc. Exp. Biol. Med., *55*:176, 1944.

92. Huggins, C., Grand, L.C., and Brillantes, F.P.: Mammary cancer induced by a single feeding of polynuclear hydrocarbon and its suppression. Nature, *189*:204, 1961.

93. Wilson, R.G., et al.: Prolactin and breast cancer. Proc. R. Soc. Lond. (Biol.), *66*:865, 1973.

94. Smithline, F., Sherman, L., and Kolodny, H.D.: Prolactin and breast carcinoma. N. Engl. J. Med., *292*:784, 1975.

95. Furth, J.: The role of prolactin in mammary carcinogenesis. *In* Human Prolactin. Edited by J.L. Pasteels and C. Robyn. Amsterdam, Excerpta Medica, 1973.

96. Adam, E., et al.: Vaginal and cervical cancers and other abnormalities associated with exposure *in utero* to diethylstilbestrol and related synthetic hormones. Cancer Res., *37*:1249, 1977.

97. Gordon, J., et al.: Estrogen and endometrial carcinoma. N. Engl. J. Med., *297*:570, 1977.

98. Scully, R.E.: Estrogens and endometrial carcinoma. Hum. Pathol., *8*:481, 1977.

99. Weiss, N.S.: Cancer risk and estrogen use in the menopause. N. Engl. J. Med., *293*:1199, 1975.

100. Greenwald, P., et al.: Cancer risks from estrogen intake. N.Y. State J. Med., *77*:1069, 1977.

101. Lippman, M.E., et al.: *In vitro* model systems for the study of hormone-dependent human breast cancer. N. Engl. J. Med., *296*:154, 1977.

102. Lippman, M.E., and Allegra, J.C.: Current concepts in cancer: receptors in breast cancer. N. Engl. J. Med., *299*:930, 1978.

103. Jensen, E.V.: Steroid hormone receptors. Adv. Pathobiol., *1*:48, 1975.

104. Bresciani, F., et al.: Early stages in estrogen control of gene expression and its derangement in cancer. Fed. Proc., *32*:2126, 1973.

105. O'Malley, B.W., et al.: Effects of steroid hormone receptors on gene transcription. Adv. Pathobiol., *6*:79, 1977.

106. Howanitz, J.H.: Hormone receptors and breast cancer. Hum. Pathol., *12*:1057, 1981.

107. Chan, L., and O'Malley, B.W.: Mechanism of action of the sex steroid hormones. N. Engl. J. Med., *294*:1372, 1976.

108. Zava, D.T., and McGuire, W.L.: Human breast cancer: androgen action mediated by estrogen receptor. Science, *199*:787, 1978.

109. Cho-Chung, Y.S., Bodwin, T.S., and Clair, T.S.: Cyclic Amp-binding proteins: relationship with estrogen receptors in hormone-dependent mammary tumor regression. Eur. J. Biochem., *86*:51, 1978.

110. Henderson, I.C., and Canellos, G.P.: Cancer of the breast. The past decade. N. Engl. J. Med., *302*:17, 78, 1980,

111. Fenoglio, C.M., Tlamsa, G., and Habif, D.V.: Pituitary-containing benign cystic teratoma of the ovary in a patient with metastatic breast cancer: a case report. Diag. Histopathol., *5*:143, 1982.

112. Tolis, G.: Prolactin: physiology and pathology. Hosp. Pract., *15*:85, 1980.

113. Antunes, C.M.F., and Stolley, P.D.: Cancer induction by exogenous hormones. Possible androgen-induced cancer. Cancer, *39*:1896, 1977.

114. Christopherson, W.M., Mays, E.T., and Barrows, G.H.: Liver tumors in young women: a clinical pathologic study in 201 cases in the Louisville registry. *In* Progress in Surgical Pathology. Vol. II. Edited by C.M. Fenoglio and M. Wolff. New York, Masson Publishing USA, 1980.

115. Kirschner, M.A.: The role of hormones in the etiology of human breast cancer. Cancer, *39*:2716, 1977.

116. Drew, S.I.: Immunological surveillance against neoplasia: an immunological quandary. Hum. Pathol., *10*:5, 1979.

117. Klein, G.: Immunological surveillance against neoplasia. Harvey Lect., *69*:71, 1974.

118. Henney, C.S., et al.: Natural killer cells. Am. J. Pathol., *93*:459, 1978.

119. Miller, J.F.A.P.: T cell regulation of immune responsiveness. Ann. N.Y. Acad. Sci., *249*:9, 1975.

120. Broder, S., and Waldmann. T.A.: The suppressor-cell network in cancer. N. Engl. J. Med., *299*:1281, 1335, 1978.

121. Siegel, B.V.: Tumor immunity. Am. J. Pathol., *93*:515, 1978.

122. Baldwin, R.W., and Price, M.R.: Immunobiology of rat neoplasia. Part I. Tumors as stimulators of the immune response. Ann. N.Y. Acad. Sci., *276*:3, 1976.

123. Snyderman, R., and Pike, M.C.: Macrophage migratory dysfunction in cancer. A mechanism for subversion of surveillance. Am. J. Pathol., *88*:727, 1977.

124. Rhodes, J., Bishop, M., and Benfield, J.: Tumor surveillance: how tumor may resist macrophage-mediated host defense. Science, *203*:179, 1979.

125. Paul, W.E., and Benacerraf, B.: Functional specificity of thymus-dependent lymphocytes. Science, *195*:1293, 1977.

126. Ishimoto, A., et al.: Mouse fetal antigens in Rauscher leukemia. Bibl. Haematol., *43*:180, 1975.

127. Prehn, R.T., and Prehn, L.M.: Pathobiology of neoplasia. Am. J. Pathol., *80*:529, 1975.

128. Rothe, J., et al.: Hormone resistance and hormone sensitivity. N. Engl. J. Med., *296*:277, 1977.

129. Karpas, A.: Viruses and leukemia. Am. Sci., *70*:277, 1982.

130. Purtilo, D.T.: X-linked lymphoproliferative syndrome. An immunodeficiency disorder with acquired agammaglobulinemia, fatal infectious mononucleosis, or malignant lymphoma. Arch. Pathol. Lab. Med., *105*:119, 1981.

131. Levine, G.D., and Rosai, J.: Thymic hyperplasia and neoplasia: a review of current concepts. Hum. Pathol., *9*:495, 1978.

132. Ames, B.N.: Identifying environmental chemicals causing mutations and cancer. Science, *204*:587, 1979.

133. Waldren, C., Jones, C., and Puck, T.: Measurement of mutagenesis in mammalian cells. Proc. Natl. Acad. . USA, *76*:1358, 1979.

134. Weisburger, J.H., and Williams, G.M.: Carcinogen testing: current problems and new approaches. Science, *214*:401, 1981.

135. Aebi, H., et al.: Study of nuclei, nucleoli and nuclear bodies in goiter and papillary thyroid cancers. Experientia, *33*:1642, 1977.

136. Moriwaki, K., and Imai, H.T.: Membranes of ploidy shift from diploidy to tetraploidy in MSPC-1 mouse myeloma. Exp. Cell. Res., *111*:483, 1978.

137. Smith, H.S., Springer, E.L., and Hackett, A.J.: Nuclear structure of epithelial cell lines derived from human carcinomas and nonmalignant tissues. Cancer Res., *39*:332, 1979.

138. Forger, J.M., Choie, D.D., and Friedberg, E.C.: Non-histone chromosomal proteins of chemically transformed neoplastic cells in tissue culture. Cancer Res., *36*:258, 1976.

139. Letnansky, K.: The phosphorylation of nuclear proteins in the regenerating and premalignant rat liver and its significance for cell proliferation. Cell Tissue Kinet., *8*:423, 1975.

140. Rowley, J.D.: Association of specific chromosome abnormalities with

type of acute leukemia and with patient age. Can. Res., *41*:3407, 1981.

141. Miles, C.P.: Non-random chromosome changes in human cancer. Br. J. Cancer, *30*:73, 1974.

142. Levan, G., and Mitelman, F.: Clustering of aberrations to specific chromosomes in human neoplasms. Hereditas, *79*:156, 1975.

143. Cohen, A.J., et al.: Hereditary renal cell carcinoma associated with chromosomal translocation. N. Engl. J. Med., *301*:592, 1979.

144. Knudson, A.G., et al.: Chromosomal deletion and retinoblastoma. N. Engl. J. Med., *295*:1120, 1976.

145. Haag, M.M., Soukup, S.W., and Neely, J.E.: Chromosome analysis of a human neuroblastoma. Can. Res., *41*:4995, 1981.

146. Golomb, H.M., et al.: Correlations of clinical findings with quinacrine-banded chromosomes in 90 adults with acute nonlymphocytic leukemia. N. Engl. J. Med., *299*:614, 1978.

147. Conforti, A., et al.: Ultrastructural changes in human leukemic cell nuclei. Virchows Arch. [Cell Pathol.], *22*:143, 1976.

148. Ghadially, F.N., and Parry, E.W.: Intranuclear annulate lamellae in Ehrlich ascites tumor cells. Virchows Arch. [Cell Pathol.], *15*:131, 1974.

149. Borek, C., and Fenoglio, C.M.: Scanning electron microscopy of surface features of hamster embryo cells transformed *in vitro* by x-irradiation. Cancer Res., *36*:1325, 1976.

150. Chen, L.B., Gallimore, P.H., and McDougall, J.F.: Correlation between tumor induction and the large external transformation sensitive protein on the cell surface. Proc. Natl. Acad. Sci. USA, *73*:3570, 1976.

151. Barnett, R.E., Furcht, L.T., and Scott, R.E.: Differences in membrane fluidity and structure in contact-inhibited and transformed cells. Proc. Natl. Acad. Sci. USA, *71*:1992, 1974.

152. Isselbacher, K.J.: Increased uptake of amino acids and 2-deoxy-d-glucose by virus-transformed cells in culture. Proc. Natl. Acad. Sci. USA, *69*:585, 1972.

153. Furcht, L.T., Scott, R.E., and Maercklein, P.B.: Independent alterations in cell shape and intramembranous particle topography induced by cytochalasin B and colchicine in normal and transformed cells. Cancer Res., *36*:4584, 1976.

154. Bales, B.L., Lesin, E.S., and Oppenheimer, S.B.: On cell membrane lipid fluidity and plant lectin agglutinability. A spin label study of mouse ascites tumor cells. Biochim. Biophys. Acta, *465*:400, 1977.

155. Willingham, M.C., and Pastan, E.: Cyclic AMP modulates microvillus formation and agglutinability in transformed and normal mouse fibroblasts. Proc. Natl. Acad. Sci. USA, *72*:1263, 1975.

156. Isselbacher, K.J.: The intestinal cell surface: properties of normal, undifferentiated, and malignant cells. Harvey Lect., *69*:197, 1974.

157. Bell, G.I.: Models for the specific adhesion of cells to cells. Science, *200*:618, 1978.

158. Dudai, Y., et al.: Purification by affinity chromatography of the molecular forms of acetylcholinesterase present in fresh electric-organ tissue of the electric eel. Proc. Natl. Acad. Sci. USA, *69*:2400, 1972.

159. Sinha, A.A., Bentley, M.D., and Blackard, C.E.: Freeze-fracture observations on the membranes and junctions in human prostatic carcinoma and benign prostatic hypertrophy. Cancer, *40*:1182, 1977.

160. Sheridon, J.D., and Johnson, R.G.: Cell junctions and neoplasia. *In* Molecular Pathology. Edited by R.A. Good, S.B. Day, and J.J. Yunis. Springfield, IL, Charles C Thomas, 1975.

161. Todaro, G.J.: Autocrine secretion of peptide growth factors by tumor cells. *In* Proceedings of Research Frontiers in Aging and Cancer, September 22, 1980. Natl. Cancer Inst. Monogr., *60*, 1980.

162. Puck, T.T.: Cyclic AMP, the microtubule-microfilament system, and cancer. Proc. Natl. Acad. Sci. USA, *74*:4491, 1977.

163. Tomiyasu, U., Hirano, A., and Zimmerman, H.M.: Fine structure of human pituitary adenoma. Arch. Pathol., *95*:287, 1973.

164. Wertzman, S., Margulies, D.H., and Scharff, M.D.: Mutations in mouse myeloma cells. Ann. Intern. Med., *85*:110, 1976.

165. Mennemeyer, R., Hammar, S.P., and Cathey, W.S.: Malignant lymphoma with intra-cytoplasmic IgM inclusions. N. Engl. J. Med., *291*:960, 1976.

166. Weisberg, J.I.: Urinary muramidase in hairy cell leukemia. N. Engl. J. Med., *293*:150, 1975.

167. Korb, J., and Riman, J.: Presence of intramitochondrial bodies in avian leukemic myeloblasts. Eur. J. Cancer, *12*:959, 1976.
168. Ghadially, E.N., and Skinner, L.C.: Giant mitochondria in erythroleukemia. J. Pathol., *114*:113, 1974.
169. Warburg, O.: On the origin of cancer cells. Science, *123*:309, 1956.
170. Brinkley, B.R., Fuller, G.M., and Highfield, D.P.: Cytoplasmic microtubules in normal and transformed cells in culture: analysis by tubulin antibody immunofluorescence. Proc. Natl. Acad. Sci. USA, *72*:4981, 1975.
171. Puck, T.T.: The role of the cell surface and the microfibrils in transformation. Adv. Pathobiol., 7:331, 1980.
172. Tok, B.H., and Muller, H.K.: Smooth muscle-associated antigen in experimental cutaneous squamous cell carcinoma, keratoacanthoma, and papilloma. Cancer Res., *35*:3761, 1975.
173. Godal, T., et al.: Altered membrane-associated functions in human lymphocytic leukemia cells. Int. J. Cancer, *21*:561, 1978.
174. Cercek, L., and Cercek, B.: Application of the phenomenon of changes in the *structuralness* of cytoplasmic matrix in the diagnosis of malignant disorders: a review. Eur. J. Cancer, *13*:903, 1971.
175. Berlin, N.I.: Tumor markers in cancer prevention and detection. Cancer, *47*:1151, 1981.
176. Fenoglio, C.M.: Antigens, enzymes and hormones. Their roles as tumor markers in gynecologic neoplasia. Diagn. Gynecol. Obstet., *2*:33, 1980.
177. Maugh, T.H.: Biochemical markers: early warning signs of cancer. Science, *197*:543, 1977.
178. Lokich, J.J.: Tumor markers: Hormone antigen and enzyme in malignant disease. Oncology, *35*:54, 1978.
179. Odell, W.D.: Glycopeptide hormones and neoplasia. N. Engl. J. Med., *297*:609, 1977.
180. Zidar, B.L., et al.: Acute myeloblastic leukemia and hypercalcemia. A case of probable ectopic parathyroid hormone production. N. Engl. J. Med., *295*:692, 1972.
181. Vaitukaitis, J.L.: Human chorionic gonadotropin—a hormone secreted for many reasons. N. Engl. J. Med., *301*:324, 1979.
182. Trump, D.L., Mendelsohn, G., and Baylin, S.B.: Discordance between plasma calcitonin and tumor-cell mass in medullary thyroid carcinoma. N. Engl. J. Med., *301*:253, 1979.
183. Weber, G.: Enzymology of cancer cells. N. Engl. J. Med., *296*:486, 1977.
184. Greenstein, J.P.: Biochemistry of Cancer. 2nd Ed. New York, Academic Press, 1954.
185. McCaffrey, R., et al.: Terminal deoxynucleotidyl transferase activity in human leukemic cells and in normal thymocytes. N. Engl. J. Med., *292*:775, 1975.
186. Ramot, B., et al.: Adenosine deaminase (AOA) activity in lymphocytes of normal individuals and patients with chronic leukaemia. Br. J. Haematol., *36*:67, 1977.
187. Yam, L.T., and Mitus, W.J.: The lymphocyte B-glucuronidase activity in lymphoproliferative disorders. Blood, *31*:480, 1968.
188. Watson, R.A., and Tang, D.B.: The predictive value of prostatic acid phosphatase as a screening test for prostatic cancer. N. Engl. J. Med., *303*:497, 1980.
189. Weinhouse, S.: Metabolism and isoenzyme alterations in experimental hepatomas. Fed. Proc., *32*:2162, 1973.
190. Nondquest, R.E., Anglin, J.H., and Lerner, M.P.: Antigen shedding by human breast cancer cells *in vitro-in vivo*. Br. J. Cancer, *37*:776, 1978.
191. Ashall, F., Bramwell, M.E., and Harris, H.: A new marker for human cancer cells. 1. The Ca antigen and the Ca1 antibody. Lancet 2:1, 1982.
192. Sell, S., and Becker, F.F.: Alpha-fetoprotein. J.N.C.I., *60*:19, 1978.
193. Gold, P., and Freedman, S.V.: Specific carcino-embryonic antigens of the human digestive system. J. Exp. Med., *122*:467, 1965.
194. Limas, C., and Lange, P.: A, B, H antigen detectability in normal and neoplastic urothelium: Influence of methodologic factors. Cancer, *49*:2476, 1982.
195. Marx, J.L.: Tumor promoters: carcinogenesis gets more complicated. Science, *201*:515, 1978.
196. Shoyab, M., DeLarco, J.E., and Todaro, G.J.: Biologically active phorbol esters specifically alter affinity of epidermal growth factor membrane receptors. Nature, *279*:387, 1979.

197. Rous, P., and Kidd, J.G.: Conditional neoplasms and subthreshold neoplastic states. J. Exp. Med., *73*:365, 1941.

198. Berenblum, I., and Shubik, P.: The persistence of latent tumor cells induced in the mouse skin by a single application of 9, 10-dimethyl-1,2-benzanthracene. Br. J. Cancer, *3*:384, 1949.

199. Goldberg, A.R., Delclos, K.B., and Blumberg, P.M.: Phorbol ester action is independent of viral and cellular *src* kinase levels. Science, *208*:191, 1980.

200. Heidelberger, C.: Chemical carcinogens. Cancer, *40*:430, 1977.

201. Gartler, S.M., et al.: Glucose-6-phosphate dehydrogenase mosaicism as a tracer in the study of hereditary multiple trichoepithelioma. Am. J. Hum. Genet., *18*:282, 1966.

202. Silver, R.T., Young, R.C., and Holland, J.F.: Some new aspects of modern cancer chemotherapy. Am. J. Med., *63*:772, 1977.

203. Perzin, K.H., Fenoglio, C.M., and Pascal, R.R.: Tumors of the large and small intestine. *In* Principles and Practice of Surgical Pathology. Edited by S. Silverberg. New York, John Wiley and Sons, 1983.

204. Fenoglio, C.M., et al.: Defining the precursor tissue of ordinary large bowel carcinoma. Implications for cancer prevention. Pathol. Annu., *12*:87, 1977.

205. Richart, R.M.: Cervical intraepithelial neoplasia. A review. Pathol. Annu., *8*:301, 1973.

206. Pierce, G.B.: Differentiation of normal and malignant cells. Fed. Proc., *29*:1242, 1970.

207. Gurdon, J.B., and Woodland, H.R.: On the long-term control of nuclear activity during cell differentiation. Curr. Top. Dev. Biol., *5*:39, 1970.

208. Mintz, B.: Malignancy vs. normal differentiation of stem cells as analyzed in genetically mosaic animals. Adv. Pathobiol., *6*:153, 1977.

209. Abercrombie, M.: Contact inhibition and malignancy. Nature, *281*:259, 1979.

210. Lipkin, G., Knecht, M.E., and Rosenberg, M.A.: Potent inhibitor of normal and transformed cell growth derived from contact inhibited cells. Cancer Res., *38*:635, 1978.

211. Voyleo, B.A., et al.: Concavalin A-mediated hemadsorption by normal and malignant human mammary epithelial cells. Cancer Res., *38*:1578, 1978.

212. Schubert, D., et al.: Alterations in the surface properties of cells responsive to nerve growth factor. Nature, *273*:718, 1978.

213. Apffel, C.A.: Nonimmunological host defenses: a review. Cancer Res., *36*:1527, 1976.

214. DeLarco, J.E., and Todaro, G.J.: Epithelioid and fibroblastic rat kidney cell clones: epidermal growth factor (EFG) receptors and the effect of mouse sarcoma virus transformation. J. Cell. Physiol., *94*:335, 1978.

215. Folkman, J.: Tumor angiogenesis factor. Cancer Res., *34*:2109, 1974.

216. Klagsbrun, M., Knighton, D., and Folkman, J.: Tumor angiogenesis activity in cells grown in tissue culture. Cancer Res., *36*:110,1976.

217. Folkman, J.: The vascularization of tumors. Sci. Am., *234*:58, 1976.

218. Auerbach, R., Kubai, L., and Sidky, Y.: Angiogenesis induction by tumors, embryonic tissues and lymphocytes. Cancer Res., *36*:3425, 1976.

219. Bots, G.: Proliferation of blood vessels and stroma in brain tumors: an enzyme histochemical study. Virchows Arch. [Pathol. Anat.], *372*:175, 1976.

220. Nicolson, G.L., and Poste, G.: The cancer cell: dynamic aspects and modifications in cell-surface organization. N. Engl. J. Med., *295*:197, 253, 1976.

221. Reich, E.: Tumor associated fibrinolysis. Fed. Proc., *32*:2174, 1973.

222. Clifton, E.E.: Effect of fibrinolysin on spread of cancer. *In* Pharmacology Symposium on the Fibrinolysin System. Presented at the 48th Annual Meeting of the Federation American Society of Experimental Biology, Chicago, IL, 1964.

223. Ushijima, K., et al.: Characterization of two different factors chemotactic for cancer cells from tumor tissue. Virchows Arch. [Cell Pathol.], *21*:119, 1976.

224. Cohen, M.D., Brozna, J.P., and Ward, P.A.: *In vitro* and *in vivo* production of chemotactic inhibitors by tumor cells. Am. J. Pathol., *94*:603, 1979.

225. Gould, V.E., Sommers, S.C., and Terzakis, J.A.: Squamous differentiation and basal lamina deposition in endometrial adenoacanthoma. Am. J. Pathol., *83*:25, 1976.

226. Pertschuk, L.P., and Rosen, Y.: An immunofluorescent study of tumors with specific antisera for squamous epithelial intercellular substance and basement membrane. Am. J. Clin. Pathol., *60*:601, 1973.

227. Hoover, H.C., and Ketcham, A.S.: Metastasis of metastases. Am. J. Surg., *130*:405, 1975.

228. Sugarbaker, E.V.: Patterns of metastasis in human malignancies. *In* Cancer Metastasis. Edited by I.J. Fidler. New York, Marcel Dekker, 1977.

229. Sindelar, W.F., Tralka, T.S., and Ketcham, A.S.: Electron microscopic observations on formation of pulmonary metastases. J. Surg. Res., *18*:137, 1975.

230. Erikson, O., Lisnell, A., and Mellgren, J.: Studies on the dissemination of tumors by the blood. Swed. Cancer Soc. Yearbook, *3*:23, 1959.

231. Herman, P.G., et al.: Microcirculation of the lymph node with metastases. Am. J. Pathol., *85*:333, 1976.

232. Galasko, C.S.B.: Mechanisms of bone destruction in the development of skeletal metastases. Nature, *263*:507, 1976.

233. Keller, A.R., et al.: Correlation of histopathology with other prognostic indications in Hodgkin's disease. Cancer, *22*:487, 1968.

234. Flores, L.: Host tumor relationships in medullary carcinoma of the breast. Surg. Gynecol. Obstet., *139*:683, 1974.

235. Carr, I., Underwood, J.C.: The ultrastructure of the local cellular reaction to neoplasia. Int. Rev. Cytol., *37*:329, 1974.

236. Ioachim, H.L.: The stromal reaction of tumors: an expression of immune surveillance. J.N.C.I., *57*:465, 1976.

237. Stutman, O., Latime, E.C., and Figarella, E.F.: Natural cytotoxic cells against solid tumors in mice: a comparison with natural killer cells. Fed. Proc., *40*:2699, 1981.

238. Hanna, N., and Burton, R.C.: Definitive evidence that natural killer (NK) cells inhibit experimental tumor metastasis *in vivo*. J. Immunol., *127*:1754, 1981.

239. Meltzer, M.S., Occhionero, M., and Ruco, L.P.: Macrophage activation for tumor cytotoxicity: regulatory mechanisms for induction and control of cytotoxic activity. Fed. Proc., *41*:2198, 1982.

240. Werkmeister, J., et al.: Tumor cell differentiation modulates susceptibility to natural killer cells. Cell. Immunol., *69*:122, 1982.

241. Salmon, S.E., et al.: Quantitation of differential sensitivity of human tumor stem cells to anticancer drugs. N. Engl. J. Med., *298*:1321, 1978.

242. Frei, III, E., and Lazarus, H.: Predictive tests for cancer therapy. N. Engl. J. Med., *298*:1358, 1978.

243. Bertino, J.R.: Toward improved selectivity in cancer chemotherapy: the Richard and Hinda Rosenthal Foundation Award Lecture. Cancer Res., *39*:293, 1979.

244. Huggins, C.: Endocrine-induced regression of cancers. Science, *156*:1050, 1967

245. Legha, S.S., Davis, H.L., and Muggia, F.M.: Hormonal therapy of breast cancer: new approach and concept. Ann. Intern. Med., *88*:69, 1978.

246. Sakai, F., et al.: Increase in steroid binding globulins induced by tamoxifen in patients with carcinoma of the breast. J. Endocrinol., *76*:219, 1978.

247. Silver, R.T., Young, R.C., and Holland, J.F.: Some new aspects of modern cancer chemotherapy. Am. J. Med., *63*:772, 1977.

248. Chabner, B.A., et al.: The clinical pharmacology of antineoplastic agents. N. Engl. J. Med., *292*:1159, 1975.

249. Weinstein, J.N.: Liposomes and local hyperthermia: selective delivery of methotrexate to heated tumors. Science, *204*:188, 1979.

250. Gale, R.P.: Advances in the treatment of acute myelogenous leukemia. N. Engl. J. Med., *300*:1189, 1979.

251. Friedkin, M.: The biochemist's outlook on cancer research. Fed. Proc., *32*:2148, 1973.

252. Schrek, R., and Stefani, S.S.: Toxicity of microtubular drugs to leukemic lymphocytes. Exp. Mol. Pathol., *34*:369, 1981.

253. Noonan, F.P., et al.: Cell-mediated immunity and serum blocking factors in cancer patients during chemotherapy and immunotherapy. Cancer Res., *37*:2473, 1977.

254. Thomas, E.D.: The role of marrow transplantation in the eradication of malignant disease. Cancer, *49*:1963, 1982.

255. Marx, J.L.: Interferon (II): learning about how it works. Science, *204*:1293, 1979.
256. Marx, J.L.: Monoclonal antibodies in cancer: clinical trials of monoclonal antibodies in cancer therapy are beginning, but the best bet for their use may be in cancer detection. Science, *216*:283, 1982.

Chapter 5

AGING

Have you not a moist eye, a dry hand, a yellow cheek, a white beard, a decreasing leg, an increasing belly? Is not your voice broken, your wind short, your chin double, your wit single, and every part about you blasted with antiquity.

—2 Henry IV, I, ii

CHARACTERISTICS OF THE AGING PROCESS

Aging is an intrinsic part of life's continuum and is inseparable from development. It is difficult to separate the pathology from the physiology of aging.[1] As measured from the adult vantage point, any significant decline in function is regarded as abnormal; yet these losses must be considered normal for the chronologic time at which they occur.

Age is a functional incapacity of all cells. It has a genetic basis, is accelerated by environmental agents, is regulated by neuroendocrine, immune, and other humoral factors, and is accompanied by structural changes in cells, tissues, and organs.

Aging may best be defined as the sum total of changes that occur in all individuals with the passage of time. The capacity of an organism to maintain its vitality progressively declines, as reflected by morphologic, physiologic, and biochemical parameters; this general decline in performance eventually leads to death.

Life Span

Some suggest that aging starts at birth, whereas others cite puberty or the end of bone growth as the point at which aging accelerates. Nevertheless, the *normal human life span* is approximately *80 to 100* years unless interrupted by accident or disease (Fig. 5–1). The human life span compares well with other species (Table 5–1). The fruit fly has a life

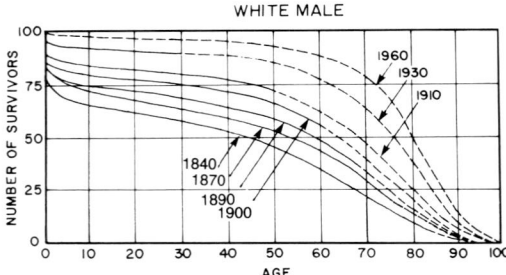

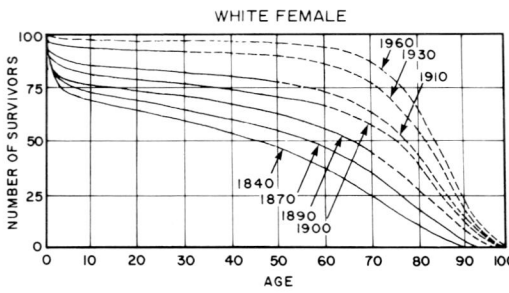

Figure 5–1. This figure shows survivors from birth to successive ages, white males and females, in the United States, by year of birth, 1840 to 1960. Note: Broken lines are based on projected mortality. (From Jacobson., P.H.: Cohort survival for generations since 1840. Milbank Mem. Fund. Q., *42*:36, 1964.)

Table 5–1. *Estimation of Life Span*

Common Name	Recorded Maximum Life Span yr
Southern wallaroo	24.5
Little brown bat	24
White-handed gibbon	31.5
Sumatran orangutan	>50
Chimpanzee	>44.5
Lowland gorilla	>39.33
Hairy armadillo	18.83
American beaver	>20
House mouse	3.5
Pack rat	7
Black rat	4.67
Guinea pig	7.5
Finback whale	>80
Sperm whale	>65
Coyote	21.83
Polar bear	34.67
Jaguar	23
Bengal tiger	26.25
Gray seal	41
Asiatic elephant	70
Mongolian wild horse	34
European wild boar	19.5
Red deer	26.5
Giraffe	36.58

(Modified from Sachar, G.A.: Mammalian life histories: their evolution and molecular-genetic mechanisms. Adv. Pathobiol., 7:21, 1980.)

span of 40 days; the mouse, 3 to 5 years; the chicken, 20 to 30 years; and the lordly tortoise may live 150 years.

Man has seemingly protected himself from injury, in the early and middle years, perhaps to his own ultimate detriment. He has succeeded in doubling his life expectancy, but not his reproductive life span, beyond the usual procreative period of approximately 40 years.

Until recently, "old age" was defined legislatively and socially in the United States as age 65, although this age did not always reflect biologic old age. The retirement age limit has recently been changed to 70. Despite health and vigor in many individuals 65 and over, many in this age group are likely to suffer from multiple chronic diseases.

As the result of improvements in sanitation, housing, nutrition, treatment of infectious disease, and medical therapy, many persons reach a near-maximal life span of 80 to 90 years. This longevity has resulted in a large elderly population, frequently with difficult socioeconomic problems.

Numerous reports exist of individuals in various populations living to 120, 140, or even 160 years of age. These include the Andean Vilcamamba tribe in Ecuador, the Hunza of Kashmir, and the Abkhasiz in the southern Soviet Union.[2] Although occasionally documented with records, most of these reports do not withstand critical analysis; the life span of most humans remains at 80 to 100 years. The mortality rate doubles every 7 years beyond the age of 30, and the rate of probability of dying increases exponentially with increasing age.[3] The leading causes of death are noted in Table 5–2.

Table 5–2. *Leading Causes of Death in the United States, 1976 and 1979*

Rank	Cause of Death	Number of Deaths	Death Rate per 100,000 Population	% 1976 Total Deaths	% 1979 Total Deaths
	All causes	1,910,440	890.2	100.0	100.0
1	Diseases of heart	723,729	337.1	37.9	37.8
2	Cancer	377,312	175.8	19.9	20.6
3	Stroke	188,623	87.9	9.9	9.1
4	Accidents	100,761	46.9	5.3	5.5
5	Influenza and pneumonia	61,666	28.7	3.2	3.0
6	Diabetes mellitus	34,508	16.1	1.8	1.8
7	Cirrhosis of liver	31,453	14.7	1.6	1.6
8	Arteriosclerosis	29,366	13.7	1.5	1.5
9	Suicide	26,832	12.5	1.4	1.4
10	Diseases of infancy	24,809	11.6	1.3	1.1
11	Homicide	19,554	9.1	1.0	1.1
12	Emphysema	17,796	8.3	0.9	1.1
13	Congenital anomalies	13,002	6.1	0.7	0.7
14	Nephritis and nephrosis	8,541	4.0	0.4	0.5
15	Septicemia and pyemia	6,401	3.0	0.3	0.4
16	Other and ill-defined	246,087	114.7	12.9	12.8

(Modified from Vital Statistics of the United States, 1976 and 1979.)

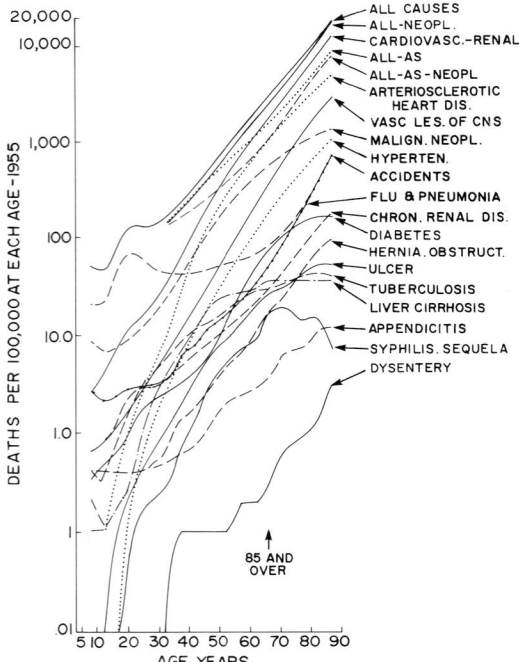

Figure 5–2. Age-specific death rates for major causes in the United States in 1955. (From Kohn, R.R.: Human aging and disease. J. Chronic Dis., *16*:5, 1963.)

Aging and Disease

When we speak of aging, we must be careful to separate those changes that are an intrinsic part of aging from those that are consequent to the process (Fig. 5–2). Similarly, the distinction between aging processes and the diseases associated with aging, such as senile dementia and atherosclerosis, is important because these and other similar diseases are not inevitable consequences of aging.

One must recall that aging lesions may resemble changes associated with specific diseases. Thus, the age-related decline in glucose tolerance, if improperly evaluated, might be diagnosed as diabetes.[4] Another age-related change that mimics a disease is an increased renin level, which can be associated with hypertension.[5] In the absence of independent markers for diabetes and hypertension, age-adjusted normal values for diagnostic tests must be developed.

Spectrum of Diseases During Life

Childhood (Birth to 14 Years)

The spectrum of disease to which an individual is most subject differs throughout a lifetime (Table 5–3). Up to the

Table 5–3. *Spectrum of Disease*

Age	Cause
0–5	Allergy
	Infection
	Neoplasia (leukemia, Wilms', medulloblastoma, retinoblastoma)
5–15	Allergy
	Diabetes (juvenile)
	Infection
	Accidents
15–30	Allergy (asthma)
	Accidents (suicide)
	Venereal disease
	Endocrine (women)
	Acne
30–40	Complications of pregnancy
	Ulcer
	Hypertension
	Suicide
	Homicide
40–60	Heart disease (infarct, hypertension, rheumatic fever)
	Liver disease (cirrhosis)
	Kidney disease (glomerular nephritis)
	Neoplasia (lung, colon, breast, ovary)
60–80	Neoplasia (lung, colon, prostate)
	Cardiovascular disease
80–100	Neoplasia (leukemia, lymphoma, prostate)
	Dementia (Alzheimer's, Parkinson's)
	Osteoporosis, osteoarthritis
	Accidents (fractures)
	Infection
	Cardiovascular disease

(Modified from King, D.W.: Health problems. *In* Young Adulthood. Edited by J. Scanlon. New York, Academy for Educational Development, 1979.)

age of five, relatively uncommon diseases include numerous *congenital disorders*, for example, storage diseases, sickle cell anemia, Down's syndrome, and cystic fibrosis. The incidence of *accidents, infections,* and *allergies* is high, with a small number of cases of *juvenile diabetes* and *neoplasia*. Except for lymphomas and leukemias, the incidence of neoplasia is low from five years of age until the late thirties and forties.[6]

Adolescence and Young Adulthood (15 to 40 years)

Accidents, mental disease (sometimes with suicide attempts), *allergies, acute infections* (often viral and sometimes with late complications), *alcoholism, venereal disease, hypertension,* and *endocrine problems* occasionally interfere with a relatively healthy life until the age of 40.

Middle Age (40 to 65 years)

In the forties and fifties, changes in diet and *endocrine balance,* and severe *cardiovascular, renal,* and *liver problems* are seen. Cardiovascular problems occur in 50% of the population.[6] Other prominent diseases in this group, besides myocardial infarcts and hypertension, with or without cerebral hemorrhage, include maturity-onset diabetes, chronic glomerulonephritis and nephrosis, cirrhosis preceded by viral or alcoholic hepatitis, and *neoplasia*.[7] Although skin tumors are the most common cancers in all age groups, these are usually not fatal. Many middle-aged women develop breast or uterine cancers. Older men develop lung, colon, or prostate cancers. Approximately 20% of males and females in this age group die of cancer.[6]

Elderly (65 to 90 years)

In the 65- to 90-year-old group, one sees progressive deterioration of the skin (wrinkles), hair (white and thin), eyes (increasing presbyopia and cataracts), ears (deafness), teeth (periodontal disease), joints (osteoarthritis), and spine (osteoporosis and herniated discs), with a marked diminution in physical abilities. Replacement of functional cells in the heart, liver, kidney, and lung by connective tissue or fat makes the individual increasingly more sensitive to various insults and injurious agents. Infection is often the terminal process leading to death[8] (see Fig. 5–2).

Role of Neoplasia and Cardiovascular Disease

In discussing this spectrum of age-related diseases, it is interesting to note that if all cancers were cured, the average projected life span of an individual would only increase by approximately 3 years. If all cardiovascular diseases were cured, the average life span would only increase by 10 years.[9] Indeed, if all diseases were cured, the life span would

Table 5–4. *Estimation of Life Span*

Cause of Death	Gain in Years in Expectation of Life if Cause was Eliminated	
	At Birth	At Age 65
Major cardiovascular and renal diseases	10.9	10.0
Heart diseases	5.9	4.9
Vascular diseases affecting CNS	1.3	1.2
Malignant neoplasms	2.3	1.2
Accidents, excluding motor vehicular	0.6	0.1
Motor vehicle accidents	0.6	0.1
Influenza and pneumonia	0.5	0.2
Infectious diseases (excluding tuberculosis)	0.2	0.1
Diabetes mellitus	0.2	0.2
Tuberculosis	0.1	0.0

(Adapted from life tables published by the National Center of Health Statistics, US Public Health Service and US Bureau of the Census, "Some Demographic Aspects of Aging in the United States," February, 1973.)

be extended by a matter of only several years (Table 5–4). It is, therefore, a reasonable premise that aging is an intrinsic phenomenon in humans that is accelerated by multiple associated factors. As the major diseases are cured, we shall still die in the 80- to 100-age range, owing to an increased incidence of accidents and infection aggravated by poor host responses (see Fig. 5–2).

THEORIES OF ETIOLOGY OF AGING

In discussing theories of aging, one must keep in mind which factors are causes and which are consequences. One theory of aging suggests a genetically programmed cell death, or cessation of all cellular growth. Accumulation of somatic mutations could result in structural and functional changes in the neuroendocrine, vascular, connective tissue, and immune systems (Table 5–5). We already accept a *mul-*

Table 5–5. *Theories of Aging*

Genetic—all cells
  Programmed in genome
  Somatic mutation
    Error-prone
    Karyotypic abnormalities

Control—homeostasis
  Neuroendocrine
    CNS, hypothalamus, first- and second-order endocrine glands
      (pituitary, ovary, etc.)
    Target-cell receptors (e.g., endometrium)
  Immune system
    Autoimmune antigen and antibody increase
    Decrease in primary B-cell response
    Decrease in natural killer cells

Extracellular—matrix components altered
  Increase in binding of collagen
  Increase in free radical effects on cells
  Mesenchymal structural alterations (fibrosis, osteoporosis)

tifactorial etiology for neoplasia and other diseases, and should adopt a similar view for the etiology of aging.

It has also been suggested that aging merely represents a summation of disease processes occurring over a lifetime, despite strong evidence for an intrinsic phenomenon that regulates the maximum life span in each particular species.[10] Multiple disease processes obviously accelerate and accentuate the aging processes and result in early deaths, sometimes in childhood, before the aged phenotype becomes manifest. Congenital abnormalities, inborn errors of metabolism, injury from various infectious agents, physical injury including radiation from the sun, nutritional excesses, deficiencies, and imbalances, drugs and pollutants in the environment, and injurious immune reactions all aggravate aging processes or, indeed, may "prematurely" terminate the life span. All these agents may produce somatic mutations or altered nucleotide sequences, but germ-cell mutations appear rare. Therefore, the effects of these injuries are not transmitted to future generations.

At present, three major areas are being investigated for their significance in the etiology of aging: (1) *genetic and environmental cellular factors,* (2) changes in cell-population-regulating *control mechanisms,* particularly the central nervous system (CNS), neuroendocrine, and immune systems, and (3) *extracellular* and vascular *degenerative* alterations.

Genetic and Environmental Cellular Factors

Those who believe that cellular factors are the basis of aging suggest that all cells wear out, and functional incapacity, if not actual cell death, eventually results. These investigators believe that cells are programmed at birth or are injured during life so as to cease division and to make errors in transcription and translation that eventually lead to atrophy or cell death, with a resultant functional deficiency of the tissue or organ. Classic examples of organs that *involute* or *atrophy* include the *thymus, testis, ovary, uterus,* and *breast.*

Programmed Aging

The evidence that each species has a given life span appears to be indisputable. Animals in the wild have a shortened life span because of natural predators. Even animals kept in a germ-free environment have a defined life span that is only slightly prolonged by low-calorie diets, antioxidants, and freedom from infection. That certain individuals have a family history of a *shorter life span* is often related to a *genetic susceptibility* to diseases such as *hypertension* and *diabetes,* which have life-diminishing effects.

Classic diseases of premature aging such as infantile progeria (Hutchinson-Gilford syndrome), adult progeria (Werner's syndrome), and, some would suggest, juvenile diabetes, exhibit striking signs of the aging phenomenon independent of environmental insults and other disease processes[11] (Table 5–6).

Hayflick's elegant demonstration in the 1960's that fibroblasts have a defined number of generations, that is, 40 to 60, must be considered to be of great significance, even though such a phenomenon has not been elucidated for epithelial cells[12,13] (Table 5–7). Aging cells in the *heart* and *brain* are *postmitotic,* and do not divide; thus their lack of remaining generations is not significant.

In experiments with transplanted bone marrow stem cells in congeneic mice, continued division occurs for at least 8 successive passages.[14] The doubling time is less in genetic diseases (Table 5–8).

Table 5–6.   *Aging Syndromes*

Down's syndrome
Werner's syndrome (adult progeria)
Cockayne's syndrome
Hutchinson-Gilford syndrome (infantile progeria)
Ataxia-telangiectasia
Seip syndrome (generalized lipodystrophy, hereditary type)
Cervical lipodysplasia, familial
Klinefelter's syndrome
Turner's syndrome
Steinert's disease (myotonic dystrophy)

(Modified from Martin, G.M.: Genetic syndromes in man with potential relevance to the pathobiology of aging. *In* Genetic Effects of Aging. Edited by D. Bergsma and D.E. Harrison. New York, Alan R. Liss for the National Foundation–March of Dimes, BD:OAS XIV(1), 1978.)

Table 5–7.   *Embryonic Fibroblasts*

Species	Range of Population Doublings for Cultured Normal Embryo Fibroblasts	Mean Maximum Life Span yr
Galapagos tortoise	90–125	175 (?)
Man	40–60	110
Mink	30–35	10
Chicken	15–35	30 (?)
Mouse	14–28	3.5

(Adapted from Hayflick, L.: The cell biology of human aging. N. Engl. J. Med., *295*:1305, 1976.)

Table 5–8.   *Population Doublings*

Syndrome	Age (yr)	No. Population Doublings in vitro
Progeria	9	2
Werner's (patient 1)	48	2
Werner's (patient 2)	48	8
Werner's (patient 3)	37	10
Werner's (patient 4)	43	4.5
Progeria	5	30

(Modified from Martin, G.M., Sprague, C.A., and Epstein, C.J.: Replicative life-span of cultivated human cells. Effects of donor's age, tissue, and genotype. Lab. Invest., *23*:86, 1970 © U.S.–Canadian Division of the International Academy of Pathology.)

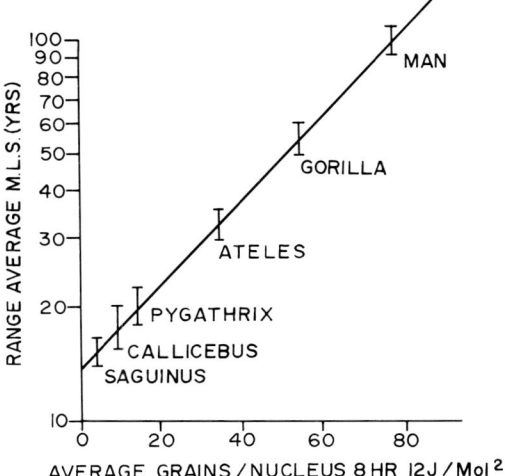

Figure 5–3. Correlation of the average number of grains incorporated per nucleus during unscheduled DNA synthesis with the maximum life span (M.L.S.) of 6 primate species. Fibroblasts from each species were irradiated with 12 J ultraviolet and incubated in the presence of 2 μC/ml ³H-thymidine and 2 mmol hydroxyurea for 8 hours. (From Hart, R.W., and Daniel, F.B.: Genetic stability in vitro and in vivo. *In* Aging, Cancer and Cell Membranes. Edited by C. Borek, C.M. Fenoglio, and D.W. King. New York, Thieme-Stratton, 1980.)

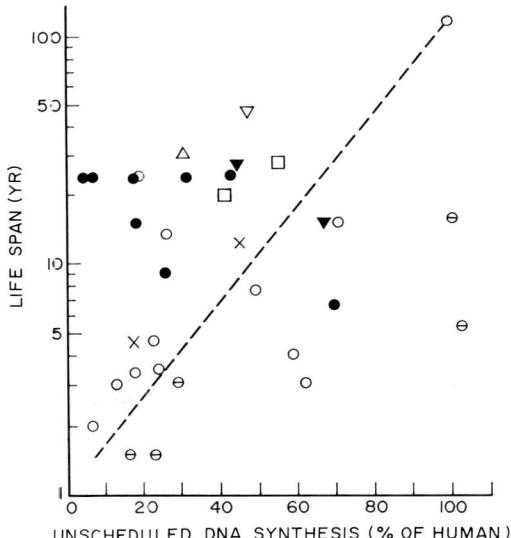

Figure 5–4. The relation of repair potential to life span in 34 species of mammals. Abscissa: unscheduled DNA synthesis (% of human); ordinate: life span (yr). The symbols denote groups of species as follows: ×, Marsupialia; ⊖, Insectivora; ●, Primates; ○, Lagomorpha; ◐, Rodentia; △ Cetacea; □ Carnivora; ▽ Perissodactyla; ▼, Artiodactyla. A broken line indicates a presumptive correlation between life span and the ability of unscheduled DNA synthesis. (From Kato, H., et al.: Absence of correlation between DNA repair in ultraviolet irradiated mammalian cells and life span of the donor species. Jpn. J. Gen., 55:99, 1980.)

It has also been suggested that rather than actual cell death or cell loss programmed in the genome, the cell's individual genetic control mechanisms proceed through a period of differentiation and development whereby at different stages in life, such as puberty and menopause, different portions of the genome are expressed. The lack of expression of some portions of the genome after a certain number of divisions, transcriptions, or control interactions may diminish function and effectiveness without causing actual cell death.

Environmental Factors Producing Somatic Mutations

With age, protein synthesis decreases in fidelity. It has been postulated that this change involves errors of tRNA (for accuracy) and rRNA (for efficiency) in protein production[15] (Figs. 5–3 and 5–4). This change may also be linked to decreased efficiency in DNA repair, with resultant errors in transcription.

The genetic "error-prone" theory suggests that somatic mutations cause errors in translational, transcriptional, and DNA repair mechanisms, all of which lead to macromolecular deficiencies.[16] The protein error-correcting machinery is in operation, but not with perfect efficiency.[17] This theory is not in favor at present.

Hart and Daniel[18] believe that a general loss of homokinesis results from defects in the DNA repair mechanism and replication, and that the accumulation of damaged DNA is not exclusively equated with mutation. Rapidly dividing intermitotic cells accumulate DNA damage and mutations, whereas postmitotic cells accumulate DNA damage, but not necessarily demonstrable mutations.

Cell Populations with Regulatory Control Mechanisms

Many investigators believe that cells and tissues of the body do not all age equally and that the major aging phenomena occur in the particular cell populations exerting control functions; included are cells of the CNS, the neuroendocrine system, and the immune system.

"Neuroendocrine" Theory of Aging

Those who support this concept suggest that a program for aging is genetically encoded in the brain and is expressed in a scheduled timetable of growth, maturation, and aging, and that controlling signals from the brain are relayed to peripheral tissue through hormonal and neural stimulation or inhibition.[19] Considerable controversy exists as to whether *increased degradation, decreased hormone synthesis* and *secretion* rate, or *decreased target organ sensitivity* (number of receptor sites, binding, or internalization) to the hormone is a general phenomenon in aging. Obvious hormonal changes are associated with puberty and with cessation of the reproductive cycle.

Denckla[20] has found that rats that have undergone hypophysectomy have an increased life span. With this evidence, he postulated the existence of a neuropituitary hormone, synthesized and released at puberty, that limits life span by impairing adversely a set of cell responses to thyroxine and other hormones.

Immune System

A second major control system of many tissues is the immune system (Table 5–9), which is an attractive target for investigation because: (1) with age, several immune functions decline; (2) the rise and fall in the activity of the immune system with age is inversely related to that of the death rate; and (3) the decline in normal functions of the immune system seems to trigger neoplastic, autoimmune, and immune complex diseases of the blood and blood vessels, which in turn have harmful secondary effects on various organs.

Table 5–9. *Changes in the Immune System with Age*

Lymphocytes	No change in total number
	Decrease in B-cell maturation
	Increase in suppressor (T) cells
	Decrease in helper (T) cells
Complement	Deficient complement levels associated with age, neoplasia, and infection
Antibody	Lack of thymic-dependent antibody response
	Decrease in primary response to new antigens
	Increase in globulins associated with secondary response and autoimmunity (benign monoclonal gammopathies)
	Increase in idiotypic antibodies to receptors
Immune Complexes (Ag, Ab, C)	Presence in all obsolescent glomeruli
	Presence in many vessel injuries
	Presence in many tissues previously injured
	Presence as amyloid either as light chains or in complexes with other protein and carbohydrates
Tolerance	Decrease in natural and acquired tolerance
Lymphoid tissue	Involution of thymus
	Loss of thymic hormones
	Atrophy, hypertrophy of some lymph nodes
	Hyperplasia of selected lymphoid elements particularly in bone marrow
	Infiltration of lymphoid tissue in various organs (e.g., thyroid)

Walford[21] has reviewed the following evidence in favor of the dominant role of the *immune response* in determining *longevity*: (1) changing the H-2 locus in congeneic mice increases their life span;[22] (2) the lower quality of nutrition seen in the aged is accompanied by a lowered immune response; (3) the lower temperature also seen in the aged lowers the immune response; and (4) the life span of experimental animals can be increased by bone marrow and thymic transplants.

Evidence against the immune system's being the determining factor in longevity includes the observation that nude mice with thymic aplasia and immune deficiencies live approximately as long as normal mice and that insects with no immune response may have a varying life span.

It is controversial whether intercurrent disease compromises normal function or whether the decline in immune function predisposes individuals to disease. The latter viewpoint is favored for the following reasons: the onset of decline in thymus-derived T-cell function occurs as early as sexual maturity with thymic involution, long before immunodeficiency states develop. *Immune deficiency, amyloid deposition,* and *autoimmunity* in mice that have undergone thymectomy neonatally can be prevented or reversed by reconstitution with *syngeneic grafts* of young thymuses.[23]

Burnet[24] has emphasized the double jeopardy of aging, which consists of a diminished immune function and an increased prevalence of forbidden clones of cells. Thus, the normal immune surveillance mechanisms are weakened just when they are needed most.

These *forbidden clones* may arise from any of the mechanisms suggested by the error theories of aging, so that either cells of a "non-self" type are produced or a misrecognition of normal for abnormal cells takes place, with the subsequent production of autoantibodies.

Another dimension is added when one considers that susceptibility to disease and immune responsiveness are governed by genes linked to the major histocompatibility complex (MHC). A number of autoimmune disorders associated with the HLA-A1-B8-DW3 linkage group have a higher incidence in females;[25] however, females live longer in all animal species, so this antigen group is not the dominant factor in longevity.

Populations of immune cells that produce humoral factors regulating coagulation, collagen synthesis, vasospasm, chemotaxis, and a host of other important reactions must also be considered in this group of controlling immune influences.

Extracellular Factors Affecting Aging Processes

Vascular System

Many investigators have suggested that aging is a direct result of *injury* to *vessels*. These researchers cite the common occurrence of arteriosclerosis in the aged, with its many complications affecting the heart, brain, kidney, and peripheral circulation. They further suggest that thickening of the arteries and arterioles decreases nutritional supplies and oxygen to the tissues as well as allows toxic metabolites such as CO_2 and lactic acid to accumulate.[26]

Changes in the extracellular environment that result from damage in the vascular compartment may alter the structural configuration, permeability, and function of the ground substance. Nevertheless, it must be recognized that capillaries and venules, in which much of the transport of nutritional substances takes place, are not affected in arteriosclerosis. Basement membranes thicken, however, with increased collagen and deposition of serum proteins, immunoglobulins, and in some cases amyloid. Although vessel disease plays an important role in diminishing an individual's life span, the removal of atherosclerosis from vessels would still not markedly increase the maximal life span.

Extracellular Matrix

Considerable discussion has revolved around the *extracellular components* in aging. Collagen is believed to have increased cross-linking, decreased turnover (although turnover is always small), and increased degradation.[27] These reactions are partially controlled by antioxidants, pH, ion concentration, and disease states. Elastin disappears from large vessels, whereas collagen, proteoglycans, and serum proteins are deposited in basement membranes. The gross effects of disorders of the ground substances, resulting in dehydration with wrinkling of the skin, are obvious. It appears unlikely that these extracellular components are the prime cause of cellular malfunction, despite problems of permeability and diffusion of substrates or metabolites. Nevertheless, the escape from cellular repair mechanisms and the general disorganization of extracellular matrices produce important lesions of aging with significant consequences. Diverticula, hernias, prolapse, rupture of intervertebral discs, cataracts, and numerous alterations of the skeletal muscular system are prime examples of defects in the extracellular matrix associated with the aging process.

MORPHOLOGIC AND FUNCTIONAL CHANGES IN CELLS AND TISSUES

General Alterations in Structure and Function

Morphologic Alterations

Aging is often represented by *cellular* and *organellar atrophy,* which includes a decrease in size or function as well as an actual loss of cells. This type of atrophy results from a

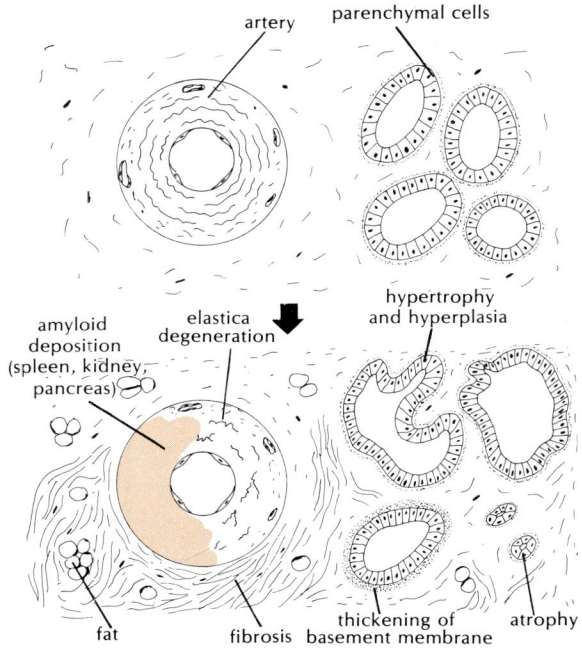

Figure 5–5. Tissue changes in aging.

lack of compensatory ability to replace structural organelles that may provide alternate pathways of intermediary metabolism for functions for which the cell is normally responsible. *Compensatory* cellular reactions, that is, *hyperplasia* and *hypertrophy*, are often followed by more abnormal responses including metaplasia, dysplasia, and occasionally neoplasia. Vacuoles, inclusions, pigment, amyloid, and immune complex deposits are all commonly associated with aged cells (Fig. 5–5).

Cell loss and random *atrophy, hypertrophy,* and *hyperplasia* of cells may interrupt architectural relationships, disorganize receptor sites, block circulatory channels needed for substrate incorporation and secretion of extracellular products, interfere with endocrine and neural control mechanisms, and inhibit cell migration in a manner that ultimately interferes with function (Table 5–10).

Table 5–10. *Cellular Alterations with Age*

Parameters Generally Increased

1. Cell size and volume
2. Nuclear size and volume
3. Nucleolar size and number
4. RNA and protein content
5. Vacuoles (lipid, glycogen, water)
6. Autophagosomes

Parameters Generally Decreased

1. DNA replication and repair
2. RNA synthesis
3. Protein synthesis

Functional Changes

Ultimately, the *functional ability* of a cell, tissue, organ, or organism is based on its ability to maintain the stability of its unit components. This maintenance is partly a function of the DNA repair mechanisms. Defective DNA repair can lead to the accumulation of lesions or mutations, which either may be lethal or may lead to an altered phenotype, as seen in neoplasia.

Of great importance in aging is the *"escape"* of extracellular components from cellular repair and controlled turnover mechanisms. Alteration in structure and disorganization in matrix patterns can cause significant functional loss.

Cell Loss and Natural Death of Cells

It is well recognized that the aged organism loses cells in every organ, either because cells die as a result of injury and are not replaced, or because cells unassociated with a specific disease process drop out. Cell loss is most common in organs composed of postmitotic cells in which cell division and replacement is impossible. That cells lost by every organ system are replaced to a varying degree by connective tissue or fat results in some disorganization of function. The presence of inflammatory foci suggests that a disease process rather than physiologic aging is the primary cause. The organs in which prominent cell loss occurs are noted in the following sections.

Heart and Cardiovascular System

The loss of myocardial cells with aging or with disease is associated with hypertrophy of the remaining cells and replacement of lost cells by connective tissue or fat.

Central Nervous System

The loss of cells in the brain is associated with a decrease in total brain weight.[28] This selective loss is not seen in all areas of the brain. Lost are norepinephrine-producing cells in the locus ceruleus, dopamine-producing cells of the substantia nigra, cholinergic cells of the hippocampus, and other neurons in different portions of the cerebral cortex and hypothalamus.[29]

Thymus and Immune System

The cell loss that occurs in the thymus with involution starting at puberty is accompanied by a decreased response to T-dependent antigens.[30] This decrease is greater than with T-independent antigens. Other effects are a decreased response to mitogenic agents, a decreased T-cell affinity for antigenic determinants with an autoidiotypic antibody to the antigen-combining site, and a postulated increase of suppressor cells. There are also increases in autoantibodies, production of immune complexes, and decreased tolerance.[31]

Ovary, Testis, and Reproductive System

In the ovary, a significant *loss* of *ova* is seen, from several hundred thousand at puberty to a few thousand postmenopausally.[32] The number of *spermatogonia* is *decreased*.[33] Target tissues, particularly the breast and endometrium, lose their hormone responsiveness, eventually leading to their atrophy.

Cell Organelle Atrophy and Degeneration

Nucleus

Aged cells often have *large nuclei* representing an attempt at compensatory repair. Although many cells have altered karyotypes, definitive alterations in banding patterns in aged cells have not been identified. A loss of the *repressed X chromosome* has been noted.[34] Although sister chromatid exchange rates are the same as in the young, the inducibility by mitogens of these rates is decreased. Hart et al.[35] have shown an in vitro *decrease* in *unscheduled DNA synthesis* representing a *decrease in efficiency* of *DNA repair enzymes;* this work is presently being carried out in vivo on experimental animals. Whether injury to DNA occurs in genetic transmission or is acquired during the life of a cell, improper repair mechanisms will have a significant effect on all cytoplasmic activities.

Cytoplasm

The cytoplasm of the aged cell often shows less organization of the *endoplasmic reticulum* (ER) and the presence of more free ribosomes. The fidelity of protein synthesis decreases, and various alterations in structure and activity of various enzymes have been noted. In particular, the adaptive enzymes glucokinase, nicotinamide-adenine dinucleotide phosphate (NADPH), cytochrome C reductase, and acetylcholinesterase are reduced. However, the glucokinase activity can be restored in vitro with the addition of corticosteroid hormones.[37]

Primary antibody synthesis is decreased, whereas autoantibody production increases. In addition, the abnormal production of excess light chains and macroglobulins are well known. The rate of *collagen synthesis* usually decreases in the aged, especially in inflammatory repair reactions, but albumin synthesis may actually increase to offset a greater protein loss from the kidneys.[38] Some *hormone synthesis* is decreased (often estrogens), although for many endocrine glands, reliable studies are not available.[39]

Mitochondria may have abnormal cristae with varying alterations in size and shape. *Lysosomes,* particularly autophagic vacuoles, may increase in aged cells. The greater number of *autophagic vacuoles* might suggest a higher protein turnover of cellular components associated with increased damage, perhaps compensated for by increased nucleolar ribosomal precursors in the nuclei. Exact turnover times in aging and disease states have not been described, however, and other factors such as hypoxia and degeneration associated with chronic disease may play a role. *Myofibrils* in muscle show a decreased ability to contract, and *microfilaments* in macrophages appear to function poorly in phagocytosis. Membrane receptors, particularly those for hormones, for example, insulin receptors, are decreased in the aged cell.

The increased numbers of *vacuoles* and *inclusions* present in aged cells are extensively discussed in Chapter 6. The aged cell has more than its share of lipid, water, glycogen, and protein vacuoles, abnormal crystals, and deposits of pigment, particularly lipofuscin and hemosiderin.

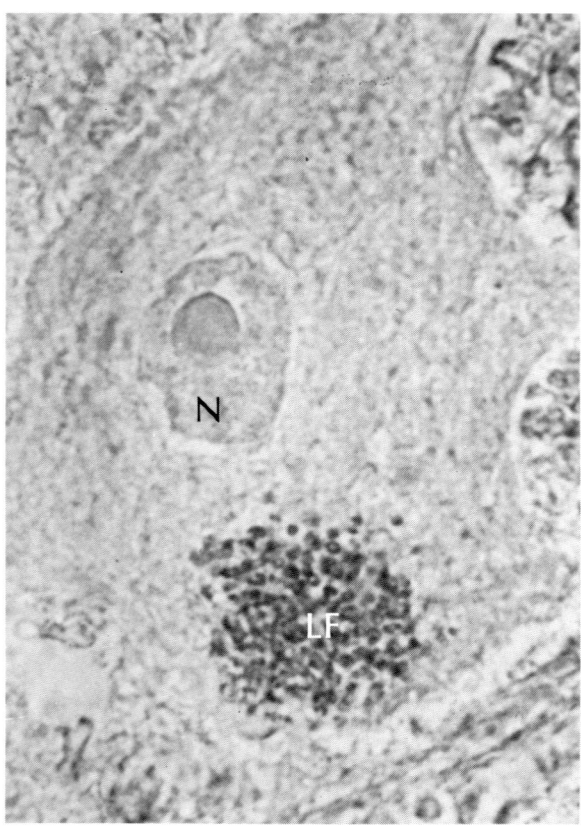

Figure 5–6. A magnocellular neuron is seen in an aging Macaca mulatta red nucleus. An unstained section examined in a bright field microscope contains a prominent nucleus (N) and a lipofuscin (LF) collection. (Courtesy of Dr. H. Barden, Psychiatric Institute, New York.)

Lipofuscin (ceroid) consists of 60% protein, 25% lipid, and 10% carbohydrate, stains with both acid-fast and sudanophilic stains, fluoresces under the polarizing microscope, and contains characteristic lysosomal enzymes including acid phosphatase and cathepsins.[40] Lipofuscin is believed to represent polymerized cellular products unable to be degraded, which are mainly lipids because lysosomes are deficient in lipases (Fig. 5–6).

Most of the cellular functional changes are probably unrelated to morphologic changes such as lipofuscin or amyloid deposits. Rather, aging changes are subtle, and the decreased function of individual cells is apparent only when they are organized into tissues and organs in which concerted action must be demonstrated. Lipofuscin levels are increased in several disease states (Table 5–11).

Table 5–11. *Disorders in which Lipofuscin Levels are Increased*

Neuronal ceroid lipofuscinosis, dominant or Parry type
Presenile dementia
Tremor of intention, ataxia, and lipofuscinosis
Abetalipoproteinemia
Amaurotic family idiocy, juvenile type
Cockayne's syndrome
Neuronal ceroid lipofuscinosis, infantile Finnish type
Down's syndrome

(Modified from Martin, G.M.: Genetic syndromes in man with potential relevance to the pathobiology of aging. *In* Genetic Effects of Aging. Edited by D. Bergsma and D.E. Harrison. New York, Alan R. Liss for the National Foundation–March of Dimes, BD:OAS XIV(1), 1978.)

Cellular Hypertrophy, Hyperplasia, Metaplasia, and Neoplasia

Cardiac cells are a prime example of cells that are unable to divide but that compensate for injury by *hypertrophy*. Skeletal and smooth muscle cells, and occasionally liver cells, also enlarge when subjected to increased stress.

Hyperplasia, an increase in the number of cells, is commonly seen in the aged bone marrow, particularly in nests of proliferating lymphocytes, which may be related to the plasma cell dyscrasias with abnormal immunoglobulins that occur more frequently in the aged population.[41] Myointimal proliferation (hyperplasia) is seen in several forms of arteriosclerosis.[42] Particularly noteworthy is the hyperplasia of the prostate present in almost all men over the age of 60. Focal collections of hyperplastic cells are also commonly seen in the endocrine glands, including pituitary, thyroid, parathyroid, adrenal, and pancreas.[43] Work from this laboratory has shown a marked increase in the calcitonin-containing C cells of the thyroid. Proliferation of bile duct epithelium in the liver and epidermidization of the pulmonary bronchiolar cells may be aging phenomena or disease-related hyperplastic lesions.

Solitary or multiple endocrine *adenomas* are occasionally associated with increased production of hormone; these growths are usually nonfunctional and are commonly seen as an extension of hyperplasias already noted.

Polyps of the colon, endometrium, and larynx are most commonly seen in the aged population. Hyperplastic reactions may sometimes become *metaplastic*, particularly in the prostate, cervix, bladder, bronchial epithelium, and endometrium. *Neoplastic* changes are most commonly seen in the skin, breast, cervix, colon, ovary, prostate, and lung.[44] Many syndromes are associated with an increased susceptibility to neoplasia (Table 5–12).

Table 5–12. *Syndromes or Lesions Associated with Increased Susceptibility to Neoplasms*

Aryl hydrocarbon hydroxylase inducibility
Cancer of the colon
Fibrocystic pulmonary dysplasia
Hashimoto's struma
Hemochromatosis, primary
Leiomyomata, hereditary multiple, of skin (and uterus?)
Polyposis, intestinal I (familial polyposis of the colon)
Polyposis, intestinal II (Peutz-Jeghers syndrome)
Polyposis, intestinal III (Gardner's syndrome)
Seborrheic keratoses
Xeroderma pigmentosum, mild type
Xeroderma pigmentosum
Ataxia-telangiectasia
Bloom's syndrome
Fanconi's pancytopenia
Werner's syndrome
Addison's disease and cerebral sclerosis
Down's syndrome
Klinefelter's syndrome
Turner's syndrome

(Modified from Martin, G.M.: Genetic syndromes in man with potential relevance to the pathobiology of aging. *In* Genetic Effects of Aging. Edited by D. Bergsma and D.E. Harrison. New York, Alan R. Liss for the National Foundation—March of Dimes, BD:OAS XIV(1), 1978.)

Extracellular Tissue Changes

Vessel Changes

The extracellular aging tissues include vessels, lymphatics, ligaments, tendons, and fascia containing collagen, elastin, proteoglycans, hyaluronic acid and other ground sub-

Table 5–13. *Components of Connective Tissue*

Collagen
Elastin
Reticulin

Glycosaminoglycans
  Sulfated
    Heparan sulfate
    Heparin
    Dermatan sulfate
    Keratan sulfate
    Chondroitin sulfate (4 + 6)
  Nonsulfated
    Hyaluronic acid

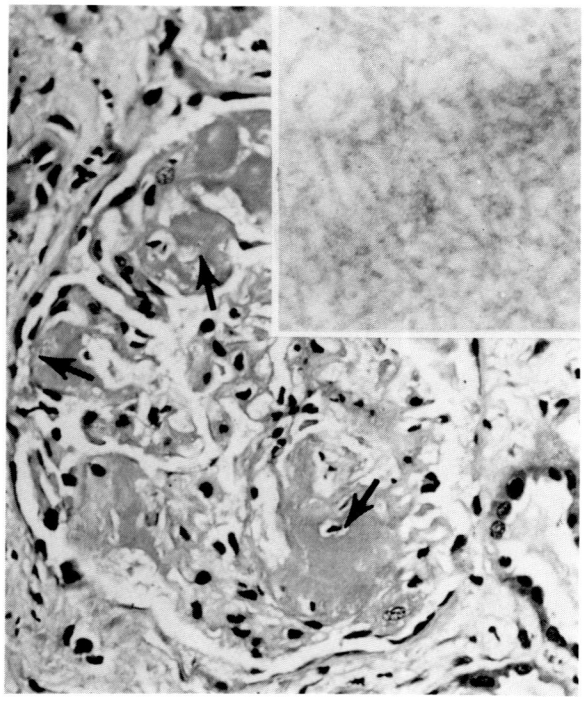

Figure 5–7. Amyloid (arrows) in kidney glomerulus. The inset is a transmission electron micrograph showing nonbranching amyloid fibrils.

stances (Table 5–13). The several types of arteriosclerosis represent a hyperplastic reaction in the intima and media, particularly of the myointimal cells, as well as deposits of lipid, calcium, and serum proteins in the walls of the vessels. The integrity of the lymphatics is particularly important when one considers the critical necessity for constant circulation of T cells in the immune defense reactions. Basement membrane thickening of capillaries occurs in aging,[45] but thickening of the basement membrane in the kidney and lung, organs most vulnerable to disease processes, may represent disease effects. Thickened basement membranes in the reproductive and endocrine glands are prominent, although their origin is obscure.

The presence of immune complexes and of amyloid deposits under the basement membrane, and sometimes in the extracellular space, is of great significance. The immune complexes are extensively discussed in Chapter 3.

Amyloidosis

This entity is associated with many disease states. The former classification of amyloidosis into primary, that is, occurring particularly in the heart and tongue, and secondary, characterized by deposits in the spleen, liver, and adrenal associated with chronic granulomatous disease states, no longer pertains because of newer knowledge on the composition of amyloid.

Amyloid is a proteinaceous aggregated substance of twisted, β-pleated sheet fibrils of great chemical diversity, but usually containing abnormal globulins. It appears as an eosinophilic homogeneous opaque mass with hematoxylin and eosin staining (Fig. 5–7).

Glenner[46] has classified amyloidosis into three major groups: (1) *acquired systemic amyloidosis*, (2) *organ-limited amyloidosis*, and (3) *localized deposition amyloidosis* (Table 5–14).

A major form of systemic amyloidosis occurs after recurrent or granulomatous infections, such as tuberculosis, or autoimmune diseases, such as rheumatoid arthritis. This amyloid type is associated with an isolated protein, which consists of a serum *protein (SAA)* with a molecular weight of 14,000 daltons that breaks down into tissue *protein (AA)* of 8,500 MW.[47] The SAA serum protein is synthesized by fibroblasts or monocytes, and hydrolytic enzymes remove 30 to 40 amino acids to produce the AA tissue protein. This altered immunoglobulin can neither be excreted nor metabolized and deposits itself in subendothelial spaces in the liver, kidney, spleen, and adrenal.

The *amyloid* associated with *immunocyte dyscrasias*, including monoclonal gammopathy, multiple myeloma, and primary macroglobulinemia, is considered to be principally a

Table 5–14. *Classification of Amyloidosis*

Clinicopathologic Process	Major Fibril Protein	Chemically Related Protein
Acquired systemic amyloidosis		
Immunocyte dyscrasias with amyloidosis	AL*	L
Primary macroglobulinemia (Waldenström's)	AL*	L
Heavy-chain disease	AL†	L*
Agammagloblinemia	AL†	L*
Other immunocytic neoplasms	AL†	†, ‡
Reactive systemic amyloidosis	AA*	A*
Acute recurrent and chronic supportive or granulomatous infections (e.g., tuberculosis)	AA*	A
Chronic inflammatory conditions (e.g., rheumatoid arthritis)	AA	A
Hodgkin's disease	AA	A
Nonlymphoid solid tumors (e.g., renal and bladder carcinoma)	‡	‡
Heredofamilial systemic amyloidosis		
Organ-limited amyloidosis		
Immunocyte-derived (diffuse or nodular)		
Respiratory tract	AL*	L*
Urinary tract; bone marrow and lymphoid system	AL†	L†
Cardiovascular ("senile" cardiomyopathy)	ASc_1	‡
Cerebral plaques; paired helical filaments	‡	‡
Cutaneous (lichenoid, macular)	‡	‡
Localized deposition		
Endocrine-organ- or tissue-associated		
Medullary carcinoma of thyroid	AE_1	Calcitonin
Insulinoma, islets of Langerhans in diabetes	‡	Insulin†
Tumors of pituitary, intestine, and pancreas (glucagonoma, gastrinoma)		Specific hormones
Plasmacytoma	AL†	L†
Conjunctival; laryngeal	‡	‡
Renal cases in "myeloma nephrosis"	AL†	L†
Specific nonlymphoid solid tumors		
Hereditary deposits		
Concretions		
In aged persons		

*Assumed initial derivation, individual exceptions may exist
†Postulated clinical derivation based on clinicopathologic evidence or preliminary chemical (non-amino-acid-sequence) data
‡No confirmed clinicopathologic or chemical evidence exists
A, amyloid; L, light chain
(Modified from Glenner, G.G.: Medical progress: amyloid deposits and amyloidosis. The β-fibrilloses. N. Engl. J. Med., *302*:1333, 1980.)

dimer of light chains with a molecular weight of 10,000 daltons × 2. These light chains are also incompletely metabolized, may be seen in plasma cells, are deposited in capillaries of several tissues, and are excreted in the urine as *Bence Jones protein*.

The third form of amyloid is deposited in localized form in various tissues, including the thyroid in medullary carcinoma and the islets of Langerhans in diabetes mellitus. It has been shown that the amyloid deposit of *medullary carcinoma* is in fact precalcitonin, and the *islet deposit* in diabetes is crystallized *proinsulin*.[48] Identity of these forms of amyloid with certain proteins suggests that any crystalline protein produced in excessive amounts, denatured and precipitated in a specific site, with characteristic electron-microscopic and histochemical characteristics, may be called amyloid.

Although the foregoing conditions are interesting and have proved to be valuable in elucidating immune mechanisms of various disease states, by far the most common ubiquitous deposits of amyloid are seen in the *aging process*. It has been suggested that the amount of amyloid increases linearly with aging, although at different rates in specific individuals. When carefully stained, cells of many individuals show some degree of amyloid deposition at death. These deposits are characteristically seen as subendothelial in the spleen, pancreas, and liver, as extracellular in the heart, where they are known as *senile cardiomyopathy*,[49] and as plaques in the cerebral vessels sometimes associated with paired helical filaments of *Alzheimer's disease*.[50] Other concretions, such as the corpora amylacea of the prostate, are also common in aged individuals.

In most instances of amyloid in the aged, although the material has both the specific histochemical staining reactions of amyloid (that is, Congo red, crystal violet, thioflavine T) and the appropriate electron-microscopic fibrillar pattern, the chemical composition has not been thoroughly investigated. It has been suggested that senile amyloid has characteristics similar to prealbumin.

Other Extracellular Changes

Changes in the ground substance, both generally and in specific sites, such as the lens protein, vitreous humor, the synovial fluid, and the nucleus pulposa of the intervertebral disc, result in specific alterations in both structure and function. Structural alterations and the consequent weakening of fascia, tendons, and ligaments increase the number of diverticula, particularly of the esophagus, colon, bladder, and kidney tubules, hernias, particularly inguinal, abdominal, and diaphragmatic, and prolapse, particularly in the rectum, bladder, and uterus.

These changes, along with bone loss and demineralization (osteoporosis), degeneration of joints, and impaired repair processes bode poorly for the aged population.

SPECIFIC ORGAN CHANGES: STRUCTURE AND FUNCTION

Many of the specific organ changes associated with the aging phenomenon are often only described at postmortem examination. In fact, a serious, documented discrepancy exists between clinical and autopsy diagnoses for many diseases (Table 5–15).

Table 5–15. *Discrepancies Between Clinical and Autopsy Causes of Death*

Category	No. of Cases per Category	No. of Diagnoses per Category	No. of Errors per Category	% of Error
Cardiovascular disorders	386	569	365	64.0
Neoplasms	230	234	85	36.3
Respiratory disorders	157	160	87	54.4
Cerebrovascular disorders	127	127	89	70.0
Renal disorders	58	69	56	81.2
Gastrointestinal disorders	53	59	29	49.1
Hepatobiliary and pancreatic disorders	49	50	39	78.0
Congenital disorders	31	34	16	47.0
Neonatal disorders	25	29	13	44.8
Systemic infections	22	22	13	59.0
Peripheral vascular disorders	17	17	4	23.5
Metabolic and endocrine disorders	18	18	7	38.9
Intracranial infections and degenerations	13	13	9	69.2
Skeletal-neuromuscular disorders	12	15	5	33.3
Autoimmune disorders	6	6	5	83.3

(Modified from Gwynne, J.F.: Death certification in Dunedin hospitals. N.Z. Med. J., 86:77, 1977.)

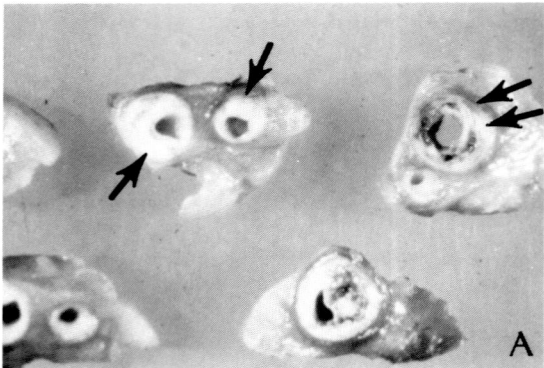

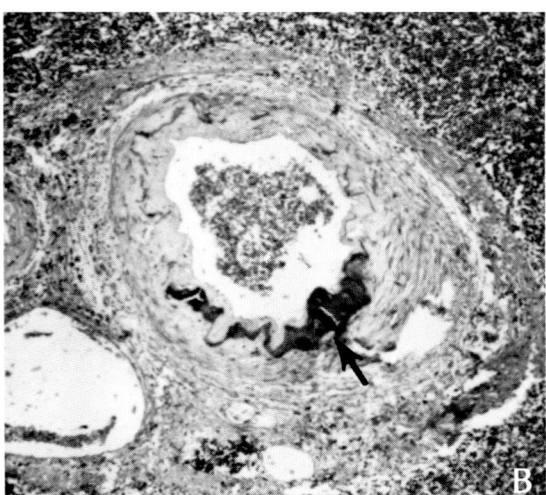

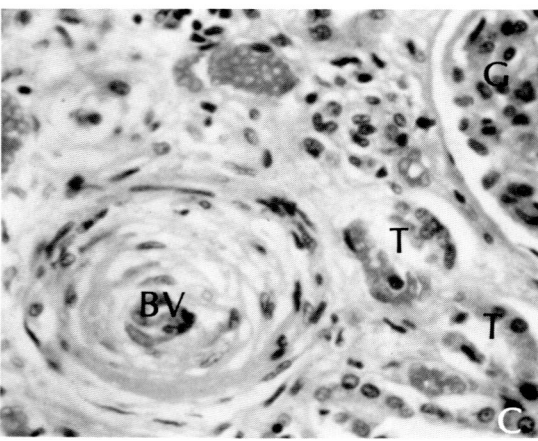

Figure 5–8. Vascular abnormalities. *A,* Atherosclerosis involving the vessels are narrowed eccentrically (arrows) and also appear laminated (double arrows). *B,* Mönckeberg's sclerosis involves a medium-sized artery. The calcified tunica media (arrow) appears basophilic using standard staining techniques. *C,* Arteriolonephrosclerosis with prominent "onion skinning" of the blood vessels (BV). Renal tubules (T) and part of a glomerulus (G) are also present.

Vascular

Arteries

Aside from the gross physical changes seen with aging, the single most prominent lesion associated with aging is arteriosclerosis. Arteriosclerosis means hardening of the arteries and is usually divided into three types: *atherosclerosis, Mönckeberg's medial calcific sclerosis,* and *arteriolosclerosis.* Nearly every organ shows some evidence of the presence of at least one type of arteriosclerosis (Fig. 5–8).

Atherosclerosis. The most important arteriosclerotic lesions are those of atherosclerosis because of the tissues they affect. Atherosclerosis affects principally the aorta and the coronary and cerebral vessels, along with other main branches of the aorta such as the iliac, renal, and carotid arteries (Fig. 5–8). The complications of myocardial infarct, stroke, and peripheral ischemia are discussed in Chapter 3.

Mönckeberg's Medial Calcific Sclerosis. This second type of arteriosclerosis affects arteries in both organs and peripheral arteries. Although histologically readily apparent in the vessels of the wrists and ankles, the deposits of calcium in the medial layers of these arteries is of little physiologic significance (see Fig. 5–8).

Arteriolosclerosis. This disorder affects the smaller arterioles and consists of proliferation of the intimal and medial layers, often with infiltration of serum proteins, including immunoglobulin (see Fig. 5–8). Arteriolosclerosis is most commonly seen in the kidney, spleen, pancreas, and periadrenal vessels. The constriction caused by thickening of the vessel walls sometimes results in ischemia and scarring of the tissue it supplies. In the kidney, this constriction may be associated with hypoxic stimulation of the juxtaglomerular apparatus to produce renin, which may eventually result in hypertension.

A fourth arterial lesion is endarteritis obliterans, seen particularly in the ovary, uterus, and the prostate with increasing age.

Veins and Lymphatics

Lesions of the veins include saphenous varicosities and hemorrhoidal varicosities of the rectum. Both often contain secondary thrombi of the vessels.

The lymphatics have not been carefully studied in aged individuals, but the lymph nodes often show atrophy and fibrosis.

Heart

Age-associated morphologic changes in the heart appear to be progressive and are generally irreversible. The changes include myofibrillar atrophy, infiltration of the interstitial tissue of the myocardium with connective tissue, fat, and sometimes amyloid, and the intracellular deposition of lipofuscin. The pericardium may show serous atrophy and focal areas of fibrosis (healed pericarditis)[51] (Table 5–16).

Table 5–16. *Cardiovascular Changes Associated with Age*

Pericardium	Fibrosis
	Serous atrophy
Endocardium and valves	Elastosis, fibrosis
	Calcification of annulus fibrosus
	Dilatation of valve ring
Myocardium	Fibrosis
	Brown atrophy
	Amyloidosis
	Hypertrophy
	Lipofuscin deposits
Coronary vessels	Atherosclerosis
	Arteriolosclerosis

Endocardium

A gray-white thickening of the endocardium that develops in the first decade is seen first in the right atrium and later progresses into both ventricles and the left atrium. With advancing age, this thickening becomes more prominent with proliferation of the elastin and collagen fibers of the endocardium. Degeneration and endocardial sclerosis may occur with: (1) fragmentation and disorganization of elastic fibers; (2) collagenous endocardial reduplication with hyaline sclerosis of the endocardium and myocardium; and (3) vacuolization and focal hypertrophy of muscle cells with lipid infiltration.

The valves of the endocardium may have *marantic vegetations* composed of edematous fibrinous excrescences on the valve edges. In addition, lipid infiltrates of the valve leaflets may become organized and calcified. A variant of atherosclerosis frequently seen with age is myxoid degeneration of the muscle cells at the base of the valve. *Floppy valves* with lack of elastic fibers are also seen.

Myocardium

Atherosclerotic or arteriosclerotic changes in the elastin fibrils of the media of peripheral arteries of the heart may increase vascular resistance, decrease oxygen perfusion, and raise blood pressure.

Myocardial ischemic changes are described in Chapter 3. In addition to the loss of myofibrils and the presence of lipofuscin, ultrastructural changes in the Z bands and, often, a decreased number of mitochondria are present.[52] Lipid vacuoles may be seen intracellularly in injured cells. An attempt at nuclear hyperplasia and persistent DNA repair mechanisms may result in hyperchromatic enlarged nuclei, sometimes with hyperdiploid chromosomes. *Amyloid* is commonly found in small quantities in and around aged myocardial cells, in the interstitial tissue, and in the walls of blood vessels.

Lung

The total lung capacity of aged individuals is not believed to be appreciably reduced when adjusted for sex and height; however, the residual volume increases and the vital capacity thus decreases with age. Moreover, numerous diseases throughout life may reduce the pulmonary reserve.[53]

The maximum oxygen uptake by the lung for transport to tissues peaks at approximately age 20 and then decreases steadily, dropping by approximately 30% by the age of 60.[54] Changes in the shape of the thorax may occur, including slight kyphosis of the spine, intervertebral disc disease, thickening of the scapular muscles, and a tendency toward a *"barrel chest."* The alveolar ducts and respiratory bronchioles may dilate at the expense of the surrounding alveoli, which become more shallow. This phenomenon, *duct ectasia,* apparently correlates well with age.

Liebow has noted alveolar epithelial proliferation with a loss of alveolar elasticity, an increased calcification of bronchial cartilage, and an increase in bronchial glands with age.

All older individuals have some degree of emphysema, known as senile emphysema[55] (Fig. 5–9). The increased interstitial fibrosis of age cannot be distinguished from that following pneumonitis. This difficulty in distinguishing aging from a postdisease state is also true of squamous metaplasia of terminal bronchioles. Carcinomas increase in incidence with age, largely in relation to smoking[56] (Table 5–17).

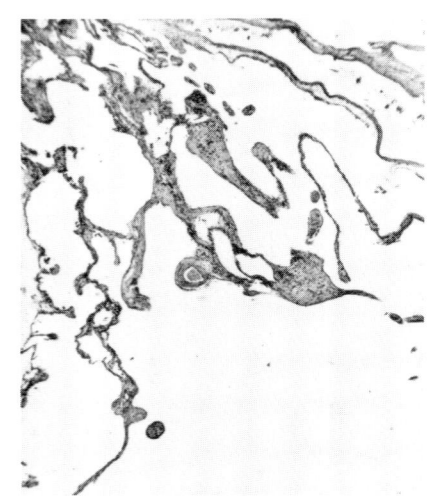

Figure 5–9. In pulmonary emphysema, the air spaces are distended and there is terminal clubbing of the ruptured alveolar septa.

Table 5–17. *Pulmonary Changes Associated with Age*

Epiglottis and larynx	Papilloma
	Amyloidosis
Lung	Bronchiolar epidermidization
	Duct ectasia
	Amyloidosis
	Fibrosis
	Senile emphysema
	Atelectasis
	Carcinoma

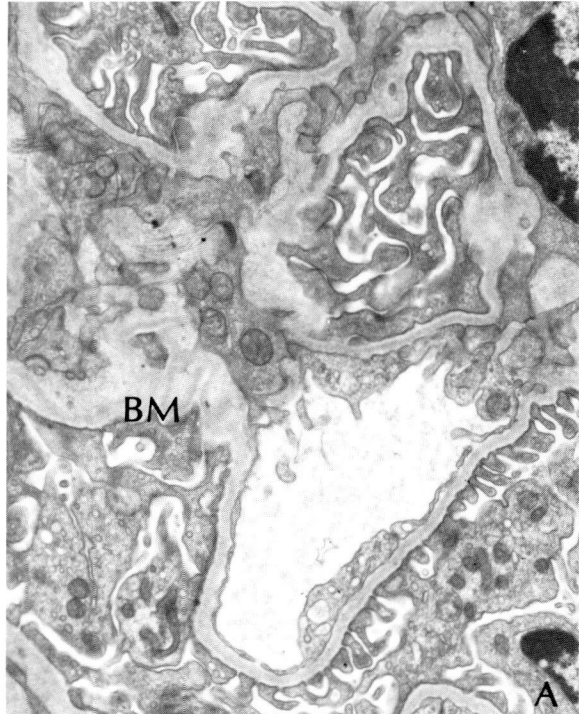

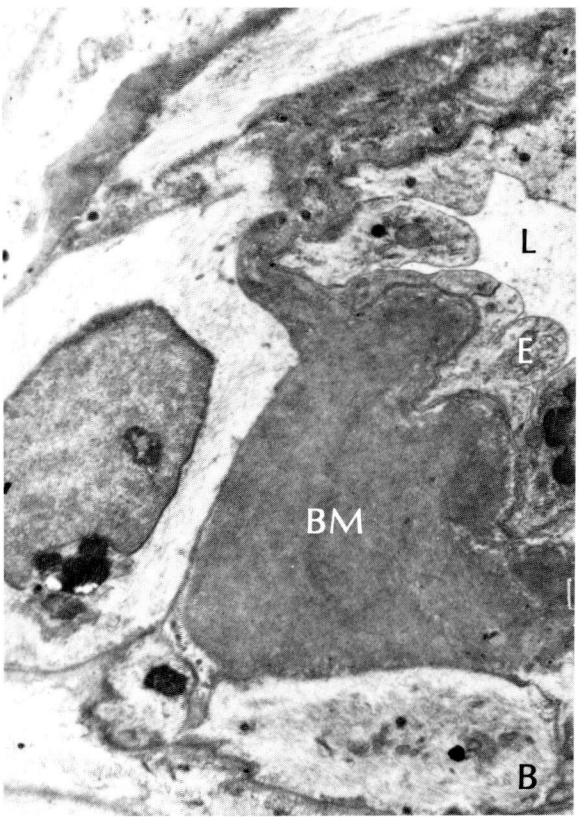

Figure 5–10. Basement membrane (BM) thickening. *A*, Renal glomerulus shows irregular thickening. *B*, Portion of a vessel shows irregular thickening of basement membrane outside the endothelial cells (E). Part of the vascular lumen (L) is also seen.

Kidney

Infections throughout life accentuate the aging process in the kidney and genitourinary tract. The kidney usually decreases in size. Its greatest weight of approximately 170 grams occurs sometime during the third or fourth decade and then drops to approximately 125 grams in the sixties[57] (Table 5–18).

Table 5–18. *Genitourinary Changes Associated with Age*

Kidney	Atrophy (cortex and medulla)
	Glomerular basement membrane changes associated with age or maturity-onset diabetes
	Amyloidosis
	Diverticula (tubules)
	Fat infiltration (medulla)
	Arteriolosclerosis
Prostate	Benign hypertrophy (lateral lobes)
	Occult cancer (posterior lobe)
Testes	Hydrocele
	Atrophy
	Thickened basement membrane
	Decreased spermatogenesis
Bladder	Cystitis cystica
	Cystocele
	Papilloma
	Carcinoma

Glomeruli and Vessels

As many as one-third to one-half of the glomeruli are lost by the seventh decade. Glomeruli represent about 18% of the cortical volume in the newborn and less than 6% in the adult.[57,58] Glomerular changes include reduplication and focal thickening of the glomerular basement membrane, and this thickening may be an index of the aging phenomenon (Fig. 5–10). As a corollary, other studies suggest that *basement membrane thickening* in diabetes may also be an index of the severity of that disease.

Some glomerular fibrosis and scarring usually result from vascular disease. *Immune deposits* associated with immunoglobulin abnormalities have also been implicated in the aging process. Proliferation of medial cells with thickening of the vessel walls are seen in many vessels.

Tubules and Interstitial Tissue

The tubules also show thickening of their basement membranes.[58] Most interesting is the marked increase in the number of distal tubular diverticuli with age. Oliver[59] has shown that *diverticula*, reported as rare findings at birth, may increase to as many as 300 per 100 nephrons at age 80. The interstitial tissue also shows an increase in collagen fibers and, sometimes, infiltration by lipid and an increase in acid mucopolysaccharide ground substance.

Function

Physiologic studies on the kidneys of older individuals often show a *decrease* in *glomerular filtration* and *ineffective renal blood flow.*[60] In addition, as the filtration fraction increases, the renal tubular function, including reabsorption, decreases with concomitant acid-base balance changes and *proteinuria.*[61] Although *nocturia* is commonly attributed to *prostatic hyperplasia,* urine retention, and bladder dysfunction, it has been suggested that the normal urine-forming cycle changes with age and increases urine production during the night.[62]

Bladder

Alterations in the bladder include an increase in edema, accentuation of rugae, round-cell infiltration, and sometimes *cystitis cystica,* that is, isolated pockets of epithelial cells forming cysts. Papillomas, generally considered premalignant, increase in frequency with age (Table 5–18).

Gastrointestinal Tract

Cellular turnover in the gastrointestinal tract is more rapid than in any tissue except skin and bone marrow. This turnover allows prompt removal of toxic substances in differentiated cells that are sloughed daily.

Esophagus

Esophagitis associated with reflux of acid, diverticula, hiatal hernia,[63] and cancer, especially in the lower two-thirds, are all more common in the elderly than in younger individuals. Small, asymptomatic hiatal hernias appear in 60% of individuals over the age of 60 (Table 5–19).

Table 5–19. Gastrointestinal Changes Associated with Age

Esophagus	Diverticula
	Hiatal hernia
Stomach	Mucosal atrophy or hypertrophy
	Polyps
	Carcinoma
Ileum	Infarcts
	Atrophy with malabsorption
	Lipoma
	Leiomyomata
Colon	Amyloid
	Diverticula
	Polyps
	Colitis
	Carcinoma
	Muscle atrophy with vessel changes
	Mucocele (appendix)
	Rectocele
	Hemorrhoids
	Amyloid
Pancreas	Atrophy
	Fatty infiltration
	Fibrosis
	Amyloidosis
	Focal hyperplasia
	Calcification
	Adenoma
	Carcinoma

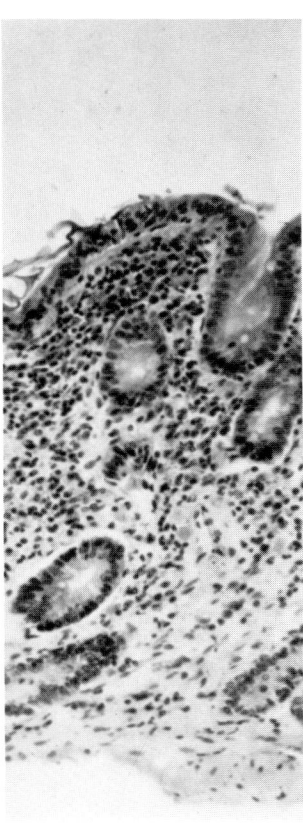

Figure 5–11. Normal *(A)* and atrophic *(B)* small intestinal epithelium. Note the well-formed villi in the normal specimen.

Stomach

The emptying rate of the stomach decreases with age. The incidence of atrophic gastritis is increased and is sometimes associated with pernicious anemia and carcinoma of the stomach.[64] The secretion of secretin, gastrin, and hydrochloric acid usually decreases. Contractile abnormalities of unknown etiology may be present.

Small Intestine

The small intestine loses motility with age. A decrease or an increase of lymphoid tissue in both Peyer's patches and in the submucosa has been described. Atrophy of both intestinal villi and cellular microvilli (Fig. 5–11) is associated with a loss of intestinal enzymes.[65] This change results in decreased absorption of amino acids, sugars, and other small molecules including vitamins, particularly vitamin B_{12}. Some vascular injury, arteriosclerosis, and venous thrombosis may be present (Table 5–19).

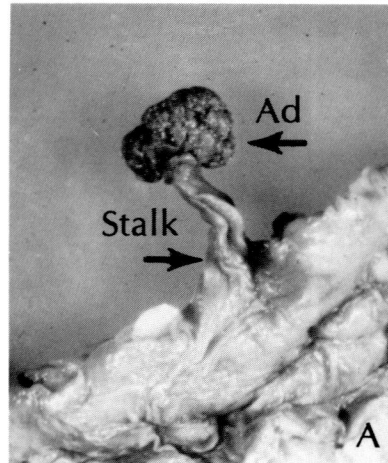

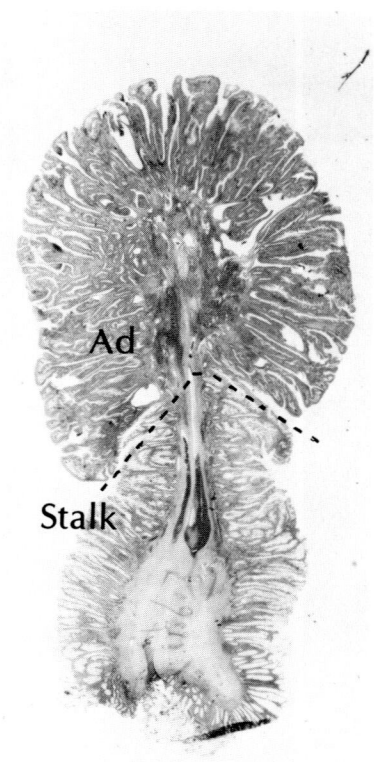

Colon

The colon is principally concerned with the absorption of sodium, chloride and water and the secretion of potassium and bicarbonate. Decreased food and fluid intake, altered electrolyte balance, insufficient bulk, and deficient motor tone may promote *constipation* in the aged. *Diarrhea* in the elderly is often due to excessive use of cathartics.[66] In addition to vascular changes already noted, peculiar angiodysplasias may be present.

Although diverticula appear in fewer than 8% of individuals under 60, 40% of people over the age of 70 have some degree of diverticulosis.[67] Infection, obstruction and gross hemorrhage are common complications. *Polyps,* 90% *hyperplastic* in type, become increasingly prominent with age (Fig. 5–12). Ten percent of the less commonly found *adenomatous polyps* show carcinomatous changes.[68]

Colon cancer, particularly of the lower sigmoid, is the most common fatal carcinoma when males and females are considered together. Nonspecific colitis is much more common than the more serious inflammatory bowel diseases such as regional enteritis and ulcerative colitis.

The most common lesion of the gastrointestinal tract is *hemorrhoids,* which are occasionally associated with portal hypertension and cirrhosis, but are usually related to inherent weaknesses in the vessel walls, possible valve defects, and stresses accumulated over time during defecation. *Rectocele* or *prolapse* is another common condition associated with aging. The rectum is an excellent site to biopsy to detect amyloid (Table 5–19).

Figure 5–12. An adenomatous polyp. *A,* Gross appearance. *B,* Microscopic appearance. The neoplastic adenomatous (Ad) tissue is present in the head of the polyp. The stalk is composed of normal mucosa.

Hepatobiliary

Liver

The aging liver changes little. Its weight may decrease, but the normal architecture appears to be well preserved. The presence of some variability in liver cell nuclear size and chromatism reflects aging *polyploidy;* some cells show tetraploid or octaploid chromosome numbers[69] (Fig. 5–13). *Proliferation* of *bile ductules,* thickening of arterioles, and an increase in type III collagen, which is unassociated with viral or alcoholic hepatitis or biliary obstruction, may be present in portal areas.[70]

Although deposits of amyloid and iron are common, these changes are usually minimal. Cytoplasmic *vacuoles* and of course, lipofuscin deposits have been noted in older individuals. Inclusions usually contain lipid, water, and occasionally glycogen, particularly if maturity-onset diabetes is present. Hepatic enzyme levels do not substantially change because of the large reserves of liver cells. Inducible enzymes, particularly the mixed-function oxidative enzymes in the smooth endoplasmic reticulum (SER), may be moderately reduced.

Morphologically, the *SER is reduced* and the number of lysosomes is increased. Albumin synthesis may be decreased suggesting altered rough endoplasmic reticulum (RER) function, or it may be increased with a greater protein loss in kidneys. With the increase in some serum globulins previously noted, the albumin-globulin ratio may change (Table 5–20).

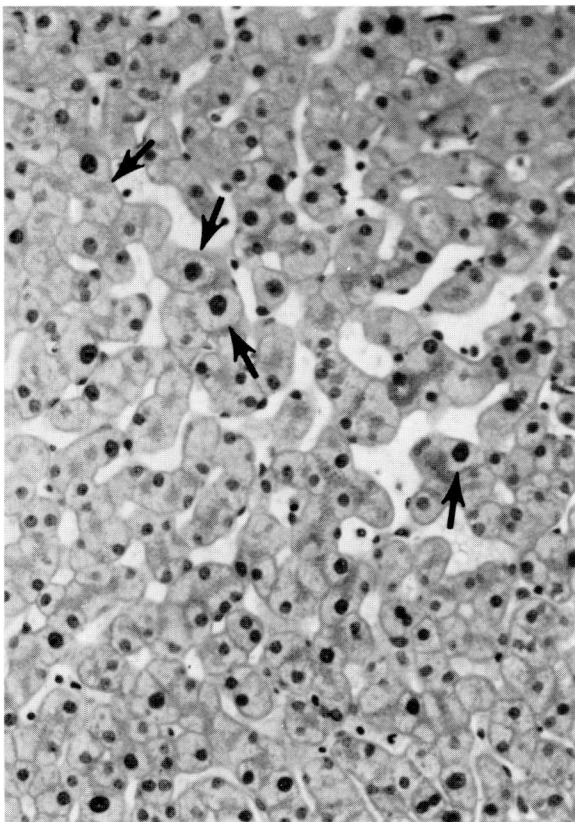

Figure 5–13. In aging polyploidy in the liver, enlarged and hyperchromatic nuclei of hepatocytes (arrows) reflect the polyploid state.

Table 5–20. *Hepatobiliary Changes Associated with Age*

Liver	Cyst
	Biliary tract adenoma
	Amyloidosis
	Hepatocarcinoma
	Fibrosis
Gallbladder	Mucocele
	Atrophy-hypertrophy with obstruction
	Cholecystitis
	Cholelithiasis
	Carcinoma

Gallbladder

The gallbladder changes associated with cholecystitis, cholelithiasis, and cholangitis, although more common in the middle and old age, are generally considered to be disease processes rather than aging phenomena.

Pancreas (Exocrine)

Endocrine changes in the islets of Langerhans are noted later in this chapter, under the discussion of the neuroendocrine system.

The pancreas is most difficult to examine in autopsy studies of the aged because of the rapid autolysis it undergoes following death. Observations of fibrosis and inflammatory infiltrates are common features of the aged pancreas and probably represent end effects of injury (Table 5–19).

Central Nervous System

Aged brains have narrowed gyri with less prominent sulci, thickened meninges, and enlarged ventricles. Many investigators have reported a 5 to 10% loss in brain weight.[28] A *20% decrease* in the *number of cells* in the cerebral cortex and a 25% decrease in cells of the cerebellar cortex have also been reported, but these results are controversial (Table 5–21).

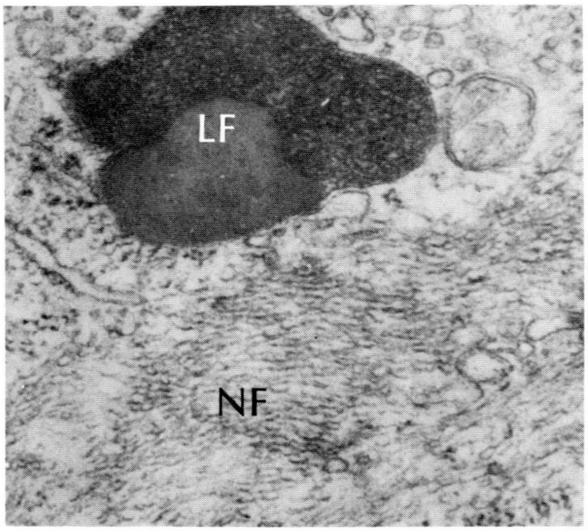

Table 5–21. *CNS and Peripheral Nerve Changes Associated with Age*

Central Nervous System	Cortical atrophy
	Lipofuscin deposits
	Alzheimer's neurofibrillary degeneration
	Parkinson's disease (changes in substantia nigra)
	Amyloidosis
	Atherosclerosis
	Aneurysm (berry)
	Thrombosis, embolism
Peripheral Nerve	Atrophy
	Amyloidosis
	Degeneration
	Myelin degeneration
	Sciatica

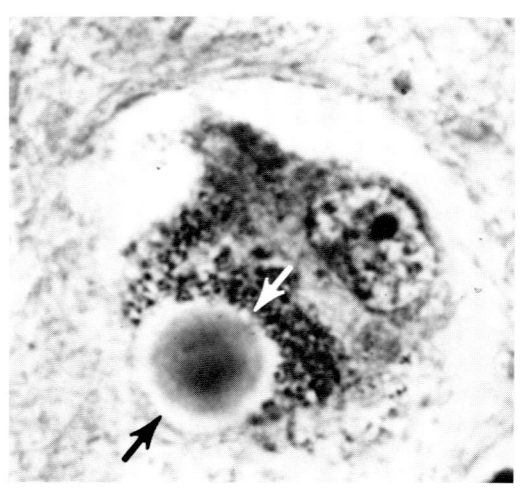

Figure 5–14. In the aging brain, lipofuscin (LF) deposits may be prominent in the neurons. The latter also contain numerous neurofilaments (NF).

Figure 5–15. In Parkinson's disease, the neurons of the basal ganglia may contain Lewy bodies (arrows).

In many diseases, neuronal degeneration and gliofibrillary replacement in the cerebral cortex have been demonstrated. Filamentous deposits of *neurotubules* and *amyloid* are described in many neurologic diseases. In addition, neuromelanin may be deposited in the dopamine-producing cells (Fig. 5–14) in small quantities in normal, aged brains. Lipofuscin may be present in neurons (Fig. 5–14).

Brains removed at autopsies from elderly people also show varying degrees of morphologic changes usually associated with arteriosclerosis, Alzheimer's disease,[71] and sometimes Parkinson's disease (Fig. 5–15). Senile dementia is severe in 5% and moderate in 10% of individuals aged 65 and over. The finding of features similar to presenile and senile dementia and *Alzheimer's disease*, namely, senile plaques, neurofibrillary deposits, and granulovacuolar degeneration, suggests a common pathogenesis of these disorders, which may be related to the aging process. *Arterio-*

sclerotic and *Parkinsonian dementias* may be encountered in the elderly, though less commonly than those dementias associated with Alzheimer's disease or idiopathic causes. Loss of initiative, poor judgment, loss of recent memory, disorientation, and other personality changes characterize the state of senility.

Neuroendocrine System

The endocrine system undergoes a progressive aging process that has long-range effects in several target tissues (Table 5–22). Changes in pituitary and hypothalamic functions are believed by some to be responsible for programming the sequences of aging.

Table 5–22. *Neuroendocrine Changes Associated with Age*

Pituitary	Cyst
	Atrophy
	Focal hyperplasia
	Adenoma
Thyroid	Focal hyperplasia
	Atrophy
	Adenoma
	Toxic and nontoxic nodular goiter
	Thyroiditis (Hashimoto's, Riedel's struma)
	Amyloidosis (aging or medullary carcinoma)
Parathyroid	Atrophy
	Cyst
	Hyperplasia
	Adenoma
Adrenal	Atrophy
	Focal hyperplasia
	Cortical adenoma
	Cortical carcinoma
	Pheochromocytoma
	Amyloidosis

The neuroendocrine system also has complex interrelationships with the immune system. The *pituitary* and the *thymus* appear to be related, and pituitary hormones influence cellular and humoral functions of immune surveillance in aged individuals. Adrenocorticotropic hormone (ACTH) and thyrotropin (TSH) as well as other hormones have effects on the maturation and senescence of cells of the immune system.

Pituitary

The basophilic cells in the anterior lobe, responsible for the secretion of gonadotropins, are occasionally vacuolated with age. Mitochondria may degenerate. The levels of pituitary hormones are variable and depend on which hormone is examined.[72] There is an age-dependent increase in follicle-stimulating hormone (FSH). High levels of cir-

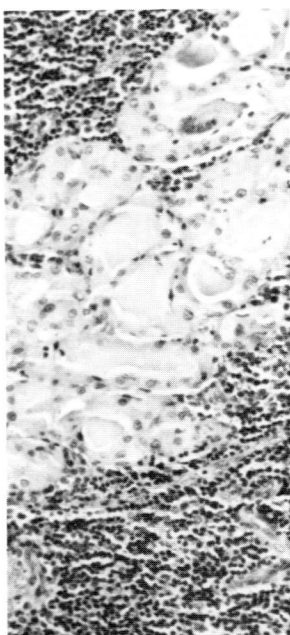

Figure 5–16. In Hashimoto's thyroiditis, the follicular epithelium has acquired Hürthle cell changes and is surrounded by a prominent lymphocytic infiltrate.

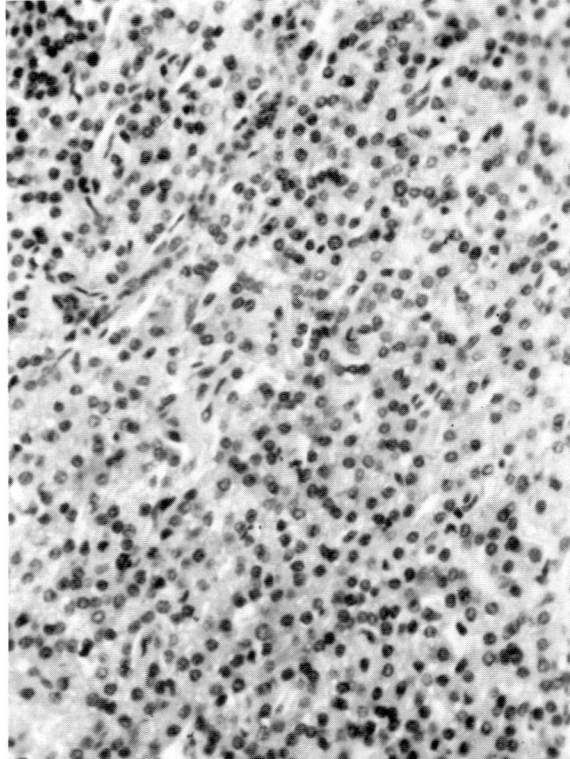

Figure 5–17. In parathyroid gland hyperplasia, there is a marked increase in the numbers of chief cells, and the normal amount of parathyroid fat is no longer present. (Courtesy of Dr. M. Grimes, Department of Pathology, College of Physicians and Surgeons, Columbia University, New York.)

culating and urinary gonadotropin may reflect the decreased level of circulating estrogens (end-organ atrophy), which fail to exert a negative feedback on their production. Frequently, no change is seen in chorionic gonadotropins, but growth hormone is decreased by one-third.[73] TSH and ACTH do not appear to *change* with age, however. The most common tumor is a neutrophilic chromophobe adenoma, usually producing prolactin. There is a significant age-related decline in growth hormone secreting cells after the age of 40.

Thyroid

Follicular atrophy, with replacement by fibrous tissue and chronic inflammatory cells, is often seen throughout the gland (Fig. 5–16), but the organ usually has reserve sufficient to maintain function. Although TSH may be released in inactive form and T_4 and T_3 have been reduced in some experiments, plasma T_4 levels often do not change, and thyroxine binding to globulin is not altered. *Nontoxic adenomas* and areas of *atrophy* and *hyperplasia* are common lesions. The calcitonin-secreting cells are present in the parafollicular regions as well as lining follicles and may undergo focal hyperplasia with age.

Parathyroid

These glands are sometimes atrophic, but hyperplastic foci are more commonly seen (Fig. 5–17). These foci are generally chief cells, occasionally oxyphil cells, and rarely clear cells (degenerated chief cells). Primary adenomas are more common in the middle-aged than in the young.

Adrenal

The weight of the adrenal has little relation to age. Increased pigmentation and proliferation of connective tissue have been noted in the medulla, along with loss of lipid in cortical cells. The latter has been correlated with decreased steroid synthesis. Glucocorticoid levels do not fall appreciably, although androgen production is diminished in males. Antidiuretic hormone (ADH) is decreased, with a corresponding loss of renal tubule sensitivity. *Adenomas,* usually nonfunctional, may be present.

Pancreas (Endocrine)

Many older individuals develop maturity-onset diabetes. In general, there appears to be no defect in the beta cells in the islets of Langerhans, and the defect apparently resides in the target tissues. Amyloid deposition appears in the islets and is believed to be crystallized proinsulin. The pancreas commonly shows arteriolosclerosis and the changes previously noted in the exocrine pancreas.

Reproductive System

Aging changes are particularly dramatic in the reproductive tract (Table 5–23).

Table 5–23. *Reproductive Changes Associated with Age*

Uterus	Atrophy (endometrium)
	Polyp (endometrial-endocervical)
	Carcinoma (endometrium)
	Retroversion
	Prolapse
	Hyperplasia
Fallopian Tubes	Fibrosis
Ovary	Atrophy (ovary and follicles)
	Cyst
	Cystadenoma
	Carcinoma
Breast	Atrophy and fibrosis
	Cystic disease
	Duct ectasia
	Intraductal papillomatosis
	Carcinoma
Testis	Atrophy
Prostate	Benign prostatic hypertrophy
	Carcinoma

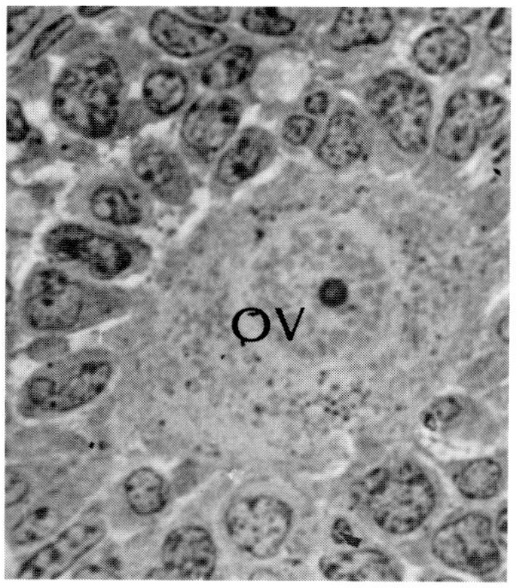

Figure 5–18. An ovum (OV) in an ovary is surrounded by supporting cells.

Ovary

The number of ova, estimated at approximately 700 thousand at birth, drops to perhaps 10 to 15 thousand at age 40 to 50 (Fig. 5–18). Ovaries examined in the 35 to 45 age group have fewer and smaller follicles; however, the hilus cells are more prominent. The ovary becomes shrunken and less responsive to gonadotropins, especially in postmenopausal women, and estrogen and progesterone synthesis decrease with age.

In contrast to the secretion of estradiol in the reproductive years, the major secretory product of the postmenopausal ovary is androstenedione. The decrease in estrogens and progesterone in females and testerone in males is partially compensated by increased adrenal synthesis. *Follicle cysts*, mucinous and serous cysts, and cancer are common lesions.

Uterus

The uterus usually becomes small and contracted with age if leiomyomata, polyps, or malignant tumors are not present. Endarteritis obliterans is found in the vessels in the myometrium. The endometrium slowly loses its ability to respond to tropic hormones. Gradual end organ failure may be reflected in a *mixed proliferative-secretory endometrium*. The glands subsequently become inactive and finally *atrophic*. The epithelium of the cervix becomes thinned and nonglycogenated. *Prolapse* and *retroversion* of the uterus are common. The incidence of endometrial *carcinoma* increases following menopause, whereas cervical carcinoma is more common in the forties.

Vagina

The vagina appears to be shorter and smaller, with loss of elasticity, increase in fibrosis, and thinning of the epithelial surface. Glycogen is absent from the atrophic epithelium. Prolapse of the vagina is not rare.

Vulva

The changes in the vulva are similar to those in the vagina. In addition, vulvar hair is lost, and other skin adnexa atrophy.

Breast

The mammary glands are gradually replaced by fibrous and fatty tissue. *Cystic disease* may also be present, with areas of dilated ducts and fibrosis. *Intraductal papillomas* and *carcinoma* are both more common in the aged.

Testis and Epididymis

In the male, the prominent spermatids seen at ages 20 to 40 decrease by 50% at ages 50 to 70. This change is associated with an exponential decrease in stem cells with age.[33] The basement membrane and tunica propria thicken, and the *Leydig cells decrease;* testosterone synthesis is thereby reduced. Changes in Sertoli cells are less evident. Growth potential is decreased, and little evidence of cell renewal exists. The epithelium of the seminal vesicles is decreased in number, and subepithelial connective tissue may replace the muscle. Lipofuscin pigment and amyloid may be noted. *Hydrocele* of the epididymis is common.

Prostate

The tubuloalveolar glands, which contribute to the formation of the ejaculate, are reduced in the aged prostate. Metaplasia of the epithelial cells, from columnar to cuboidal, and replacement of glands and muscle by collagen are noted. Hypertrophy and hyperplasia of the glands and stroma, known as *benign prostatic hypertrophy*, may result in prominent nodularity and a predisposition to obstruction and subsequent infection (Fig. 5–19). *Occult carcinomas*, as well as clinically significant carcinomas, of the aged are common[74] (Fig. 5–20).

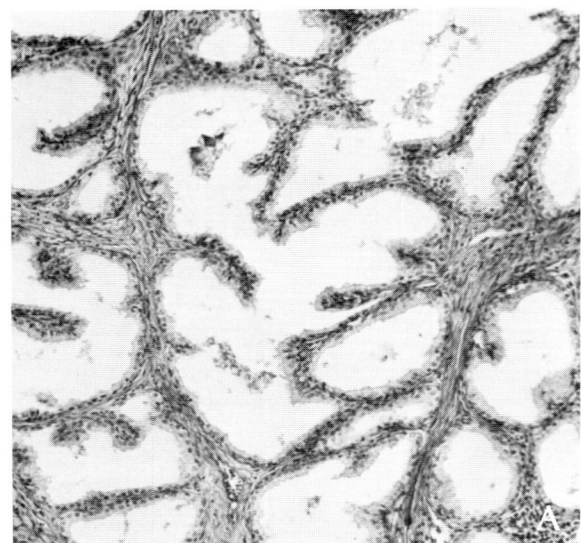

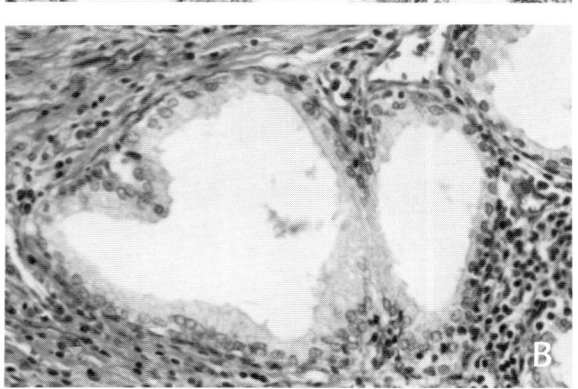

Figure 5–19. Benign prostatic hypertrophy. *A*, Proliferation of benign prostatic glands is present. *B*, Hypermagnification illustrates the regular nonpleomorphic cells lining the gland lumina. (Courtesy of Dr. M. Melicow, College of Physicians and Surgeons, Columbia University, New York.)

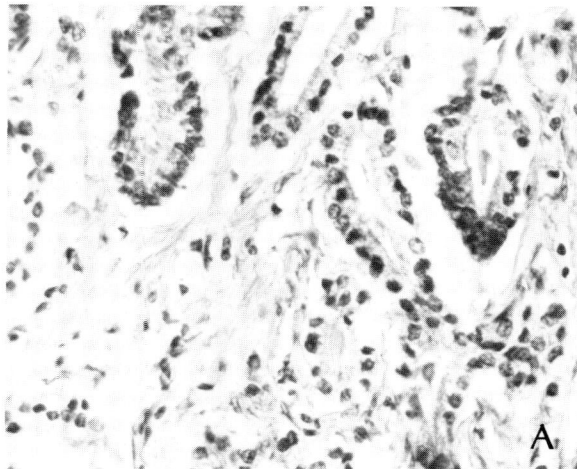

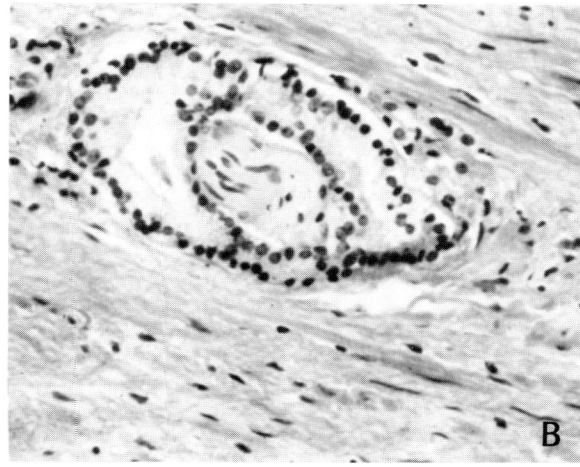

Figure 5–20. Prostatic carcinoma. *A*, Carcinoma of prostate. *B*, Same tumor involving a nerve. (Courtesy of Dr. M. Melicow, College of Physicians and Surgeons, Columbia University, New York.)

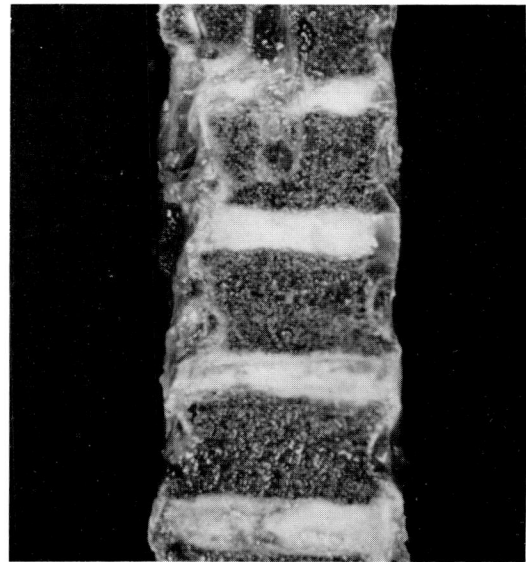

Figure 5–21. Osteoporosis of lumbar spine.

Penis

With age, fibroelastosis of the trabeculae and the corpus spongiosum increases. Progressive sclerosis with narrowing and obliteration of arteries and veins may occur.

Bone and Joints

The predominant skeletal lesions in aging are *osteoporosis*[75] (Fig. 5–21) and *osteoarthritis.* It has been suggested that the arthritides of old age are not only the result of wear and tear on the joints, but also are due to a metabolic disequilibrium in joint tissues. Chondrocytes react to certain hormones with increased cellular proliferation and a greater production of collagen. These have an arthrosis-promoting effect and, together with secondary effects of estrogen, thyroxine, and somatotropin, may induce calcification.

Another common lesion of the aged is *intervertebral disc degeneration* of the *anulus fibrosus* with *herniation* of the *nucleus pulposus.* This disorder results in impingement on nerve roots and causes pain, as in sciatica. Pathologic fractures, including osteoporotic compression fractures and fractures due to metastatic carcinoma, are much more common in the aged. Fibrogenesis increases, and osteogenic replacement occurs at a reduced rate.

In the oral cavity, gum tissue is more friable, some bone is lost, and *periodontal disease* may occur, with infection that often results in the need to replace teeth with dentures.

Lymphoreticular System

The bone marrow of aged individuals may exhibit general *hypoplasia,* but lymphoid elements show *hyperplastic foci.* Severe anemia, leukopenia, and thrombocytopenia are uncharacteristic of the elderly and peripheral blood counts are comparable to those of younger age groups (Table 5–24). As with other cells, the reserve and compensatory cellular responses to stress and infection are reduced. The elderly may respond poorly with an inadequate leukocytosis to bacterial infections.

Table 5–24. *Lymphoreticular Changes Associated with Age*

Lymph nodes, spleen, bone marrow, thymus, Peyer's particles	Atrophy or hypoplasia
	Hyperplasia (particularly lymphoid elements)
	Thymic involution (puberty)
	Myasthenia gravis or thymoma
	Myelofibrosis
	Leukemia (particularly chronic lymphocytic leukemia)
	Lymphoma
	Multiple myeloma
	Amyloidosis

The peripheral lymphoid tissue is often *atrophied,* sometimes *fibrosed* as a result of infections throughout life, but sometimes it is *hyperplastic.* In particular, proliferation of lymphoid cells appears to occur in the bone marrow and sometimes in the gut, lung, thyroid, and other organs; this proliferation may be indicative of the increased autoimmune state.

Antibody synthesis, cell-mediated immunity, and mitogen responses all decline with age. The decreased affinity of lymphoid cell membranes for antigenic determinants may be associated with the known autoidiotypic antibody to the antigen combining site.[76]

Thymic-dependent antibody responses decline sooner and faster than thymic-independent ones. Thymic hormones are lost with involution of the thymus.[77] The *depressed immune* response may be associated with an age-dependent increase in suppressor T-cell activity, and alterations in specific T-cell function (helper or suppressor) appear to be critical in the pathogenesis of aging. The percentage of B and T cells does not change much.

With the increase of effective suppressor T cells, abnormal immunoglobulin synthesis (benign monoclonal gammopathies) increases, as does the level of autoantibodies, which is associated with increased deposits of antigen-antibody complexes. Acquired tolerance is also lost by some of the mechanisms previously discussed.

Muscle

Changes in muscle with age include *atrophy* (Table 5–25) with a rapid decline in motor tone and some loss of contractility. Muscle tissue is controlled by neuronal, hormonal, and vascular factors. Neural innervation and effects on membrane receptors are both important in progressive changes with age. Muscular involution (decline in muscle mass), with increased extracellular water and potassium, constitute important problems for the aged. These problems are compounded by the replacement of competent cells with connective tissue and fat, which are not contractile.

Ultrastructurally, the number and size of myofibrils are reduced, and synthesis of myofibrils is abnormal. The basement membrane is thickened and shows protrusions of the

Table 5–25. *Musculoskeletal Changes Associated with Age*

Muscle	Degeneration or atrophy
	Dystrophy
	Amyloidosis
Bone and Joint	Osteoarthritis
	Rheumatoid arthritis
	Osteoporosis
	Paget's disease
	Intervertebral disc rupture
	Fractures

sarcolemma. Chromatin marginates and clumps at the periphery of the nucleus. An increase in DNA results from attempts at repair. More nucleoli are often seen, but fewer satellite nuclei. *Lipofuscin* deposits may be present, along with an increase in *autophagic lysosomes*. The changes seen in myofilaments with aging are not as severe as those in the atrophy associated with muscular dystrophy, but they are similar.[78]

Aging muscle fibers are associated with a decreased number of motor end plates and nerve fibers. The motor unit is smaller, the primary synaptic clefts appear enlarged, and the basement membrane is thickened. Although the action potential is not altered much, contraction time, latency period, and relaxation period are prolonged, and the maximum rate of tension developed is decreased. Muscle strength decreases linearly with age. The ability to engage in physical exercise decreases with age in concert with the diminished capacity of the cardiovascular system to deliver oxygen.

Few changes are noted in muscle enzymes, although some decrease in glycolytic and oxidative enzymes has been reported.

Skin

Epithelium

The skin of the aged individual shows marked changes, particularly around the face and neck[79] (Table 5–26). Wrinkles appear and are associated with atrophy of the epidermis and changes in the underlying dermis, fat, and muscle. The dermis is thickened with aggregation of collagen fibrils, elastin may be altered, and elastosis becomes more apparent. *Decreased* numbers of *melanocytes* in hair follicles result in graying of hair.[80] Conversely, a focal increase in melanocytes in the skin of the hands and legs results in pigmented age spots.

Table 5–26. *Common Aging Changes in the Skin*

Seborrheic keratosis
Solar (actinic) keratosis
Nevus
Melanoma
Hemangioma
Sweat gland adenoma
Sebaceous adenoma
Squamous cell carcinoma
Basal cell carcinoma
Atrophy, elastosis

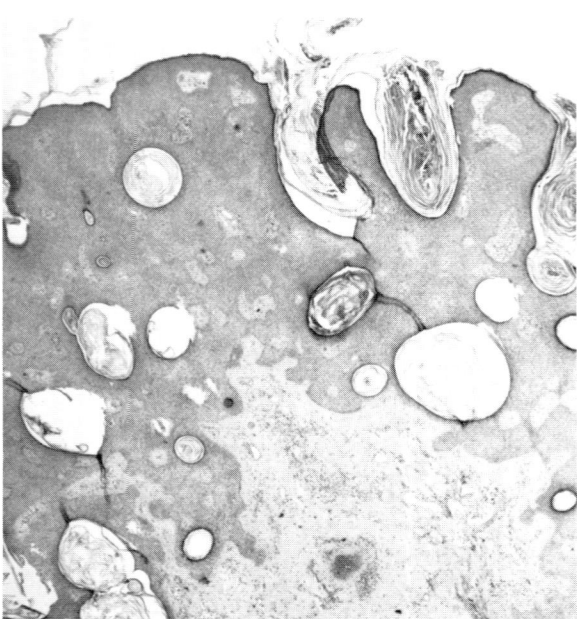

Figure 5–22. Section of a seborrheic keratosis, a common lesion of the face or trunk in middle age and later. The epidermis is thickened and shows cystic inclusions of horny material (pseudohorn cysts).

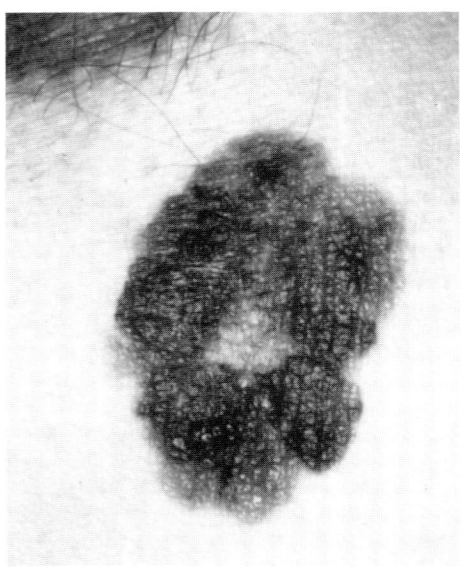

Figure 5–23. In malignant melanoma, note the irregular border of this pigmented tumor.

The *benign proliferations* of the skin more prevalent in the aged include epidermal seborrheic keratosis (Fig. 5–22), keratoacanthoma, subepidermal fibrosis, vascular angiomas, solar (actinic) keratosis, and leukoplakia. Bowen's disease, occasionally epidermoid and basal cell *carcinoma*, and malignant *melanocytic* lesions (Fig. 5–23) may be seen in the elderly.

Dermal Connective Tissue Changes

Considerable controversy exists concerning the changes in connective tissue in aged individuals. The normal *dermis* contains ground substance with *collagen fibers* and a semi-solid matrix of *elastin, glycoproteins, proteoglycans,* and *hyaluronic acid.* This macromolecular network reacts with the fluids and solids that permeate it through the basal lamina.

Studies on aging have concentrated on changes in collagen synthesis, secretion, and polymerization. The first step in *cross-linking* of immature collagen fibrils involves lysyl oxidase, which requires the presence of copper, and results in an oxidative deamination of lysyl and hydroxylysyl groups to form reactive aldehydes. The hydroxylysine then reacts with galactose and glucose and links collagen with carbohydrates. With age, hexose moieties increase, and collagen becomes more resistant to action by proteolytic enzymes. The question of increased cross-linkage of collagen fibrils with age is still controversial.[81] Collagen fibrils and soluble elastin enclosed in fibrous sheaths show some change in cross-linking, but the nature of the linkage is unresolved.

Recently, changes in the content of collagen pyridinoline have been demonstrated. This stable cross-linking amino acid for collagen fibers increases in amount from infancy until age 30, when it declines again. Moriguchi and Fujimoto[82] have advocated measuring the amount of this amino acid as an index of stable, mature collagen cross-links and the aging phenomenon. In discussing hepatic fibrosis, Rojkind and Dunn[83] suggest that evaluation of prolyl hydroxylase activity, at least in the liver, may be of value in assessing injury or the pathogenesis of fibrosis.

EFFECT OF INJURY ON AGING

Genetic Factors

Basically, each mammalian species has a specific range of life span. Humans with long-lived parents usually have a long life span. Females live longer than males.

In several major diseases, the life span is shortened[11] (see Table 5–6). In *infantile progeria (Hutchinson-Gilford syndrome),* the child exhibits signs of aging by age 10. These signs include graying of the hair, wrinkles, stunted growth, an increased incidence of diabetes and malignant disease, and the development of arteriosclerosis. In *adult progeria (Werner's syndrome)*, similar abnormalities appear in the patient's late thirties or early forties. In addition, in a variety of congenital abnormalities the life span appears to be shortened, not only by the increased susceptibility to infection and neoplasia, but also because of an actual acceleration of the aging process. These abnormalities include Down's syndrome, juvenile diabetes, congenital heart disease, and multiple endocrine adenomatosis.

Physical Factors

The effect of oxygen on the life span of the individual has been studied frequently. Some of the longest-lived populations reside in high-altitude areas (in the Soviet Union, Peru, and the United States[2]) where the oxygen content is reduced. These people apparently do not have an increased incidence of myocardial infarcts, despite the acknowledged fact that patients with myocardial ischemia, associated with atherosclerosis and coronary artery thrombosis, have a more limited life span.

Actuarial statements often correlate the rate of aging with increasing temperature. Those populations living in warm climates around the equator have a shorter life span than those in the moderately temperate region. The Eskimo, however, does not have a long life span, owing to infectious disease and other causes.

The fruitfly (Drosophila) has an increased life span associated with depressed body temperature. One species of hibernating pocket mouse, with a low body temperature and metabolic rate, lives five to eight years longer than other comparable species. In larger hibernating animals such as bears, the depression of body temperature and metabolic rate is appreciably smaller in relation to total body size, and these animals do not live appreciably longer than their counterparts. Thus, in some species, temperature plays a significant role, but it is probably less important in the human.

The effect of exercise on life span is of great interest today. A recent Harvard study has shown that graduates who underwent moderate exercise throughout their lives had a decreased incidence of cardiovascular disease and lived longer.

Nutritional Factors

The classic studies of McCay[84] some 40 years ago showed that rats given a *total caloric diet reduced 45%* had a *25% increase in life span*. In addition, the incidence of *progressive glomerular nephropathy*, a disease in rats often correlated with the aging process, was reduced by a diet restricting total calories, protein, and carbohydrate; this diet was also associated with a decreased metabolic rate.

The correlation between low, but not deficient caloric

intake, if restricted early in life, and longevity appears to be strong. Obesity commonly correlates with a shorter life span, particularly in patients with cardiovascular disease. The criteria used by insurance companies to set premium rates have been recently challenged by Andres,[85] who cited nine separate studies. He noted that individuals who were 10% *overweight* according to standard weight tables actually *lived longer.*

In addition to a reduction in total calories, the aged population often has a decreased intake of iron, thiamine, riboflavin, niacin, calcium, and vitamin A. Burkitt et al.[86] suggested that an increased intake of meat, decreased fiber, and increased sugar and fat intakes correlated with the increased incidence of colon neoplasia in Western cultures.

The number of *calories* needed by aging persons fall from approximately *4000* in younger years to as low as *2000* per day. With less exercise, anorexia, loss of weight, and decreased motility of the gastrointestinal tract, constipation may result. Wounds heal more slowly when calories are restricted, perhaps as a result of a delay in collagen cross-linking and decreased immune responses. The effect of *antioxidants* on aging, including vitamin E and mercapto-ethylamine (MEA) 2-hydrochloride, remains controversial.

Infectious Factors

With poor nutrition, poor immune responses, and the presence of increased somatic mutations, infections become a significant hazard to the older age group.

Elderly people differ from the young in their susceptibility and response to certain infectious agents. Respiratory viral disorders common in young people are often seen as a secondary complication to other disease in the elderly. *Gram-negative* and other bacterial infections, in part secondary to a decline in immune function, are more common. The aged are prone to obliterative vascular disease that causes ulcers of the skin with subsequent infection and invasion by bacteria. *Benign prostatic hypertrophy* in men predisposes them to *urinary infections* due to obstruction of the urinary system.

Valenti et al.[87] studied the factors that predispose aged individuals to infection, particularly by gram-negative bacilli. He found that bladder incontinence, inability to walk well, and inability to perform other activities of routine daily life all contributed to infection. Underlying respiratory disease and a bedridden state are significant detrimental factors.[87]

Bacterial infections in the aged are commonly caused by pneumococcus, staphylococcus, and streptococcus. More unusual bacteria, including *mycobacteria,* are increasingly virulent in the aged and may result in debilitation and sometimes widespread dissemination. Similarly, the cardiovascular and CNS manifestations of tertiary *syphilis* are more prominent in older age groups.

Historically, older individuals with cardiac or renal failure have been noted to be particularly prone to pneumonia caused by influenza virus with secondary bacterial infection. *Hepatitis* in aged individuals tends to pursue a more serious course than in younger people (Fig. 5–24).

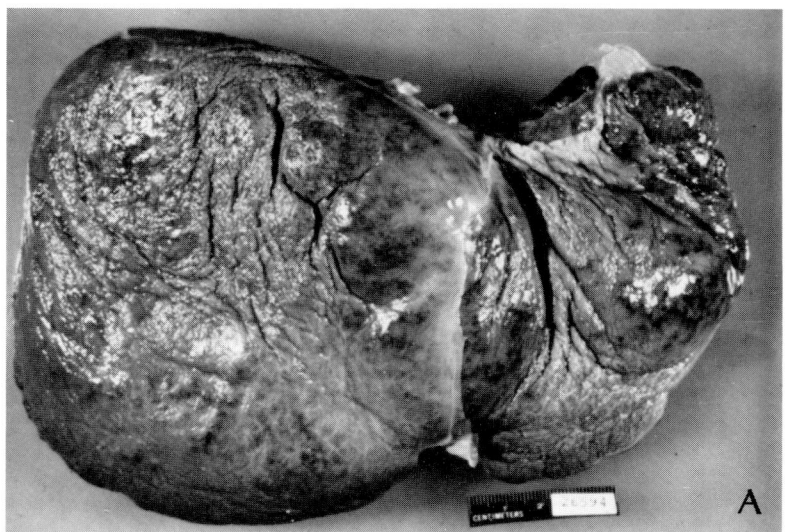

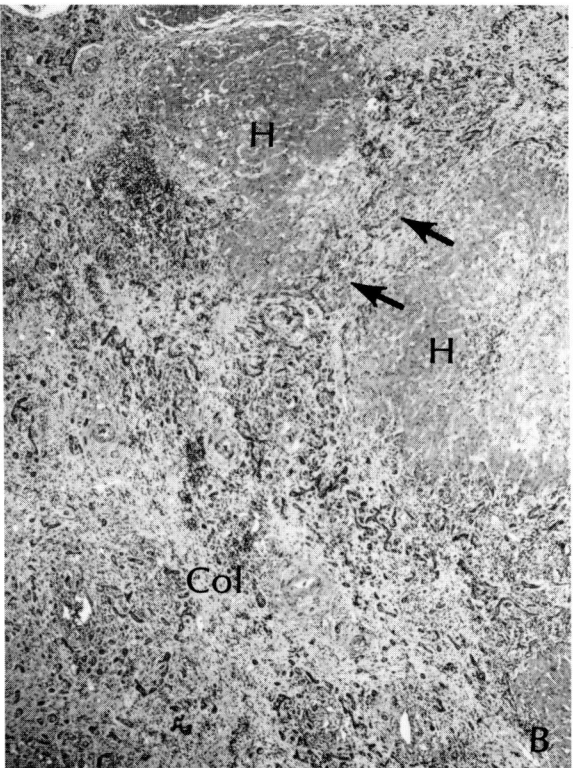

Figure 5–24. The liver of a 62-year-old woman who died of fulminant viral hepatitis. *A*, Grossly, the liver shows a marked reduction in weight and capsular wrinkling due to the loss of the underlying hepatic parenchyma. *B*, Histologic section shows massive hepatic necrosis with extensive areas of collapse (Col), bridging hepatic necrosis (arrows), and small islands of surviving hepatocytes (H).

Diseases caused by slow viruses, including Creutzfeldt-Jakob disease, kuru, and progressive multifocal leukoencephalopathy, manifest themselves mainly in middle-aged and elderly people. In the aged population there are often immune deficiencies, and along with bacterial and viral infections, there is a susceptibility to fungal infections. These infections are particularly prominent when patients are being treated with heavy doses of broad-spectrum antibiotics or immunosuppressive drugs.

Chemicals, Hormones, and Drugs

We have previously commented that aging appears to be associated with marked changes in hormone synthesis and control mechanisms. These effects are most prominently associated with reproductive organ changes. With a *decrease in estrogen* levels in women, changes are not only physically apparent in the hair and skin, but also in an *increased incidence of atherosclerosis.* Experimentally castrated male rats live longer than females, perhaps owing to the absence of the detrimental *labilizing effect* of *testerone* on lysosomal membranes.

Many drugs affect the aging process, but their synergistic mechanisms are largely unknown. In the extremes of youth and age, drugs may also have atypical effects. Thus, toxicity, untoward effects, and dosage must be carefully considered. The aged are also more likely to take a combination of drugs, which may interact with each other in detrimental ways.[88]

Cortisone and *gold* are used in the treatment of *arthritis.* Both the local and the systemic effects of these agents on the immune response and renal function must be further investigated. *Antihypertensive agents,* while providing a vital cardiovascular protective effect, may also produce *toxic effects* in the older population using them. Electrolyte problems can occur with the use of diuretic agents, and the development of chronic liver disease and cirrhosis has been noted with one antihypertensive drug, alpha-methyldopa. The widespread use of *antibiotic agents* decreases the synthesis of vitamin K and promotes malabsorption. Aspirin and alcohol may worsen the hypertrophic gastritis sometimes seen in the aged or may cause erosive gastritis. *L-DOPA,* a drug used in the treatment of human Parkinson's disease, prolongs life in albino mice, but may have serious toxic effects both in animals and in humans.

The effect of long-term exposure to environmental toxic agents, including *nicotine* and hydrocarbons, on the development of carcinoma of the colon, bladder, and pancreas has not yet been proved, but evidence that hydrocarbons cause lung cancer appears to be strong.

Immune Reactions and Products

We have already noted that the primary antibody response to antigenic stimulation may be decreased with age, although secondary anamnestic responses still occur. Secondary responses, with the resultant accumulation of antibodies over a lifetime, raise the globulin content of the aged population. Prominent autoimmune diseases such as lupus erythematosus, rheumatoid arthritis, scleroderma, dermatomyositis, and Hashimoto's disease have been discussed.

It is increasingly well recognized that most diseases, regardless of their etiology, develop some autoimmune components over a long time. Immune complexes may thereby be deposited in organs and vessels and may perhaps contribute to the pathologic picture of aged organs. When assays for circulating (nondeposited) immune complexes were performed in different aged populations, it was noted that few complexes were detectable prior to age 60. Between the ages of 60 and 70, the incidence was 20%. This increased to 33% in individuals between 70 and 75 years of age, and rose to 40% in individuals over age 76.[89]

Aging is a predictable event. The decrease in function of cells, tissues, and organs associated with quantitative changes in physiologic and biochemical parameters, as well as prominent intracellular and extracellular structural alterations, is an individual phenomenon within a general range of maximal life spans for each species. Aging, therefore, has a definite genetic basis that may be influenced by environmental agents such as geography, climate, socioeconomic status, and life style.

REFERENCES

1. Ludwig, F.C.: Senescence. Pathology facing medicine's ultimate issue. Arch. Pathol. Lab. Med., *105*:445, 1981.
2. Blumenthal, H.T.: Aging: biologic or pathologic? Hosp. Pract., *13*:127, 1978.
3. Friese, J.F.: Aging, natural death, and the compression of morbidity. N. Engl. J. Med., *303*:130, 1980.
4. Reaven, G.M.: Does age affect glucose tolerance? Geriatrics, *32*:51, 1977.
5. Laragh, J.H., Sealey, J.E., and Brunner, H.R.: The control of aldosterone secretion in normal and hypertensive man: abnormal renin-aldosterone patterns in low renin hypertension. Am. J. Med., *53*:649, 1972.
6. National Center for Health Statistics: Monthly Vital Statistics Report, Final Mortality Statistics, 1978. DHHS Publ. No (PHS) 80–1120, Vol. 29, No. 6, Supplement (2). Bethesda, MD, 1978.
7. Reff, M.E., and Schneider, E.L. (eds.): Biological Markers of Aging. Bethesda, MD, U.S. Department of Health and Human Services, NIH Publication No. 82-2221, April, 1982.
8. Youmans, G.P., et al. (eds.): The Biologic and Clinical Basis of Infectious Diseases. Philadelphia, W.G. Saunders Co., 1975.
9. Hayflick, L.: The biology of human aging. Adv. Pathobiol., 7:80, 1980.
10. Sachar, G.A.: Mammalian life histories: their evolution and molecular-genetic mechanisms. Adv. Pathobiol., 7:21, 1980.
11. Martin, G.M.: Genetic syndromes in man with potential relevance to the pathobiology of aging. Birth Defects, *14*:5, 1978.
12. Hayflick, L.: The limited in vitro lifetime of human diploid cell strains. Exp. Cell Res., *37*:614, 1965.
13. Hayflick, L.: The cell biology of human aging. N. Engl. J. Med., *295*:1302, 1976.
14. Harrison, D.E.: Lifespans of immunohemopoietic stem cell. Adv. Pathobiol., 7:187, 1980.

15. Mariotti, D., and Ruscitto, R.: Age-related changes of accuracy and efficiency of protein synthesis machinery in rat. Biochim. Biophys. Acta, *475*:96, 1977.
16. Orgel, L.E.: The maintenance of the accuracy of protein synthesis and its relevance to aging. Proc. Natl. Acad. Sci. USA, *49*:517, 1963.
17. Orgel, L.E.: The maintenance of the accuracy of protein synthesis and its relevance to aging: a correction. Proc. Natl. Acad. Sci. USA, *67*:1476, 1970.
18. Hart, R.W., and Daniel, F.B.: Genetic stability *in vitro* and *in vivo*. Adv. Pathobiol., *7*:123, 1980.
19. Everitt, A.V., and Burgess, J.A.: Hypothalamus, Pituitary and Aging. Springield, IL, Charles C Thomas, 1976.
20. Denckla, W.D.: Aging, dying and the pituitary. *In* Biological Mechanisms in Aging. Edited by R.T. Schimke. Bethesda, MD, National Institute on Aging, NIH Publication No. 81-2194, June, 1981.
21. Walford, R.L.: Immunology and aging. Am. J. Clin. Pathol., *74*:247, 1980.
22. Smith, G.S., and Walford, R.L.: Influence of the H-2 and H-1 histocompatibility systems upon lifespan and spontaneous cancer incidence in congenic mice. Birth Defects, *14*:281, 1978.
23. Bliznakov, E.G., et al.: Partial reactivation of impaired immune competence in aged mice by synthetic thymus factors. Biochem. Biophys. Res. Comm., *80*:631, 1978.
24. Burnet, F.M.: Immunology, Aging and Cancer. San Francisco, W.H. Freeman, 1976.
25. Greenberg, L.J., and Yunis, E.J.: Histocompatibility determinants, immune responsiveness and aging in man. Fed. Proc., *37*:1258, 1978.
26. Kohn, R.R.: Principles of Mammalian Aging. Englewood Cliffs, NJ, Prentice-Hall, 1978.
27. Harman, D.: The aging process. Proc. Natl. Acad. Sci. USA, *78*:7124, 1981.
28. Pearl, R.: The Biology of Death. Philadelphia, J.B. Lippincott, 1922.
29. Finch, C.E.: Neuroendocrine mechanisms and aging. Fed. Proc., *38*:178, 1979.
30. Weksler, M.E.: The senescence of the immune system. Hosp. Pract., *16*:53, 1981.
31. Siskind, G.W., et al.: Immunological aspects of aging. *In* Proceedings of the Conference on Biological Mechanisms in Aging (sponsored by NIA), June 23 to 25, 1980. Bethesda, MD, U.S. Department of Health and Human Services, Public Health Service, National Institutes of Health, National Institute on Aging, 1980.
32. Durbin, P., et al.: Development of spontaneous mammary tumors over the lifespan of the female Charles River (Sprague-Dawley) rat. Influence of ovariectomy, thyroidectomy, and adrenalectomy-ovariectomy. Cancer Res., *26*:400, 1966.
33. Sasano, N., and Ichijo, S.: Vascular patterns of the human testis with special reference to its senile changes. Tohoku J. Exp. Med., *99*:265, 1969.
34. Fang, J.W., et al.: Aging and X chromosome loss in the human ovary. Obstet. Gynecol., *45*:455, 1975.
35. Hart, R.W., et al.: Pathology of DNA and the biology of aging. *In* Proceedings of the Conference on Biological Mechanisms in Aging (sponsored by NIA); June 23 to 25, 1980. Bethesda, MD, U.S. Department of Health and Human Services, Public Health Service, National Institutes of Health, National Institute on Aging, 1980.
36. Florini, J.R., et al.: The influence of aging on protein synthesis. *In* Proceedings of the Conference on Biological Mechanisms in Aging (sponsored by NIA), June 23 to 25, 1980. Bethesda, MD, U.S. Department of Health and Human Services, Public Health Service, National Institutes of Health, National Institute on Aging, 1980.
37. Roth, G.S.: Receptor changes and the control of hormone action during aging. Adv. Pathobiol., *7*:228, 1980.
38. Tonna, E.A.: Aging of skeletal-dental systems and supporting tissues. *In* Handbook of the Biology of Aging. Edited by C.E. Finch and L. Hayflick. New York, Van Nostrand Reinhold, 1977.
39. Andres, R., and Tobin, J.D.: Endocrine systems. *In* Handbook of the Biology of Aging. Edited by C.E. Finch and L. Hayflick. New York, Van Nostrand Reinhold, 1977.
40. Barden, H.: Interference filter brain microfluorometry of neuromelanin and lipofuscin in human. J. Neuropathol., *39*:598, 1980.
41. Osserman, E.F., et al.: Plasma cell dyscrasias: general considerations, plasma cell myeloma: primary macroglobulinemia, amyloidosis, heavy

chain diseases. *In* Hematology. Edited by W.J. Williams et al. New York, McGraw-Hill, 1972.

42. Martin, G.M., and Sprague, C.A.: Symposium on *in vitro* studies related to atherogenesis: life histories of hyperplastoid cell lines from aorta and skin. Exp. Mol. Pathol., *18*:125, 1973.

43. Burrow, G.N., et al.: Microadenomas of the pituitary and abnormal sellar tomograms in an unselected autopsy series. N. Engl. J. Med., *304*:156, 1981.

44. Cutler, S.J., and Young, J.L., Jr.: 1975 Third National Cancer Survey Incidence Data. Natl. Cancer Inst. Monogr., No. 41, 1975.

45. Xi, Y-P, et al.: Age-related changes in normal human basement membrane. Mech. Ageing Dev., *19*:315, 1982.

46. Glenner, G.G.: Amyloid deposits and amyloidosis. The β-fibrilloses. N. Engl. J. Med., *302*:1283, 1980.

47. Rosenthal, C.J., et al.: Isolation and partial characterization of SAA—an amyloid relative protein from human serum. J. Immunol., *116*:1415, 1976.

48. Tischler, A.S., and Compagno, J.: Crystal-like deposits of amyloid in pancreatic islet cell tumors. Arch. Pathol. Lab. Med., *103*:247, 1979.

49. Shtrashburg, S., et al.: Demonstration of AA-protein in formalin-fixed, paraffin-embedded tissues. Am. J. Pathol., *106*:141, 1982.

50. Shirahama, T., et al.: Senile cerebral amyloid. Am. J. Pathol., *107*:41, 1982.

51. Kohn, R.R.: Heart and cardiovascular system. *In* Handbook of the Biology of Aging. Edited by C.E. Finch and L. Hayflick. New York, Van Nostrand Reinhold, 1977.

52. Limas, C.J.: Aging of the myocardium. Acta Cardiol. [Brux.], *26*:249, 1971.

53. Klocke, R.A.: Influence of aging on the lung. *In* Handbook of the Biology of Aging. Edited by C.E. Finch and L. Hayflick. New York, Van Nostrand Reinhold, 1977.

54. Sorbini, C.A., et al.: Arterial oxygen tension in relation to age in healthy subjects. Respiration, *25*:3, 1968.

55. Fletcher, C., et al.: The Natural History of Chronic Bronchitis and Emphysema. London, Oxford University Press, 1976.

56. Auerbach, O., et al.: Smoking habits and age in relation to pulmonary changes. N. Engl. J. Med., *269*:1045, 1963.

57. Goldman, R.: Aging of the excretory system: kidney and bladder. *In* Handbook of The Biology of Aging. Edited by C.E. Finch and L. Hayflick. New York, Van Nostrand Reinhold, 1977.

58. Darmady, A.J., Offer, J., and Woodhouse, M.A.: The parameters of the aging kidney. J. Pathol., *109*:195, 1973.

59. Oliver, J.R.: Urinary system. *In* Problems of Ageing: Biological and Medical Aspects. Edited by E.V. Cowdry. Baltimore, Williams & Wilkins, 1939.

60. Davies, D.F., and Shock, N.W.: Age changes in glomerular filtration rate, effective renal plasma flow, and tubular excretory capacity in adult males. J. Clin. Invest., *29*:496, 1950.

61. Adler, S., et al.: Effect of acute acid loading on urinary acid excretion by the aging human kidney. J. Lab. Clin. Med., *72*:278, 1968.

62. Lobban, M.C., and Tredre, B.E.: Diurnal rhythms of renal excretion and of body temperatures in aged subjects. J. Physiol., *188*:48P, 1967.

63. Wolf, B.S., Brahms, S.A., and Khilnani, M.R.: The incidence of hiatal hernia in routine barium meal examinations. Mt. Sinai J. Med., *26*:598, 1959.

64. Isokoski, M., et al.: Parietal cell and intrinsic factor antibodies in a Finnish rural population sample. Scand. J. Gastroenterol., *4*:521, 1969.

65. Sayeed, M.: Age related changes in intestinal phosphomonoesterases. Fed. Proc., *26*:259, 1967.

66. Manier, J.W.: Diarrhea and constipation: mechanism and treatment. Semin. Drug. Treat., *3*:321, 1974.

67. Manousos, O.N., Truelove, S.C., and Lumsden, K.: Prevalence of colonic diverticulosis in general population of Oxford area. Br. Med. J., *3*:762, 1967.

68. Fenoglio, C.M., et al.: Defining the precursor tissue of ordinary large bowel carcinoma: implications for cancer prevention. Pathol. Annu., *12*:87, 1977.

69. Carr, R.D., Smith, M.J., and Keil, P.G.: The liver in the aging process. Arch. Pathol., *70*:15, 1973.

70. Schaffner, F., and Popper, H.: Non-specific reactive hepatitis in aged and infirm people. Am. J. Digest. Dis., *4*:389, 1959.

71. Ball, M.J.: Alzheimer's disease. Arch. Pathol. Lab Med., *106*:157, 1982.
72. Finch, C.E.: Neuroendocrine and autonomic aspects of aging. *In* Handbook of the Biology of Aging. Edited by C.E. Finch and L. Hayflick. New York, Van Nostrand Reinhold, 1977.
73. Vidalon, C., et al.: Age-related changes in growth hormone in non-diabetic women. J. Am. Geriatr. Soc., *21*:253, 1973.
74. Harbitz, T.B., and Haugen, O.A.: Histology of the prostate in elderly men. Acta Pathol. Microbiol. Scand., *80A*:756, 1972.
75. Riggs, B.L., et al.: Effect of the fluoride/calcium regimen on vertebral fracture occurrence in postmenopausal osteoporosis. N. Engl. J. Med., *306*:446, 1982.
76. Goidl, E.A., et al.: Studies on the control of antibody synthesis. XV. Effect of nonspecific immunodepression on antibody affinity. Cell Immunol., *47*:293, 1979.
77. Weindruch, R.H., and Walford, R.I.: Aging and functions of the RES. The ontogeny and phylogeny of the reticuloendothelial system. *In* The Reticuloendothelial System: A Comprehensive Treatise. Vol. 5. Edited by N. Cohen. New York, Plenum Publishing, 1980.
78. Hanzlikova, V., and Gutmann, E.: Ultrastructural changes in senile muscles. *In* Impairment of Cellular Functions During Aging *in vitro* and *in vivo*. Edited by E. Holeckova and V.J. Cristofalo. New York, Plenum Publishing, 1975.
79. Domonkos, A.N.: The aging skin. Cutis, *4*:539, 1968.
80. Fitzpatrick, T.B., Szabo, G., and Mitchell, R.E.: Age changes in the human melanocyte system. *In* Advances in Biology of Skin. Vol. 6. Edited by W. Montagna. Oxford, Pergamon Press, 1965.
81. Bailey, A.J., Robbins, S.P., and Balian, G.: Biological significance of the intermolecular cross-links of collagen. Nature, *251*:105, 1974.
82. Moriguchi, T., and Fujimoto, D.: Age-related changes in the content of the collagen crosslink, pyridinoline. J. Biochem., *84*:933, 1978.
83. Rojkind, M., and Dunn, M.A.: Hepatic fibrosis. Gastroenterology, *76*:849, 1979.
84. McCay, C.M.: Chemical aspects of ageing and the effect of diet upon ageing. *In* Cowdry's Problems of Ageing. Edited by A.I. Lansing. Baltimore, Williams & Wilkins, 1952.
85. Andres, R.: Influence of obesity on longevity in the aged. Adv. Pathobiol., *7*:238, 1980.
86. Burkitt, D.P., Walker, A.R.P., and Painter, N.S.: Effect of dietary fibre on stools and the transit-times, and its role in the causation of disease. Lancet, *2*:1408, 1972.
87. Valenti, W., Trudell, R.G., and Bentley, D.W.: Factors predisposing to oropharyngeal colonization with Gram-negative bacilli in the aged. N. Engl. J. Med., *298*:1108, 1978.
88. Levine, R.R.: Pharmacology. Drug Actions and Reactions. Boston, Little, Brown, 1973.
89. Rosenthal, M.: Lebensalter und Immunitat III. Zirkulierende Immunkomplexe in verscheidener alterogrupper. Blut, *37*:271, 1978.

In an earlier chapter, the major classes of agents injurious to the cell and various diseases associated with each of these agents were introduced. In this chapter, the effects of specific agents on particular cell organelles and intermediary pathways are examined in greater detail.

As has been noted, changes at the subcellular level are often reflected as alterations in the structure and function of tissues, organs, and the organism. These changes are based upon the unique roles subserved by cellular organelles (Fig. 6–1). In the *cell membrane*, the primary barrier to many agents of injury, synthetic product transport and intercellular communication take place. Within the cytosol, the *microtubular and microfibrillar* systems provide a basis for a *cytoskeleton*, for movement, and for contraction. Enzymatic pathways in the *smooth* and *rough endoplasmic reticulum* (SER and RER) are involved in synthetic and detoxification processes. Transport and modification of cellular products in this system are related to passage through the *Golgi* apparatus and various cytoplasmic vesicles, including the cell's degradative organelles, the lysosomes. The *mitochondria* provide energy for many of these cellular functions.

Directing the complex activities of the cell is the *nucleus*, the nucleic acid content of which ensures inheritance of the cell's varied structural and functional characteristics by succeeding generations. The changes imposed upon these cellular substituents produce "*cellular injury*," which is dis-

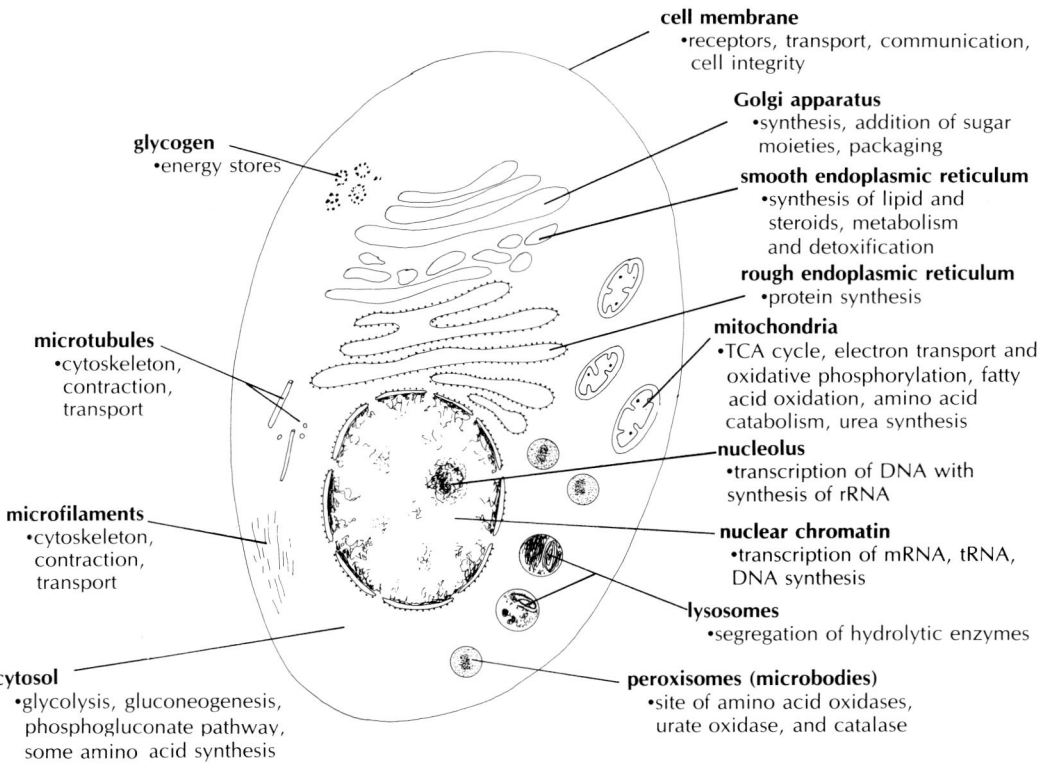

cell membrane
•receptors, transport, communication, cell integrity

Golgi apparatus
•synthesis, addition of sugar moieties, packaging

smooth endoplasmic reticulum
•synthesis of lipid and steroids, metabolism and detoxification

rough endoplasmic reticulum
•protein synthesis

mitochondria
•TCA cycle, electron transport and oxidative phosphorylation, fatty acid oxidation, amino acid catabolism, urea synthesis

nucleolus
•transcription of DNA with synthesis of rRNA

nuclear chromatin
•transcription of mRNA, tRNA, DNA synthesis

lysosomes
•segregation of hydrolytic enzymes

peroxisomes (microbodies)
•site of amino acid oxidases, urate oxidase, and catalase

glycogen
•energy stores

microtubules
•cytoskeleton, contraction, transport

microfilaments
•cytoskeleton, contraction, transport

cytosol
•glycolysis, gluconeogenesis, phosphogluconate pathway, some amino acid synthesis

Figure 6–1. The structure of the cell and the functions of organelles.

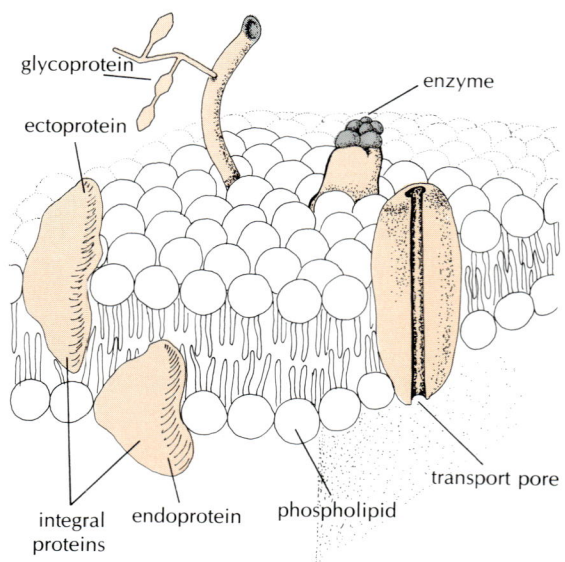

Figure 6–2. Fluid mosaic model of membrane structure; some of the structural and functional components are indicated.

The labels in the figure read:
glycoprotein
ectoprotein
enzyme
integral proteins
endoprotein
phospholipid
transport pore

cussed in this chapter in relation to normal organelle structure and function (Fig. 6–1).

PLASMA MEMBRANE

Fluid Mosaic Model of Membrane Structure

The *fluid mosaic* model of cell membranes suggested by Singer and Nicolson in 1972[1] is now widely accepted (Fig. 6–2). It allows us to understand how membrane modulations permit cellular responses that reflect the state of differentiation, stage in the cell cycle, cell function, and interactions with environmental agents.

The three-layered (trilaminar) membrane, approximately 75 to 100 Å thick, consists of a hydrophobic bipolar lipid core, as well as inner and outer layers with traversing hydrophilic protein moieties (Fig. 6–2). The central core lipids are primarily neutral fats, phospholipids, and cholesterol. Phospholipids, the major lipids in all cell membranes, are asymmetrically distributed on the two sides of the membrane. Phosphatidylethanolamine and phosphatidylserine are preferentially located on the inner part of the membrane, and lecithin and sphingomyelin are found on the outer part.[2,3]

The physical state of membrane lipids depends on temperature. Phospholipids change from a liquid gel to a liquid crystalline state at what is called the *"transition temperature."* A definite relationship exists between cellular temperatures and fatty acid composition. This relationship helps to determine membrane fluidity and permeability.

Glycoproteins and lipoproteins, known as *integral proteins,* pass partly or entirely through the membrane. Like the lipids, these proteins are asymmetrically distributed in membranes.[5] Two types of integral proteins may be distinguished. *Ectoproteins* have a substantial hydrophilic mass projecting beyond the outer surface of the lipid bilayer. Examples include the glycoprotein spikes on enveloped viruses (influenza), histocompatibility antigens, glycophorin, and intestinal brush border hydrolases. *Endoproteins* do not project beyond the cytoplasmic face of the bilayer, and the majority of their mass may be associated with the cytoplasmic side of the membrane.

Integral proteins interact with both the hydrophilic and hydrophobic portions of the membrane and are intercalated into the lipid bilayer to differing depths; some span the entire membrane. Protein location is determined by the amount of folding and critical amino acid composition of the protein.[6] The interactions with spanning integral proteins such as *glycophorin* may affect both intra- and extracellular events.

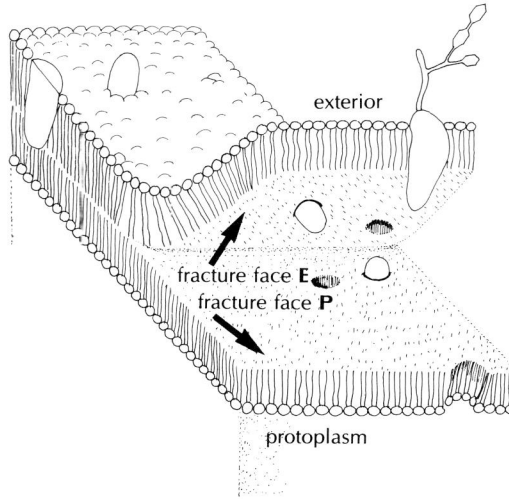

Figure 6–3. The process of freeze-fracture splits the membrane down the center of the lipid bilayer, thereby exposing two fracture faces. (Modified from Weissmann, G., and Claiborne, R. (eds.): Cell Membranes: Biochemistry, Cell Biology, and Pathology. New York, HP Publishing, 1975.)

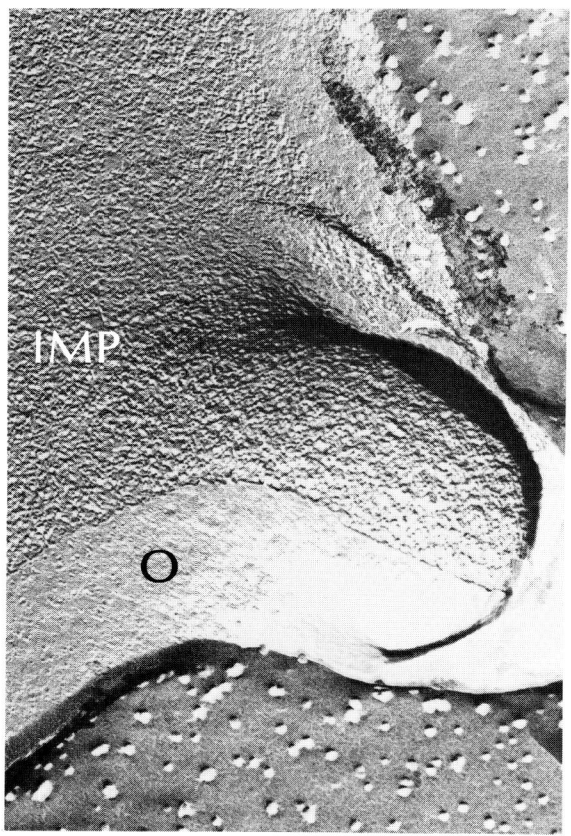

Figure 6–4. In this freeze-etch of a human red blood cell, the part in the middle has intramembranous particles (IMP). The outside surface (O) is etched and has no intramembranous particles. (Courtesy of Dr. Leo Furcht, Department of Pathology, University of Minnesota.)

One way to visualize the integral proteins is to freeze-fracture the membrane, a procedure by which it is split through the center of the lipid bilayer (Figs. 6–3 and 6–4). One half is called the *E surface* (external); the other half is the *P surface* (protoplasmic). The P half is closest to the cytoplasm, and the E half is closest to the external, or exoplasmic space. If an integral protein or complex lipid is present, the fracture passes around it, so that the internal lipid portion appears smooth, whereas the integral proteins appear in cross-section as *intramembranous particles (IMP)*.

In the red blood cell membrane, the IMP are rod-like structures 100 to 1000 Å long and 70 Å in diameter and are related to membranous *glycophorin, band 3 protein,* and cytoplasmic protein *spectrin.*[7] The IMP may function in ion transport by forming ion pores, it may represent unique membrane proteins with high affinity receptors for antigens and lectins, or it may transmit signals across the membrane affecting other organelles.[8]

Membrane Fluidity

We have stated that the membrane exists in a fluid mosaic state. This concept is substantiated by functional studies including membrane fusion, aggregation, disaggregation of IMP with freeze-etch techniques, and the redistribution or capping of membrane markers. Normally, membrane composition and fluidity change during cellular growth and differentiation,[9] but are also controlled by serum components[10] and by temperature.[11]

The classic demonstration of membrane mobility was by Frye and Edidin,[12] who fused mouse and chicken cells to form *heterokaryons.* These cells were labeled with differently colored fluorescent antibodies to mouse and chicken membrane antigens. A complete mixing of the mouse and chicken surface components was seen in 40 minutes.

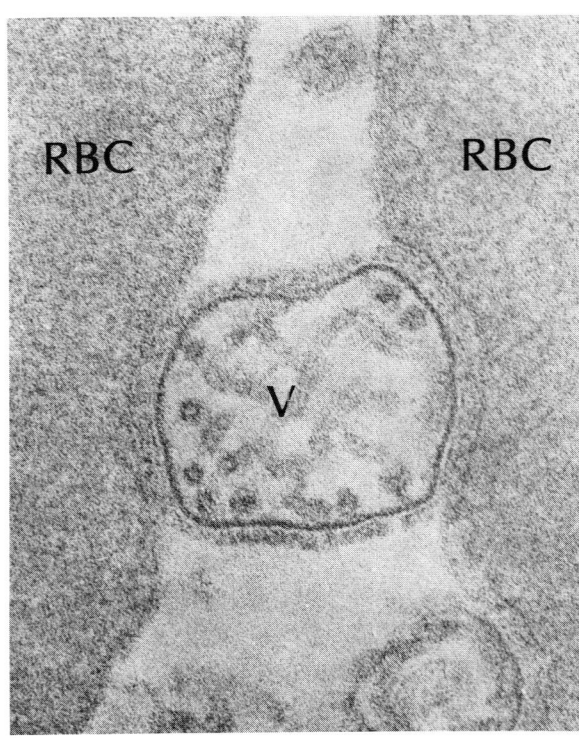

Figure 6–5. Fusion of two red blood cells (RBC) by Sendai virus (V).

Membrane fusions normally occur during exocytosis, when vacuole membranes fuse with the plasma membrane, and during fusion of lysosomes with phagocytic vacuoles. Membrane fusion is also critical during fertilization. Investigators have studied specific membrane events that take place during the experimental fusion of two mammalian cells facilitated by *Sendai virus* (Fig. 6–5) or *polyethylene glycol (PEG)*.[13] A generalized increase in membrane potential[14] and membrane resistance with resultant ion leakage[15] are seen. Fusion of the membrane occurs, with subsequent intermixing of membrane components.

The best experimental demonstration of the cell's ability to move membrane determinants is the *capping* phenomenon. In this process, a membrane receptor complex, or an antigen in combination with its complementary antibody, undergoes an energy-dependent topographic redistribution from a randomly dispersed pattern to localization at one pole. This process is followed by internalization (endocytosis) into cytoplasmic vesicles, which may later fuse with lysosomes.[16]

Membrane Stability

Although we have stressed the fluid nature of the plasma membrane, we have not mentioned those aspects that lend it stability. In the red blood cell, glycophorin appears to be held in place by a fibrillar network of contractile proteins located on the inner face of the membrane. This network consists of actin and a myosin-like material known as *spectrin*.[17] The interacting proteins glycophorin, spectrin, actin, and band 3 protein appear to form a cytoskeleton that regulates red blood cell shape.[18,19] Antispectrin antibodies exclusively localize spectrin to cell membrane sites related to *glycophorin*.[20] Mg^{++}-dependent adenosine triphosphatase (ATPase) also functions in maintaining the cellular shape.[21] Similar actin-myosin microfilamentous frameworks have been associated with plasma membranes of many other cell types.[22,23]

Tubulin, normally found in microtubules, may also be tightly bound to this cytoskeleton. Researchers have associated intriguing paracrystalline arrays of membrane-to-membrane cross bridges with the inner surface of plasma membrane.[24] The exact significance of these structures is unclear, and they may be related to the cytoskeletal framework previously described.[25]

Cell Surface Coats

Surface coats, which are present on the plasma membrane of many cells, contain glycoproteins, glycolipids, and other protein molecules externally bound to the bimolecular lipid layer of the plasma membrane. In some situations, surface coats appear to be a permanent part of the cell structure, whereas in others, they appear to be external. The *glycocalyx,* a term meaning "sweet husk," comprises all the components external to the plasma membrane and always contains carbohydrate and usually sialic acid (Fig. 6–6). It may contain surface antigens, receptor sites, and substances involved in cell adhesion, absorption, movement, protection, and shape.[26]

The appearance and thickness of the *glycocalyx* varies with the cell type. Intestinal cells have a readily observable glycocalyx that covers the intestinal microvilli and consists of closely packed filamentous material varying in thickness from 0.1 to 0.5 mm. Following its secretion by the Golgi apparatus, the glycocalyx is transported to the cell surface, but its exact method of incorporation is unclear. The distribution of the cell surface coat varies along the membrane, is modified in relation to cell recognition events, and is usually absent from junctional areas.

Cell Cohesion and Adherence

Cellular cohesion is partially a function of the cell surface. Cells can adhere to each other as well as to a substratum, and the latter is especially important for mobility along a surface. When cells in suspension encounter a surface, they develop numerous membranous extensions to overcome electrostatic forces. The cell surface, particularly the *microvillus,* carries negatively charged carboxyl groups in neuraminic acid, glycoproteins, and glycolipids which aid cellular cohesion and adherence.

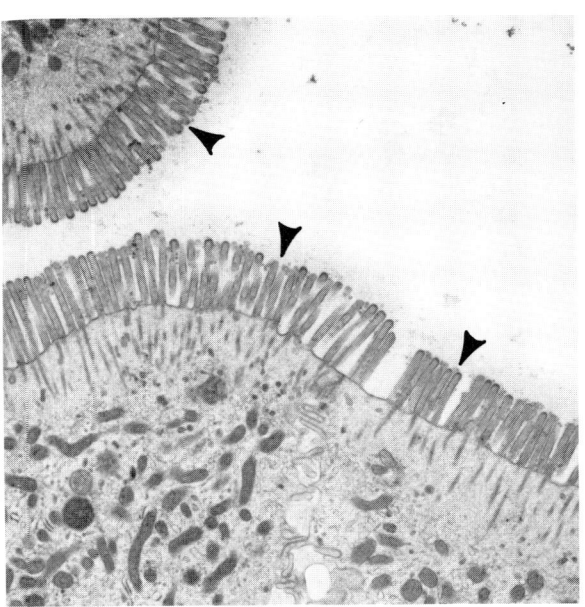

Figure 6–6. Transmission electron micrograph shows glycocalyx covering cells. The thickness of this coat is indicated by the arrow heads.

Membrane-associated Enzymes

Membrane-associated enzymes (Table 6–1), whose active sites exclusively face the external environment rather than the cytoplasm, are known as *exoenzymes*. Other enzymes have active sites both on the membrane and in the cytoplasm.

Certain specialized membranes contain moieties important in their functional activities. For example, membrane proteins at cholinergic synapses appear to undergo phosphorylation as a result of receptor interactions with neurotransmitters. These changes regulate ionic permeability, so that specific cellular events may occur.

Table 6–1.   *Enzymes With Activity Confined to the Membrane*

Enzymes of nucleotide metabolism
   2' 3' Cyclic adenosine monophosphate (cAMP) cyclic nucleotide 3' phosphohydrolase
   Adenyl cyclase
   Uridine triphosphatase (UTPase)
   5 Adenosine monophosphate (AMP) phosphatase

Adenosine triphosphatases (ATPases)
   ATPases not linked to fibrous membrane proteins
   Mg^{+2} ATPase
   Na^+, K^+ ATPase ouabain inhibited
   Ca^{+2} ATPase inhibited by Mg^{+2}

Enzymes of carbohydrate metabolism
   Neuraminidase
   Cytosine monophosphate (CMP) N-acetylneuraminic acid glycoprotein sialytransferase
   N-acetyl β-glucosaminidase
   α-, β-D glucosidase
   α-, β-D galactosidase
   α, β-L fucosidase
   β-D-xylosidase
   α-D-mannosidase
   N-acetyl-β-D-galactosaminidase
   β-Glucuronidase
   N-acetyl-galactosaminyl transferase

Phosphatases
   Vitamin B_6 phosphate phosphatase
   Mg^{+2}-dependent phosphoprotein phosphatase

Proteinases
   3 Proteinases (pH optima 7.4, 7.4, 3.2)
   2 Proteinases (pH optima 3.4, 7.4)

Protein kinases
   Cyclic adenosine monophosphate (cAMP) independent, stimulated by mono- and divalent cations to phosphorylate band 2 spectrin proteins
   cAMP stimulated Ca^{+2} inhibited, monovalent cation inhibited

Miscellaneous
   Nicotinamide-adenine dinucleotide (NAD^+) glycohydrolase (DPNase)
   Nicotinamide-adenine dinucleotide phosphate ($NADP^+$) glycohydrolase (TPNase)
   Reduced nicotinamide-adenine dinucleotide (NADH) acceptor oxidoreductase

(Modified from Schrier, S.L.: Human erythrocytic membrane enzymes: current states and clinical correlates. Blood, 50:229, 1977.)

Membrane fractions enriched with acetylcholine (ACh) receptor sites also contain a protein kinase responsible for the phosphorylation of endogenous membrane polypeptides. This event is responsive to ACh binding, perhaps by altering the conformational structure of the receptor. Erythrocyte membranes contain an endogenous protein phosporylating system, the protein kinases.[27] These kinases are both dependent upon, and independent of, adenosine 3'5'-cyclic monophosphate (cAMP) and appear to regulate a variety of membrane properties.[28]

Membrane-associated Receptors

Many cells possess surface molecular units that extend through the external portion of membranes and serve as specific recognition units. These structures, known as *receptors* (Table 6–2), are mobile and can be modulated or induced by a variety of agents, including the substrate for the receptor. They are often found on the external portion of the integral proteins.

Table 6–2. *Examples of Membrane Receptors*

Hormone Receptors
    Polypeptides (e.g. insulin)

Neurotransmitter Receptors
    α and β noradrenergic transmitters
    Dopamine
    Cholinergic (acetylcholine) transmitters

Immune Receptors
    Antigen receptors on B cells (IgM, IgG, IgE, IgA, IgD)
    Complement receptors
    Ia receptors (B, null cell, activated T cells)
    T-cell receptors for unsensitized red blood cells

Infectious Agent Receptors on Host Cells
    Bacteria (exotoxins)
    Viral membrane components (hemagglutinin)
    Parasites (Duffy blood group factor)

Lectin and Mitogen Receptors
    Phytohemagglutinin
    Concanavilin A

Drug Receptors
    Anesthetics (halothane)
    Analgesics (opiates, endorphins, enkephalins)
    Antibiotics (penicillin)
    Chemotherapeutic agents (nitrogen mustard)
    Others (digitalis, colchicine)

Molecular and Macromolecular Receptors
    Amino acids, sugars, fatty acids
    Low-density lipoprotein
    Growth-factor receptors

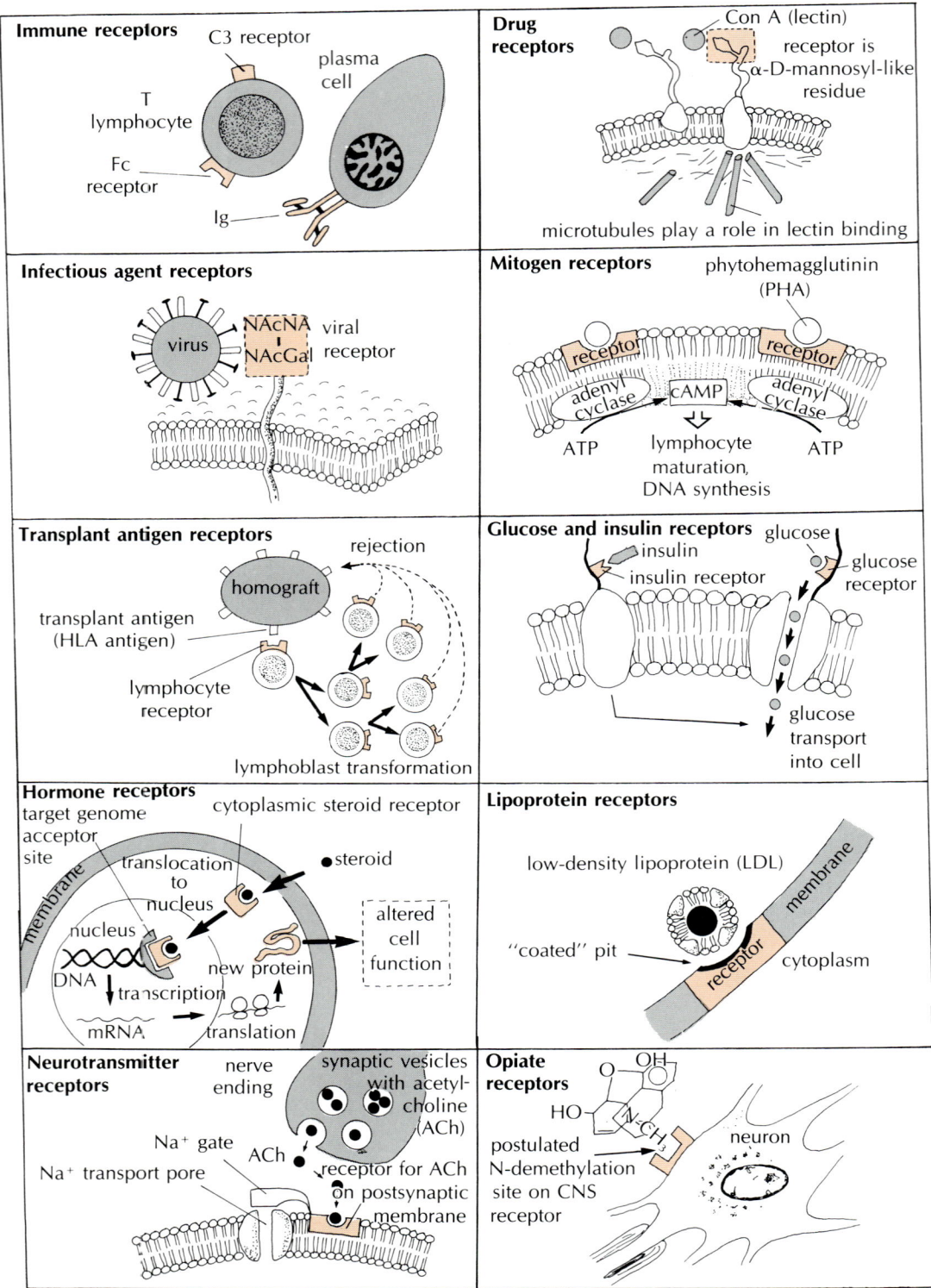

Figure 6–7. Cell surface receptors and some of their functions.

Membranes have receptors for hormones, neurotransmitters, infectious agents, microbial synthetic products, drugs, lectins, low-density lipoproteins, antigens, antibodies, complement, and numerous other substances (Fig. 6–7).

Not enough is known about receptor synthesis. Receptors are probably made in the endoplasmic reticulum (ER) and are later inserted into the membrane.[29] Once on the cell surface, they may be changed and modulated by enzymatic degradation, pinocytosis, and in situ phosphorylation, or they may be transported intracellularly. Under special situations, receptors may be induced on cells that do not ordinarily have them.

Hormone Receptors

Certain hormone receptors (Table 6–3) can recognize and selectively bind specific hormones or neurotransmitters, thereby activating adenylate cyclase and generating cAMP, which in turn initiates a series of events leading to specific biologic responses.

Table 6–3.   *Examples of Internalization of Receptors with Coated Pits*

Transport protein receptors
Low-density lipoprotein
Transferrin
Transcobalamine
Hormone receptors
Epithelial growth factor
Nerve growth factor
Melanotropin
Human chorionic gonadotropin
Insulin
Other receptors
α_2 macroglobulin
Maternal immunoglobulin α_2
Lysosomal enzymes
Asialoglycoprotein

(Modified from: Symposium on Research Frontiers in Aging and Cancer: International Symposium for the 1980's. Cancer Inst. Monogr., *60*, 1980.)

The majority of *peptide hormone receptors* are on the plasma membrane, but some binding sites have also been identified on the intracellular membranes of the SER, RER, Golgi apparatus, mitochondria, and nuclei.[30] Even those hormones that usually react with a cytoplasmic receptor, such as estrogen, may enter target cells by an initial interaction with the plasma membrane. Although it is controversial, specific receptor components have been demonstrated for *estradiol*-17β on the surfaces of estrogen-responsive cells.[31]

Most *hormone receptors* appear to be *intrinsic membrane proteins.*[32] They may be proteins, glycoproteins, lipoproteins, or glycolipoprotein molecules that exist in equilibrium with the rest of the membrane components. A phospholipid portion seems to be important for *adrenocorticotropic hormone*. *Thyroid-stimulating hormone, insulin, luteinizing hormone,* and *human chorionic gonadotropin* appear to have important carbohydrate components in their receptors.[33]

Infectious Agent Receptors

Receptors for certain infectious agents and microbial products have been found in many cells (Table 6–2), including those for *diphtheria, malaria,* and *influenza* (see Chap. 3). Specific receptors have been identified for numerous viruses.[34] These receptors aid in the attachment of the viral particle to the target cell. The best-studied example is influenza virus, in which the receptor on red blood cells is located on an integral host protein that also has receptors for blood groups and other substances of the glycophorin molecule.

A receptor for the *malarial* parasite appears to exist on *red blood cells* of patients with the *Duffy blood type*.[35]

Receptors also exist for specific microbial products including diphtheria, cholera, and tetanus *toxins*. The enterotoxin choleragen of Vibrio cholerae binds to a glycolipid receptor, which activates the adenylate cyclase system.[36]

Immune Receptors

A complex of *membrane components* on *lymphocytes, monocytes, macrophages,* and *granulocytes* is concerned with *antigen recognition* and subsequent specific cellular differentiation. Some aspects of these events are discussed in detail in Chapter 2.

Lectin Receptors

Lectins are glycoproteins that are specifically directed against certain oligosaccharide sequences in the cell membrane (Table 6–2). They have hemagglutinating properties and are used as probes of membrane structure. Lectins also have blastogenic effects,[37] which are discussed in Chapter 2.

Pharmacologic Receptors

An exceptionally interesting drug receptor is that for *opiates*, which interacts in a stereospecific fashion with these compounds (Table 6–2). This receptor mediates the major pharmacologic actions of opiates and of the endogenous opiate-like substances known as endorphins and enkephalins.[38] *Endorphins* refer to peptides produced by the pituitary, whereas *enkephalins* are endogenous pentapeptides found in the brain. The target neurons with receptors for endorphins are present in high density in pain pathways.

Preliminary data suggest that the receptor molecule contains cerebroside sulfate,[39] and this molecule may exist in several conformations that are influenced by salt concentration.[40] When endorphins, or drugs such as *morphine*, bind to these receptors, they change ion permeability, increase cAMP,[38] and initiate a series of subsequent physiologic changes that mediate the perception of pain.

Work on the receptor protein for *digitalis* has suggested ATPase as a candidate. A strong correlation exists between binding of digitalis to the cell membrane and the pharmacologic effects of ATPase, but definitive proof of this relationship remains to be established.[41]

Low-density Lipoprotein (LDL) Receptors

Receptors for these substances bind the major cholesterol-carrying lipoprotein of plasma *(LDL)*, regulate the rate at which this lipoprotein transfers cholesterol into the cell, and are present within *coated pits* (Table 6–3). Like the insulin receptor, its activity is under feedback control; the amount of cholesterol entering the cell is inversely proportional to the intracellular cholesterol concentration. LDL binds to the receptor and enters the cell by absorptive endocytosis.[42]

Function of the Cell Membrane

The membrane acts as a protective barrier to the outside environment and allows cellular organelles to perform integrated functions. In order for the cell to obtain necessary nutrients, secrete needed products, excrete toxic substances, and remain under homeostatic control, the cell membrane must constantly change. The five major functions of the membrane are listed in Table 6–4.

Table 6–4. *Membrane Functions*

Structure
  Containment of cellular organelles
  Maintenance of relationship with cytoskeleton, endoplasmic reticulum, and other organelles
  Maintenance of ion and substrate balance

Protection
  Barrier to toxic molecules and macromolecules
  Barrier to foreign organisms and cells

Activation of Cell
  Hormones—regulation of cell activity
  Mitogens—cell division
  Antigens—antibody synthesis
  Growth factors—proliferation and differentiation

Transport
  Diffusion and exchange diffusion
  Endocytosis, pinocytosis, and phagocytosis
  Exocytosis—secretion
  Active transport

Cell-Cell Interaction
  Communication between cells through junctions
  Symbiotic nutritive relationships
  Release of enzymes and antibodies to environment
  Relationships with extracellular matrix

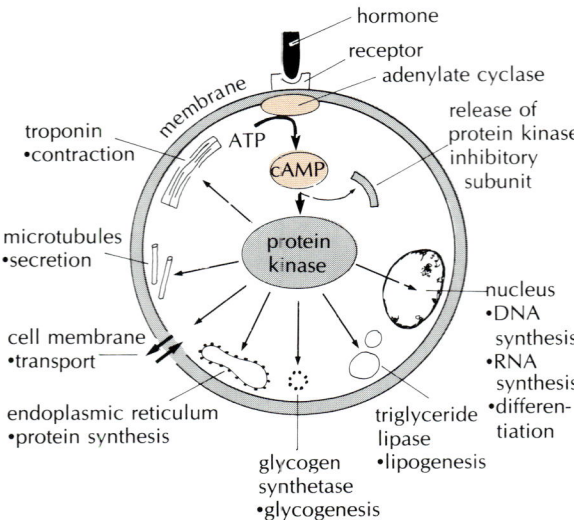

Figure 6–8. The biologic effects of cyclic AMP (cAMP) rest in its ability to activate the enzyme (or enzymes) known as protein kinase, which in turn activates or inactivates other enzymes by phosphorylation.

Role of Cyclic Nucleotides

One of the more extensively studied forms of communication between the plasma membrane and the cell interior is the adenyl cyclase-cAMP system (Fig. 6–8 and Table 6–5). It remains unclear how surface receptors communicate with the cyclase system because each probably lies on opposite sides of the plasma membrane.[43]

Table 6–5. *Second Messenger for Polypeptide and Catecholamine Hormones*

Hormones That Stimulate Adenylate Cyclase	Hormones That Do Not Stimulate Adenylate Cyclase
Adrenocorticotropic hormone	Angiotensin
Calcitonin	Catecholamines (α-adrenergic)
Catecholamines (β-adrenergic)	Chorionic somatomammotropin
Chorionic gonadotropin	(placental lactogen)
Follicle-stimulating hormone	Epidermal growth factor
Glucagon	Fibroblast growth factor
Luteinizing hormone	Growth hormone
Luteinizing-hormone releasing	Insulin
factor	Insulin-like growth factors
Lipotropin	Multiplication-stimulating activity
Melanocytic stimulating hormone	Oxytocin
Nerve growth factor	Prolactin
Parathyroid hormone	Prostaglandin F_2
Prostaglandin F_1	Somatomedin
Thyrotropin-releasing hormone	Somatostatin
Vasopressin	
Thyrotropin-stimulating hormone	

(Modified from Kolodny, E.H.: Current concepts in genetics. Lysosomal storage diseases. N. Engl. J. Med., 294:1217, 1976.)

The cAMP system has been divided into four functional phases: *activation, synthesis, effector,* and *degradation.* The *activation phase* begins when a receptor becomes occupied and activated. A signal is transmitted by an unknown means from the receptor to adenyl cyclase located on the inner surface of the membrane. In the *synthesis phase,* Ca^{++}-dependent *adenyl cyclase* is activated; this process may require guanosine triphosphate (GTP) and results in the synthesis of *cAMP from ATP.* In the *effector phase,* cAMP cellular responses are mediated by a group of enzymes known as *protein kinases.* The enzymes appear to consist of two subunits: *catalytic* and *cAMP-binding* regulatory units. By binding to the regulatory subunit, cAMP promotes the dissociation of the two subunits that results in the conversion of an inactive complex to the active enzyme. This enzyme is then capable of phosphorylating other enzymes. *Degradation,* the final phase of the cAMP system, inactivates cAMP by hydrolysis to 5′ adenosine monophosphate. The reaction is catalyzed by phosphodiesterase (Fig. 6–8).

The *cyclase system* primarily affects general cell functions, such as transport of amino acids and synthesis of protein. This system also mediates certain unique functions such as the production and release of insulin by beta cells, the production of thyroxine by thyroid cells, and the regulation of glycogen metabolism by the liver (Table 6–5).

Cyclic guanosine monophosphate (cGMP) and *cAMP* interact with each other and have *opposing effects,* which are best illustrated in cells capable of antagonistic events, for example, contraction and relaxation, glycogen synthesis and glycogen breakdown, and proliferation and contact inhibition. Cyclic GMP is usually present in cells at one tenth the concentration of cAMP.[33]

How do proteins as ubiquitous as adenyl cyclase and cAMP regulate so many specialized functions? In any given cell, cAMP can only be recruited by a specific signal at a specific site, that is, the receptor. The second part of the specificity lies in the responses of the cell to the signal. These are the unique function of the specialized enzymatic machinery of a particular, differentiated cell.[44]

Cellular Transport and Effect of Ions on Membranes

Water moves freely by *passive diffusion* through functional or structural molecular pores of the membrane. Normally, *channels* within integral proteins are capable of transporting ions through the membrane.[45] Ion permeability is probably also related to membrane fluidity.[46]

Because the cell membrane is essentially a lipid structure and constitutes an initial barrier to water-soluble materials of low molecular weight, specific transport processes are required for their passage. There may be, in many instances, a transient interaction with specific membrane components known as *carriers,* which transport small substrates such as amino acids and sugars and require energy.

The movement of a given substrate depends upon the substrate concentrations at both sides of the membrane, the affinity of the carrier for the substrate, and the metabolic requirements of the cell.

Cations have a crucial role in determining both the structural and functional characteristics of the membrane, especially in cells concerned with electrical excitation or transmitter release. Inorganic cations also help to determine the configuration of lipid arrays and the excitability of the membrane.[47] Changes in temperature may aggregate the membrane proteins in such a way that new hydrophilic pathways are generated, allowing for increased ion and nonelectrolyte transport mechanisms.

In general, *cationic transport* requires the production and maintenance of opposing gradients of Na^+ and K^+. These gradients are generated by the sodium-potassium pump in the membrane. The energy needed for the cationic pumping is generated by the splitting of ATP by a Mg^{++}-dependent activated ATPase.

The role of ions in membrane function is exemplified by muscle cells, which are specialized for the purpose of contraction. The excitation and contraction depends on the

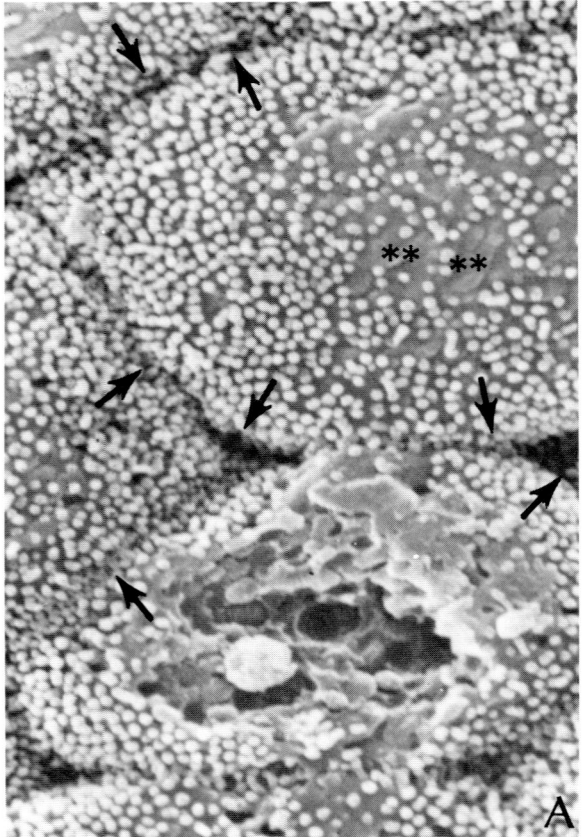

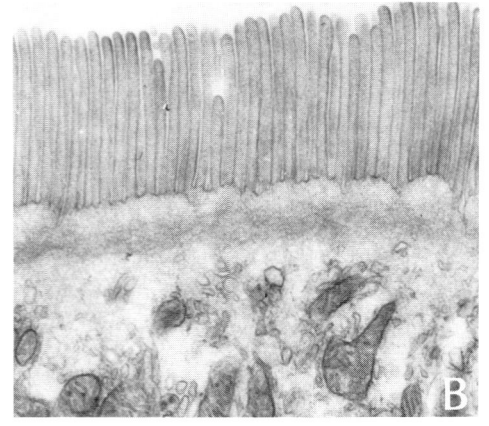

Figure 6–9. *A,* This scanning electron micrograph shows endocervical mucin-secreting cells covered by microvilli. Dark areas (arrows) represent the intercellular spaces. Mucin can be seen swelling up from inside the cell to partly conceal the microvilli (**). A gap is present in the apical surface where mucin has already been secreted from the cell. *B,* In this transmission electron micrograph, intestinal absorptive cell is covered with a lush microvillous surface.

integrity of all the membrane systems, and Ca^{++} is thought to be the link between stimulating events, which occur at the cell surface, and contraction, which takes place at the sarcomere level. The calcium must move to the *troponin* Ca^{++}-binding site for contraction, and it must be removed for relaxation. A variety of *calcium "sinks"* store excess Ca^{++}.[48] The function of both muscle and nerve cells depends upon the action potentials generated; the majority of energy required for these events comes from the splitting of ATP to adenosine diphosphate (ADP).

Movement of material into the cell occurs by *endocytosis (pinocytosis or phagocytosis)*. Solutes or secretions may be *exported* by the process of *exocytosis* or *emiocytosis*. (Fig. 6–9). Cells export substances such as hormones, colostrum, mucin, proteoglycans, enzymes, antibodies, and collagen.

Epithelial function in large part concerns transport of materials into and from the cell, and a number of morphologic adaptations, usually with extensive surface folding, accommodate this function. Specialized areas of the plasma membrane concerned with inward transport are found on the membranes of many cell types. *Microvilli* are the most common of these specialized structures. The microvillus structure is moderately complex in terms of both its morphologic arrangement and its enzymatic content. For example, the microvillous border of intestinal cells contains a number of *hydrolytic enzymes,* including disaccharidases and dipeptidases, *synthetic enzymes,* such as glycosyltransferases, and *carrier proteins* for amino acid and sugar transport.

Protection from the Environment

The third major function of the cell membrane is to protect intracellular reactions, macromolecules, and organelles from direct contact with injurious agents in the extracellular environment. The *modulation of membrane receptors* may hinder passage of infectious agents, toxins, and drugs into the cell and may enhance and guide useful substrates, hormones, and other substances to appropriate synthetic or degradative sites and organelles.

Intercellular Communication

Most cells in tissues are not isolated from their neighbors; therefore, they need to communicate with one another. Communication usually occurs in one or more of four general *ways:* by *membrane receptors,* by *humoral* substances, by *electrical impulses,* or through *intercellular junctions* (Table 6–6). These last structures are specialized areas on the cell membrane where cells are joined. At this point, the membranes of the two apposed cells are specialized and allow the passage of molecules from one cell's interior to the other's. These junctional areas, more permeable than the

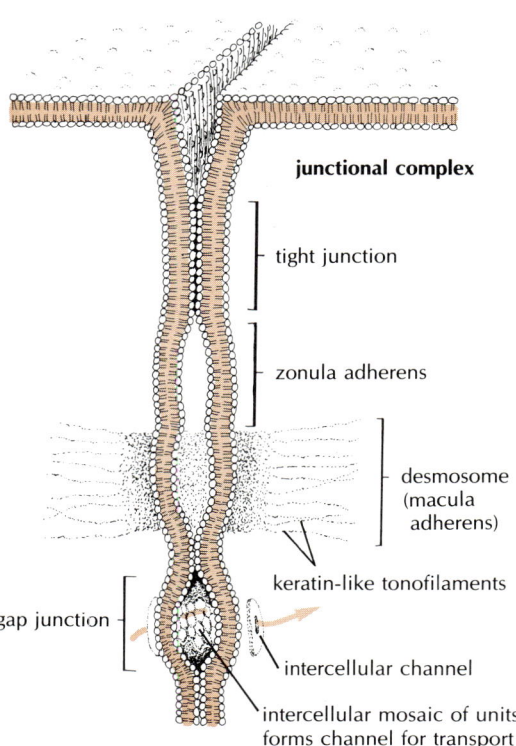

junctional complex

tight junction

zonula adherens

desmosome (macula adherens)

keratin-like tonofilaments

gap junction

intercellular channel

intercellular mosaic of units forms channel for transport

Figure 6–10. Structural components of the junctional complex. A gap junction is also shown at bottom.

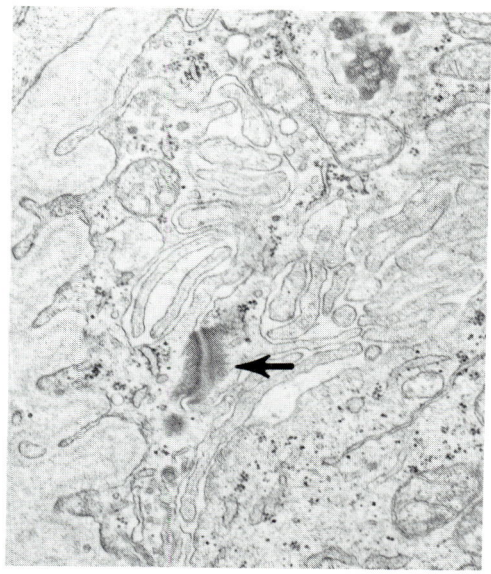

Figure 6–11. Desmosomal attachment between two adjacent cells (arrow).

Table 6–6. *Classification of Junctional Complexes*

Tight junctions
Intermediate junctions (zonula adherens)
Desmosomes (macula adherens)
Hemidesmosomes
Septate junctions
Gap junctions

rest of the cell membrane, are controlled by a process known as gating.

Gating is primarily controlled by calcium ions. If the cytoplasmic calcium level rises, the permeability of the junctional areas decreases. This gating mechanism plays an important role in cellular injury because it allows uninjured cells to *"seal themselves off"* from damaged neighbors. A damaged cell releases calcium into the environment of its noninjured neighbor. The increased calcium ion concentration decreases the permeability at the junction of the uninjured cell, and it is sealed off from the injured neighboring cells.

Structure and Function of the Junctional Complex

The *junctional complex*, first described by Farquhar and Palade,[49] is a complex specialization of the epithelial cell surface membrane and consists of three parts (Fig. 6–10): (1) *the tight junction (zonula occludens)*, a barrier to cellular diffusion; (2) the *zonula adherens*, an intermediate junction; and (3) the *macula adherens*, otherwise known as a *desmosome* (Fig. 6–11).

The junctional complex is the most elaborate area of contact between mammalian epithelial cells. The *zonula adherens* is usually the site of insertion for the *terminal web*.[50] The epithelial *desmosome* acts as a system of braces for cell stabilization. Desmosomes are occasionally found intracellularly, especially in epidermal tumors and in virally infected cell cultures. *Hemidesmosomes* may also be present and are located along basal aspects of cells in the plane of apposition to the basal lamina.[51]

Gap Junctions

Gap junctions (Fig. 6–10) are common between many types of adult and embryonic cells and are believed to have a role in differentiation.[52] They frequently accompany the junctional complex; these junctions may also occur as independent structures. Gap junctions are considered to be the morphologic counterpart of low-resistance pathways between cells, and they allow intercellular exchange of low-molecular weight metabolites and ions, thereby facilitating *electrotonic coupling* of cells.[53]

Septate Junctions

These junctions are uncommon in human cells, but often occur in insects. They resemble pleated ribbons or a series of flattened, hexagonal units.[54] Septate junctions have been identified in the cerebellum and ovary.[55] Like gap junctions, they are believed to be sites of electrotonic coupling.

T-Tubule System

One other membrane structure that deserves brief mention is the *T system* of tubules, which invaginates from the plasma membrane of striated muscle. These tubules appear to be responsible for conducting the surface activation signals into the cell and thereby play an important role in the coupling of excitation and contraction reactions.[56]

Agents of Injury: General

The cell membrane is the first cellular barrier to the environment. Therefore, it is susceptible to many noxious materials. These agents may change the basic chemical structure of the membrane or its fluidity and may thus alter receptors, enzymes, or other membrane-associated determinants. Because such changes are intimately concerned with cellular recognition events, the cell may lose the discriminatory powers that usually enable it to respond to external stimuli. The transport properties of the membrane may also be altered. Some injurious agents may punch discrete holes in the membrane or may lead to nonspecific changes in surface structure, for example, complement-mediated cell-membrane lysis.

Genetic Factors

Genetic disorders may affect the plasma membrane by altering its structure and shape, its receptors, or its transport properties (Table 6–7).

Sickle cell anemia, Huntington's disease, muscular dystrophy,[57] and *abetalipoproteinemia* are genetic disorders with profound associated structural membrane changes reflected in red blood cell structure. In sickle cell anemia (see Chap. 3), the

Table 6–7. *Genetic Diseases Associated with Alterations in Membrane Structure and Function*

Sickle cell disease
Huntington's disease
Muscular dystrophy
Familial hypercholesteremia
Fanconi's syndrome
Aminoaciduria
Cystinuria
Hartnup's disease

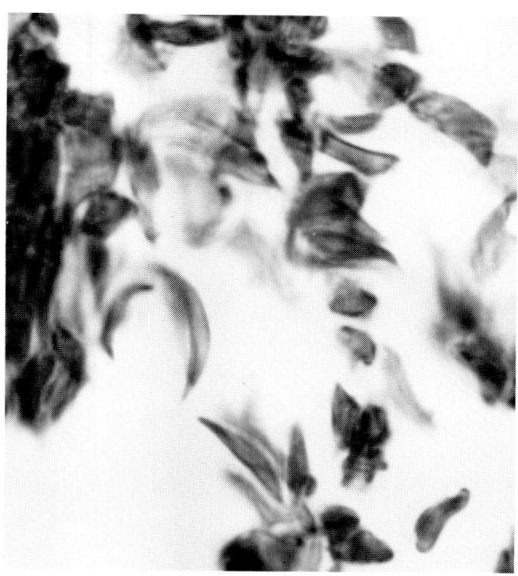

Figure 6–12. This light micrograph of red blood cells from a patient with sickle cell disease shows the change in red blood cell morphology that gives the disease its name.

polymerized abnormal HbS molecules bind to the actin-spectrin lattice and distort the shape of the red blood cells[58] (Fig. 6–12). This change results in deformability, altered surface area, ion transport, and fragility. The erythrocytes in patients with Huntington's disease, an autosomal dominant disorder of the central nervous system, have an increased number of stomatocytes or prickle cells; this phenomenon suggests an alteration in the state of the membrane lipids.[59]

In *congenital muscular dystrophy,* many cells are affected by alterations in membrane fluidity. Changes in lymphocytes are reflected by abnormalities in the ability to cap.[60]

Congenital deficiency of serum LDL leads to an abnormality in the sphingomyelin-lecithin content of erythrocyte membranes and decreases their membrane fluidity. The *spur cells* formed as a result of these abnormalities are more easily phagocytosed in the lymphoreticular system, and hemolytic anemia develops.

Other genetic diseases are associated with abnormalities of specific receptors. For example, *familial hypercholesterolemia* is an autosomal genetic disease associated with a defect in the *LDL* receptor. The disease is characterized by hypercholesterolemia and premature coronary artery disease.[61]

Type II hyperlipoproteinemia shows three distinct autosomal dominant disorders of the receptor. One type of patient totally lacks the receptors, another has defective receptors, and in the third group, the gene controlling internalization of the receptor in the coated pit is defective.[62] The coated pit contains an aggregate of receptors appropriate for a specific substance or organism[63] (see Table 6–3).

Genetic enzyme defects may lead to abnormalities in membrane transport. *Cystinuria, Hartnup's disease,* and *iminoglycinuria* all show defective transport processes.[64] Others are listed in Table 6–7.

Other heritable enzyme defects in membranes lead to different diseases. For example, the absence of lactase in the brush border of intestinal cells causes lactose intolerance in infancy; this disease is also occasionally seen in adults.

Nutritional Factors

The most striking cell membrane changes associated with altered nutritional states are reflected in the erythrocytes of patients with severe *hepatic dysfunction.* The disordered plasma lipoprotein metabolism seen in such diseases causes abnormalities in red blood cell shape, with the appearance of *spur cells.* This process occurs in two separate and sequential steps. The first is a modification of membrane architecture and composition, including the selective acquisition of cholesterol. In the second step, the nonspecific loss of membrane surface area leads to the formation of spurs and bizarre, irregular contours. Hemolysis results as the cells become trapped and phagocytosed in the lymphoreticular system of the spleen and lymph nodes.

Membrane function can be affected experimentally by the addition of certain nutritional substances. For example, alterations in the plasma membrane transport processes and concurrent changes in Ca++ permeability are believed to play a role in cell death following *galactosamine* administration.[65]

The in vitro administration of *polylysine* and *polyarginine* in high concentrations agglutinates cell membranes. Excessive amounts of *vitamin A* induce *lysis* of *plasma cell membranes* and, in other concentrations, affect *lysosomal membranes* by releasing hydrolases.[66]

Physical Agents

The effects of temperature, radiation, pressure, and hypoxia on the membrane are briefly considered (Table 6–8).

We have already noted that changes in *temperature* affect membrane fluidity by altering lipid organization. The exchange of phospholipids from the plasma and the movement of phosphatidylcholine across the red blood cell membrane are temperature dependent. Furthermore, thermal injury induces *electrolyte* and *water shifts*.[67]

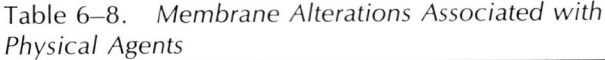

Table 6–8. *Membrane Alterations Associated with Physical Agents*

Physical Agent	Alteration
Temperature	cold: ↓ transport warm: ↑ transport and flux and mobility of lipoprotein components
Radiation	↑ membrane permeability ↑ osmotic lability ↑ K+ loss
Pressure	loss of microvilli
Hypoxia	↑ permeability ↑ Na+, H₂O influx ↑ K+ efflux

Radiation increases *membrane permeability*, osmotic fragility, and potassium loss from the cell. It also alters the lipid composition of the membrane by the formation of lipid peroxides.[68] Finally, radiation may alter cellular shape and topographic features.

Increased pressures in obstructive processes cause the loss of surface microvilli in structures secondarily affected. For example, the tight junctions become irregularly shaped, and gap junctions are lost from bile canaliculi in large *bile duct obstruction* by *stones* or surgical ligation[69] (Fig. 6–13).

Hypoxia eventually produces *leaky cell membranes* with swelling and rupture, accompanied by the aggregation of

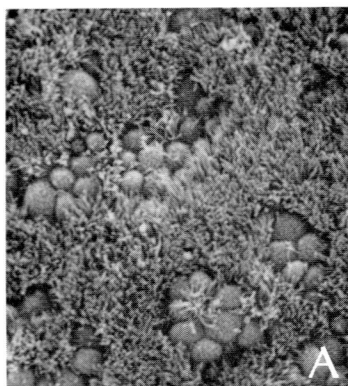

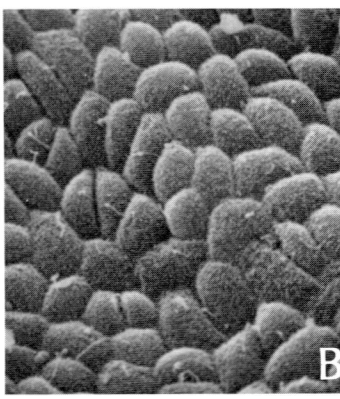

Figure 6–13. The effect of pressure on the cell surface. *A,* The lining epithelium of normal fallopian tube has numerous microvilli and cilia. *B,* In hydrosalpingitis, the fluid accumulations cause the disappearance of microvilli and cilia.

IMP[70] and alterations in the cyclic nucleotides. Because of permeability changes, *cytoplasmic enzymes* diffuse into the circulation. Such a hypoxic mechanism is at work to increase the serum level of creatine phosphokinase *(CPK)*, the classic clinical enzyme marker of *myocardial infarction*.

Hypoxia may also lead to osmotic lysis of erythrocytes by producing slits and holes 100 to 1000 Å long in the membrane that intercommunicate and are permeable to large molecules.[71]

Infectious Agents

Infectious agents may also induce membrane abnormalities (Table 6–9).

Table 6–9. *Membrane Alterations Associated with Infectious Agents*

Infectious Agent	Alteration
Viruses	Cytolysis
	Giant cell fusion (herpes, measles)
	Appearance of new viral membrane antigens
Bacteria	Cytolysis
	Enzymes (protease)
	Toxins (lecithinase: Clostridium perfringens)
	Phagocytosis (meningococcus, Mycobacterium tuberculosis, gonococcus)
Fungi	Phagocytosis (Candida albicans, yeast form)
Parasites	Endocytosis following attachment to parasites (Duffy receptor malaria parasite)
	Exocytosis of parasites following rupture of red blood cells

Viruses. We have previously noted that cell membranes have receptors for infectious agents. When viruses fuse with the membrane following interaction with their receptors, changes in the orientation of the fatty acids alter the fluid bilayer structures.[72] The severity of these disturbances varies with the virus. The effects of *Newcastle disease virus* are far more pronounced than those of *influenza virus*. In the latter case, however, the degree of distortion of the bilayer is related to the status of the hemagglutinin in the viral membranes. The infectious influenza virus contains the hemagglutinin in the cleaved form necessary for viral penetration[73] (Fig. 6–14).

The fusion of the viral membrane with host cell membranes damages the normal ionic barrier, but this damage is repaired once fusion is completed.[14] The cytolysis seen in some viral infections may result from membrane damage subsequent to cytoplasmic and lysosomal enzyme release. In some viral infections, a decline in membrane phospholipid synthesis coincides with the release of cytoplasmic enzymes.[74]

The attachment of viruses and membrane fusion with host cells may also induce *giant cell formation*. This effect has been seen with measles, influenza, herpes simplex, and

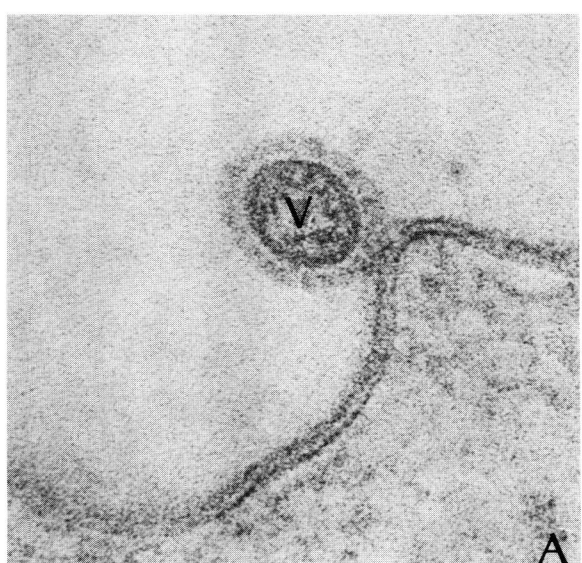
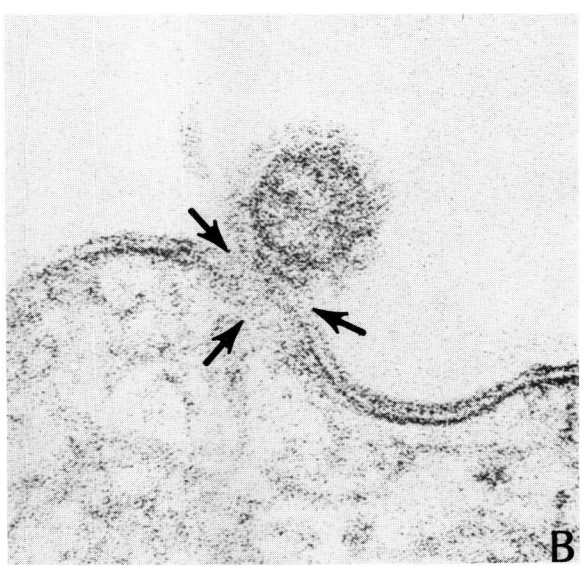

Figure 6–14. *A*, Viral (V) attachment to a cell. *B*, As the process proceeds, the membrane of the infected cell undergoes focal dissolution (arrows).

vesicular stomatitis viruses and appears to be generally associated with enveloped viruses.

New membrane surface components may appear following integration of viral genetic material into the host cell genome.[75] These virally related *membrane antigens* may stimulate immunologically mediated membrane damage by means of direct cytotoxic reactions or antibody reactions with complement.[76]

Bacterial Toxins. The synthetic products of infectious agents may also damage membranes. Bacterial toxins exemplify this phenomenon; they may damage cells either directly or indirectly. *Colicins* are toxic proteins synthesized by Escherichia coli, each of which is determined by a single gene.[77] Colicin E_2 damages DNA, E_3 damages ribosomes, and E_1 and K block the active transport of lactose, amino acids, and K^+.

Toxins from Clostridium perfringens and Clostridium tetani are anticholinergics. Phospholipase C lecithinase from C. perfringens opens channels in the cell membrane and allows the diffusion of small ions. These channels are opened by the cleavage of phosphorylcholine, a substance possibly covering a Na^+ gate.[78]

Vibrio cholerae also produces a highly toxic exotoxin. Patients first have acute, severe diarrhea and abdominal pain. They may pass as many as 20 liters of "rice water" stools per day. The toxin increases the intestinal active transport of Na^+, Cl^- and H_2O by increasing cellular levels of cAMP through stimulation of adenyl cyclase.[79]

Drugs and Chemicals

Many drugs interact with the cell membrane and alter its basic structure (Table 6–10). Local *anesthetics* asymmet-

Table 6–10. *Effects of Drugs on Membrane Structure and Function*

Agents	Effects
Mitogens	Stimulation of division and in vitro
Concanavilin A	capping
Phytohemagglutinin (PHA)	
Hormones	Regulation of receptor sites on membranes
Peptides	
Catecholamines	
	Changes in membrane cytoskeletal networks
Cytochalasin	Microfilaments
Colchicine	Microtubules
	Changes in transport processes
Digitalis	Na^+, K^+-ATPase and active transport ↑
Cyanide	Respiratory burst of phagocytosis ↓
Procaine	Intercalation with lipoproteins and binding
	Changes in surface morphology
Alcohol	Clubbing of microvilli
Lithium	Clubbing of microvilli
Mercury	Cell-surface vesicle formation

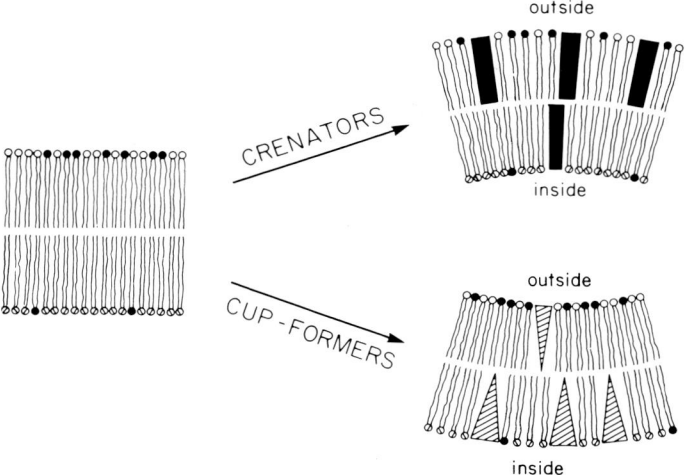

Figure 6–15. Diagram of the proposed mechanism of drug-erythrocyte interactions according to the bilayer-couple hypothesis. It is proposed that different agents intercalate into the two halves of the bilayer to different degrees. Crenators concentrate in the outer half; cup-formers concentrate in the inner half. (From Singer, S.J.: Structure of membranes. *In* Cell Membranes. Structure, Receptors, and Transport. Edited by C. Fenoglio, C. Borek, and D. W. King. New York, Stratton Intercontinental Medical Book, 1975.)

rically intercalate into the membranes. If they intercalate into the external portion, they preferentially expand that layer and crenate the cells. Conversely, if these agents intercalate into the inner leaflet, cuplike forms result. This differential expansion of the plasma membrane is reflected in alterations in fluidity, shape, and chemical structure[80] (Fig. 6–15).

Anesthetics may also alter lectin-binding sites by changing the cytoskeletal components, that is, through the loss of membrane-associated microfilaments and microtubules. Similar changes are made by cytochalasin and colchicine through an effect on the microfilaments and microtubules, respectively.[81] The appearance of *microappendages, blebs,* and *ruffles* dramatically demonstrates the altered membrane structure.[82]

The classic example of a drug-induced membrane change is *carbon tetrachloride toxicity* in which extensive *lipid peroxidation* results in abnormal cell function, including transport.[83] Intracellular accumulation of calcium and decreased levels of ATP are changes on the membrane surface that culminate in cell death.

Transport can be altered by other drugs. *Ouabain* inhibits phosphoglycerate kinase-mediated ATP synthesis[84] and thereby decreases ion transport. *Digitalis* binds and inhibits a specific sarcolemmal T-system receptor thought to be Na^+, K^+-ATPase.[41] That metabolic inhibitors such as *cyanide* enhance the uptake of certain drugs suggests the presence of a drug permeability barrier. This barrier can be modulated by differences in intrinsic protein phosphorylation.[85]

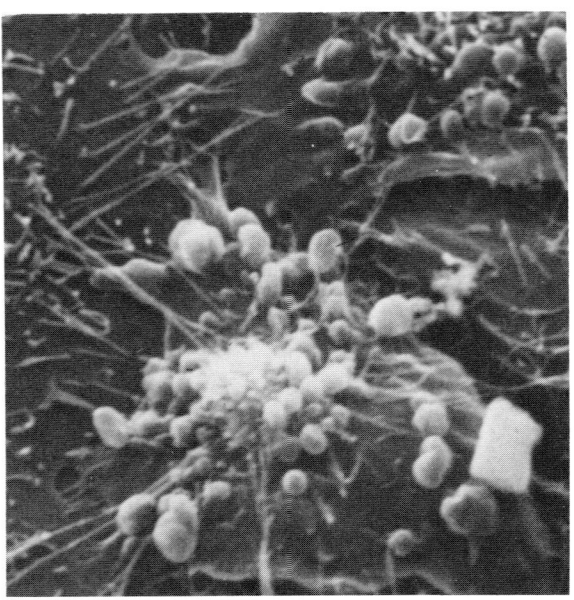

Figure 6–16. This scanning electron micrograph of cells grown in tissue culture demonstrates membrane shedding. This event is most striking over the central parts of the cell.

Other substances such as *alcohol* and *lithium* cause swelling, clubbing, and loss of microvilli at transport surfaces. At higher concentrations, these drugs produce irregular, shaggy holes in the cell surfaces.[86] Alcohol may affect membrane fluidity as well, but if cells are exposed to it for a long time, they become tolerant to this effect. Other membrane-lytic agents are listed in Table 6–10.

Membrane blebbing or shedding (Fig. 6–16) is a reversible physiologic response of the cell to various changes in its environment.

A unique type of surface vesicular injury is produced by sulfhydryl-blocking agents, such as *mercury*, that promote random formation of cell surface vesicles.[87]

It has recently been found that some chemicals can *induce* the formation of gap *junctions*. These drugs include the potassium conductance blockers, *tetraethylamine* and *4-aminopyridine*. Cultured muscle cells treated with these agents become mechanically active and spontaneously contract.

Immune Agents

Many cell membranes are injured by *direct contact* with lymphocytes and macrophages, as well as by *humoral substances* such as histamine, proteases, antibodies, lymphokines, and complement (Table 6–11). These components frequently act in concert with one another. The precise *interactions* among *host cells*, soluble *mediators*, and *immunoglobulins* and the *interactions* among *B cells*, *T cells*, *macrophages*, and killer *null cells* are currently unclear. However, we do know that intimate intercellular contact is required for many of these reactions to occur.

Studies using the lymphocyte-mediated cytolysis system have shown that the initial target cell-lymphocyte interac-

Table 6–11. *Membrane Alterations Associated with Immune Reactions*

Cytolysis
  Cell-cell interaction
  Cell-ADCC interaction
  Complement (antibody-independent) lysis

Blastogenesis
  Cell membrane changes
  "Rounding" of cell

Secretion of light chains
  Myeloma cells (with exocytosis and distorted microvilli)

Capping
  Induced by antigens and lectins

E, EA, EAC
  Rosettes with unsensitized and sensitized RBC reacting with B and T cells and macrophages

Alteration in receptors
  Myasthenia gravis: acetylcholine receptors decreased
  Maturity-onset diabetes: insulin receptors decreased

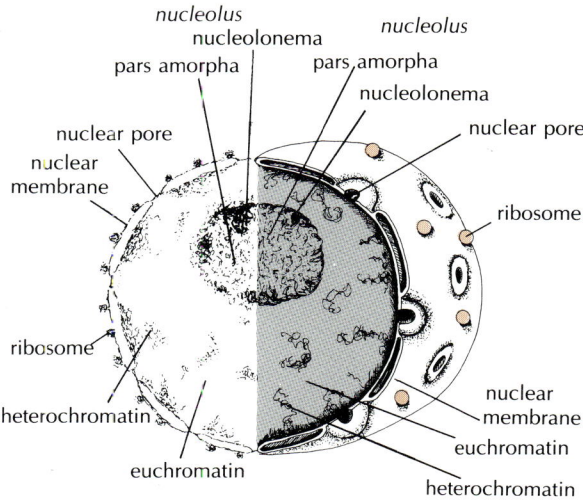

Figure 6–17. The structure of the nucleus. At right is a schematic, three-dimensional representation; at left is the schematic of the structures with transmission electron microscopy.

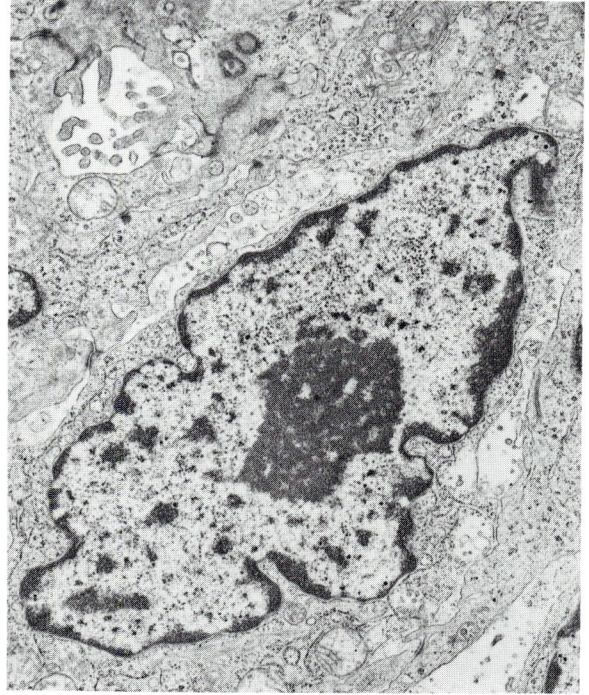

Figure 6–18. The nucleus often demonstrates prominent peripheral chromatin clumping and a nucleolus.

tion and subsequent target cell destruction are separate events. The initial interaction is an energy-dependent, temperature-independent event, whereas the target cell destruction is energy independent and temperature dependent.

Immune cytolysis involving antibody binding to membrane antigen in the presence of complement frequently damages the membrane directly. In studies by Hammer et al.[88] using antibody and complement-mediated immune hemolysis, three types of membrane changes were produced: surface rings, globular aggregates within the membrane, and transient openings.

Complement is responsible for many of the membrane abnormalities associated with immune injury. The insertion of C5b or the C7 subunit of the C5b to C7 complex into the phospholipid bilayers of the membrane[88] is particularly important in membrane damage. C5b and C7 have hydrophobic polypeptide chains that become exposed when C5b and 6 react with C7 to form the C5b, 6, 7 complex. These hydrophobic molecules, which include C8 and C9, react with other hydrophobic molecules in the lipid center of membranes and produce a transmembrane channel with high permeability to water and ions.[89] C3b and C6b form a stable, hydrophilic complex with the plasma membrane. The C5b to C9 complex on red blood cells is a thin-walled, 150-Å cylinder rimmed by an annulus at one end. Its internal diameter is 100 Å.[90] The classic complement rings seen on membranes after complement lysis may represent these complexes. This feature is associated with rapid leaking of K^+ and large cytoplasmic macromolecules, along with the rapid influx of water.

Antibodies may interact with membranes in a way that does not destroy them, but merely interferes with their functions. Examples include those diseases in which antibodies bind to receptor molecules, such as certain forms of diabetes mellitus and myasthenia gravis. Certain antibodies may also bind, block, or destroy cell junctions and may thus interfere with intercellular communication. In *pemphigus*, autoantibodies to desmosomes cause their dissolution and separation, resulting in a lack of cellular adhesion.[91]

NUCLEUS

Normal Structure and Function

The nucleus is a complex structure, the components of which constantly undergo active physiologic, morphologic and functional alterations (Figs. 6–17 and 6–18 and Table

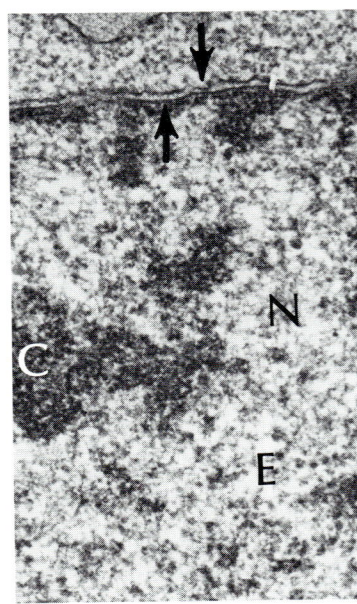

Figure 6–19. The nucleus (N) contains heterochromatin (C), which is condensed, and euchromatin (E), which is dispersed. The double-layered nucleus membrane (arrows) separates the nucleus from the rest of the cell.

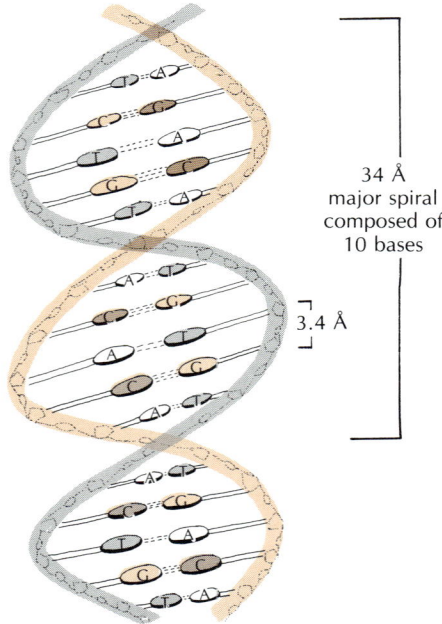

34 Å major spiral composed of 10 bases

3.4 Å

Figure 6–20. Double helix of DNA.

6–12). It is extremely sensitive to a multitude of injurious agents. In this section we consider the components of the nucleus, including *chromatin, nucleolus, nuclear envelope, nuclear fibrous lamina,* and *nucleoplasm.* Because the nucleus contains the cellular genetic constituents, it is not surprising that some injurious agents irreversibly damage the cell and produce heritable changes known as mutations.

Table 6–12. *Nuclear Structures*

Chromatin
Nucleolus
Nucleoplasm
Nuclear bodies
Nucleolar channel system
Nuclear inclusions
Fibrous lamina
Nuclear membrane
Nuclear pore complex

Chromosomes and Chromatin

Chromosomes carry the genetic information and undergo complex alterations throughout the cell cycle. They are visible only during mitosis. At this time, each chromosome consists of two arms (sister *chromatids*) united by a *centromere* called a *kinetochore* when attached to the spindle fiber during division. During interphase, one can see that, ultrastructurally, most regions of the chromatin appear condensed. These regions are known as *heterochromatin.* The dispersed portion is known as *euchromatin* (Fig. 6–19).

The constant, reversible transformations that occur between the condensed heterochromatin and the dispersed euchromatin depend upon cellular metabolism, the state of differentiation, and the stage of the cell cycle. Active euchromatin regions are transcribed or replicated. Inactive chromatin refers to areas not undergoing active transcription. In most cell nuclei, about 80 to 90% of the chromatin at any one time is inactive heterochromatin.

Chromatin Components. Chromatin consists of *DNA, RNA,* and *proteins.* DNA contains two purines, adenine and guanine, and two pyrimidines, cytosine and thymine (Fig. 6–20). Each is linked to a deoxyribose sugar forming a compound known as a *nucleoside,* which becomes a *nucleotide* when a phosphate group is added. RNA also contains two purine and two pyrimidine bases, but uracil is substituted for thymine and the pentose ribose forms the nucleoside. DNA is arranged in a specific configuration in chromatin. Recently, a new structure of DNA was described with a zigzag, sugar phosphate background. This has been called Z-DNA and is an attractive candidate for a regulatory role in genetic activity.[92]

Chromatin contains two major classes of protein: (1) basic proteins known as *histones* and (2) the nonhistone proteins, a heterogeneous group of *acidic proteins*. Histones are divided into five main classes, each coded for by specific histone genes. These classes are known as H_1, H_2A, H_2B, H_3 and H_4 and they differ in size, charge, and amino acid composition.

The histones appear to organize the long DNA molecules into a more compact form (Fig. 6–21). This effect is partially achieved by electrostatic interactions between the positively charged basic amino acid groups in the histones and the negatively charged DNA phosphate groups.

The *nonhistone* chromatin proteins are *acidic proteins* with an affinity for nucleohistones; these proteins bind to DNA and interact with it preferentially at the A-T base and single-stranded DNA regions. Increasing evidence suggests that the nonhistone proteins are partially responsible for the regulation of gene expression, especially transcription, by affecting the binding of DNA to histones.[93]

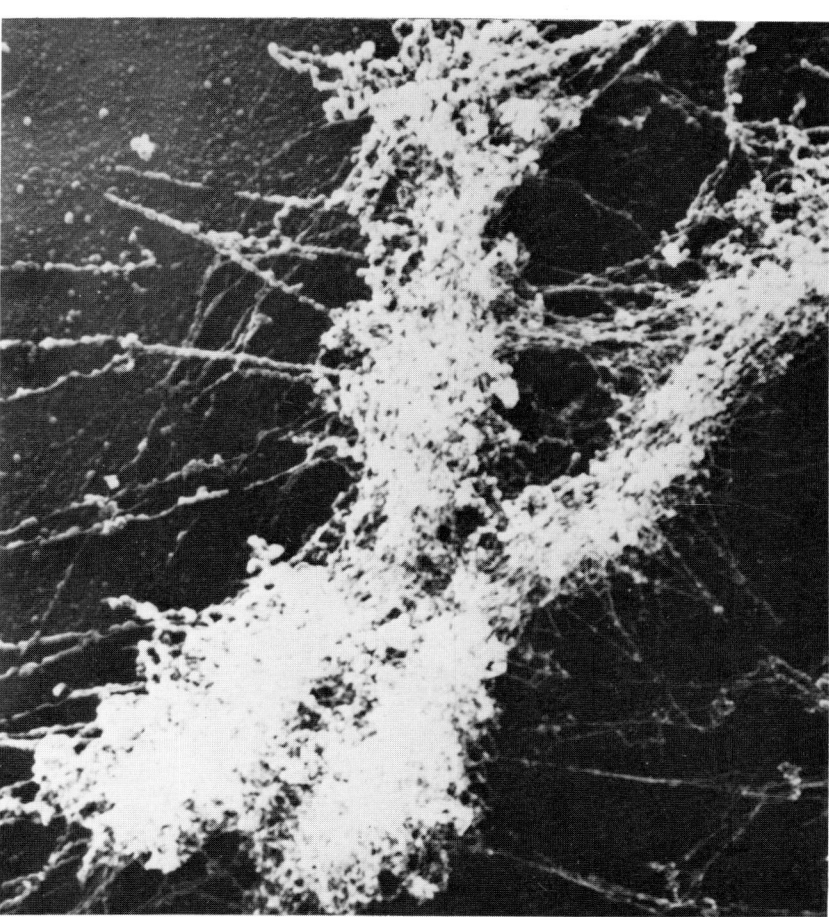

Figure 6–21. Scanning electron micrograph showing the fibrillar nature of a chromosome. (Courtesy of Professor C. Mouriquand, Université Scientifique et Médicale de Grenoble, France.)

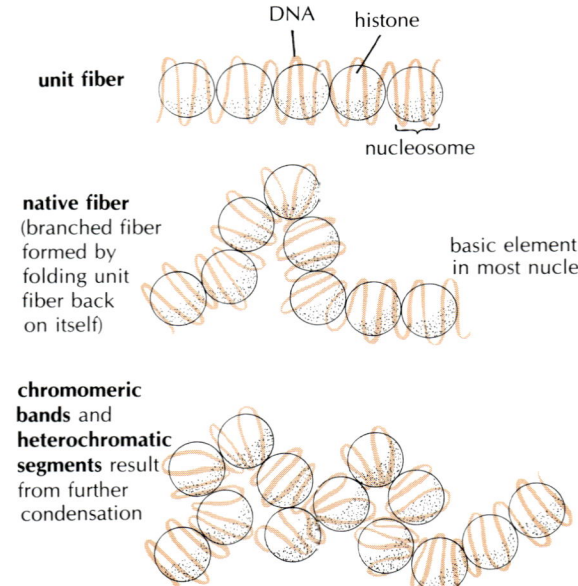

unit fiber

DNA   histone

nucleosome

native fiber
(branched fiber
formed by
folding unit
fiber back
on itself)

basic element
in most nuclei

chromomeric
bands and
heterochromatic
segments result
from further
condensation

Figure 6–22. Chromatin exists as a regularly repeating structure resembling beads on a string. Various condensations of the unit fiber result in different chromatin conformations in nuclei.

Chromatin Structure. Eukaryotic chromatin exists as a regularly repeating structure that resembles beads on a string (Fig. 6–22). The repeating subunits, *nucleosomes (nubodies)*, contain 140 to 200 base pairs of DNA hexagonal crystals, cylinders, or arc-like arrays.[94] The nucleosomes have been visualized as 7.0- to 8.5-nm globular particles. Under a bright-field microscope, one may see an intense peripheral density with a central light core.[95]

The DNA in the nucleosome appears to be tightly folded around a core of histone molecules,[96] which are arranged as an octomeric complex of 2 of each of the histones H_2A, H_2B, H_3, and H_4.[97] The *nucleosomes* are separated by 40 to 60 base pairs of double-stranded DNA associated with histone H_1. The H_1 fraction probably has the leading role in determining the coiling or folding of nucleosomal chains arranged in tandem to form the 200- to 250-Å chromatin fibers that are seen in chromosomes.[98] This fraction also probably helps to stabilize chromosomal structure. *Internucleosomal spacer* DNA is of variable lengths and is probably symmetrically coiled between 2 adjacent nucleosomes.[99]

Ris[100] has described a hierarchy of chromatin organization. In his model, the first level of organization is the *unit fiber*, in which the histones condense the DNA approximately 7 times into a 10-nm fiber. This fiber folds back on itself and gives rise to the branched native fiber, and forms the *supercoil*, which is 20 to 30 nm wide. The native fiber is assumed to be the basic element in most nuclei. With further condensation, the native fiber becomes organized into *chromomeric bands, heterochromatic segments,* and during mitoses, *chromonema,* which form the helix of the mitotic chromosomes.

Chromatin Banding. Chromosomes can be stained with a variety of substances to produce characteristic banding patterns that reflect the underlying molecular organization (Table 6–13).

Table 6–13. *Classification of Banding*

Type of Band	Stain	Area or Components Stained
Q	Quinacrine	Adenine and thymidine regions
G	Giemsa	Heterochromatin (H_1, H_2) region
C	Fluorochrome dyes	Paracentromeric region
R (reversible)	Immunofluorescent Ab	Guanine and cytosine regions

Many of the common banding techniques employ fluorochrome dyes specific to DNA, especially at the A-T regions. The dye is quenched in the guanine-rich regions, and the result is a characteristic C banding pattern.

Heterochromatin, especially the histone fractions (H_1 and H_2A), appears to be responsible for banding with the *Giemsa stain.*[101] Reverse banding *(R banding)* is obtained with guanosine- and cytosine-specific nucleotide.

In addition, a group of repetitive DNA molecules is known as satellite DNA.[102] Heterochromatin and centromere regions are enriched with this material.

Nonchromatin DNA. Cytoplasmic membrane-associated DNA *(cmDNA)* differs from DNA in chromatin or mitochondria. It is thought to be synthesized in the nucleus and transported to cytoplasmic membranes. The hybridization studies that demonstrate repeated sequences of cmDNA in the heterochromatin areas of chromosome 9 in man prove its nuclear origin.[103] *DNA* is also associated with *centrioles* and *mitochondria.*

Chromatin Activation. The activation of chromatin involves a series of structural changes, especially the unraveling of the native fiber to that of the simpler unit fiber, and then to a single nucleotide chain, single because only one strand is transcribed.

It is assumed that the factors that turn on transcription and unravel the native fiber also change the DNA-histone binding and thereby lead to an unraveling of the DNA and RNA polymerase attachment.

Replication and Repair

Eukaryotic chromosomes replicate by *semiconservative division:* each daughter cell in the new chromosome receives half of the old DNA and half that is newly synthesized (Fig. 6–23). DNA strands in replication separate at several points, and complementary bases are added. Replication takes place simultaneously at 1000 or more loci, principally during the S period of the cell cycle.[104]

Following cell injury, *repair* processes are carried out by *exo-* and *endonucleases, trimming enzymes, polymerases* (Table 6–14), DNA *ligase,* and rarely, *deoxynucleotidyl transferase.*[105] These repair reactions maintain genetic stability throughout the life of the cell.

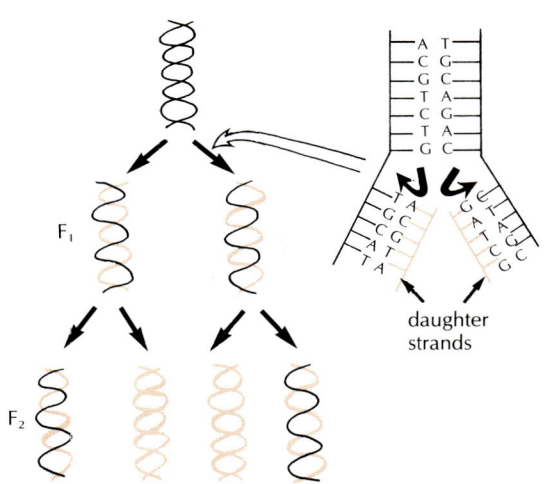

daughter strands

Figure 6–23. Semiconservative replication of DNA. In the first daughter DNA (F₁), each double strand contains a parent strand. In the F₂ double strands, there are two hybrids and two newly synthesized double strands. Opening up of parent double-stranded DNA (upper right) serves as a template for new strand synthesis.

Table 6–14.   *Classification of Human DNA Polymerases*

New Name	Previous Name	Site	Molecular Weight
Polymerase α	DNA polymerase I DNA polymerase II DNA polymerase C Cytoplasmic DNA polymerase	Cytoplasm	1.3×10^6
Polymerase β	DNA polymerase II DNA polymerase I Mini DNA polymerase DNA polymerase VI	Nucleus or cytoplasm	0.4×10^6
Polymerase γ	DNA polymerase III R DNA polymerase A DNA polymerase	Unknown	$\sim 10^6$
Viral DNA polymerase	Reverse transcriptase	Cytoplasm	1.3×10^6

(Modified from Todaro, G.J.: Type C virogenes: genetic transfer and interspecies transfer. Adv. Pathobiol., 4:38, 1976.)

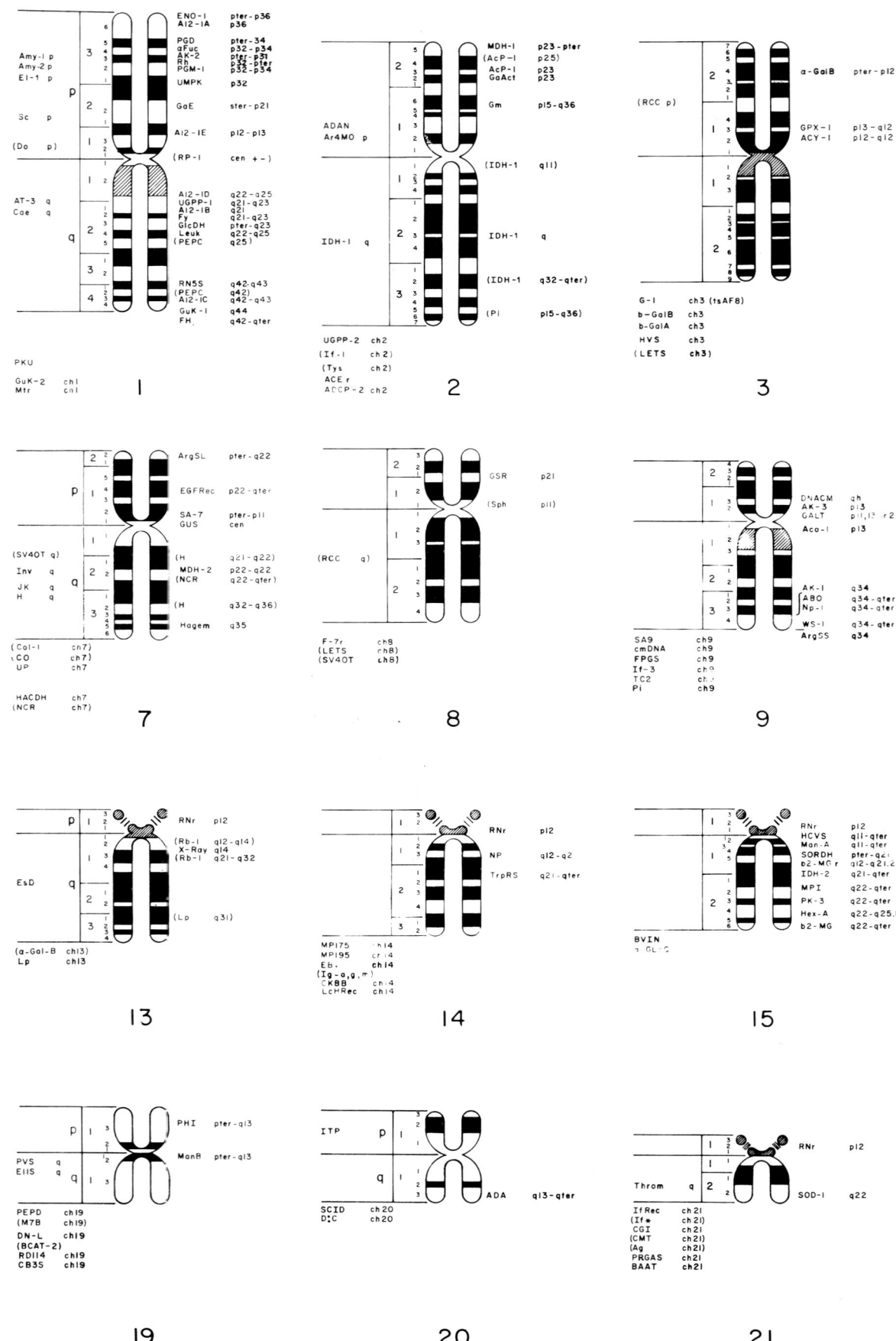

Figure 6–24. Chromosome map. (Courtesy of Dr. F. Ruddle, Department of Biology, Yale University.)

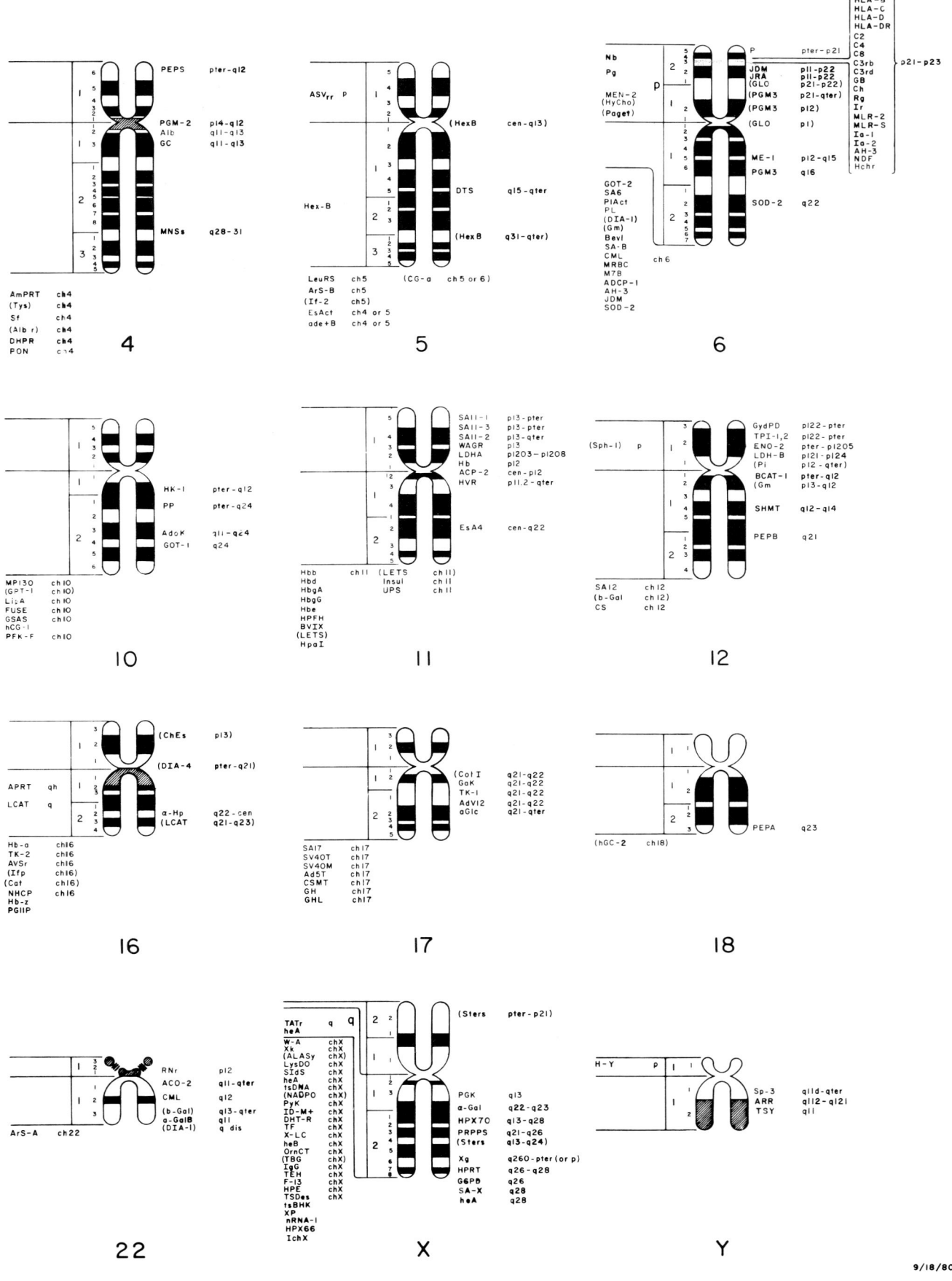

Figure 6–24 *continued.*

Transcription

In mammalian cells, DNA is over a meter long and codes for approximately 50 to 100 thousand proteins. Over 400 genes have now been mapped on the human chromosome[106] (Fig. 6–24 and Table 6–15). Nuclear DNA transcribes 4 major classes of RNA, 3 of which *(rRNA, tRNA, mRNA)* actively participate in protein synthesis.

Ribosomal RNA (rRNA) is transcribed from nucleolar DNA. Two major classes *(18S* and *28S)* are derived from a larger *45S RNA* molecule. The rRNA links with 20 to 30 proteins to form a ribosomal structural unit that provides the mechanism by which the gene product can be translated and amplified.

Transfer RNA (tRNA) has at least 60 types, one of which binds to a specific activated amino acid and transfers it to the ribosome, where protein synthesis occurs. Transfer RNA is rich in minor base modifications of which methyl-

Table 6–15. *Examples of Chromosomal Gene Map**

Blood Groups	ABO (9)	Rogers (6)
	Rh (1)	Duffy (1)
	Chido (16)	
Proteins and Glycoproteins	Major histocompatibility complex (6)	
	β-2 Microglobulin (15)	
	Immunoglobulin κ chain (6)	
	λ chain (16)	
	Heavy chain (16)	
	α-Haptoglobulin (16)	
	Complement (6)	
	Properdin B (6)	
Hormones	Insulin (11)	
	Human chorionic gonadotropin (17)	
	Somatotropin (placental lactogen) (17)	
	Prolactin (6)	
Soluble enzyme	Glucose-6-phosphate dehydrogenase (X)	
Mitochondrial enzymes	Citrate synthetase (12)	
	Isocitrate dehydrogenase (15)	
	Malate dehydrogenase (7)	
Lysosomal enzymes	Superoxide dismutase (2) (6)	
	Peptidase A (18), B (12), C (1), D (19)	
	Amylase (1)	
	α-Galactosidase (Fabry's) (X)	
	β-Galactosidase (22)	
Membrane components	Hexokinase (10)	
	α-Fetoprotein (5)	
	B-cell receptor (6)	
	Receptor C3d (6)	
	Glycophorin (11)	
Nuclear components	Ribosomes (12) (1) (7)	
	5S RNA (1)	
	Ribosomal RNA (13), (14), (15), (21), (22)	
	Thymidine kinase (17)	
Others	Interferon (2), (5), (9), receptor (21)	
	Hageman factor (7)	

*Number in parentheses indicates chromosome number.

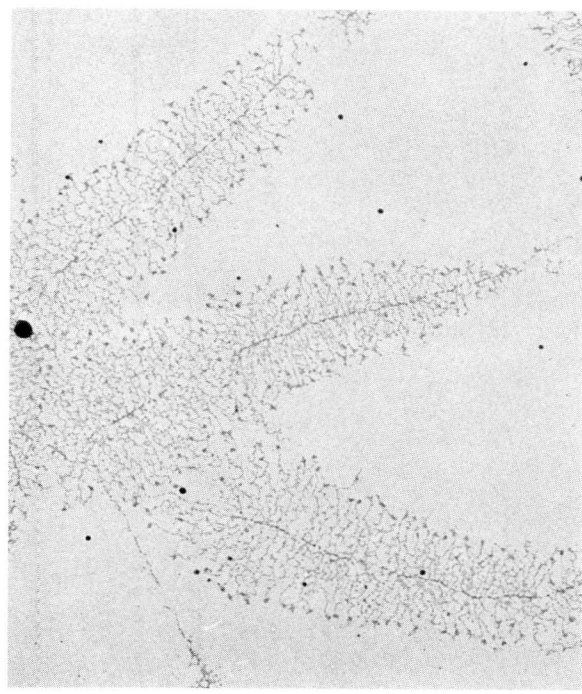

Figure 6–25. Extrachromosomal nucleolar genes isolated from oocytes of the spotted newt *Triturus viridescens.* (Courtesy of O.L. Miller, University of Virginia.)

ation is the most common. This process occurs in all 4 major bases and changes the tertiary structure of the tRNA.[107] Methylation may be important for the proper functioning of tRNA in amino acetylation, in binding to ribosomes, and in recognition of specific *codons* by the *anticodon* amino acid determinants.

The third class of RNA is *heterogeneous RNA (HnRNA)*. This RNA molecule is much larger than the others and may be the precursor of mRNA; it also contains nonfunctional nucleotides.

The fourth class, *messenger RNA* (mRNA), codes for structural, enzymatic, and exported proteins. The structural genes from which mRNA is synthesized are few. For example, only two to four copies of structural genes have been identified for two major proteins, hemoglobin and immunoglobulin.

Complexes of RNA transcripts may be generated on DNA "hairpin loops" to yield a periodic, beaded structure. Nuclear transcriptional complexes are seen rarely in rat liver cells by electron microscopy. Two different morphologic patterns are distinguishable: multiple "Christmas tree"-like figures (Fig. 6–25), probably related to rRNA transcription, and *twisted fibrils* in single units along the DNA molecule, related to non-nucleolar transcription.[108]

Humans have approximately 3.3×10^9 base pairs in their genome, and the possibility of 2×10^6 genes of approximately one kilobase each. The number of active genes has been estimated to be between 50 and 100 thousand. This indicates that there is a great redundancy or that an appreciable quantity of DNA is inactive, is used in regulation or differentiation, or is merely part of the structural component of the chromosome.

Mammalian genes consist of coding portions of DNA called *exons*, interspaced with *intervening sequences* of silent DNA called *introns*.[109] The introns all start with GT, end with AG, and are AT rich. They vary between 10 and 10 thousand nucleotides in number. Over 60 separate introns are present in chick collagenase genes. Most mammalian genes contain at least one intron, but neither the histone gene of drosophila nor any genes in bacteria contain introns. The coding portions of a particular polypeptide lie in noncontiguous segments. We have previously discussed (see Chap. 2) the *minigenes* (that is, variable, constant, J, and D genes) separated by intervening sequences that code for different immunoglobulin polypeptides.[110] The intervening sequences may be removed either by minigene recombination within the genome or by RNA splicing following transcription.

On each site of the coding sequences (exons) are long portions of flanking DNA. Before the cap site of the first coding sequence on the 5' end, several hundred nucleotides are found. At the -27 nucleotide site, the TATAA or "Hogness box" is believed necessary to initiate transcription in vitro, but not necessarily in vivo. At the -80 nucleotide site, the "CCAAT box" is believed to be nonessential for transcription in vitro, but important for thymidine kinase transcription in vivo. On the 3' flank of DNA, the termination site for transcription has not yet been identified.

Exons inserted within introns have the possibility of *recombination, mRNA splicing,* and *somatic mutation.* These gene variations offer enormous evolutionary advantage in improving gene structure and function with time. In regard to amplification, the gene coding for dihydrofolate reductase is increased a thousand times in response to methotrexate induction.[111] The position of genes is altered in immunoglobulin synthesis with movement of the D and J gene and C_H switching. Multigene systems have recently been identified in humans for a number of systems (Table 6–16).

Table 6–16. *Informational Multigene Systems in Humans*

Structural proteins
    Actin*
    Keratins*
    Collagens*
    Chorionic proteins*

Serum proteins
    Hemagglutinins*
    Serine esterase*
    Complement components*

Developmental systems
    T allele
    Transcriptional signals
    Translational signals

Membrane systems
    Immune response genes
    Membrane receptors (hormone, cAMP)
    Membrane transport systems
    Embryonic antigens
    Blood cell antigens

Nervous system
    Membrane molecules mediating specific cell-cell interactions
    Information storage

*These proteins exist in multiple structural forms.
(Modified from Hood, L.: The evolution of multigene families. Adv. Pathobiol., 6:51, 1977.)

Transfection experiments with *recombinant DNA* have made it possible to introduce genes into various mammalian cells in vitro and to amplify them in *bacterial plasmids* to produce appreciable quantities of gene products, particularly hormones, enzymes, and antibodies. Many genes cannot be amplified to make a particular, identifiable product. In order for gene amplification to take place, the following are required: a *DNA vector* to introduce the foreign DNA into the genome; a *means of recombination;* a system to facilitate *replication* of the vector; and a *gene identification schema,* to identify the gene or the gene product.

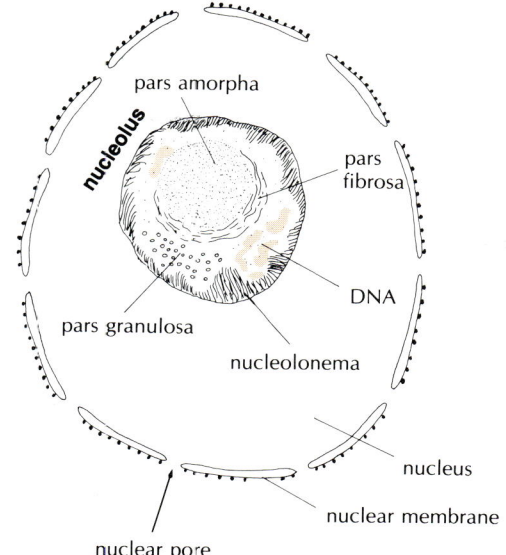

pars amorpha

nucleolus

pars fibrosa

DNA

pars granulosa

nucleolonema

nucleus

nuclear membrane

nuclear pore

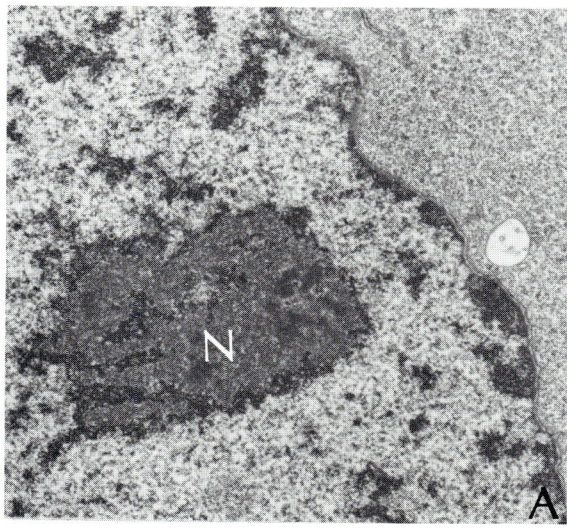

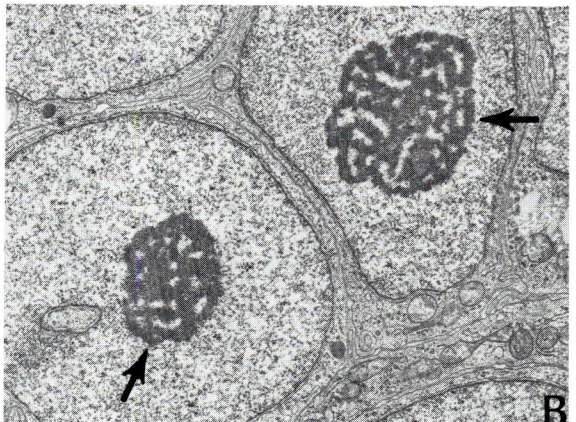

Figure 6–27. The nucleolus may have several configurations. *A,* Compact nucleolus (N) with prominent pars fibrosa and pars granulosa. *B,* Thread-like nucleolonemas comprise the nucleolus in these cells (arrows).

The vector is often a virus introduced into a mammalian cell. A second vector may be a *phage* introduced into a *bacterial plasmid.* The latter is an extrachromosomal piece of DNA able to replicate in bacterial cells. The foreign DNA is obtained from mammalian DNA by the use of a series of *restriction endonucleases* that make breaks at particular nucleotide sequences. The insertion into plasmids by recombination, of approximately 1×10^6 MW fragments of DNA, allows the accumulation of a *plasmid bank* or *library,* each containing only one gene.[112]

Following multiple replication of the one plasmid containing the one gene of interest, the probe for identification of the gene is a cDNA copy of known mRNA. After replication of cells, the DNA of the colonies is transferred to a nitrous filter paper laid over the colonies and is hybridized with known mRNA. Identification of DNA by this method is called the *Southern blot* technique, whereas identification of RNA is called the *Northern blot* technique.

Nucleolus

The *nucleolus* is the second major component of the nucleus. In normal cells, one or two nucleoli are usually present and function as organizing units for ribosomal precursors. A nucleolus consists of four major components: (1) the *DNA* that codes for rRNA, (2) the *pars amorpha,* (3) the *pars fibrosa,* and (4) the *pars granulosa* (Figs. 6–26 and 6–27).

The *pars amorpha,* the fibrillar center of nucleoli, is a low-density structure seen by light and electron microscopy that contains fibrils resistant to pepsin and RNAase digestion. This component persists throughout mitosis, is closely associated with the chromosomes, and is composed of proteins and small amounts of DNA.[113]

The *pars fibrosa* or fibrillary structure is approximately 50 Å in diameter and 300 to 400 Å in length. Its light and dense fibrillar components both consist of ribonucleoprotein (RNP).

The last component, the *pars granulosa,* contains granular particles 150 to 200 Å in diameter. Radioautographic studies that showed that uridine incorporated into rRNA first appeared in the fibrillar component and later in the granular portion suggest a pathway of ribosomal RNA development.

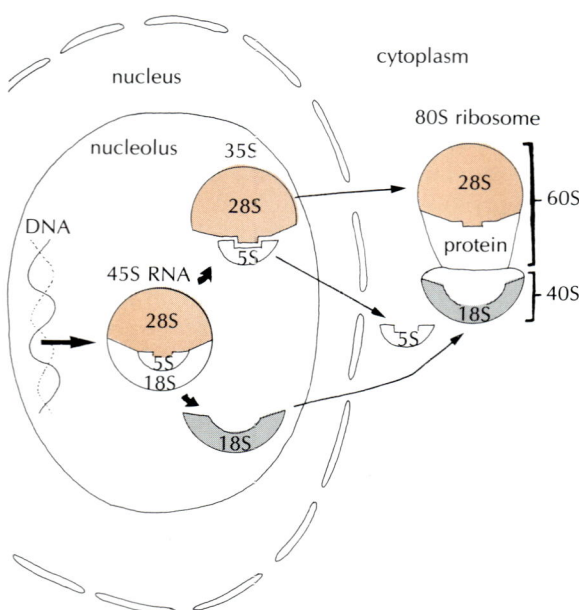

nucleus

cytoplasm

nucleolus

80S ribosome

DNA

45S RNA

35S

28S

28S

5S

28S

5S

18S

18S

protein

28S

5S

18S

60S

40S

Figure 6–28. Synthesis of ribosomal RNA takes place in the nucleolus with assembly of 80S ribosomes in the cytoplasm after passage of components through nuclear pores.

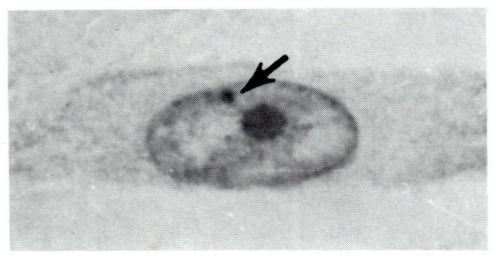

Figure 6–29. Barr body (inactivated X chromosome at arrow) in a neuron.

DNA genes for ribosomal RNA are unique in that their transcription occurs in the nucleolus. The morphologic features, including size, of nucleoli are good cytologic indicators of rRNA synthesis. Ribosomal RNA, mRNA, and tRNA are transcribed as larger precursor molecules, which are then cleaved by ribonuclease to smaller, mature products. Genes coding for ribosomal RNA initially produce a *45S RNA* that breaks to a *35S (32S) RNA* and an *18S RNA*. The *18S RNA* is incorporated into the *40S protein* subunit of the 80S cytoplasmic ribosome. The *35S RNA* in the nucleolar granule breaks down into *28S RNA*, which appears in the *60S protein* component of the *80S complete ribosome*. A *5S* RNA is also transported to the cytoplasm (Fig. 6–28).

Ribosomal proteins appear to be synthesized on cytoplasmic ribosomes and transported into the nucleolus, where they are complexed with RNA to form *preribosomal particles*. In addition to ribosomal structural proteins, protein elongation factor[114] and endogenous protein kinase have been found in the nucleus. This finding suggests that some translation may occur in the nucleus. An additional part of the nucleolus is the *nucleolar organizer* region, which is near certain chromosome sites responsible for the formation of nucleoli.[115]

Other Nuclear Structures

We think of the nucleus as the site of the nucleolus, chromatin, and little else. Other structures do contribute to nuclear morphology, however. These include *Barr bodies,* the *nuclear membrane* with its adherent ribosomes, *membrane pore complexes,* the dense *fibrous lamina,* the *nuclear matrix,*[116] and *intranuclear channel system,* and the *nucleoplasm* with its variety of enzymatic and structural proteins. In this section, we briefly discuss these often neglected structures.

Barr Bodies

Barr bodies represent *inactivated* condensed *X chromosomes* in the female (Fig. 6–29). They sometimes disappear with age. Recent evidence suggests that this chromosome may have a limited transcriptional function.[117]

Nuclear Membrane

The nucleus is covered by 2 adjacent *membranes* that are usually separated by a 100- to 600-Å perinuclear space (Fig. 6–30). Each membrane is a trilaminar structure, approximately 80 to 90 Å thick, that fuses at irregular intervals to form the *nuclear pore complex*. Attached to the outer nuclear membrane are ribosomal granules. The inner surface of the nuclear membrane is associated with fibrous material. This *fibrous lamina* may have a structural or transport role.

The nuclear envelope contains many different types of proteins, phospholipids, nonpolar lipids, enzymes, and perhaps, small amounts of RNA and DNA. Because of the number of oxidative enzymes associated with the nuclear surface (Table 6–17) and because of the special properties of the associated ATPase, it has been suggested that the nuclear envelope may function minimally in electron transport and oxidative phosphorylation. This structure also contains *receptors* and is a binding site for lectins and insulin.[118]

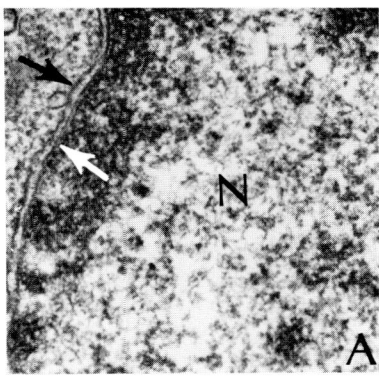

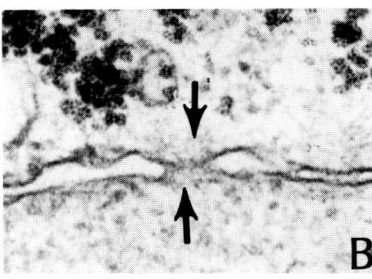

Figure 6–30. Nuclear membrane. *A,* The double-layered nuclear membrane (arrows) separates the nucleus (N) from the cytoplasm. *B,* This membrane becomes focally obliterated to produce the nuclear pore (arrows).

Table 6–17.   *Enzymes of Nuclear Membrane*

ATPase
NADH
NADH⁺ oxidase
Cytochrome C reductase
Cytochrome C oxidase
Cytochrome B5
Microsomal enzymes

The *membrane* is permeable to many macromolecules as well as to small organic molecules. Macromolecular components appear to pass through the nuclear pores, but may also be exchanged by vesicles. Materials of low molecular weight also freely diffuse through the membrane or travel by sodium-dependent transport processes.

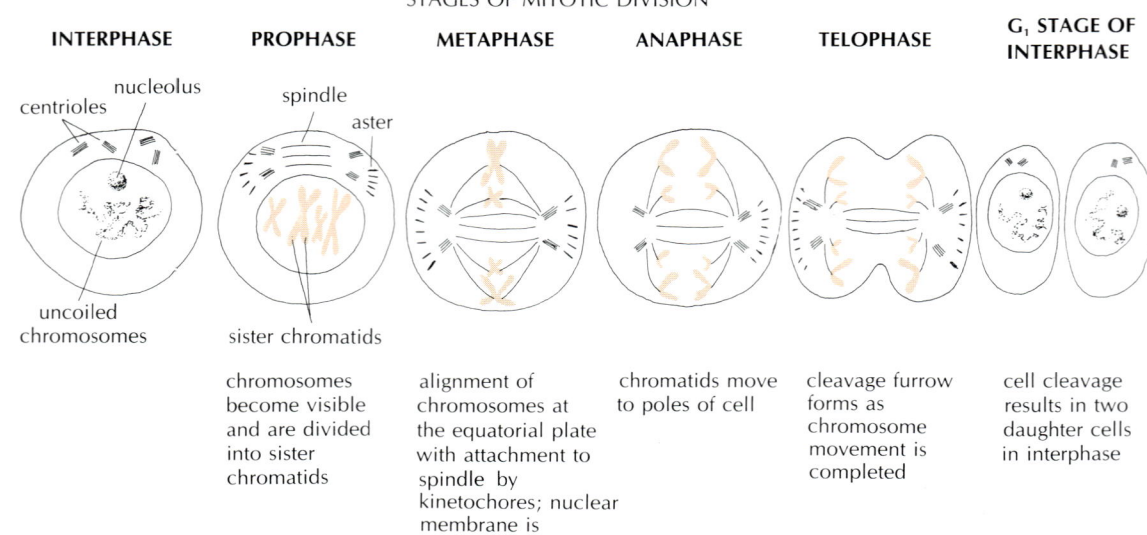

INTERPHASE	PROPHASE	METAPHASE	ANAPHASE	TELOPHASE	G₁ STAGE OF INTERPHASE

centrioles — nucleolus

spindle — aster

uncoiled chromosomes

sister chromatids

| | chromosomes become visible and are divided into sister chromatids | alignment of chromosomes at the equatorial plate with attachment to spindle by kinetochores; nuclear membrane is broken down | chromatids move to poles of cell | cleavage furrow forms as chromosome movement is completed | cell cleavage results in two daughter cells in interphase |

Figure 6–31. Stages of mitosis.

During mitosis (Fig. 6–31), as the cell proceeds into prophase, the nuclear envelope disappears by breaking down into small vesicles or large sheets that retain pore complexes. During anaphase and early telophase, membrane fragments coalesce on the surface of condensed chromatin. These membrane fragments are derived from the endoplasmic reticulum or from pieces of the previous nuclear envelope.

Nuclear Pores

Nuclear pore complexes are intricate structures thought by some investigators to be distinct cellular organelles involved in intracellular transport because they remain intact and attached to the nuclear lamina after the complete removal of the nuclear membrane.[119] Once the membrane is removed, the pores are observed as isolated intact ring structures containing annular subunits.[120]

Chromatin fibers within the nucleus attach to the nuclear envelope through the annular material of the pore, and it is felt that these attachment sites are necessary to maintain interphase chromatin fibers in fixed positions. A second function of these attachment sites is to serve as initiating points for DNA synthesis.[121]

Nuclear Bodies

Two major types of *nuclear bodies* occur in mammalian nuclei: *simple* and *granular*. The simple type appears to be composed chiefly of protein, whereas the granules of the granular type contain ribonucleoprotein. The simple bodies, 0.3 to 0.5 μ in size, are probably a constant feature of the nucleus, but are only detected in about 10 to 15% of nuclei examined. The number of granular nuclear bodies is increased in hyperactive states and pathologic conditions.

General Effects of Injury

The extent of nuclear injury depends upon the dose and the route of the particular agent involved, the virulence (if an infectious agent), and the cell's response. The stage of the cell cycle may be critical in determining both the effect of the agent and the ability of the cell to respond. Numerous substances are known to influence cell growth as well as the cell's ability to respond with division and synthesis.

The nucleus may have several responses to injury, for example, *karyorrhexis* (nuclear fragmentation), *karyolysis* (nuclear swelling), or *pyknosis* (nuclear condensation). These alterations may be secondary to changes in nuclear membrane permeability with accompanying ion and water shifts. Injury may also be reflected in changes in specific nuclear components, especially in the chromatin and nucleolus.

A *chromosomal break* is one that affects both strands of the chromosome and usually occurs during G_1. A *subchromatid break* may result from injury in late G_1, S, or G_2 periods. It affects only one strand and thus only one chromatid. Subchromatid breaks usually occur during prophase and affect small portions of the chromatid. Some injurious agents, such as radiation and some drugs, are known to affect particular parts of chromosomes. *Radiation* and *bleomycin* cause immediate chromosomal damage that may be repaired within one hour. Exchanges cannot be repaired, but gaps may heal.

Damage to *chromosomes* often results in *mutations*. In certain cases, phenotypic changes may be present without any grossly discernible chromosomal abnormality, as in sickle cell anemia. Conversely, gross chromosomal abnormalities may occur in up to 1% of live births, with minimal or no phenotypic alterations. Abnormal chromosomes are present in a group of diseases, however. These chromosomal aberrations appear as *breaks, gaps, exchanges, translocations, additions, deletions, bridges,* or *rings* and are readily recognized using standard karyotype analysis or the newer banding techniques.

Gene mutations are permanent, heritable changes in the genetic material of cells and consequently in their structure or activities. Radiation-induced mutations differ from spontaneous mutations only in their much higher frequency. Both *chromosome mutations* and *point mutations* have been described with respect to radiation. Chromosome aberrations represent changes in the number of genes by inclusion of extra chromosomes or sets of chromosomes in the nucleus, or addition or loss of small parts of chromosomes. Point mutations represent changes in the nature of genes by small changes in DNA, such as loss or substitution of nucleotides and base pairs. Damage to cells is lethal if many alterations occur in many sites on DNA with resultant loss of large amounts of genetic material and proliferative capacity. Point mutations and losses of only small amounts of genetic material are generally not lethal.

Damaged DNA may be measured following injury by thymidine incorporation (unscheduled DNA synthesis), which measures the activity of the cellular complement of ligases and exo- and endonucleases that act to repair altered regions.[105] *"Error-prone"* repair occurs in those instances in which no complementary strand is left, or when genetic information has been copied inaccurately. In these cases, the new DNA differs from that which was damaged and is then edited by 3' exonuclease. This exonuclease scans the new DNA for errors. A variation in the amount of editing by exonuclease is related to the frequency of spontaneous mutations.[122]

When *nucleoli* are *injured*, they generally go through an ordered sequence of events as follows: (1) *formation* of a compact *sphere*, (2) *segregation* of the *four nucleolar components*, (3) *degranulation*, which leaves (4) a *residual fibrillary* proteinaceous *mass* of material.

Genetic Factors

Diseases due to mutant genes are conventionally divided into *recessive, dominant,* and *X-linked disorders.* In recessive disorders, the single mutant gene responsible for the disease must be present in both members of the chromosome pair, that is, it must be homozygous, for the disease to become manifest. Heterozygous individuals with only one mutant gene in the chromosome pair do not usually express the disorder. On the other hand, a mutant gene that is always expressed, whether homozygous or heterozygous, is responsible for diseases with dominant inheritance, with

Table 6–18. *Examples of Alterations in Chromosomes in Genetic Diseases*

Alterations in karyotype (cytogenetic diseases)
  Autosomes
    Down's syndrome (trisomy 21)
    Cri du chat syndrome (deletion 5)
    Wilms' tumor (deletion 11)
    Retinoblastoma (deletion 13)
  Sex chromosomes
    Klinefelter's syndrome (supernumerary X)
    Turner's syndrome (XO)

Alterations in gene (inborn errors without karyotypic changes)
  Hemoglobinopathies (sickle cell disease)
  Carbohydrate glycogen storage diseases (Pompe's disease)
  Amino acid deficiencies (phenylketonuria)
  Lipid storage disease (Nieman-Pick disease)
  Mucopolysaccharide disease (Hurler's syndrome)
  Nucleic acid deficiency (orotic aciduria)
  Collagen disorders (Marfan's syndrome)
  Cell transport disorders (Fanconi's syndrome)

or without variable penetrance. X-linked diseases are those conditions determined by mutant genes on the X chromosomes. Some classic sex-linked and autosomal abnormalities are shown in Table 6–18.

Examples of diseases associated with defective genes include xeroderma pigmentosum (XP), Fanconi's anemia, Bloom's syndrome, and ataxia-telangiectasia.[123] In these disorders, defective DNA repair mechanisms lead to a pathobiologic spectrum including cell death, neoplasia, and early senescence.[124]

Physical Agents

Hypoxia. Decreased oxygen concentration *(hypoxia)* may produce chromosomal breaks and abnormal chromosomal figures. A deficiency in oxidative phosphorylation and a subsequent lack of ATP inhibits DNA and RNA synthesis, as well as cell division and transport processes.

Temperature. High temperatures of 42 to 43°C result in *"stickiness"* of the telomeric ends of the chromosomes, so that chromosomal bridges form and chromosomal components clump together.[125] Heat injury probably uncoils at least a segment of the DNA.[126] Some cells grow in vitro at 41°C, but undergo nucleolar degranulation that affects the synthesis of RNA. At 44.5°C, the internucleolar chromatin retracts and leaves the fibrillary component condensed and closely packed.

Low temperatures (27°C) inhibit DNA, RNA, protein synthesis, and mitosis and have been used to produce parasynchrony in vitro. Parasynchrony is the state whereby the majority, but not all, of the cells enter the S phase simultaneously.

Radiation. The effects of *radiation* have been extensively studied, especially with respect to chromosomes and DNA repair enzymes (Table 6–19). The radiation may be in the form of x rays, ultraviolet (UV) light, radioisotopes, alpha particles, or neutrons. The effects are generally related to dose, dose rate, time, and type of radiation. The injurious effects are usually enhanced with increased oxygen levels and higher temperatures, which may produce more free radicals.

Table 6–19. *DNA Repair Mechanisms*

Photoreactivation, which requires high monomerization (no excision)

Base excision repair (glycosylases, apurine endonucleases, and insertases)

Nucleotide excision repair (error free)
  long patches (ultraviolet)
  short patches (mitomycin C)

Postreplicative repair (error prone)
  no excision repair, operative by recombination

Repair of single strand breaks

Inducible repair

Ionizing radiation produces at least three different types of DNA damage: (1) strand breaks, (2) damage of the heterocyclic bases, and (3) cross-links. The large repertoire of radiation-induced chromosomal injuries in many cell systems includes breaks, gaps, bridges, rings, dicentric chromosomes, acentric fragments, and multipolar abnormalities with chromatin exchanges.[127]

UV light produces cyclobutane rings (thymine dimers) between two adjacent thymine bases on the same DNA strand. Recognition of a dimer initiates nearby single-strand scission of the DNA by a specific endonuclease. This change is followed by excision of the defective nucleotide sequence by an exonuclease. A new portion is synthesized, using polymerase and the complementary strand as a template, and the free ends are joined to the preexisting strand by a ligase[128] (Fig. 6–32).

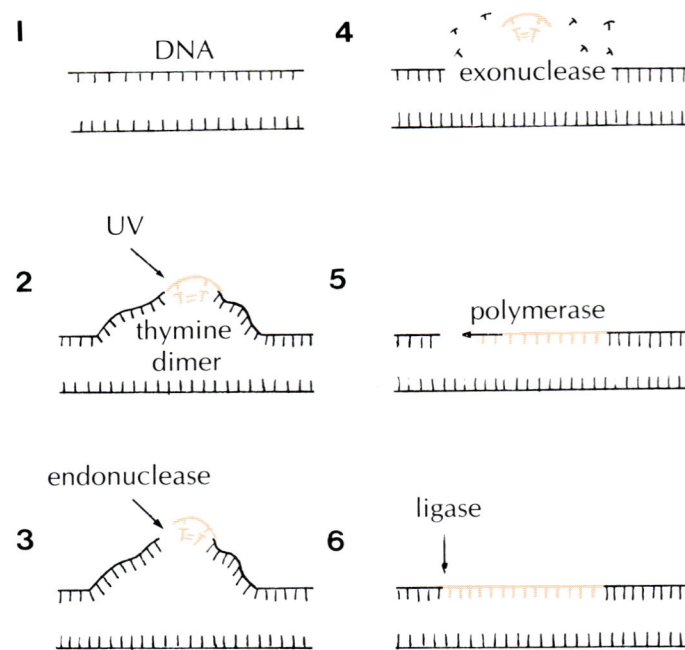

Figure 6–32. Mechanism of repair of ultraviolet (UV)-induced thymine dimers in DNA.

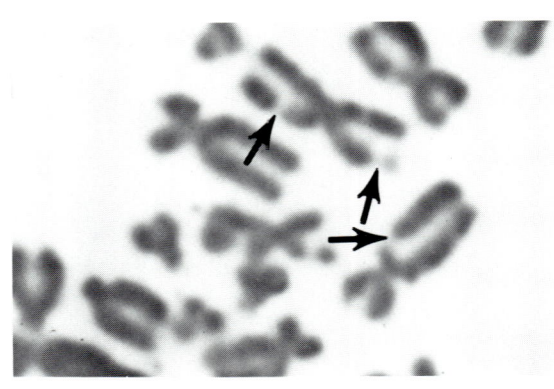

Figure 6–33. Chromosomal breaks induced by radiation. (Courtesy of Dr. T. Puck, University of Colorado, Denver.)

UV light can induce neoplastic transformations in vivo or in vitro in cells with intact DNA repair mechanisms. It has been postulated that the transformation results from an *error-prone* postreplication repair process.[129]

Death of irradiated cells may be secondary to mitotic inhibition, destruction of genes (Fig. 6–33), or cytolysis. This last factor may result from membrane damage and altered permeability.

Nutritional Factors

Nutritional deficiencies may be associated with chromosomal and nucleolar abnormalities and abnormal DNA synthesis. Thymine deficiency leads to *"thymineless death."* This phenomenon results in a block at the beginning of the "S" period, so that protein synthesis continues and the cell enlarges; no division may take place, however, and the cell eventually dies.[130]

Single amino acid deficiencies may halt synthesis of DNA; this change leads to metaphase breaks, chromatid exchanges, and alterations in the chromosomes similar to the *"pulverization"* (formation of small chromosomal fragments) process seen with viral infections.[131] Changes in other molecules, such as anions or cations, may also damage the nucleus. An example is calcium deficiency, in which abnormal chromosome segregation may occur[132] because of this cation's role in the function of the mitotic apparatus.

Amino acid deficiencies may also lead to *nucleolar damage.* Chick embryo cells grown in an arginine-deficient medium have nuclei that contain beaded structures 5.2 μ long called *"nucleolar necklaces."*[133] Nucleolar atrophy and ring forms are seen during starvation.

Infectious Agents

Chromosomal Effects. Chromosomal alterations have been reported following bacterial, viral, and mycoplasmal infections, but the literature has been most extensive with regard to viral infections (Fig. 6–34). *Viral infections* may produce cell death, genetic damage, changes in chromosome number, sister chromatid exchanges, and mutations with or without viral genome incorporation.[134] Viruses can replicate in host cells in several ways. Their genetic material can be *inserted* into the host genome and replicated, being distributed to each daughter cell at the time of division, or viruses may establish themselves in the cytoplasm and *replicate independently* of the host cell's cycle.

Chromosomal abnormalities may result from the virus itself, or they may relate to events occurring with viral synthesis. Persistence of the viral genome may produce instability of the host genome. A virally synthesized or directed enzyme may inhibit host DNA synthesis. Cell damage has also been attributed to interference with protein synthesis, host replicative processes, or a diversion of precursor metabolites from the host to viral nucleic acid and protein synthesis. Viral replication is not necessary for host chromosomes to be damaged. Gaps, breaks, and chromatin exchanges are commonly seen in vitro with infections with simian virus 40 (SV40), adenovirus, polyomavirus, and Shope, rubeola, and rubella viruses. Rings or dicentric forms are sometimes seen.

Chromosomal *"pulverization,"* characteristic of viral infection,[131,135] results in fragmentation and despiralization

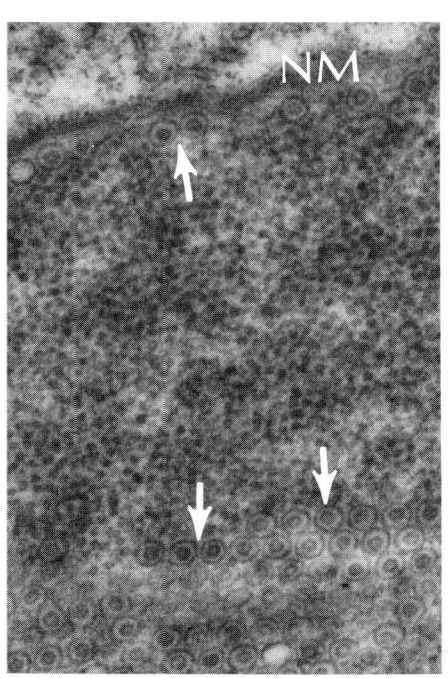

Figure 6–34. Transmission electron micrograph showing herpesvirus particles (arrows) in nucleus. They line up under the nuclear membrane (NM) just prior to release.

of chromatin and is caused by herpes simplex, herpes zoster, adeno-12, yellow fever, Newcastle, Sendai, measles, papova-, pox-, and other viruses.

Infection of human cells with adenovirus 12 leads to a high frequency of *breaks* in chromosome 17. Chromosomal breaks have been seen in human fetuses after *rubella* or *hepatitis* infection.[136]

Viruses also alter the mitotic spindle; these alterations result, for example, in syncytial *giant cell formation.* Tripolar mitotic figures with a shared spindle may also develop, and such cells have abnormal chromosomes and nuclei.

Nucleolar Effects. Bacteria, viruses, and mycoplasmas all produce *nucleolar segregation.* Segregation of nucleolar components is clearly seen with *herpesvirus* and *Coxsackie virus* infections. Identical changes are produced by *actinomycin D,*[137] *aflatoxins,* and *mitomycin C,* substances that inhibit DNA and RNA transcription. These agents, both viral and chemical, are thought to mediate their effects by binding to the DNA with subsequent inhibition of RNA polymerase. Ribosomal RNA appears to be more sensitive to these agents than tRNA and mRNA.

The *exotoxin* of Bacillus thuringiensis also produces *nucleolar segregation.* In addition, ring-shaped nucleoli, micronucleoli, dense plaques at the periphery of the nucleolus, and degranulation of the nucleolus have been noted with this toxin.[138]

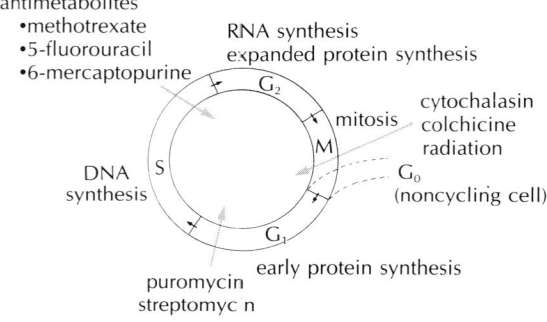

Figure 6–35. Actions of drugs and radiation in the inhibition of phases of the cell cycle.

Drugs and Chemicals

Numerous chemicals produce nuclear abnormalities by inhibiting nucleic acid synthesis or by damaging the chromosomes or nucleoli (Fig. 6–35 and Table 6–20). These compounds are important because they provide molecular tools for dissecting steps in cell and DNA replication and because they are commonly used in medical therapy, particularly as antineoplastic agents.

Table 6–20. *Effects of Drugs on DNA of Chromosome*

S-Bromodeoxyuridine (BUDR), floxuridine (FUDR), aminopterin	Inhibits DNA synthesis, allows RNA and protein synthesis
Doxorubicin (Adriamycin)	Binds to DNA, inhibits its synthesis
5-Azacytidine	Inhibits RNA, DNA and protein synthesis
Azaserine	Interferes with nucleic acid synthesis
6-Mercaptopurine	Interferes with nucleic acid synthesis
Ethionine	Ethyl analogue of methionine, interferes with nucleic acid synthesis and increases methylation of the bases of tRNA
Nitrosoureas	Cross-links, alkylates, or carbamylates DNA
Methotrexate	Folic acid antagonist, inhibits DNA synthesis
Fluorouracil	Pyridine analogue, binds thymidylate synthetase, inhibits DNA synthesis
Cyclophosphamide	Yields numerous antimetabolites that inhibit DNA synthesis

Antineoplastic Drugs. Certain antibiotics used in the treatment of cancer may have adverse nuclear effects (Fig. 6–35). *Actinomycin D,* one of the most prominent cytopathic antibiotics currently in use, interferes with DNA transcription. This drug was used in classic experiments to produce nucleolar segregation.

Bleomycin inhibits the progression of cells through the premitotic (G_2) and mitotic (M) phases of the cell cycle.[139] Secondary effects may also be mediated by the increased presence of chalones, a natural growth inhibitor in bleomycin-treated cells.[140]

Antimetabolites. The *antimetabolites* are another major category of drugs used in therapy of cancer because of their ability to inhibit DNA synthesis. An example is *5-azacytidine.* Although several mechanisms have been proposed for this drug, the favored theory is that as 5-azacytidine becomes integrated into the DNA, the DNA becomes less stable, and chromosome breaks develop.[141]

Ethionine, the ethyl analogue of methionine, combines with adenine to form *S-adenosyl ethionine.* The resulting decrease in available adenine leads to ATP deficiency. Following ethionine treatment, electron-dense opaque masses appear in the nucleolus as fragments.

Methotrexate, an analogue of folic acid, is a metabolic poison that acts during the S phase of mitosis.[111] This drug inhibits dihydrofolate reductase and deprives malignant cells of tetrahydrofolic acid, which is an essential cofactor for purine and DNA synthesis. In chemotherapy with methotrexate, later administration of citrovorum results in *"citrovorum rescue"* and stops unnecessary damage to normal cells by supplying the needed folate.

Other Therapeutic and Experimental Drugs. *Ethidium bromide* interacts with nucleic acids or chromatin by intercalating between the base pairs of the nucleic acids or by electrostatic binding to the outer phosphate groups. Treatment with ethidium bromide also causes nucleolar segregation and degranulation.[142]

Isoniazid, a drug used successfully in the treatment of tuberculosis, induces a lupus-like syndrome in some patients. This agent is capable of inducing antibodies to nuclear components, including histones.[143]

One group of drugs interferes with chromosome replication by acting primarily on the mitotic spindle. *Colchicine* blocks mitosis in prometaphase and also causes the formation of *micronuclei.* This agent inhibits the polymerization of tubulin and thus solubilizes spindles and prevents new spindle formation. High doses of colchicine produce *intranuclear vacuoles* and *blebbing* of the nuclear membrane.[144] *Vincristine* and *vinblastine* also inhibit spindle formation.

Chemicals in Foods. A number of naturally occurring compounds that are sometimes found in food may affect chromosome structure. *Aflatoxins,* in high concentrations in contaminated ground nuts, peanuts, and other foodstuffs, decrease DNA, RNA, and protein synthesis and produce abnormal chromosomes. *Amanitin,* found in some mushrooms, interferes with transcription by inhibiting RNA polymerase II. Unlike actinomycin D, the segregation of the nucleolus and condensation of the chromatin occur as two separate steps.[145]

Hormones

Hormones are capable of producing characteristic changes in nuclear morphologic features. The well-known *Arias-Stella* reaction of *endometrial cells* during early pregnancy results in the presence of cells with nuclear pleomorphism.

The steps in steroid hormone effects are as follows: the hormones bind to a cytoplasmic receptor and the resultant hormone-receptor complex is translocated to a specific nuclear or chromatin receptor molecule. In the case of *estrogens,* this translocation induces synthesis of RNA, DNA, and protein and eventually leads to cell proliferation.[146] *Progesterone* can induce a peculiar organelle in the nucleus known as the *"nucleolar channel system"* or the *"nucleolar basket."*[147] This structure, like the intranuclear annulate lamellae, is thought to function in nuclear-cytoplasmic exchanges.

Immunologic Agents

The group of disorders known as *"collagen vascular diseases,"* including systemic lupus erythematosus (SLE), rheumatoid arthritis, scleroderma, and mixed connective tissue disease, frequently feature prominent antinuclear reactions (Table 6–21) and heightened immune reactions.[148] In SLE, following initial cellular injury by a variety of agents, nucleoprotein released into the circulation stimulates *antibody* production, particularly against *DNA-protein complexes.*[149] The *hematoxylin body* and the *LE cell* represent phagocytized material consisting of denatured, clumped chromatin released from cells following injury. Patients with SLE display other abnormal antibodies as well.

In other collagen vascular diseases, such as rheumatoid arthritis and the mixed connective tissue diseases, *antibodies*

Table 6–21. *Diseases in which Immune Products React with Chromatin or DNA*

Disease	Immune Reaction
Systemic lupus erythematosus	LE cell containing phagocytized nucleus Antibodies against DNA demonstrated in cells
Rheumatoid arthritis	IgM antibody demonstrated against DNA IgM-IgG complexes
Chronic hepatitis	Core Ag (HBcAg) and Ab demonstrated in nuclei C1q complement fraction present

modifies protein secretory products and materials incorporated from the extracellular space. Cells with large quantities of *SER* usually have an *eosinophilic* appearance when stained, in contrast to the *basophilic* appearance of cells rich in *RER*.

Cells such as hepatocytes appear to have equal amounts of both SER and RER. The amount of SER and RER in a given cell reflects its functional role. ER content appears to vary diurnally, although the significance of this observation is unknown.[158.]

Ultracentrifugation of cell homogenates allows the separation of an RNA-rich fraction, the *microsomal fraction,* that represents fragmented membranes of both SER and RER. Ultrastructurally, this fraction contains membrane vesicles with or without ribosomes.

Golgi Apparatus

The *Golgi apparatus* was first seen with a metallic impregnation technique in 1898. This structure is important in the secretion of proteins and is found in virtually all cells. Its presence was confirmed ultrastructurally in 1952, when parallel arrays of membranes with closely associated vacuoles were demonstrated.[159] In *nonglandular cells,* the Golgi apparatus is *juxtanuclear;* in *glandular* epithelial cells, where it is especially well developed, it is supranuclear and often *apical* in location.

The Golgi apparatus typically consists of stacked, flattened, membranous sacs or cisternae 150 Å in diameter. These are composed of 60 Å membranes. Usually, 4 to 8 cisternae of variable length are present, separated by about 200 to 300 Å. This group of cisternae has 2 *"faces,"* an outer one nearest to transitional elements of the RER where substrates enter, and an inner face from which *condensing vacuoles* bud. The *outer face* is also known as the *entry, cis,* or *immature face,* and the *inner face* is known as the *exit, trans,* or *mature face.* The inner Golgi face is associated with condensing vacuoles 400 to 800 Å in diameter. These two faces have a functional directionality that is reflected by biochemical heterogeneity (Table 6–22 and Fig. 6–38C).

Table 6–22. *Characteristics of the Cis and Trans Faces of the Golgi Apparatus*

Enzyme Present	Cis	Trans
5'-nucleotidase	+	+
Adenylate cyclase	+	+
Periodic acid (silver methenamine)	+	+
Osmic acid impregnation	+	−
Acid phosphatase	−	+
Thiamine pyrophosphatase	−	+
Glucose-6-phosphatase	−	−

The directionality in synthesis and processing of substrates within the ER-Golgi system, as well as the heterogeneity within it, has been shown by cytochemical reactions and electron-micrographic studies. In the formation of certain secretory products, it is seen that mannose is usually added to a protein substrate early in the proximal ER cisternae (farthest from the Golgi), whereas galactose moieties are added in the Golgi apparatus.

The Golgi apparatus is the site of sugar assembly and packaging as well as secondary sulfation.[160] Chondroitin sulfate is also synthesized there. Thiamine pyrophosphatase (TPP), glycosyl transferase, and sulfation enzymes are localized to the Golgi apparatus; TPP is particularly prominent in hepatocytes and neurons. Proteolysis, as in the conversion of proalbumin to albumin, also occurs in this organelle. Interesting data[159] suggest that the Golgi apparatus plays a role in reprocessing membrane fragments of secretory granules, once exocytosis has occurred. Either by endocytic vesicle movement to the Golgi apparatus or incorporation of fragments into lysosomes with subsequent movement to the Golgi apparatus, or both, such fragments ultimately would appear in the dilated rims of Golgi cisternae at the mature face.

The transition region between the RER and the Golgi apparatus contains transitional vesicles 10 to 12 nm in diameter that arise from the smooth surface of the RER and transport substrates synthesized in the RER to the Golgi apparatus for further modification.

Granular Endoplasmic Reticulum Lysosomes (GERL)

An intermediate organelle that appears to be a connecting link between the ER, Golgi apparatus, and lysosomes is known. It appears as an acid phosphatase-rich area of SER located at the inner or "trans" aspect of the Golgi apparatus. *Four types* of *lysosomes* arise from the *GERL:* (1) *residual bodies* containing residual material incapable of further digestion; (2) *coated vesicles,* which carry lysosomal hydrolases to other cell structures such as phagosomes; (3) *type I autophagic vacuoles* containing fragments of cytoplasm and organelles; and (4) *Type II autophagic vacuoles* containing mostly myelin figures. A clear-cut functional and morphologic division into these four types is often difficult.

Some investigators consider the *condensing vacuoles* or nascent granules to be expanded parts of the GERL.[152] The GERL may also internalize lectins in neurons of dorsal root ganglia. After endocytosis, membrane-bound lectin receptor complexes have been identified in acid phosphatase-rich tubules and vesicles (GERL) located at the "trans exit" aspect of the Golgi apparatus.[152]

Steps in Protein Synthesis

Protein synthesis occurs on either membrane-bound or free ribosomes in four stages: (1) *activation of amino acids,* (2) *initiation* of the polypeptide chain, (3) *elongation,* and (4) *termination* (Table 6–23 and Fig. 6–39).

Dallner, Siekevitz, and Palade suggested that, in general, ribosomes attached to ER are active in the synthesis of

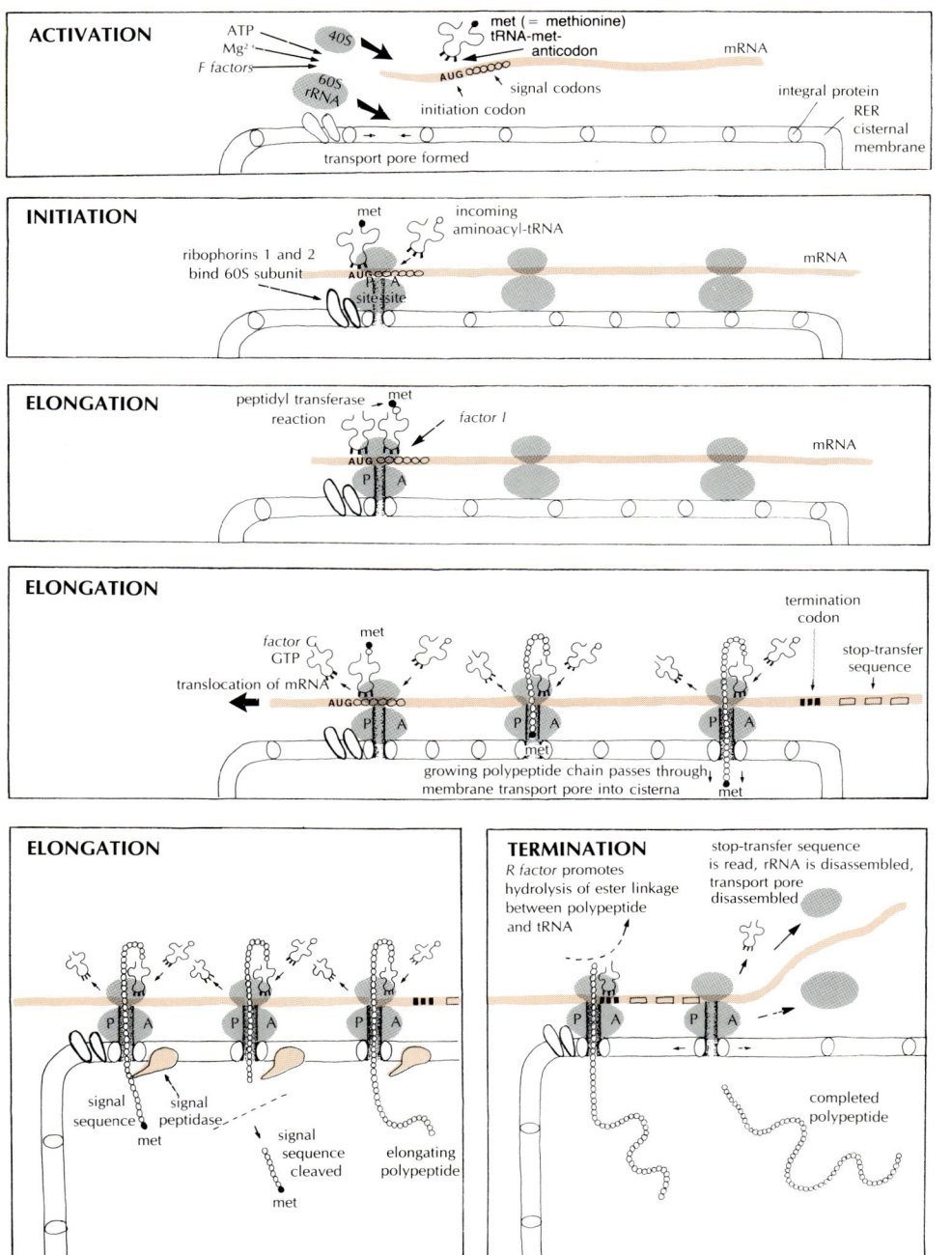

Figure 6–39. Steps in protein synthesis (see the text for discussion).

Table 6–23. *Components Required in the Four Major Stages of Protein Synthesis*

Stage	Components Required
Activation of amino acids	Amino acids tRNA Aminoacyl-tRNA synthetases ATP Mg^{2+}
Initiation of polypeptide chain	Initiating aminoacyl tRNA (met) mRNA GTP Mg^{2+} Initiation factors (F factors) 40S ribosomal subunit 60S ribosomal subunit Ribophorin 1 and 2 (ER membrane-binding proteins for binding 60S rRNA)
Elongation	Aminoacyl tRNA specified by codons Mg^{2+} Factor T GTP Factor G Signal peptidase
Termination	Termination codon in nRNA Polypeptidase release factor R Stop-transfer sequence (for disassembly of rRNA and transport pores)

secretory proteins, and those that are free in the cytoplasm are concerned with the synthesis of nonexportable proteins.[161]

In the case of membrane-bound ribosomes, small and large subunits of rRNA are bound to membranes of ER cisternae. Messenger RNA is threaded along the cleft between the two subunits, and the growing peptide chain is extruded into the cisternal lumen. This chain undergoes subsequent modifications by passing through transitional ER vesicles to the Golgi apparatus and the secretory vacuoles. The growing peptide chain may be inserted into the ER membrane rather than into its lumen. The subsequent fusion of membrane vesicles with the plasma membrane is known as cotranslational transfer.

In contrast to secretory and membrane proteins, *nonexported proteins* are synthesized on *free ribosomes* in the cytosol. By the process of post-translational transfer, *nonexported* proteins are inserted into or on the membranes of their final localization site. Recent evidence indicates that exceptions are seen in which *free ribosomes* are the sites of synthesis of certain *exportable proteins*, including the peroxisomal proteins, catalase, and urate oxidase, as well as diphtheria and cholera toxins.[162]

Activation

In the first stage of protein synthesis, activation, amino acids are esterified to their corresponding tRNA by the action of enzymes known as aminoacyl-tRNA synthetases, which use ATP for energy and require the presence of Mg^{2+}. Each tRNA possesses four functionally active sites: (1) *the anticodon site,* which is the specific nucleotide triplet complementary to codon triplets in mRNA; (2) *the amino acid binding site,* specific for a given amino acid; (3) *the amino acid activating enzyme site,* to which the specific aminoacyl-tRNA synthetase is bound; and (4) the ribosomal *recognition site.*

Initiation

During initiation of protein synthesis, which proceeds from the 5' to the 3' end of the mRNA,[163] dissociated 40S and 60S rRNA subunits are assembled; mRNA threads through a cleft between them, first binding to the 40S subunit. The 60S subunit is bound to the membrane surface of an ER cisterna by two integral membrane proteins, *ribophorin 1 and 2.* Randomly dispersed membrane proteins rearrange to form transport pores beneath the 60S central channel, through which the growing peptide chain can gain access to the cisternal lumen. With the addition of initiation factors *(F factors), GTP and Mg^{2+},* the structural requirements for a protein synthetic assembly line have been met. The complete 80S rRNA complex bears a *P site* for the elongating peptidyl tRNA and an *A site* for incoming aminoacyl tRNA.[164]

Initiation is begun when the mRNA initiation codon AUG is read by the complementary incoming tRNA, which is bound to methionine. This first aminoacyl tRNA is bound at the P site as an N-acyl derivative to insure availability of its COOH group for interaction with the NH_2 group of the next amino acid entering at the A site (Fig. 6–39).

Elongation

Elongation proceeds when an incoming aminoacyl tRNA binds to the *A site* positioned at the next codon of the mRNA. This binding requires GTP and T factor. It appears that the first 20 triplet codons, following the initiation codon AUG, code for a 20-amino-acid *"signal peptide."* This peptide is subsequently cleaved from the ultimate protein product by *"signal peptidase,"* an enzyme thought to be present in the inner portion of the ER membrane. Jackson and Blobel[165] postulated the existence of 4 signal peptides, 4 signal peptidases, and 4 signal receptors for cleavage in the protein synthetic apparatus associated with 4 membranes, namely, the ER, inner mitochondrial, plasma, and lysosomal membranes.

After binding, a 60S-bound peptidyl transferase catalyzes the peptide bond formation between the amino group of the newly arrived amino acid and the carboxyl group of the preceding methionine. When this peptide bond has been made, the growing peptidyl tRNA is then in the A site; for further elongation to occur, peptidyl tRNA and mRNA must be physically translocated or moved along the ribosome to bring the next codon into position. The "empty" tRNA is thus displaced from the P site, leaving the A site empty.

The entire sequence occurs with hydrolysis of GTP and mediation by a specific protein called *G factor*. This elongation sequence continues as mRNA "tracks" through the cleft between the ribosomal subunits. The growing peptide chain, with its leading NH_2 group, is directed down through the 60S central channel into the ER lumen.[166]

Termination

Termination, the event that results in the release of the polypeptide from its ribosomal-bound tRNA, occurs when specific mRNA termination codons UAA, UAG, and UGA are reached. Certain release factors *(R factors)* are required for this event, and a *"stop-transfer"* sequence in the mRNA may play a role in disassembly of ribosomal subunits and in dispersion of intramembranous transport pore proteins.[167]

Polypeptides delivered to the interior of the RER are subsequently segregated into transitional vesicles, which bud off and merge with the outer (cis) face of the Golgi apparatus. A continuous intramembranous system is then maintained as the protein passes (with modifications occurring such as *sulfation* or *glycosylation*) through the *Golgi apparatus,* into amorphous *condensing vacuoles,* into mature *secretory granules,* and to the cell surface for exocytosis.[159]

During synthesis along the RER, integral membrane proteins are inserted into the ER membrane itself, rather than the cisternal lumen (Fig. 6–40). On completion of such a polypeptide, the amino terminal projects into the lumen; the majority of the protein spans the membrane and the carboxyl group extends into the cytoplasm.[168] By subsequent fusion with a portion of plasma membrane in which a new integral protein is required, the NH_2 group is located on the luminal surface of the membrane, and the carboxyl group is embedded in the cytoplasm. This mechanism seems to be logical for membrane protein synthesis because this amino-exterior, carboxyl-interior polarity is maintained in virtually all membrane proteins currently examined.

Products of the Synthetic Apparatus

Labor is divided among the cellular organelles engaged in synthetic processes. It is acknowledged that proteins for export, including albumin, immunoglobulins, pancreatic enzymes, collagen, and lysosomal hydrolases are synthesized on polysomes attached to the ER membrane. These cells are often basophilic and are associated with the presence of abundant RER; however, they may undergo subsequent modification in other organelles. For example, it

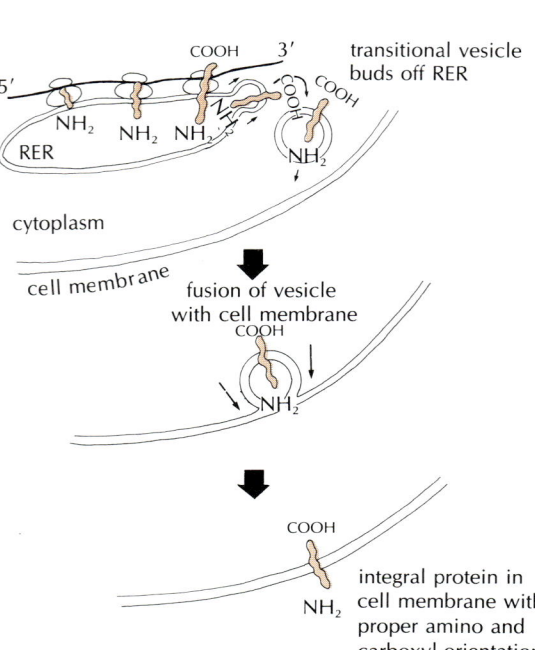

Figure 6–40. The mechanism of the synthesis and insertion of proteins destined to be integral proteins of the cell membrane involves vesicle migration and fusion with the membrane, so that the amino terminal end projects to the cell's exterior and the carboxyl terminal is embedded in the cytoplasm.

was only recently clarified that a *preproalbumin* peptide arrives at the ER cisternae where 18 amino acids are cleaved and that the resultant proalbumin is further processed in the Golgi apparatus, where another 6 amino acids are removed.

Intracellular proteins such as hemoglobin, mitochondrial inner-membrane respiratory enzymes, and structural proteins are synthesized on free ribosomes in the cytoplasm. A few extracellular proteins for export, including diphtheria toxin, are also synthesized on free ribosomes.

Cells engaged in *steroid, lipid, glycogen,* or *pigment synthesis* are *acidophilic* when seen by light microscopy because of the abundant SER present. Examples include cells of the adrenal cortex (steroids), hepatocytes (glycogen), and retinal cells (pigment).

Summary Model of Secretion

Work by Jamieson and Palade with the pancreatic acinar cell provides an elegant and insightful model of the secretory process[169] (Figs. 6–39 and 6–41). It may be summarized as follows:

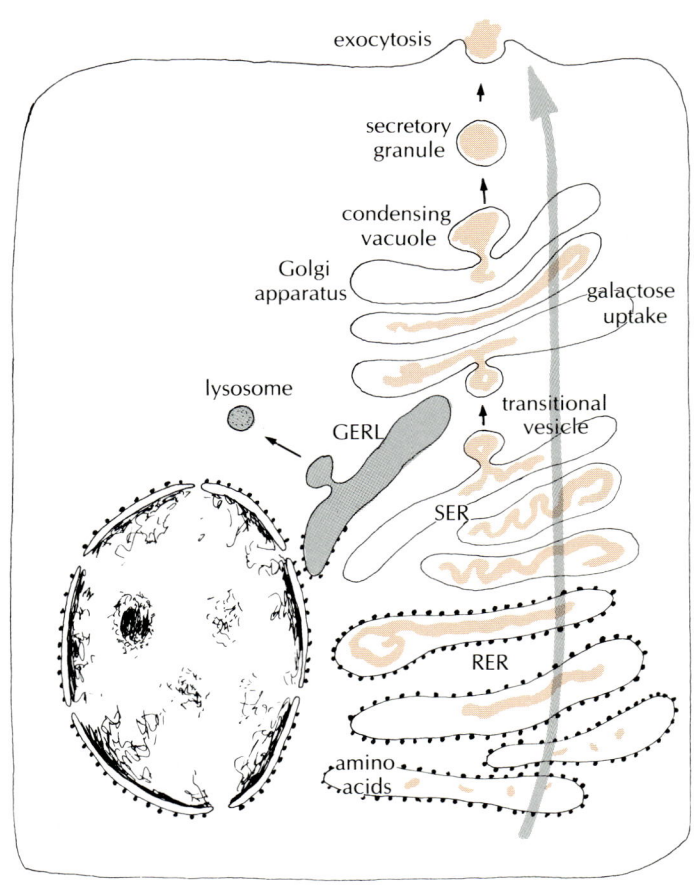

Figure 6–41. Sequence of events in protein synthesis.

1. Protein synthesis on ribosomes. Segregation follows in the intracisternal space of the ER. Cotranslational activities, including signal peptidase activity, catalysis of disulfide bonds, addition of oligosaccharides, and hydroxylation of lysine and proline in collagen-synthesizing cells, also occur here.
2. Movement of the protein moiety into transitional elements of RER and SER in which they become associated with specific receptors.
3. Transfer of protein by small vacuoles to the Golgi apparatus by continuous membrane fusion.
4. Concentration-sulfation-glycosylation-proteolysis at the level of the Golgi complex.
5. Accumulation of secretory products in the Golgi apparatus.
6. Budding of condensing vacuoles from the Golgi apparatus with secretory granule movement to the apex of the cell, followed by plasmalemma fusion and exocytosis.

General Effects of Injury

The ER undergoes five major responses when injured: (1) *swelling,* (2) *disruption* and *disorganization,* (3) *hypertrophy,* (4) *atrophy,* and (5) the formation of *inclusions* (Fig. 6–42).

Swelling is due principally to the influx of water and sodium. Areas of *"cloudy swelling"* seen by light microscopy represent swollen ER cisternae. *Hydropic degeneration* occurs when ER cisternae become ruptured to form larger vesicles. The initial stages of ER swelling can only be appreciated ultrastructurally.

A second major response may be *disruption* and *disorganization* of the various components of the ER, including the ribosomes. Hydropic dilatation of ER and disruption of the RER frequently occur together.

Because the RER is the major site of cellular amino acid incorporation and protein synthesis, its disruption and the subsequent loss of synthetic capabilities may lead to secondary cellular damage and, ultimately, to cellular death, if the initial cause of injury is not removed or inactivated.

Compensatory *hypertrophy* of ER components often occurs in response to a drug that requires metabolic detoxification or degradation. Damaged ER that cannot undergo hypertrophy may *atrophy.*

A fifth major response is *sequestration* with *inclusion formation.* Such inclusions may contain infectious agents such as viruses and bacteria, protein, glycogen, lipid, pigment, or various combinations of these substances, either in membrane-bound cisternal or vacuolar units.

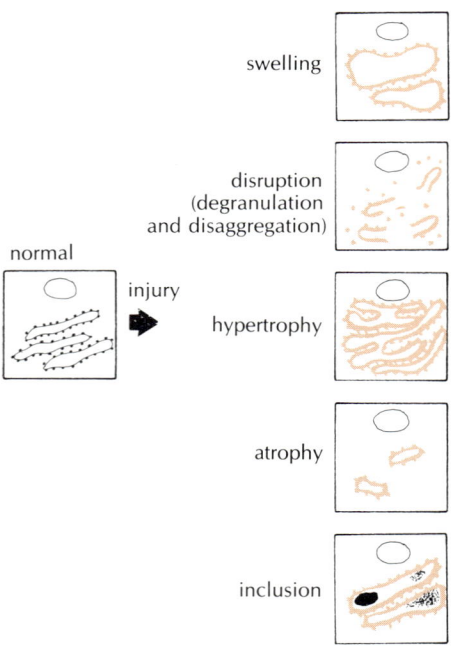

Figure 6–42. The general effects of injury on the endoplasmic reticulum.

Genetic Factors

Among the genetic disorders attributed to gene mutations and characterized by an accumulation of products in the ER, lysosomes, and cytosol are the lipid storage, glycogen storage, and protein storage diseases.

A protein storage disorder that is associated with a serum enzyme deficiency is *alpha-1-antitrypsin (AAT) deficiency.* In this disorder, accumulations of AAT in the RER and SER of hepatocytes appear prominent in some cases of emphysema and hepatic cirrhosis (Fig. 6–43).

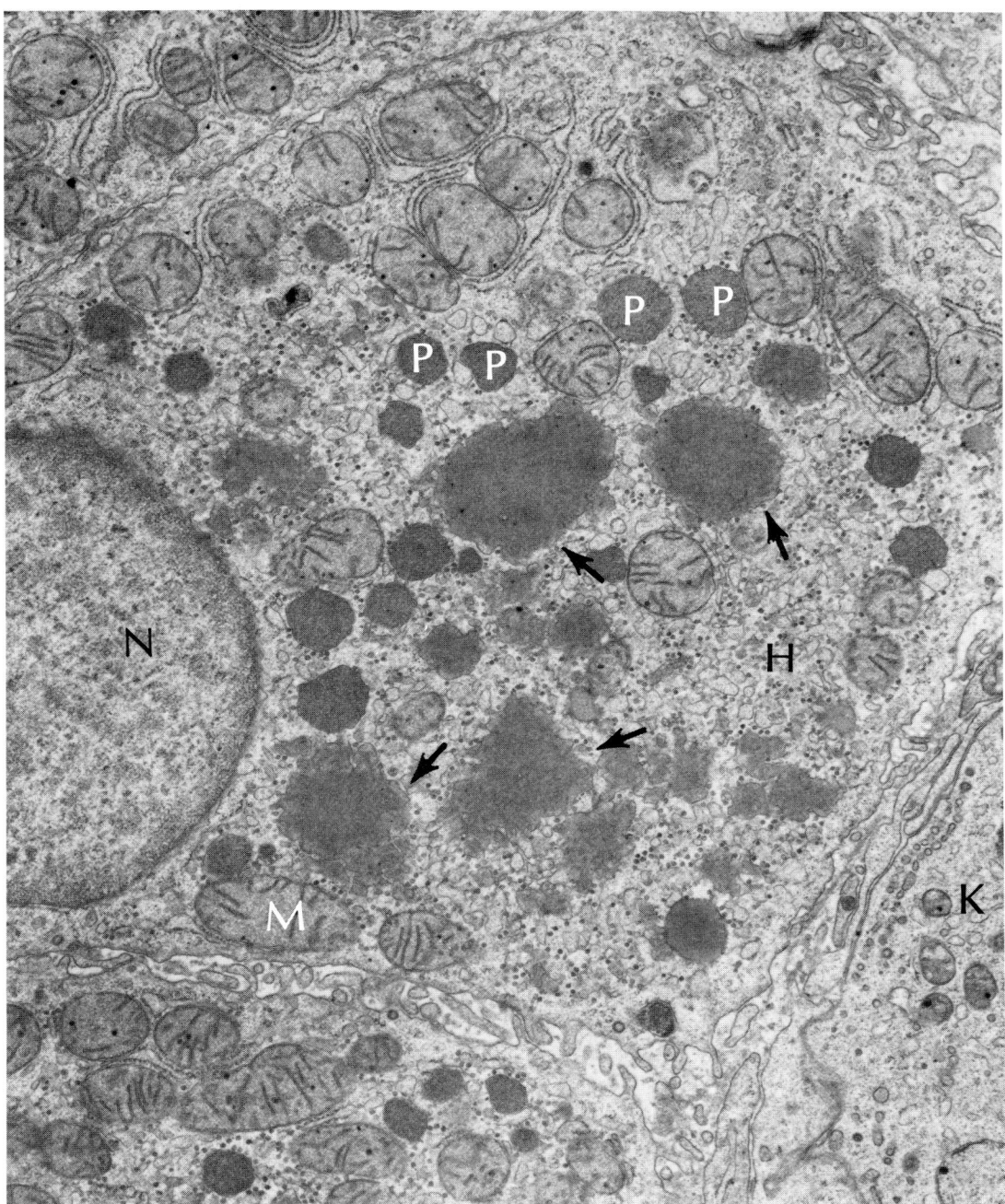

Figure 6–43. In this transmission electron micrograph of the liver from a patient with alpha-1-antitrypsin deficiency, the hepatocyte (H) contains globules of alpha-1-antitrypsin (arrows) in dilated endoplasmic reticulum cisternae. Other organelles are present, including peroxisomes (P), nucleus (N), and mitochondria (M), and an adjacent Kupffer cell (K) is seen. (Courtesy of Dr. F. Schaffner, Department of Medicine, Mount Sinai School of Medicine, New York.)

The retention of this enzyme in the ER has been related to an abnormal glycoprotein portion of the alpha-1-antitrypsin molecule in which one sees a deficiency of sialic acid, galactose, and N-acetylglycosamine and an almost twofold increase in mannose residues. These biochemical abnormalities probably lead to a lack of appropriate secretion signals or receptor interactions, so that the enzyme is not transported out of liver cells. Its absence in serum allows increased activity of proteolytic enzymes that mediate tissue damage, especially in the lung. The retained protein globules in the liver stain with periodic acid-Schiff (PAS) and resist diastase digestion. The protease inhibition (Pi) system has defined individuals who are homozygous (PiZZ) as well as heterozygous (PiMZ)[170] for this disorder.

The reticuloendothelial cells of individuals with the *Chédiak-Higashi syndrome* have a hypertrophic GERL containing crystalline deposits.[171]

Physical Agents

Hypoxia, radiation, and the increased *pressure* due to obstructive phenomena all produce dilatation, swelling, and degranulation of the ER.

Hypoxia leads to precipitous falls in ATP and to associated defects in the synthetic process associated with mRNA, and possibly in the mRNA itself. Ribosomes become separated from ER membranes, decreased in number, less aggregated, and less efficient in carrying out protein synthesis. The number of active units is reduced, and the ribosomal readout process is slowed, so that the ischemic cell is less responsive to added mRNA.[172]

Oxygen toxicity damages cells, partly by the effects of lipid peroxidation. Biomembranes and subcellular organelles are the major site of this damage, especially mitochondrial and microsomal membranes, because they contain large amounts of polyunsaturated fatty acids in their phospholipids.[173]

Hypertrophy or increased activity of the Golgi apparatus has been observed in different kinds of *radiated* cells, and histochemically detectable acid phosphatase activity is increased in the Golgi vacuoles of these cells. This activity precedes the formation of numerous autophagosomes.[174] Distension and fragmentation of the Golgi apparatus may occur as well.[175]

Temperature may also affect the ER. Hypothermia has been shown to induce helical polysomes and ribosomal crystalline arrangements.

Nutrition and Growth States

Differentiating or *regenerating* tissues characteristically have a *hypertrophied RER* and large polysomal clusters to accommodate the increased requirements for protein synthesis. Similarly, the Golgi apparatus and ER may be prominent in active, protein-secreting cells. In certain states, such as *pregnancy,* these changes may be marked.

The influence of dietary amino acids on cellular components, especially polysomes, involved in protein synthesis, is significant. Diets rich in amino acids increase the rates of synthesis.[176] The number of ribosomes in any cell is subject to nutritional modulation, and in starvation, ribosomal loss is rapid.[177] *Starvation* can reduce hepatic ribosomes up to 50% without altering either the fraction of rRNA relative to total RNA or the distribution of free and membrane-bound ribosomes. Eventually, the ribosomes dissociate. Lysine deficiency causes severe involution of Leydig cells. The SER of these cells becomes vesicular and regressive, and androgen production is lost.[178]

Choline deficiency is associated with the presence of liposomes (fat-containing vesicles), a disrupted and dilated Golgi apparatus, decreased numbers of secretory vesicles, and dilated, fragmented RER. These changes account for the abnormal intracellular transport and defective protein synthesis occurring in this state.[179]

Vitamin C deficiency may result in a breakdown of polysomes to ribosomes, that is, *disaggregation,* without dissociating ribosomes from the RER, a process known as *degranulation.* Other nutritional effects on the ER are shown in Table 6–24.

Table 6–24. *ER Alterations Associated with Nutritional Factors*

Effect	Protein-Free Diet	Control Diet*
Hepatic polyribosomes:		
Shift to heavier aggregates	Slow	Rapid
Reaggregation of:		
Total polyribosomes	Present	Present
Free polyribosomes	Present	Present
Bound polyribosomes	Present	Present
Hepatic protein synthesis:		
Interval required for increased		
in vivo and in vitro incorporation	Long	Short

*Control diet consisted of complete diet, complete amino acid mixture, or tryptophan

(Modified by permission from Sidransky, H.: Regulatory effect of amino acids on polyribosomes and protein synthesis of liver. Prog. Liver Dis., 4:31, 1972.)

Infectious Agents

Many *infectious agents* alter the ER as part of the general cellular response to the injury (Table 6–25). The presence of infection may stimulate specific cells to respond by *ER hypertrophy*, which reflects the roles played by them in combating infection. There is increased synthesis of *lytic enzymes* in macrophages and leukocytes, *immunoglobulins* in plasma cells, and *lymphokines* in lymphocytes. As granulation tissue forms in healing from an injury, hypertrophy of the RER and Golgi apparatus in fibroblasts is associated with increased synthesis and assembly of *collagen* precursor molecules.

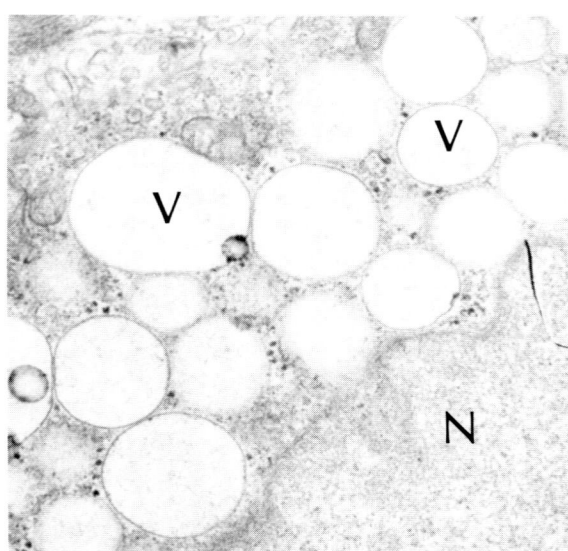

Figure 6–44. Water-filled vacuoles (V) fill the cytoplasm of the cell. The nucleus (N) is seen in one corner.

Table 6–25. *Endoplasmic Reticular (ER) Alterations Associated with Infectious Agents*

Toxic reactions
    cloudy swelling and hydropic degeneration (bacteria)
    coagulation necrosis and Councilman body (virus)

Presence of agent in cisternae and lysosomes

Interference with host protein synthesis
    diversion of protein synthesis from host to viral products
    blockage of host protein synthesis (diphtheria toxin)

Hypertrophy
    increase in lysosomal enzymes in phagocytes
    production of immunoglobulins in lymphocytes and plasma cells
    production of collagen by fibroblasts in repair process

A common feature of infection by many viruses is an altered pattern of protein synthesis in the infected cells. Some viruses inhibit macromolecular synthesis, whereas others enhance it.[180] Viruses may interfere with the protein-synthesizing ability of the cell during the uncoating, synthesis, and assembly process of the virus, either in the cytosol or ER cisternae. Furthermore, the viruses may form inclusions in the cisternae of the ER.

Alterations of the ER in viral hepatitis have been extensively studied, and the effect of the virus on the function and structure of the ER is important in the pathogenesis of this disease. The ER becomes progressively swollen and disaggregated, and degranulated ribosomes are present. The liver acquires large amounts of water in the dilated cisternae and gives rise to the classic picture of *"cloudy swelling"* (Fig. 6–44). This water accumulation can progress as the ER ruptures further, and swelling of mitochondria contributes to the ballooned cellular appearance called *"hydropic degeneration."*

As the liver cell in viral hepatitis progressively loses its water and becomes dehydrated, the ER degranulates, collapses, and with other cell constituents, condenses to a concentrated, eosinophilic mass of protein. This *"mummified" hepatocyte* is known as an acidophilic or *Councilman-like* body (Fig. 6–45).

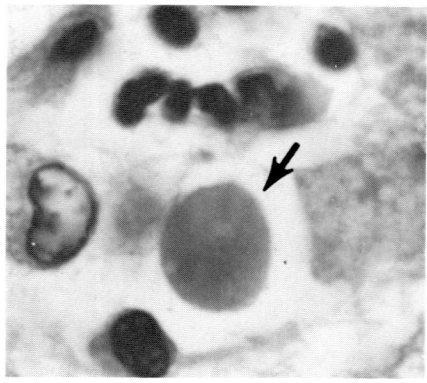

Figure 6–45. An acidophilic body (arrow) is seen in the liver.

An interesting and specific ribosomal abnormality is seen in some cells of patients with diphtheria. The *diphtheria* bacillus, Corynebacterium diphtheriae, produces an *exotoxin* that contains two *subunits, A* and *B*. The B subunit of the exotoxin binds to a specific membrane receptor and mediates transport of the entire peptide into the cell, where it is actually split into its A and B units. Fragment A *inactivates* the free form of *elongation factor 2* required for the translocation of peptidyl tRNA from the acceptor to the donor site of the ribosome. The modified form of the elongation factor can still attach to ribosomes and can bind GTP, but its translational activity is disturbed.[181]

Drugs and Chemicals

Many drugs and chemicals have been studied in relation to their effect on the ER and Golgi apparatus (Table 6–26). The majority of these agents interfere with protein synthesis. Others cause lipid peroxidation or inhibit transport, and some cause hypertrophy of the SER and Golgi region. Still other drugs and chemicals disturb other organelle functions that are secondarily reflected in the ER and Golgi apparatus. Disruption of mitochondrial respiration by cyanide or microtubule function by colchicine secondarily affects ER structure and function.

Drugs that inhibit protein synthesis include puromycin, chloramphenicol, cycloheximide, thiopseudourea, verrucarin A, actinomycin D, anisomycin, and carbon tetrachloride.

Table 6–26. *Morphologic or Functional Alterations in Ribosomes, Endoplasmic Reticulum (ER), and Golgi Apparatus with Drugs and Chemicals*

Structure and Agent	Change
Ribosomes	
Puromycin	Substitution for aminoacyl and RNA
Chloramphenicol	Binding to 55S mitochondrial ribosomes
Cycloheximide	Binding to 80S cytoplasmic ribosome
Thiopseudourea	Cross-linked complexes with ribosomes
Verrucarin A	Polysome disaggregation
Actinomycin D	Degradation of ribosomal protein
Anisomycin	Inhibition of binding of 60S subunits
Ethionine	Formation of S-adenosylethionine as competitor for methionine
ER	
Carbon tetrachloride	ER lipid peroxidation and degranulation ER (liver)
Insulin	RER hypertrophy (breast)
Hydrocortisone	RER hypertrophy (liver)
Prolactin	RER hypertrophy (breast)
Antigen	RER hypertrophy (lymphocyte)
Barbiturate	SER hypertrophy (liver)
Dieldrin	SER hypertrophy (liver)
Golgi Apparatus	
Ionophore (X537A)	Dilatation and hypertrophy
Amino nucleosidase	Hypertrophy

RER Effects. *Puromycin* disrupts the Golgi apparatus, ER, and ribosomes and interrupts peptide chain elongation by substituting aminoacyl tRNA with a form of peptidyl puromycin. *Chloramphenicol* inhibits protein synthesis by binding mitochondrial ribosomes, although the 80S cytoplasmic ribosome complex is unaffected. *Cycloheximide*, on the other hand, inhibits protein synthesis by binding 80S cytoplasmic ribosomes, but not 70S mitochondrial ribosomes (mitoribosomes). This drug causes severe degranulation of the ER.[182]

Thiopseudourea and *verrucarin A* both interact with *ribosomes.* Thiopseudourea produces aggregation of ribosomes by forming cross-linked complexes with ribosomal protein moieties, and it also inhibits translation. It appears, however, that these aggregates can still carry out transpeptidation and protein synthesis.[183] *Verrucarin A* causes "ribosomal run-off," that is, extensive polysome disaggregation with blocking of steps subsequent to the formation of the 80S initiation complex.

Actinomycin D in low doses inhibits rRNA synthesis and causes a preferential degradation of newly synthesized ribosomal proteins in regenerating liver.[184] *Anisomycin* is an antibiotic that reversibly inhibits the binding of mature 60S subunits to the met-tRNA-mRNA-40S initiation complex.[185] Other inhibitors of protein synthesis include ethionine, 4-α-naphthyl, dimethylnitrosamine, and vincristine.

Carbon tetrachloride (CCl$_4$) causes ER membrane lipid peroxidations and changes similar to those seen in oxygen toxicity. CCl$_4$ breaks down to the free radical CCl$_3$· and produces degranulation and disaggregation of polysomes, and sometimes, further breakdown to ribosomal subunits; it may also cause membrane dissolution. Microsomal enzymes are decreased in number, particularly cytochrome P450, although nicotinamide-adenine dinucleotide phosphate (NADP), cytochrome C reductase, and cytochrome B5 do not change. Subsequent peroxidation and lipid changes also occur with CCl$_4$ toxicity.[186]

SER Effects. Some of the most striking drug-induced changes in the SER are those seen in hepatocytes after the administration of *barbiturates.* These agents cause pronounced eosinophilia of the cell and induction of the mixed-oxidative microsomal system[187] (Fig. 6–46). Other chemicals, such as the pesticide *dieldrin,*[188] are associated with hypertrophied SER and a lower functional capacity.

Calcium can induce changes in membrane lipids and may alter their structural conformations and transport properties. Increased Ca^{++} levels interfere with peroxidation of liver microsomal membranes, presumably by altering their phospholipid content.[189]

Golgi Effects. The ionophore X537A causes dilatation and swelling of cisternae and vesicles of the Golgi apparatus in parathyroid cells, smooth muscle, intestinal epithelium, plasma cells, and cells of the pituitary. These changes may

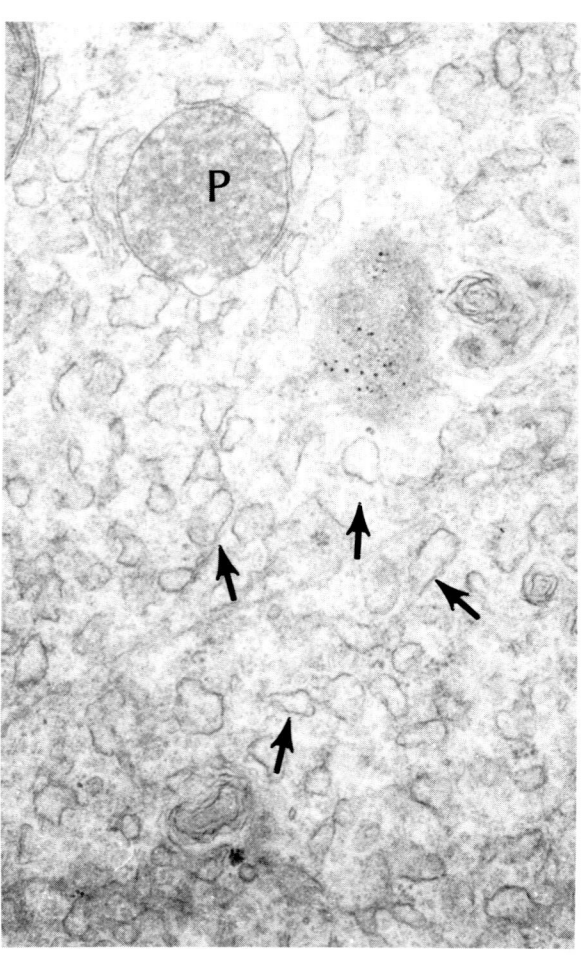

Figure 6–46. This smooth endoplasmic proliferation (arrows) is caused by "SER drug induction" in a patient taking phenobarbital. A peroxisome (P) is also seen.

be secondary to the accumulation of osmotically active substances in the Golgi apparatus.[190] This generalized effect is seen with all the ionophores. They cause striking alterations in the Golgi apparatus by interfering with the usual flow of materials among the RER, Golgi apparatus, and plasma membrane.

The Golgi apparatus hypertrophies after treatment with aminonucleosides. The enlargement is mainly due to a proliferation of a network of fine tubules associated with the Golgi system and, to a lesser extent, to an increase in the diameter of the cisternae. The surface volume of the Golgi complex doubles, with a corresponding increase in galactosyl transferase, a membrane-associated enzyme specific for the assembly of galactose in glycoprotein.[191]

Hormones

Proliferation of the ER in cells is normally induced by certain natural, hormonal stimulatory pathways. For example, ER in breast epithelium hypertrophies under insulin, hydrocortisone, and prolactin stimulation. Binding sites for hormones are found on the membranes of the ER as well as on the plasma membrane, including receptors for human chorionic gonadotropin, cAMP, and cGMP. In similar fashion, injection of thyroxine and somatotropin is associated with increased incorporation of amino acids into microsomal proteins and of glycerol into membrane lipids.

Immunologic Agents

The ER is stimulated in many immune reactions, particularly when immunoglobulin is being formed. When *lymphocytes* become *activated* by *mitogenic* agents such as *phytohemagglutinin* (PHA), 70% of the ribosomes that were inactive and free are converted to active polysomes. This process occurs by the activation of preexisting ribosome subunits, rather than by the synthesis of new ones.

Antibodies may be synthesized against *organelles* that serve as antigens. Ribosomal nucleoproteins may serve as one source of antigens in several autoimmune diseases, including Hashimoto's thyroiditis, SLE, and chronic active hepatitis. Approximately 1% of patients with SLE have antibodies directed against ribosomes, although the predominant antibodies are directed against nucleoproteins. Antibodies against the microsomal fraction may be present in chronic active hepatitis.[192]

Because the RER and Golgi apparatus are most prominent in secretory cells, it is not surprising to find that plasma cells, secreting immunoglobulin, normally display many of these organelles (Fig. 6–47). In multiple myeloma, the secretion of great amounts of immunoglobulin results in large intracisternal accumulations of protein known as *Russell bodies*. These appear as large, acidophilic, cytoplasmic and extracellular droplets by light microscopy.

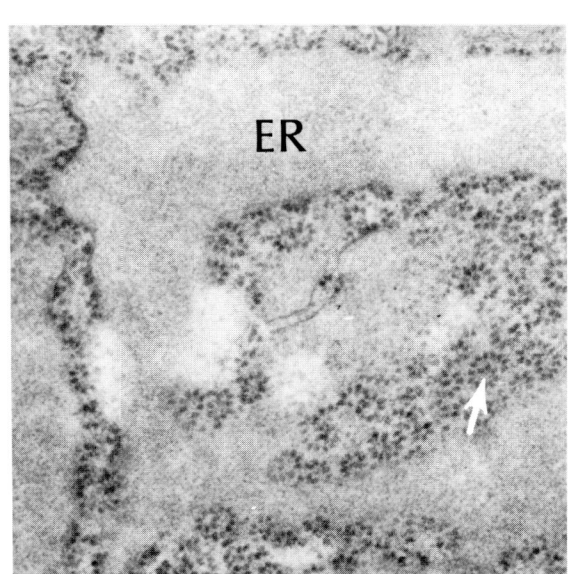

Figure 6–47. A portion of a plasma cell engaged in antibody synthesis. The cisterns of the endoplasmic reticulum (ER) are filled with electron-dense material. Polysomes (arrow) are prominent.

CYTOSKELETAL AND ANCILLARY STRUCTURES

General Characteristics of the Cytoskeleton

The endoplasmic reticulum forms a major part of the structural framework of the cell but various cells have several other important structures, including *myofibrils, microfilaments, microtubules, centrioles, basal bodies, cilia,* and *flagella,* that contribute, in a concerted fashion, to the cytoskeleton (Table 6–27). They influence the cell's size, shape, mobility, division, and transport processes, including absorption and secretion.

Table 6–27.   *Cell Structures Functioning in Contraction and Transport*

Cell membrane
Purkinje myofilament system
Microtubules (MT)
Microfilaments (MF)
Intermediate filaments (IF)
neurofilaments, tonofilaments
Microtubular- and microfilament-containing special structures
sperm tails, flagella, cilia, centrioles, basal bodies, mitotic spindle of dividing cells, desmosomes of epithelial cells
fibrillary microfilamentous structure of Porter

Myofibrils are a special class of intracytoplasmic fibrils found in muscle cells. Comprised of a thick myosin filament and a thin filament made up of actin and tropomyosin B, myofibrils provide the basic mechanism for muscle contraction.

Microfilaments are found throughout the cytoplasm and nucleus of most cells and consist principally of actin with a minor myosin component of perhaps 10 to 15%. Cellular contraction mediated by these filaments is responsible for the *amoeboid motion* in *phagocytosis.* The mitotic microfilaments attach to the spindle and cause *chromosome segregation.* Other microfilaments are important in altering the topographic distribution of membrane proteins, thereby mediating subsequent changes in cell shape. A new fibrillary microfilamentous structure has been described by Porter.[193]

Intermediate filaments of variable consistency are found in specialized cells, especially nerve and muscle, and have particular functions.

Microtubules found in both the cytoplasm and nucleus are largely composed of two types of *tubulin.* Microtubules are intimately involved in basic cellular structure, *movement* of phagocytic particles with fusion to lysosomes, and *transport* of secretory granules from the ER to the cell membrane; they are also the most important component of the *mitotic spindle.*

Centrioles act as the organizing centers and *poles* of the *mitotic spindle* and, perhaps, of other microtubules. *A basal* body is essentially a *ciliated centriole* composed of microtubules capable of spontaneous self-assembly. Basal bodies contribute to the formation of *cilia* in human cells, including bronchial and fallopian tube epithelium. A single, large cilium is called a *flagellum.* In sperm, this flagellum is its major motile force.

Myofibrils

Structure

These fibrils are composed of thick *(myosin)* and thin *(actin and tropomyosin)* filaments located in parallel arrays in skeletal muscle. Under polarizing light, myofibrils have alternating bright anisotropic *(A bands)* and dark isotropic *(I*

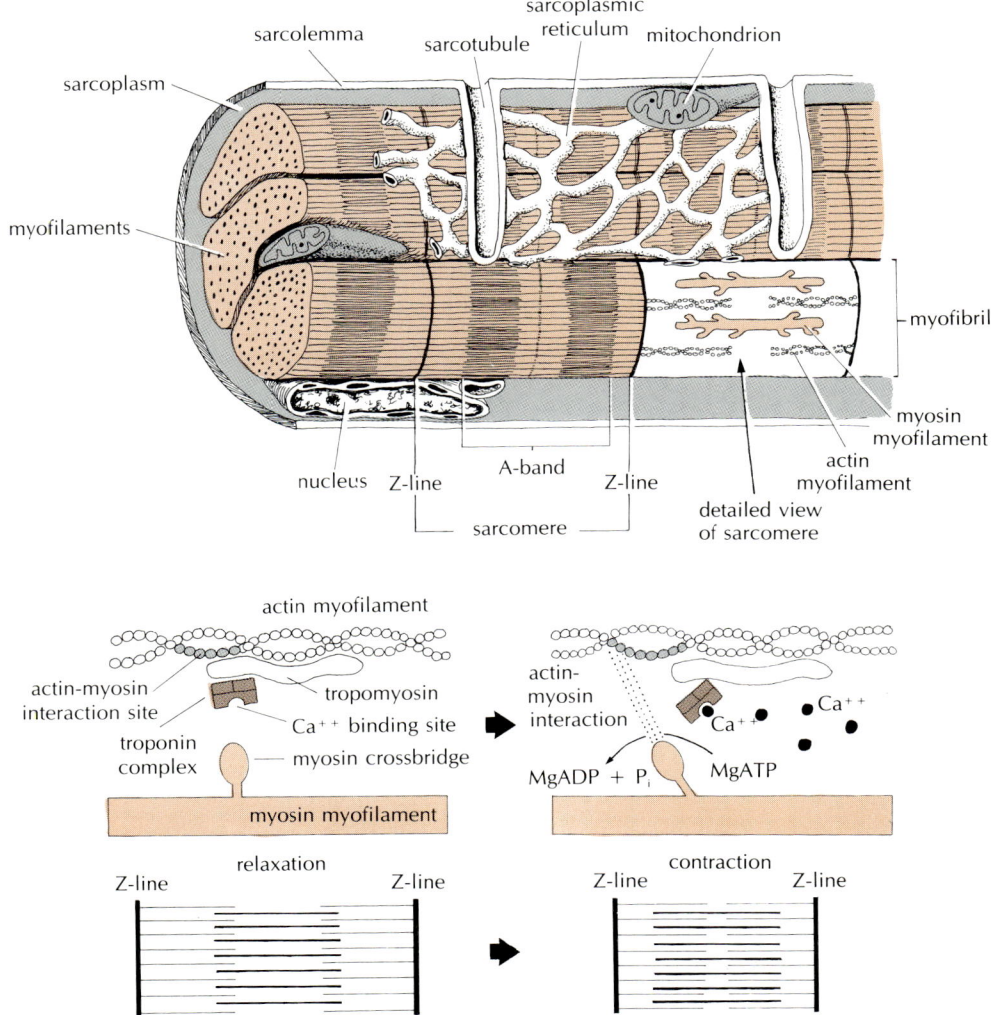

Figure 6–48. The structure of cardiac muscle is shown at the top. At the bottom, the events in muscle contraction are shown. In the relaxed state (diastole), the tropomyosin-troponin proteins inhibit interactions between actin and myosin. With systole and influx of calcium from the sarcoplasmic reticulum, calcium binding to troponin releases inhibition and allows the actin-myosin interaction to occur. (Modified from Braunwald, E. (ed.): The Myocardium: Failure and Infarction. New York, HP Publishing, 1974.)

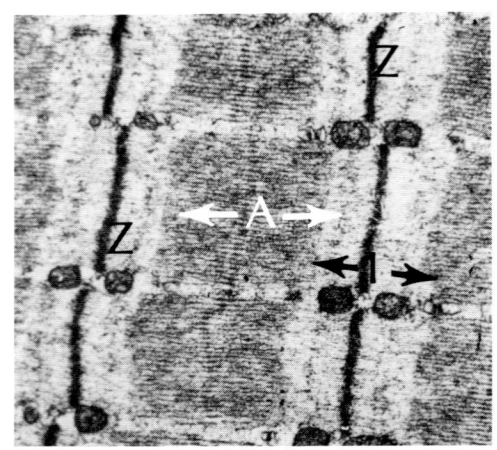

Figure 6–49. Electron micrograph of normal muscle cell shows prominent I bands (I), A bands (A), and Z lines (Z).

band) bands. The *Z band* traverses the middle of the I band, the *H band* bisects the *A band,* and the *M line* traverses the center of the H band. Skeletal muscle fibers contain a contractile unit known as a *sarcomere,* bounded by *Z lines* to which actin filaments from adjacent sarcomeres are attached (Figs. 6–48 and 6–49).

Four proteins function in the process of contraction. *Actin* and *myosin* are the contractile proteins, whereas *tropomyosin* and *troponin* act as regulatory proteins.[194] The myosin molecule contains two globular heads, the *heavy* and *light meromyosin* components (Figs. 6–48 and 6–49).

Function in Contraction

Before contraction, actin and myosin molecules are primed for action, but their interaction is blocked by the presence of tropomyosin molecules at several reactive sites on actin. When Ca^{++} ions stored in the sarcoplasm become available, they bind to the troponin complex on actin. Conformational changes that follow in the tropomyosin molecules allow the actin to react with heavy meromyosin (ATPase), and cross-bridges form.[195]

Sarcoplasm

The *sarcoplasmic reticulum* is a membrane system that envelops the myofibrillar bundles and consists of a sarcotubular network and the subsarcolemmal cisternae.[196] In muscle fibers, the tubular *T-system* is open to the extracellular space at the sarcolemmal surface of the muscle fiber. The T tubules allow the spread of electrical excitation from the cell surface to all parts of the sarcomere.

Microfilaments

Structure

Electron-microscopic examinations of almost all cells show *microfilaments* 5 to 7 nm (40 to 70 Å) in diameter.[197] Micro-

Table 6–28. *Cellular Proteins Associated with Microfilaments*

Filamin
Myosin
Vinculin
α-Actin
Actin
Fimbrin
Tropomyosin
Calmodulin
α-Kinin
Fragmin
Gelsolin

filaments are composed of actin-myosin complexes and provide the mechanical and chemical basis for many cellular activities. Actin, a ubiquitous protein, usually appears in greater concentration than myosin; that is, the actin:myosin ratio is 10:1. The well-known *sliding actin-myosin model* of muscle contraction need not, however, be the contractile model operative in other cells.[198,199] Other proteins associated with microfilaments are shown in Table 6–28.

Site

Microfilaments permeate the cytoplasm and nucleus. Interconnecting long and short filaments surround all cellular organelles including microtubules and polyribosomes.[200] Microfilaments are also associated with desmosomes, mitochondria, and occasionally peripheral elements of the RER. Microfilaments are primarily located beneath the plasma membrane in the *terminal web*. They may extend into microprojections such as *filopodia* and *microvilli*[201] (Fig. 6–50). They may be present singly, in bundles known as *stress fibers*, or as part of a microfilamentous network. Microfilaments also form at the transitory cytoplasmic con-

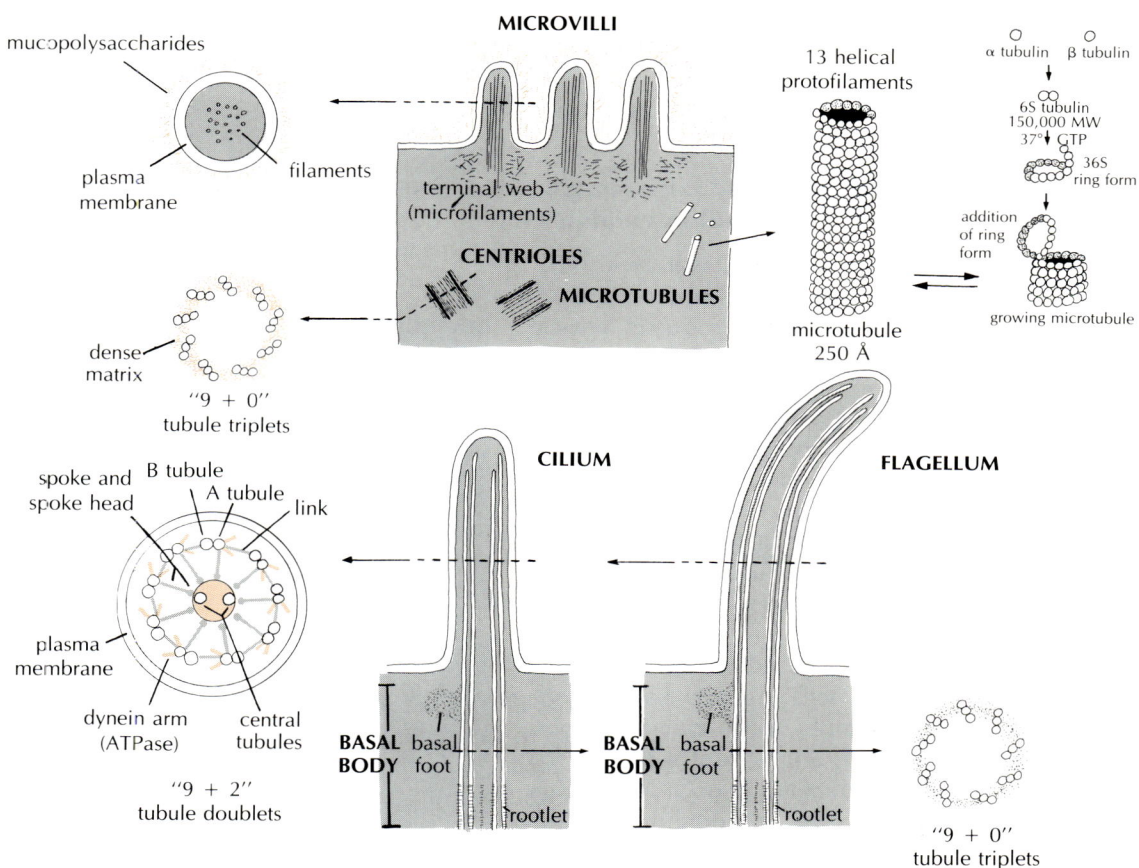

Figure 6–50. Schematic comparison of the structure of microvilli, microtubules, centrioles, cilia, flagella, and basal bodies.

after treatment with colchicine. Microtubules may also facilitate the fusion of lysosomes with *phagosomes*, as well as the extracellular release of enzymes.[214] Networks of microtubules and microfilaments have been seen in areas of

tractile ring of dividing cells, they accumulate in large numbers at the plasma membrane in areas of active phagocytosis, and they appear in the region between the mitotic spindle poles and chromosome during mitosis.[202]

Other (Intermediate) Filaments

membrane contact between macrophages and foreign particles.[215,216]

The release of many hormones, for example, insulin, involves the interaction of microtubules and microfilaments. An accumulation of calcium in a critical cellular site, possibly located in the cytosol of the pancreatic beta cell,[217] may trigger *insulin secretion* by activating a microtubular-microfilamentous system that is involved in the translocation and exocytosis of secretory granules. Microtubules, located in juxtanuclear and Golgi regions, may form cross-bridges to secretory granules and may serve as a guiding cytoskeleton for the migration of the granules to the surface web area of the cell. There, a microfilamentous network may control the access of the secretory granules to sites of exocytosis at the cell membrane.

Experiments with cytochalasin B, which interferes with microfilaments, show that this substance enhances insulin release in response to a variety of insulinotropic agents. This finding suggests that the cell web may act as a sphincter, being both barrier to and effector of exocytotic insulin release.

The biphasic insulin secretion response may then be postulated as follows (Fig. 6–53): After glucose and calcium stimulation, secretory granules are released in close proximity to the cell web. In the second part of the biphasic response, a part requiring baseline glucose levels, insulin granules from the deeper pool are mobilized along microtubular transport systems (an ATP-dependent process) to the area of the cell web for exocytosis.

Microtubules are similarly responsible for the migration of other membrane-bound substances such as melanosomes in melanophores.

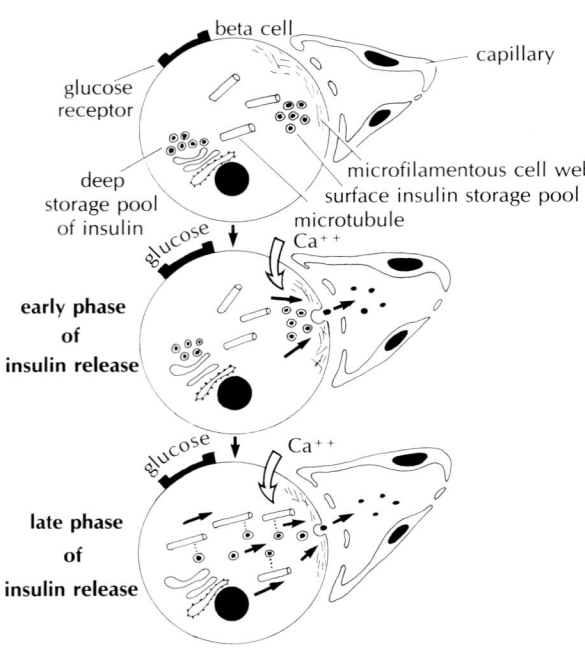

Figure 6–53. Phases of insulin secretion. Secretory granules in surface and storage pools are released to the vascular compartment through transport processes mediated by cytoplasmic microtubules and surface microfilaments that serve contractile functions.

Mitotic Spindle in Division

Microtubules of the mitotic apparatus resemble those found elsewhere in the cytoplasm (Fig. 6–54). They have a dense cortex, a light center, and amorphous material adherent to their surfaces.[218] In some species, microfilaments have been identified with microtubules in the spindle, but these findings are not constant in all cells.

Two classes of *spindle microtubules* exist: those bound to chromosomes, known as chromosomal fibers, and those running between the centrioles. Chromosomal movement may occur either by controlled shortening, lengthening, and sliding of spindle fibers or by changes in the assembly of microtubules within the spindle fibers.

Bajer has proposed a *"zipper hypothesis"* to explain the mechanisms of chromosome movement and the function of the spindle. This hypothesis suggests successive lateral attachments of kinetochore microtubules to the spindle.[219] Nicklas has proposed that poleward sliding of antiparallel microtubules and end assembly and disassembly of all microtubules occur constantly throughout mitosis.[220]

The first trace of spindle formation is observed in *prophase*. The spindle forms between the centrioles, usually on one side of the nucleus, while the nuclear membrane is still intact. Ultrastructural studies show that the ends of many nonchromosomal tubules near the poles do not reach the *metaphase plate;* some end at the plate, and some extend a good distance into the opposite half of the spindle.

At the start of *anaphase,* most filaments retract to the centriolar poles. The chromatids separate. The sister chromosomes move near the poles in opposite directions, and a larger fraction of the chromosome-attached tubules runs all the way to the poles, as if the chromosome fiber had been pushed poleward. At *midanaphase,* the chromosomes move close to the poles, and the spindle elongates as the sister chromatids move apart. As the cells pass through anaphase, the filaments near the nucleus become progressively disorganized, undergo dissolution, and disappear.[221] By *late anaphase,* the chromosome tubules have shortened, and the chromosomes have been drawn up around the poles.

The energy source for these processes is being investigated. The presence and requirement of *dynein,* other ATPases, and actin-like fibers in the mitotic spindle are debated. An ATPase has been described, and actin, as defined by the cell binding of heavy meromyosin, has been identified.[222]

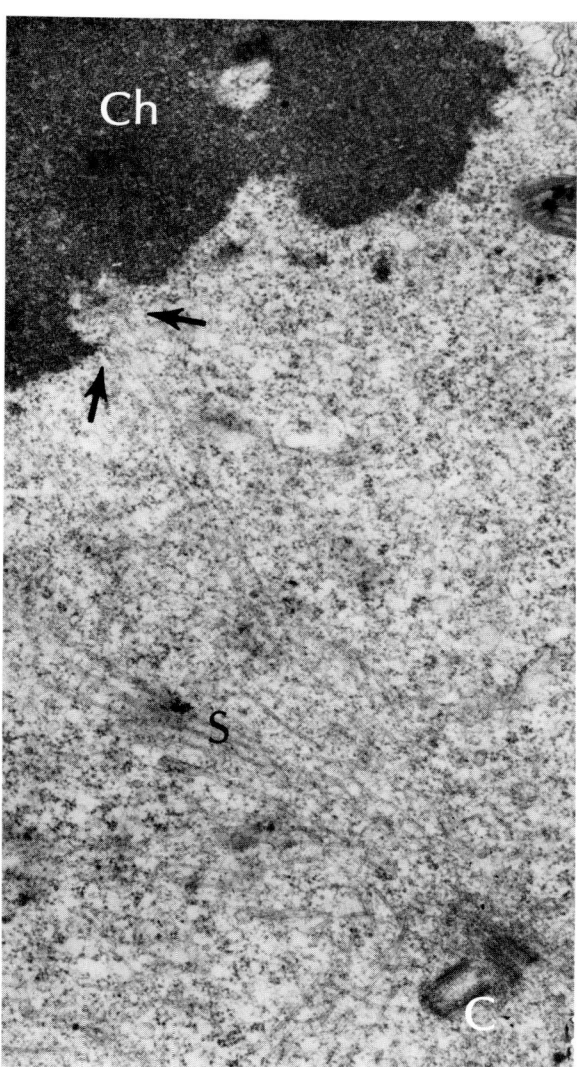

Figure 6–54. Filaments of the mitotic spindle (S) attach to the centriole (C) as well as to the chromosomes (Ch) (arrows).

Centrioles and Basal Bodies

Centrioles, kinetosomes, and *basal bodies* belong to a class of cellular organelles that have a cylindrical structure containing nine sets of three tubules or fibers. These triplets are arranged in a helical pattern. The cylindrical part of the structure is often associated with accessory structures[223] (Figs. 6–50, 6–55, 6–56, and 6–57).

Our understanding of the function of these organelles is incomplete. Centrioles act as microtubule-organizing centers and pole determinants in the mitotic spindle. Both basal bodies and kinetosomes are associated with cilia formation and ciliary motion.

Centrioles

The molecular genesis of centrioles is controversial, but they apparently can form from preexisting centrioles.[224] Centrioles are surrounded by an electron-dense *"amorphous cloud"* known as the *pericentriolar material.* This material is associated with smaller electron-dense spheres known as pericentriolar satellites (see Fig. 6–50).

Most authors believe that the centriole determines the *spindle poles* and is intimately involved in the assembly and organization of spindle microtubules into *"aster formations."* Centrioles contain DNA, which appears to be necessary to initiate aster formation.

Other postulated functions for centrioles include the generation of cilia and flagella in primitive eukaryotic cells and a possible role in the transport of materials to cilia.

Basal Bodies

A *basal body,* essentially a *"ciliated" centriole,* is principally composed of microtubules that are able to undergo spontaneous self-assembly (see Figs. 6–50 and 6–55). The basal body is usually short, approximately 0.5 μ long. It has a complicated set of associated accessory structures, and its component fibers are dispersed in an amorphous, electron-dense matrix. The diameter of the *rootlet,* which is the cytoplasmic end of the basal body, decreases as it passes deeper into the cytoplasm. The basal foot is a conical structure 150 μ wide and 130 μ long. Its base is attached to 2 or 3 of the triplet sets of the basal body.[225,226]

Basal bodies begin as *procentrioles,* which consist of a ring of amorphous material approximately 400 Å thick. Isolated microtubules appear within this amorphous ring and eventually increase to a total of 9 around the cylinder. At this point, spokes develop around the procentriole and may help to orient the assembly of the tubules.

Basal bodies are apparently necessary for the formation of the ciliary motile apparatus. They also function in the genesis of the flagella of sperm tails and as organizing centers for cytoplasmic microtubules.[227]

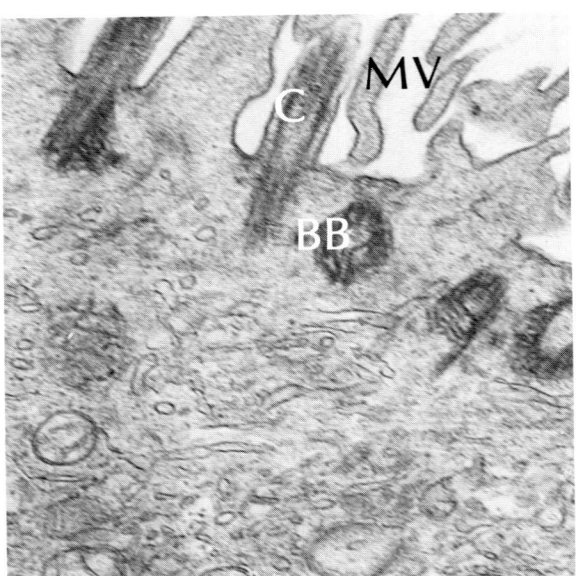

Figure 6–55. Electron micrograph showing a ciliated fallopian tube cell with prominent basal bodies (BB), cilia (C), and microvilli (MV).

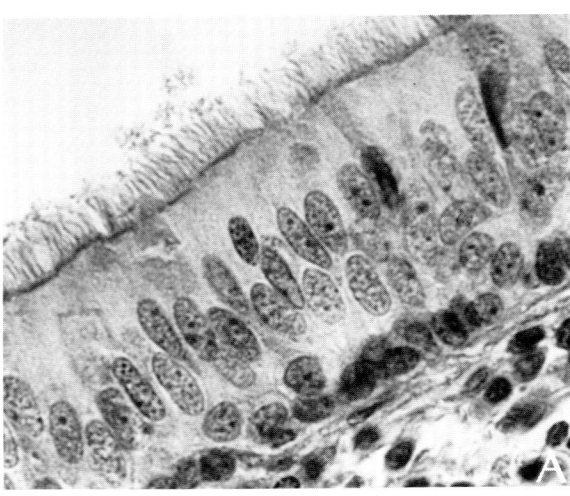

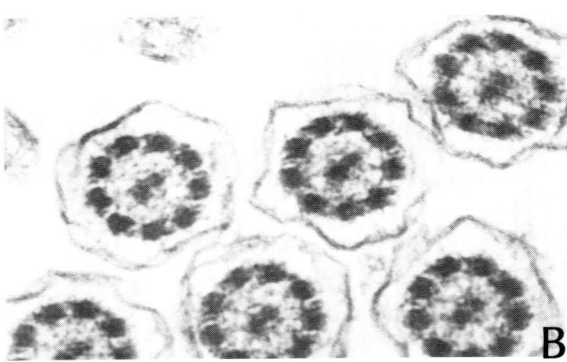

Figure 6–56. Cilia. *A,* Bronchial lining cells have prominent cilia. *B,* Electron micrograph of cross section of cilia shows the "9 + 2" configuration with nine outer doublets surrounding the central two single microtubules.

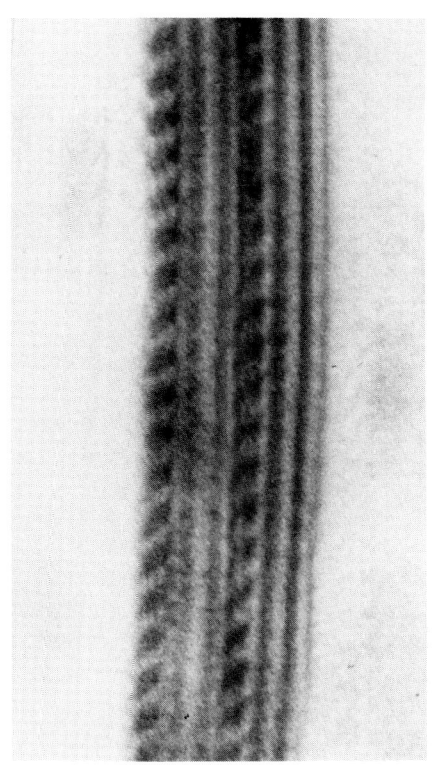

Cilia and Flagella

Some human cells are ciliated. These cilia have long axial *fibrils* and measure approximately 5 to 10 μ in length and 0.25 μ in width. *Sperm* have a *single cilium* or a *flagellum* that is 150 μ long. Cilia are attached to a basal body, and flagella are attached to an axial microtubule. Both cilia and flagella consist of a sheaf of microtubules arranged in the classic 9 +2 configuration, with 9 doublets surrounding a central pair of singles.[228] This sheaf is known as the *axoneme* (see Figs. 6–50 and 6–56).

The mechanism that enables the cilia and flagella to beat is an interaction between the axonemal doublet microtubules known as the *"sliding-microtubule"* hypothesis. This microtubule sliding occurs when the dynein arms of one doublet cyclically interact with sites of the microtubule lattice of the adjacent B subfiber.[229] When the doublets slide relative to each other, the position of the radial spokes changes[230] (Fig. 6–57).

Figure 6–57. Electron micrograph showing dynein arms from tetrahymena cilia. (Courtesy of Professor Fred D. Warner, Syracuse University.)

Agents of Cytoskeletal Injury

Table 6–30 summarizes the agents and effects of injury on the cytoskeleton.

Table 6–30. *Agents of Injury*

Agent	Microtubules (MT) Affected	Microfilament (MF) Affected
Genetic		
Muscular dystrophy	disorganized	—
Chédiak-Higashi syndrome	disorganized	—
Sickle cell disease	disorganized	—
Physical		
Hypoxia	↓ MT	↓ MF
Radiation	↑ MT in epithelium	—
Chemical		
Cytochalasin	—	inhibits MF organization stimulates contraction
Nemaline	—	disrupts MF
Amanitin	—	↑ actin
Colcemid	—	concentration ↑, intermediate 100-Å filament ↑
Colchicine	inhibits tubulin polymerization	—
Podophyllotoxin	inhibits tubulin polymerization	—
Alkaloids	inhibits MT assembly	—
Griseofulvin	affects assembled MT	—
Steganacin	inhibits tubulin assembly, depolymerizes MT	—
Immune		
Myasthenia gravis	antibodies to smooth and skeletal myofibrils	antibodies to MF
Chronic active hepatitis	—	antibodies to MF

Genetic Factors

In a variety of inherited muscle diseases, the myofibrillar components are defective. Depending upon the severity and extent of the defect, clinical signs of muscle weakness and dysfunction may be seen.

Myotubular myopathy is a disease that is sometimes genetic in nature. Nuclei with prominent nucleoli assume a central position in some cells; in others, these nuclei appear in their normal, subsarcolemmal position. Type I muscle fibers display granular degeneration and severe atrophy. Central vacuolization and glycogen deposition are also present with extensive proliferation of endomysial connective tissue.[231]

Muscular dystrophy is a genetic disorder of skeletal and smooth muscle[232,233] also characterized by nuclear centralization. Each fiber has either a single nucleus in its center or several nuclei situated in rows. *Disorganization* in the subsarcolemmal zones, with *gaps* in the *sarcomere, fragmentation* of the *myofibrils,* and *alterations* in the *Z band* with rodlike formations are noted, with loss of cross-striations and interstitial edema.[234] *Myelin figures* are often associated with the disrupted filaments.[235] It was previously believed that muscular dystrophy represented a complete failure of the regenerative capacity of the muscle fiber. This hypothesis does not appear to be true unless severe atrophy is present.

A genetic human disease with *"immotile cilia"* has been described. Patients with this disease have recurrent pulmonary infections because of poor clearance of material from the pulmonary tree by these defective cilia. Males are also infertile because their sperm are immotile.[236] A large percentage of these males have *Kartagener's syndrome* (Fig. 6–58), which is characterized by situs inversus, chronic sinusitis, and bronchiectasis. The sperm and cilia of these patients lack the dynein arms that normally form the crossbridges between ciliary microtubules that are believed to generate ciliary motion.[237]

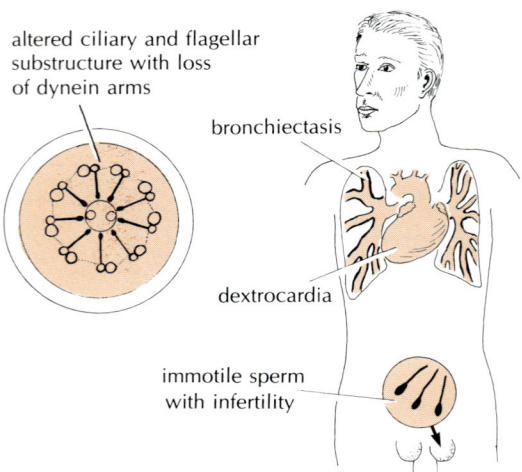

altered ciliary and flagellar substructure with loss of dynein arms

bronchiectasis

dextrocardia

immotile sperm with infertility

Figure 6–58. In **Kartagener's syndrome,** a triad of bronchiectasis, dextrocardia, and infertility result from defective ciliary and flagellar structure and function.

Physical Agents

Hypoxia. This injurious state has been well studied with regard to myofibrillar damage of the heart. Hypoxia produces marked degeneration of the fibrils, sarcoplasmic reticulum, and mitochondria. *"Stone heart"* represents an acute complication of cardiac operations in which fatal ischemic contracture of the left ventricle occurs, with irreversible myocardial damage.

Specific antibodies to cardiac myosin have been localized in areas of repeated infarction.[238] Striking degenerative processes involving contractile elements are also seen with marked myocytolysis and severe vacuolization of the mitochondria.

Both cardiac and striated muscles react to ischemia with profound histologic and ultrastructural alterations. The fibers may become *hypertrophic* as a compensatory response.

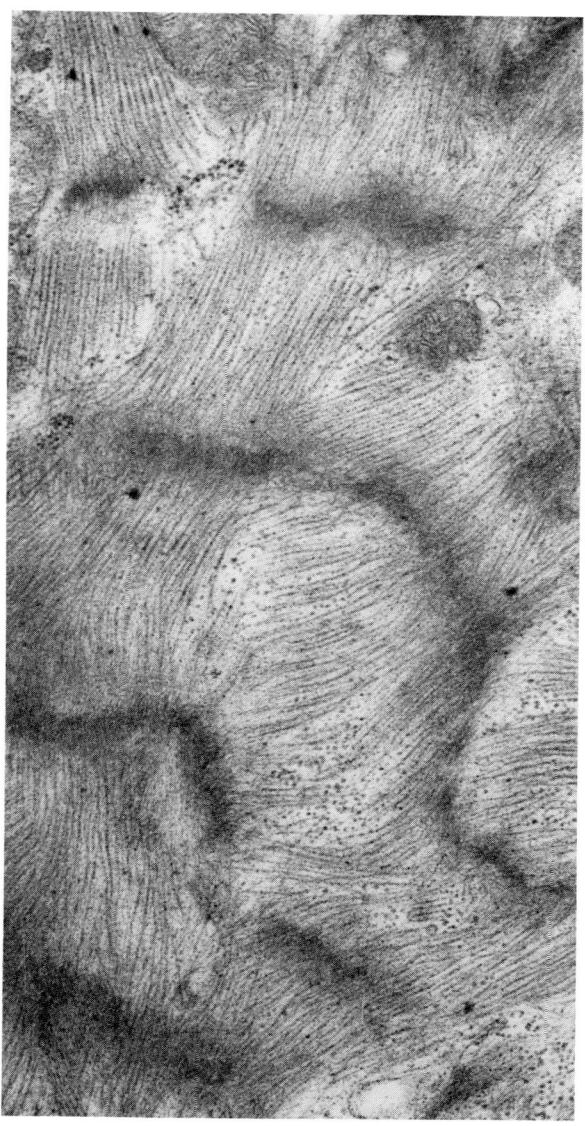

Figure 6–59. This electron micrograph of myocardium from a patient with obstructive cardiomyopathy showing marked disarray of myofibrils. (Courtesy of Professor Anton Becker, Academish Ziekerhuis Biu de Universiteit van Amsterdam, Netherlands.)

When myocardium hypertrophies, myofibrillar protein often increases and myocardial contractility decreases. This finding suggests that specific changes in the contractile proteins may alter myocardial function. It is unclear how altered myosin function changes contractile protein interaction.[239]

Biochemical abnormalities accompanying hypertrophy include increases in amino acid transport, RNA and DNA synthesis, and protein synthesis.[240] The increased oxygen consumption is probably related to the increase in the number of mitochondria. Synthesis of contractile proteins occurs following mitochondrial and ER hypertrophy.[241] A defect in ATPase activity is seen in purified myosin preparations. The intercalated discs become widened, more numerous, and probably stimulate formation of new sarcomeres.[242]

In cardiac hypertrophy associated with valvular disease marked loss and degeneration of myofilaments in the muscle are seen. In *idiopathic hypertrophic stenosis (asymmetric septal hypertrophy)*, the histologic pattern is striking because hypertrophic myofibrils run randomly rather than in parallel. It has been postulated that this disorganization results from abnormal contraction stresses. Myofibrils and myofilaments are in disarray (Fig. 6–59). In its severest form, this occurs throughout the cell. Occasionally there is criss-crossing and cross-weaving of the filaments with insertion into the wrong Z bands. Sometimes the myofibrils appear to be branched. The intercellular junctions in these areas are abnormal with side-to-side and end-to-side apposition, instead of the normal end-to-end relationship. Z-band material is increased and split. The T tubules are distorted and often contain myofibrils 100 to 300 Å in diameter.[243] Similar changes are sometimes associated with other diseases showing abnormal contraction patterns.

Radiation. Radiation produces focal myofibril lysis, myofibrillar degeneration with loss of entire myofibrils, lipid bodies, and abnormal lysosomes in muscle cells. Z-band thickening or disruption is not apparent, but the intercalated disc may be disrupted.[244]

Temperature and Other Agents. Elevated temperatures may exert harmful effects on cells because the equilibrium between tubulin dimers in microtubules is temperature-sensitive. The desynchronization of chromosomal movement is associated both with the rearrangement of kinetochore fiber microtubules into hexagonally packed structures and with the disappearance of nonkinetochore microtubules.[245]

Microtubules are easily disrupted following increased pressure, decreased temperature, or osmotic alterations. Electrical injury to the heart, as in countershock cardioversion, leads to myofibrillar degeneration and abnormalities of associated mitochondria.[246]

Nutritional Factors

Animals fed a diet deficient in *selenium* and *vitamin E* often die from acute *cardiac failure*. This disorder is associated with myofibrillar degeneration with hypercontraction bands. The pathogenesis of the injury may be related to the lack of protection by glutathione and the antioxidant vitamin E; damage by lipid peroxidation is thus allowed.[247]

Malnutrition results in muscle atrophy with degeneration of myofibrils. Specific muscle dysfunction has been noted in *beri beri* heart disease caused by *thiamine deficiency*.[248] Nutritional deficiency may also produce cardiac hypertrophy associated with a 20% increase in the size of myocytes.

Infectious Agents

In 1975, Dales reported that *adenovirus* type 5 and *reovirus* type 3 bind to microtubules during their replication in vitro. An alteration in microtubules is associated with cytopathic effects in poliovirus, adenovirus, and herpesvirus infections. The early proteins of both adeno- and herpesvirus adversely affect the host's cytoplasmic microtubules.[249]

Ultrastructural studies on virally transformed fibroblasts have shown that extrusion of viruses is associated with cellular processes containing bundles of microfilaments. In particular, *mouse mammary tumor virus (MMTV)* release is associated with extrusion from long microvilli that contain prominent microfilamentous bundles. Recent data from purified MMTV have identified a protein that co-migrates on gels with actin. This protein is an internal protein of the virion, not a contaminant of the virus isolation procedure. It has been suggested that this protein is derived from microfilaments of the host microvilli.

Actin has also been identified in cells infected by other viruses.[250] In *Reye's syndrome* following *measles viral infection,* myofibrils often accumulate *lipid* vacuoles.[251] Acute myositis often occurs after influenzal infections with significant reversible myofibrillar degeneration (Fig. 6–60).

Trichinella is a *parasite* that typically encysts in muscle and causes local damage.

Chemical Agents

Toxic Drugs Affecting Microtubules. The chemical agents originally known as *mitotic spindle poisons,* including *colchicine, colcemid,* the vinca alkaloids *vinblastine* and *vincristine,* and *podophyllotoxin,* share the ability to disrupt the assembly and function of microtubules.[252] *Tubulin* often acts as a *specific drug receptor,* and the treatment of cells with these agents reorganizes the microtubular elements; this process sometimes results in the formation of highly ordered paracrystals.[253] These birefringent crystals consist of hexagonally packed tubules, 320 Å in diameter, of linearly arranged tubulin.

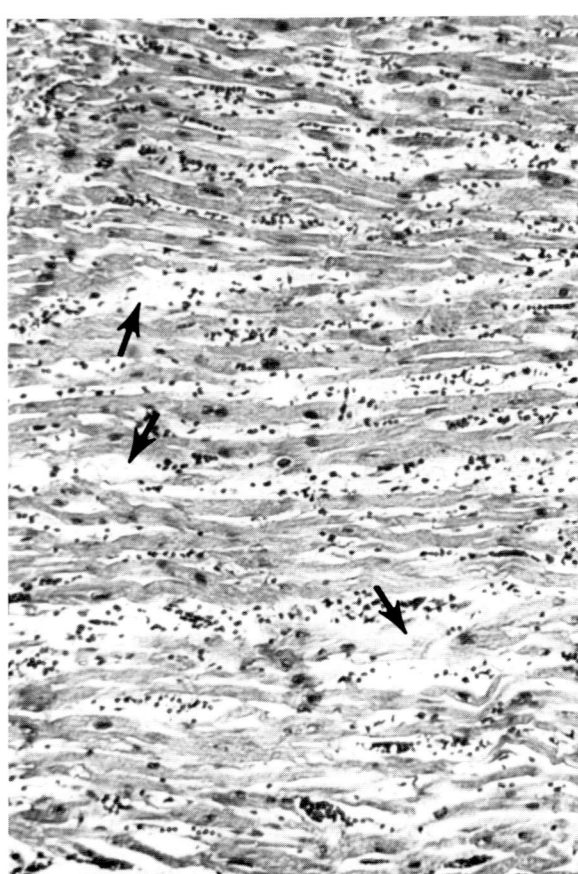

Figure 6–60. In viral myocarditis, myofibrillar degeneration is present (arrows) as well as many inflammatory cells. (Courtesy of Dr. J. Fenoglio, Dept. of Pathology, Columbia University.

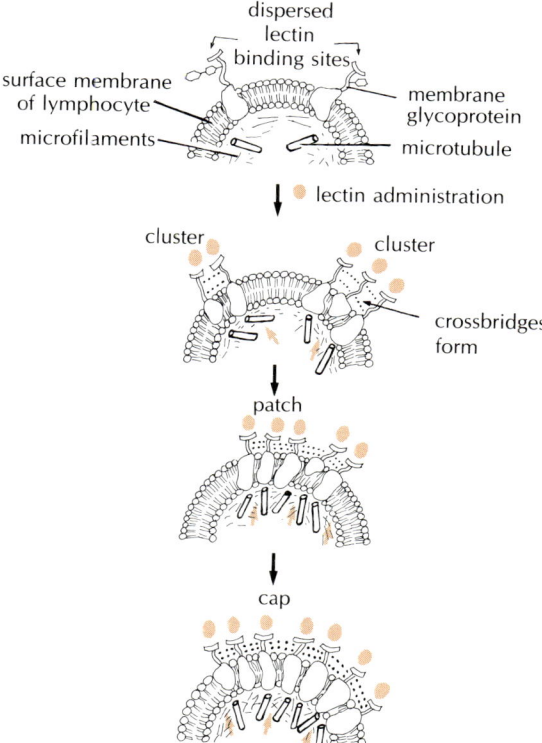

Figure 6–61. The lymphocyte phenomenon of "capping" is based on microtubule-mediated movement of cell surface lectin binding sites. With lectin administration, clusters, patches, and caps form through microtubule-directed surface changes. The process is inhibited by colchicine, an inhibitor of microtubules.

Colchicine. Incubation of a solution containing tubulin with tritium-labeled colchicine results in noncovalent colchicine binding at a protein interaction site on tubulin. Two mechanisms of microtubule disruption are postulated. Colchicine could attach to each tubulin dimer directly, thereby causing tubulin to dissociate. More likely, colchicine *binds to soluble tubulin* and *prevents* the assembly of microtubules.[254] Microtubule-dependent functions such as capping (Fig. 6–61) are inhibited by colchicine.

Podophyllotoxin. This agent binds to the same tubulin site as does colchicine. Their mechanisms of binding are different, however.[255]

Steganacin. This newly isolated antitumor agent also functions at the microtubule level. It inhibits the polymerization of tubulin and causes the slow depolymerization of preformed microtubules.[256]

Vinca Alkaloids. Tubulin binding sites of both high and low affinity have been postulated for the vinca alkaloids. Binding to the high-affinity sites on tubulin, and preventing its polymerization, may induce the formation of tubulin dimers (6S tubulin). The microtubules disappear, and crystals of protein composed of tubulin complexed to vinblastine appear. Like colchicine, the vinca alkaloids disrupt microtubules by preventing tubulin assembly, rather than by disrupting preformed microtubules. Lithium and Mg^{++} protect against the depolymerizing effects of colchicine or vinblastine and promote polymerization of tubulin.

Many spindle poisons have other actions. Both vinblastine and colchicine inhibit lymphocyte mitogenesis induced by Con A and PHA.[257] Many cells treated with these agents lose normal cell functions, become rounder, and sometimes lose cytoplasmic processes.[258] Locomotion, phagocytosis, cytoplasmic streaming, and transport[259] are defective, as are many secretory activities of cells.[254]

Toxic Drugs Affecting Microfilaments: Cytochalasin. *Cytochalasin B,* an antibiotic produced by molds, causes the disappearance of *"cables"* or *"stress fibers"* composed of actin, myosin, tropomyosin, and actinin. Cytochalasin A breaks these cables into actin-containing, rod-like structures that have been postulated to be subunits of the original microfilamentous bundles.[260] The actin-like material becomes rearranged into dense, star-like aggregates of filamentous material.

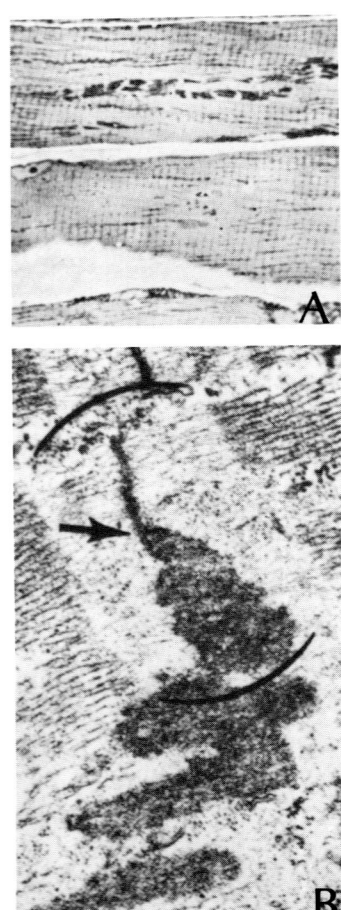

Figure 6–62. Nemaline myopathy. *A,* Phase micrograph of muscle fiber shows numerous rod-like structures. *B,* Electron micrograph shows myofibrillary destruction with accumulation of excessive Z-band material at arrow.

Administration of cytochalasin B also reversibly inhibits the mobility of sperm by decreasing the frequency of flagellar contraction. The disruption of the actin filaments associated with the plasma membrane interferes with normal membrane function.[261] Cytochalasin D causes zeiotic blebs on the surfaces of cells secondary to altered cellular microfilament function.[262]

Toxic Drugs Affecting Myofibrils. Severe myopathies may be associated with the administration of certain drugs. *Nemaline,* an anesthetic, is associated with marked myofibrillar degeneration and fragmentation (Fig. 6–62). Abnormal Z-band configurations are present, and myofilaments are inserted into the wrong Z band.[263] Actin filaments constitute the backbone of the characteristic nemaline myopathy rods.[264]

Isoproterenol causes myofilament fragmentation and contraction band formation. *Chloroquine* causes progressive proximal muscle weakness and a reversible granulovesicular myopathy.[265]

Cardiomyopathies have been described following the administration of the antineoplastic antibiotics *daunomycin and doxorubicin (Adriamycin)*. They are characteristically associated with dose-related myofiber degeneration, necrosis, and myocytolysis.[266]

The contractility of myofibrils can be stimulated by *cAMP* through augmented membrane phosphorylation. *Catecholamines* also augment contractility by first increasing levels of cAMP.[267]

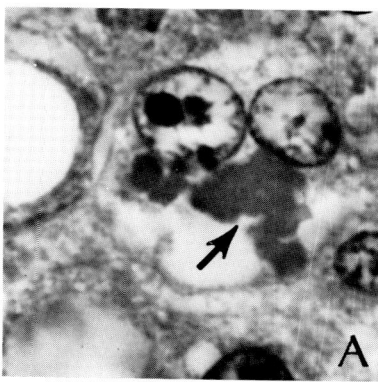

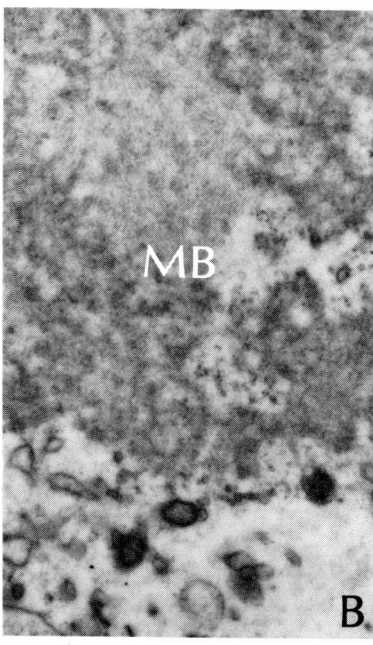

Figure 6–63. Mallory body. *A,* Light micrograph of an hepatocyte with a large, irregular Mallory body (arrow). *B,* Electron micrograph of part of a Mallory body (MB) shows its fibrillar nature.

Drugs Affecting Microfilaments and Microtubules

Alcohol. Numerous reports have shown that *Mallory bodies* (alcoholic hyalin) consist of *filaments* ranging between 5.5 and 20 μ in diameter. Antiactin antibodies bind to alcoholic hyalin. Other cellular microfilaments and intermediate filaments may be directly contiguous with the Mallory body filaments[268] (Fig. 6–63). The abnormalities in the filaments in patients with alcoholic liver disease are not confined to cells containing Mallory bodies. Cells lacking alcoholic hyalin have prominent bundles of filaments in the cytoplasm, many of which are attached to the *desmosomes* of these cells. Microtubules are also increased in number, but do not appear to be the predominant component.[269] Alcohol may also have a directly toxic effect on muscles that leads to a severe myopathy.

Griseofulvin and Phalloidin. Long-term administration of these agents experimentally produces intermediate filament hyperplasia and Mallory bodies. Mallory bodies induced in this way do not contain microfilaments, as evidenced by lack of binding by antiactin antibodies or heavy meromyosin.[270]

Hormones. Cyclic variation in the number of ciliated cells is seen in the fallopian tube and endometrium. *Ciliated cells* increase during the proliferative phase of the menstrual cycle and are prominent in states of unopposed estrogen and in estrogen-dependent lesions such as *cystic glandular* and *adenomatous hyperplasia.* Furthermore, ciliogenesis can be induced by exogenous estrogens.[271] *Tubulin synthesis* may also be under hormonal control because the amount of myometrial tubulin is increased tenfold in the preimplantation stage of pregnancy.

Role of Microtubules and Microfilaments in Inflammatory and Immune Responses

At high concentrations, *cytochalasin B*[272] suppresses leukocyte phagocytosis, exocytosis, and chemotaxis,[215] whereas in lower concentrations, it stimulates the same processes. Both cytochalasin and colchicine bind to the plasma membrane: colchicine alters membrane structure, whereas cytochalasin B inhibits membrane transport and suppresses glycolysis.

Phagocytosis. Resting cells have few assembled microtubules, but phagocytosis induces a cycle of rapid assembly and disassembly. Assembly is initiated by particle contact with the membrane and is maximal after a few minutes of phagocytosis.[216]

Phagosomes, like secretory vacuoles, are moved through the cell by microtubules. Antitubulins inhibit both the chemotactic movement of polymorphonuclear leukocytes (PMN) and the release of chemotactic factors from leukocytes.[273] Similarly, agents that inhibit microfilament function, such as cytochalasin B, inhibit the phagocytic responses of inflammatory cells.[274] It is interesting that the doses of cytochalasin B that inhibit phagocytosis in macrophages do not inhibit pinocytosis.[275]

Chédiak-Higashi Disease. In this disease, *impaired bacteriocidal* activity occurs, apparently related to *delayed fusion* of lysosomes with the phagosome. Delayed fusion is probably secondarily related to malfunctions in microtubular assembly. Degranulation of phagocytes is regulated by the microtubules, which are, in turn, regulated by cyclic nucleotides. Cyclic GMP increases microtubular function, whereas cAMP inhibits microtubular assembly.[276]

Movement of Cells, Chemotaxis, and Migration. The *motile activity* of cells depends upon the cytoplasmic contractile systems, including both *microtubules* and *microfilaments*. When either of these structures is disrupted with drugs, not only are the intracellular motile events disturbed, but also the locomotion of the cell itself. When both microtubular and microfilament systems are disrupted simultaneously by the use of cytochalasin B and colchicine, however, some cells, including macrophages, do not become totally motionless. Rather, they exhibit a special form of surface motion known as *zeiosis (blebbing)*. Ultrastructurally, the zeiotic blebs are free of organized contractile structures.[262]

Granulation Tissue and Repair. One of the interesting facets of the inflammatory response and the subsequent formation of granulation tissue is the adaptive development of contractile capabilities of fibroblasts. These cells, termed *myofibroblasts*, progressively develop thick bundles of fibrils containing actin and myosin and are believed to play an important role in connective tissue contraction and wound healing.[277] Another cell type with adaptive contractile function, the *myointimal* cell, is derived from myoblasts. These cells migrate into the intima in atherosclerosis, in which they synthesize collagen as well as participate in the organization of thrombi.

Cytotoxic Reactions and Grafts

The interaction between sensitized lymphocytes and antigen-bearing target graft or tumor cells is manifested by the adherence of *lymphocytes* to *target cells*. This attachment appears to be by pseudopodia, and microfilaments are frequently present near the areas of cellular contact of target cells by lymphocytes. Altered-cell antigen may be presented because of impaired membrane modulation, altered cellular motility, or altered cytoplasmic streaming.

Heart: Myocardial Infarction. Anticardiac muscle myofibrillar or sarcolemmal *antibodies* are demonstrated in 1 to 2% of patients with acute *myocardial infarctions*. These antibodies also appear following heart operations in 53% of those patients who had no antibodies before operation.[238]

Liver: Chronic Active Hepatitis. *Antimyosin antibodies* are frequently present in a variety of liver diseases that are thought to be immunologically perpetuated. These antibodies were first found in patients with *chronic active hepatitis* (CAH). Sera from patients with CAH selectively binds to the Z bands of isolated skeletal muscle fibers. The reactivity is absorbed with purified skeletal muscle actin, tropomyosin complex, purified troponin, or purified tropomyosin.[278]

Sera from CAH patients also reacts with smooth muscle, thymic, myoepithelial, and parietal cells, with hepatocytes, and with fibrils of cells in the renal tubules. The reactivity is removed by absorption with actin, but not with myosin, tropomyosin, or troponin.

Anti-smooth-muscle antibodies have been demonstrated in heroin addicts.[279] Another cytoskeletal abnormality in such patients is the presence of abnormal parallel tubular arrays, which have been identified in peripheral blood lymphocytes in the pericentriolar and peri-Golgi regions. These arrays contain tubules that are slightly larger than the usual microtubules.

Central Nervous System: Multiple Sclerosis. *Smooth-muscle antibodies* are present in the serum and cerebrospinal fluid (CSF) of patients with *multiple sclerosis* and chronic *lymphocytic meningoencephalitis*. That the CSF antibody levels are two to four times higher than serum levels suggests local antibody synthesis or concentration within the CNS.[280]

ANNULATE LAMELLAE

Morphology

Annulate lamellae were discovered in 1952. This structure, which consists of an array of double membrane sheets, is usually seen in the cytoplasm and occasionally in the nucleus. Annulate lamellae are most commonly seen in the cytoplasm of human oocytes and spermatocytes, but they have also been identified in both normal and neoplastic somatic cells.

Annulate lamellae appear as rows of vesicles, the number of lamellae arranged in a single stack being variable. Rarely, only a single lamella, known as a single cytoplasmic pore, is present; occasionally, clusters of 50 to 100 lamellae may be seen. Most commonly, 2 to 12 lamellae are present. Each individual lamella consists of 2 parallel membranes interrupted by pores or discontinuities that are indistinguishable from the nuclear pore complex.

Once annulate lamellae have formed and are no longer useful to the cell, they are degraded, perhaps in residual bodies. This process must occur during the cell cycle, for annulate lamellae are present in reduced numbers at the time of mitosis.[281]

Biogenesis

A number of theories regarding the biogenesis of this organelle have been advanced. In human cells, the annulate lamellae appear to arise from the nuclear envelope. Maul, however, cites evidence in human melanoma cells that the annulate lamellae represent transformed, fenestrated cisternae of Golgi apparatus.[282] It has also been suggested that annulate lamellae may be an intermediate stage in the formation of more typical ER.

Function

Intranuclear annulate lamellae are usually present at the periphery of the nuclei, and some communication exists with the internal nuclear envelope and nucleolus. Electron-dense granules, sensitive to ribonuclease digestion and associated with nucleoli, have been seen at the periphery of the annulate lamellae and measure 150 Å.

The cisternae of the annulate lamellae are continuous with the perinuclear space, which is known to communicate with the ER. Annulate lamellae may, therefore, transfer information from the nucleolus to the cytoplasm or vice versa. The majority of evidence indicates that the major function of this transitory organelle is related to protein synthesis and that some forms can be converted to RER if necessary.

Another role postulated for intranuclear annulate lamellae has been initiation of DNA synthesis and RNA transcription, especially since chromatin appears to be attached to both sides of the annulate lamellae. In early prophase, the chromatin starts to condense near the pores of the intranuclear annulate lamellae, and there appear to be sites where the replicated chromatin preferentially attaches.

Vinblastine increases the number of annulate lamellae.[283] These structures can also be induced in cells treated with other antimetabolites and metabolic inhibitors and are seen in some virus-infected cells. Finally, annulate lamellae are seen in human tumor cells including pituitary adenomas, leiomyomas, leiomyosarcomas, rhabdomyosarcomas, and malignant melanomas.[284] This finding is not surprising because neoplasms are rapidly proliferating tissues, where annulate lamellae are more likely to be found.

MITOCHONDRIA

General Characteristics

Origin

The term *mitochondrion* is derived from the Greek *"mitos,"* a *thread,* and *"chondros,"* a *grain.* Mitochondria are present

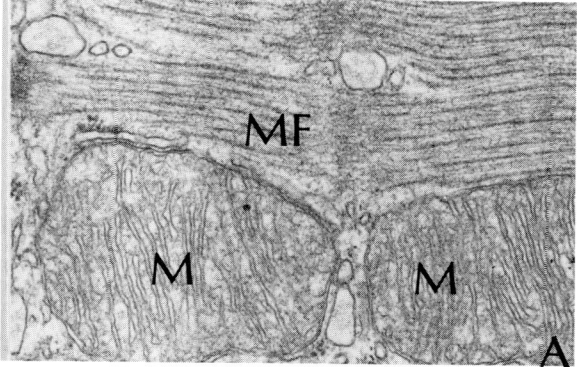

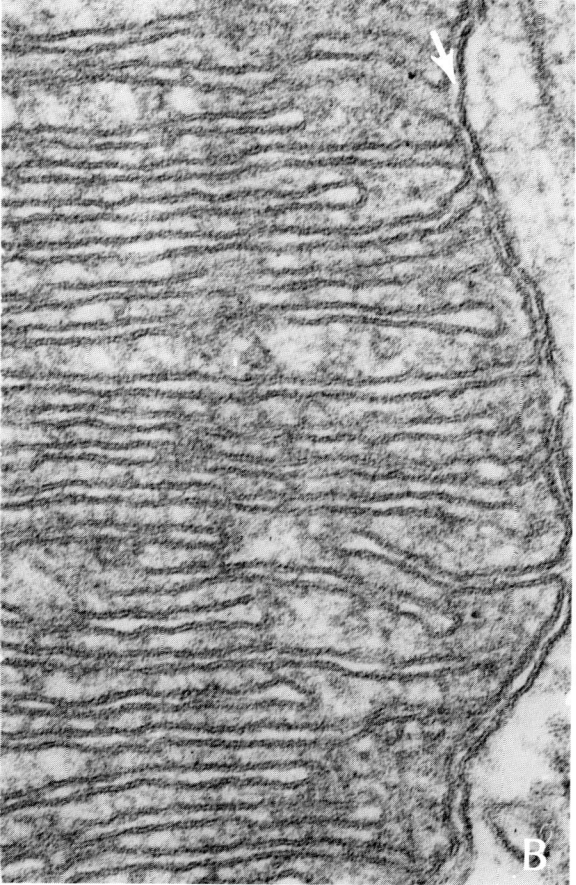

Figure 6–64. Mitochondria. *A,* Portion of cardiac muscle showing myofibrils (MF) adjacent to mitochondria (M). *B,* The continuity of the inner mitochondrial membrane with the cristae (arrows) is evident.

in all animal cells. These cellular organelles are the chief energy sources of the cell and are the major site of cellular respiration. Over 90% of total body oxygen is consumed within mitochondria.

Two suggestions have been made as to the *origin* of mitochondria: they arose (1) from compartmentalization of nuclear DNA within the cytoplasm or (2) from free-living forms that established a symbiotic relationship with host cells.[285] The second theory is most favored principally because of a distinct difference in base ratios between mitochondrial and nuclear DNA.

Mitochondria have a *half-life* of between 7 and 13 days, depending upon species type. They vary in number, size, shape, and distribution in different mammalian cells, but they *number* approximately *2000* in human liver cells and represent approximately 22% of the cytoplasmic volume. The position of mitochondria in the cell is often determined by the functional characteristics of the cell. In the *renal tubular* epithelial cell, mitochondria are found in the *basal portion* near the site of active transport.[286] In *muscle,* they are *near myofibrils* that require generation of ATP for contraction. In nerve cells, mitochondria *travel,* and their ultimate location depends upon the functional energy requirement of microtubules.[287]

Size and Shape

Classically, the mitochondrion has been described as a *rod-* or *sphere-shaped* structure (Fig. 6–64). This concept is being challenged by electron-micrographic serial sections and reconstruction techniques, however. Some models have shown a branching tubular network of large mitochondria that are present in smaller numbers than usual.[288]

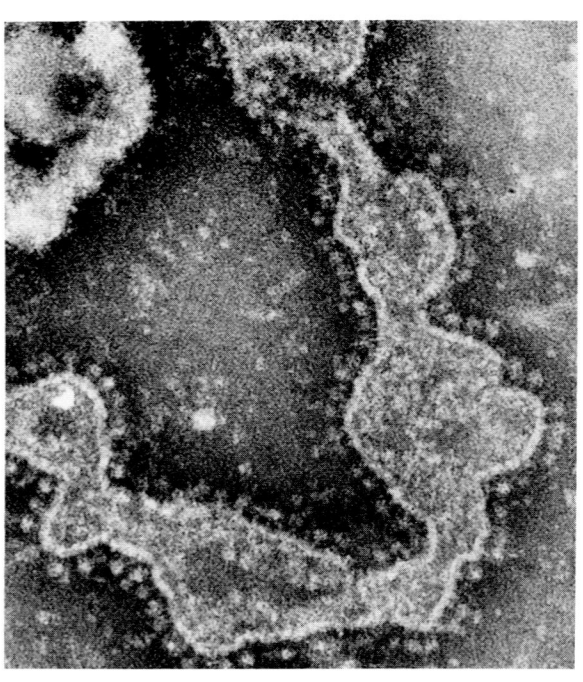

Figure 6–65. Negatively stained mitochondrion from liver showing granules called elementary particles.

The size, shape, and location of mitochondria may differ from tissue to tissue, but their basic architecture remains the same. Tight infolding of the inner membrane cristae increases the surface area where the enzymes of oxidative phosphorylation are located (Fig. 6–65). It is interesting that mitochondrial structure changes in animals whose metabolic rate fluctuates with the seasons. Frog kidney mitochondria have few cristae during the winter, whereas in the summertime, the cristae are increased in number and are tightly packed.

Dramatic changes in number of mitochondria occur throughout the cell cycle. As the cell divides, the number of mitochondria is halved. During the G_1-S transition, mitochondrial *fission* again increases the number.[289] Mitochondria are degraded by lysosomes in a manner similar to other organelles. In addition, the presence of a protease on the inner mitochondrial membrane suggests that this enzyme may participate in mitochondrial membrane hydrolysis.

DNA, RNA, and Proteins

The *DNA* of mitochondria has a circular form,[290] is not associated with histones, has a nucleic acid base ratio separate and distinct from the nuclear DNA, and appears to be attached to the inner mitochondrial membrane.[291] Unlike nuclear DNA, mitochondrial DNA replication occurs throughout the cell cycle.[292] Mitochondrial RNA and protein synthesis take place slightly after cellular DNA synthesis.[293]

The DNA is capable of transcribing tRNA, mRNA, and rRNA. Mitochondrial tRNA has an unusual distribution of methylated nucleosides, in comparison to other cellular tRNA.[294] Mitochondrial ribosomes *(mitoribosomes)* appear to be similar to the ribosomes of bacteria; that is, they have 55 to 70S rather than the 80S cytoplasmic ribosomal particles characteristic of mammalian cells.[295]

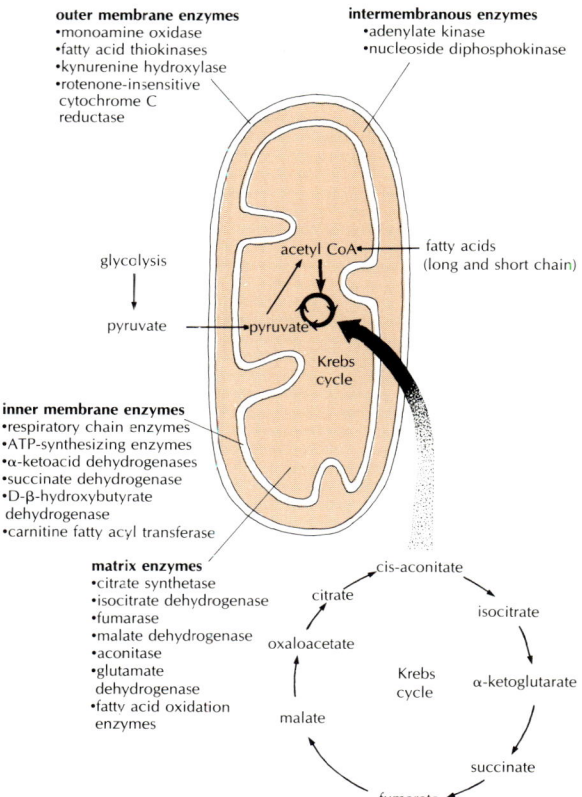

outer membrane enzymes
•monoamine oxidase
•fatty acid thiokinases
•kynurenine hydroxylase
•rotenone-insensitive
cytochrome C
reductase

intermembranous enzymes
•adenylate kinase
•nucleoside diphosphokinase

glycolysis

pyruvate

acetyl CoA•

fatty acids
(long and short chain)

pyruvate

Krebs
cycle

inner membrane enzymes
•respiratory chain enzymes
•ATP-synthesizing enzymes
•α-ketoacid dehydrogenases
•succinate dehydrogenase
•D-β-hydroxybutyrate
dehydrogenase
•carnitine fatty acyl transferase

matrix enzymes
•citrate synthetase
•isocitrate dehydrogenase
•fumarase
•malate dehydrogenase
•aconitase
•glutamate
dehydrogenase
•fatty acid oxidation
enzymes

cis-aconitate

citrate

isocitrate

oxaloacetate

Krebs
cycle

α-ketoglutarate

malate

succinate

fumarate

Figure 6–66. Mitochondrial enzyme distribution.

Although mitochondrial *DNA* may *code* for as many as *50 proteins*, most of the mitochondrial proteins are synthesized in the cytoplasm. These include the proteins of the inner membranes, functional proteins including cytochrome C, and proteins used in replication, transport, and electron transfer[296] (Table 6–31 and Fig. 6–66).

Table 6–31. *Location of Mitochondrial Enzymes*

Outer membrane
  Monoamine oxidase
  Fatty acid thiokinases
  Kynurenine hydroxylase

Space between membranes
  Adenylate kinase
  Nucleoside diphosphokinase

Inner membrane
  Respiratory chain enzymes
  ATP-synthesizing enzymes
  α-Ketoacid dehydrogenases
  Succinate dehydrogenase
  D-β-Hydroxybutyrate dehydrogenase

Matrix
  Citrate synthase
  Isocitrate dehydrogenase
  Fumarase
  Malate dehydrogenase
  Aconitase
  Glutamate dehydrogenase
  Fatty acid oxidation enzymes

(Modified from Lehninger, A.L.: Biochemistry. 2nd Ed. New York, Worth Publishers, 1975.)

Structure

Outer Membrane

Mitochondria have a double membrane encircling the matrix. The outer membrane is 70 Å thick and contains fatty-acid-activating enzymes and monoamine oxidase. The external membrane can be removed, leaving an inner membranous structure, *the mitoplast*. This external membrane has a lattice structure and is responsible for maintaining the shape of the organelle; the inner membrane has more flexibility and allows the cristae to expand and contract.

Inner Membrane

The inner membrane contains enzymes involved in *respiration, oxidative phosphorylation, electron transport,* and *ATP synthesis*.

Approximately 20 to 25% of the total mitochondrial proteins are present on the inner membrane. One of these proteins is found in spherical, electron-dense granules or knobs called *elementary particles* or intramembrane spheres.

These particles cover the inner surface of the membrane and are connected to it by narrow stalks. They are believed to be the F_1 *coupling factor* necessary for oxidative phosphorylation (Fig. 6–65).

It has been suggested that the architecture of the inner membrane is designed so that the respiratory components are arranged in self-contained loops as units for respiratory assemblies. According to this scheme, cytochrome C is midway on the respiratory chain, forms the back of the loop, and is located on the outer surface of the inner membrane. Succinic dehydrogenase, which is the point of entry from the Krebs cycle, is on the inner surface, as is cytochrome A3. The reactions in oxidative phosphorylation take place at three different locations on the electron-transport chain.

Matrix Proteins

The *matrix* contains proteins, lipids, *enzymes* of the *Krebs cycle*, pools of *nucleotides* (ADP and ATP), and various *coenzymes* (NAD, NADP, and coenzyme A [CoA]). Mitochondria are permeable to water, ions, urea, glycerol, and short-chain fatty acids, but all lipids are synthesized outside the mitochondria. An intimate relationship exists between the inner membrane and the matrix. The intracristal space contains a series of channels that allow metabolic substrates free and rapid access to and from the inner membrane.[297]

Function

Genes

Mitochondrial DNA is divided into two groups of genes: *MIT* and *SYN* (Fig. 6–67). The MIT group codes for four protein products with respiratory activity, and the SYN group codes for mitochondrial rRNA and tRNA. These two systems are quite distinct from one another. They are physically separated, but do appear to share some components. The enzymatic proteins, polymerase and ligases, which function in replication, transcription, and translation, are encoded in the nucleus.[298]

The DNA genome of the nucleus and the DNA of the mitochondria have different base ratios. No evidence suggests that mRNA transcribed on the mitochondrial DNA is translated by cytoplasmic ribosomes; conversely, DNA from the nucleus is probably not translated on mitochondrial mitoribosomes. It is not known how these two genetic systems are coordinated in vivo.

Synthesis, Assembly, and Transport of Proteins

Mitochondrial proteins appear to have a dual origin and are formed as the result of the close cooperation of two genetic systems. One of these is the conventional nuclear-

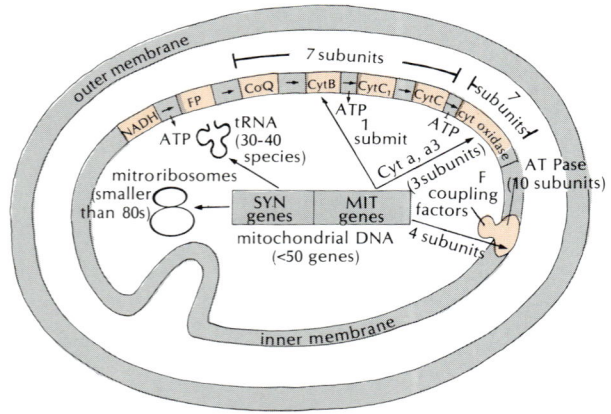

Figure 6–67. Schematic diagram of mitochondrial respiratory chain protein synthesis. The fewer than 50 mitochondrial genes are divided into SYN and MIT subgroups. SYN genes code for mitochondrial ribosomes and tRNA involved in protein synthesis. MIT genes code for inner membrane proteins involved in respiratory activity. Certain subunits of the respiratory chain proteins are known to be synthesized in the cytoplasm.

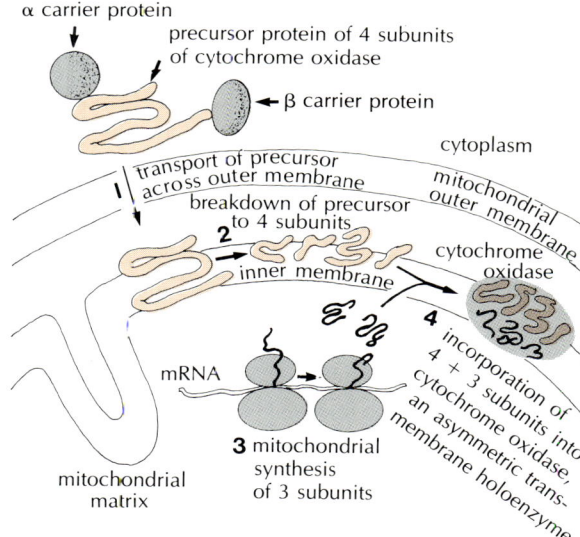

α carrier protein

precursor protein of 4 subunits of cytochrome oxidase

β carrier protein

cytoplasm

transport of precursor across outer membrane

mitochondrial outer membrane

breakdown of precursor to 4 subunits

2

inner membrane

cytochrome oxidase

4

4 + 3 subunits into cytochrome oxidase, an asymmetric trans-membrane holoenzyme

incorporation of

mRNA

3 mitochondrial synthesis of 3 subunits

mitochondrial matrix

Figure 6–68. Mitochondrial and cytoplasmic synthesis of cytochrome oxidase.

cytoplasmic system, involving nuclear DNA and the protein-synthesizing ribosomal apparatus of the extramitochondrial cytoplasm. The other system is located within the mitochondria and consists of their small amount of DNA and accompanying transcription and translation machinery.

It is believed that the mitochondria produce only about 5 to 15% of the mitochondrial protein mass; yet, these proteins are indispensable for the assembly of an intact, functional mitochondrion.[299] Mitochondria probably synthesize no more than a dozen hydrophobic polypeptides; three of these are associated with *cytochrome oxidase*, four with an *ATPase*, and one with *cytochrome B*. Detailed studies of cytochrome oxidase have shown that this enzyme consists of seven subunits. Three of these are made in mitochondria, and four are synthesized in the cytoplasm (Fig. 6–68).

One of the problems that continues to plague investigators is the means of transport of proteins synthesized in the ER from the ER to the mitochondria. In isolated yeast, mitochondrial membranes are closely bound to cytoplasmic ribosomes. It has been suggested that the mitochondrial proteins synthesized in the cytoplasm are synthesized by a special class of ribosomes located on the mitochondrial surfaces. Newly synthesized polypeptides could then be discharged across the mitochondrial membranes; this process is analogous to the transport occurring during synthesis in certain regions of the ER.[293]

Ion Transport

Mitochondria have *specific transport mechanisms* for sodium, potassium, magnesium, chloride, and bromide ions. Ion transport is respiration-dependent, and respiration is accentuated by Ca^{++}, Mn^{++}, and Sr^{++}. The membrane also transfers nitrous oxide, small substrates such as sugars and amino acids, and particular cofactors, for example, NAD, NADP, NADPH, ADP, ATP, and CoA esters.

Calcium readily accumulates in mitochondria and represents an internal reserve pool for the cell. Mitochondrial calcium ions may be concentrated up to 200 times the cellular calcium level by a specific calcium system that has both low- and high-affinity binding sites.

Calcium may precipitate as calcium phosphate hydroxyapatite, the presence of which inhibits oxidative phosphorylation. Calcium transport is inhibited experimentally by 2,4-DNP and cyanide.[300]

Metabolism and Respiration

Normally, a six-carbon glucose molecule is broken into a three-carbon pyruvate molecule by glycolysis in the cytosol. Pyruvate is converted to lactate or lactic acid, or it is oxidized to CO_2 and water by the Krebs cycle enzymes.

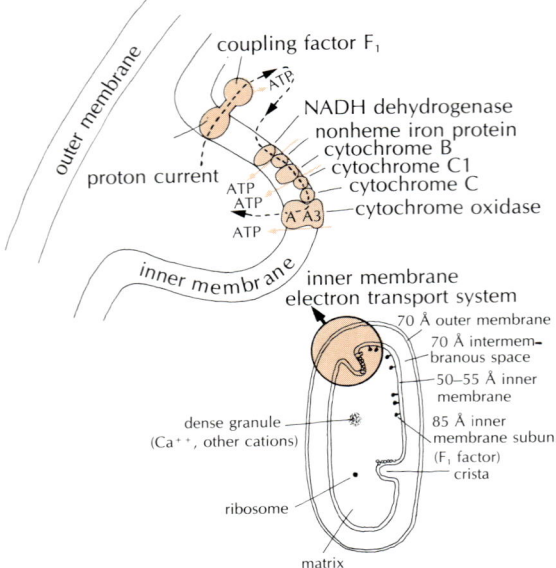

Figure 6–69. In the chemiosmotic hypothesis of oxidative phosphorylation, protons (H⁺) are transported between the matrix and the intermembranous space, giving rise to a membrane potential. The F₁ proton pump ensures continuity of the system. ATP is generated by the proton pump and along the respiratory chain at points indicated by arrows. (Modified from Racker, E.: Inner mitochondrial membranes: basic and applied aspects. *In* Cell Membranes: Biochemistry, Cell Biology, and Pathology. Edited by G. Weissmann and R. Claiborne. New York, HP Publishing, 1975.)

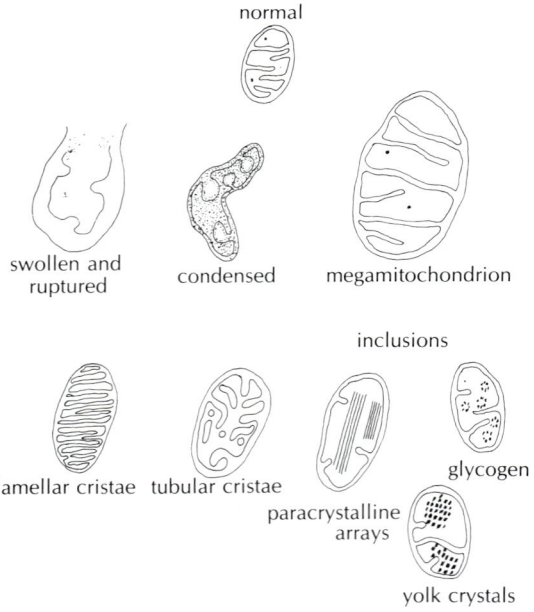

Figure 6–70. Variations in mitochondrial morphology.

Substrates of the Krebs cycle are oxidized at four points in mitochondria: (1) isocitrate, (2) alpha-ketoglutarate, (3) malate, and (4) succinate.

Hydrogen ions are released and transferred first to NAD and second to NADH; then they are released free in the medium or transferred to flavin adenine dinucleotide (FAD), producing $FADH_2$. Reduced NADH, $FADH_2$, and reduced coenzyme Q transfer electrons through various cytochromes and finally react with O_2 to form water. In liver cells, for example, over 20,000 such complete respiratory assemblies are found.

Oxidative Phosphorylation

The coupling of oxidative phosphorylation with the respiratory process provides the main source of energy for the cell. A total of 16 ATP molecules is produced for each molecule of pyruvate oxidized to CO_2 and water. Glycolysis produces 4 ATP molecules per mole of glucose, but 2 are used, leaving a net of 2. Respiration produces 32 ATP molecules per 2 moles of pyruvate, and a total of 36 ATP molecules per mole of glucose is obtained by the cell.

Mitchell[301] described the *chemiosmotic theory*, which defines the major pathway of oxidative phosphorylation (Fig. 6–69). In this scheme, mitochondrial charge plays a direct role. The inner membrane is impermeable to hydrogen ions that transport electrons along the carriers of the respiration chain. This impermeability generates a hydrogen gradient across the membrane that is a form of high energy leading to ATP synthesis.

The *ATP* produced by mitochondria is used as energy for transhydrogenation, transport, synthesis, secretion, absorption, and many other cellular functions. The ATP carrier, adenine nucleotide transferase, present on the inner membrane of the mitochondria, binds ATP and ADP and transfers ATP to the cytosol and ADP into mitochondria.

General Effects of Injury

Morphology

The general structural manifestations of mitochondrial injury include *swelling, contraction*, the formation of different and *unusual structural forms*, and the presence of *inclusions* (Fig. 6–70). One of the problems in evaluating mitochondrial injury is the presence of an innately heterogeneous population. Three-dimensional structural reconstruction studies on normal rat hepatocytes have shown two morphologic types of mitochondria, one rod-shaped and the other V-shaped.[302] These and other intermediate forms may be confused with mitochondria seen in injurious states.

Membrane Permeability

A sensitive index of injury is the permeability of the mitochondrial membrane. The intact inner mitochondrial membrane limits the rate at which nitroblue-tetrazolium and phenazine methosulfate can reach succinate dehydrogenase. Injured mitochondria allow these reagents to reach the enzyme more rapidly, to form microscopically observable formazan granules.[303]

Shrinkage and Swelling

Mitochondria undergo *contraction* and shrinkage with condensation of matrix proteins before swelling becomes irreversible.[304] One must distinguish the increased swelling associated with terminal, irreversible, and end-stage dissolution from the earlier, low-amplitude swelling associated with reversible damage.

Swelling (Fig. 6–70) is brought about either passively by a change in osmolarity or actively as a result of a deficient electron transport system. Large-amplitude swelling occurs as the result of the failure of respiratory ATP-dependent mechanisms and has been called "energized swelling." It involves an influx of salts and water into the inner mitochondrial membrane. This lesion is initially reversible by ATP, but the swollen mitochondria are incapable of oxidative phosphorylation.[305]

Large-amplitude swelling may be induced by calcium phosphate, hormones, CCl_4, Clostridium perfringens exotoxin, and cholera exotoxin. It has also been seen in hypoxia, starvation, and infection. As water enters the cell, mitochondrial membranes stretch and become distended; the outer membrane eventually ruptures.

Hypertrophy, Megamitochondria, and Abnormal Forms

Mitochondria can undergo *hypertrophy,* and this phenomenon is seen in cardiac muscle fibers before hypertrophy of myofibrils takes place. Mitochondrial hypertrophy is also prominent following digoxin and thyroxine administration. In salivary gland oncocytes, mitochondria appear hyperplastic and are increased in number.[306] Giant *megamitochondria* have been noted in the adrenal following hypersecretion and in protein or nutritional deficiency, chronic alcoholism, obstructive jaundice, myeloid leuke-

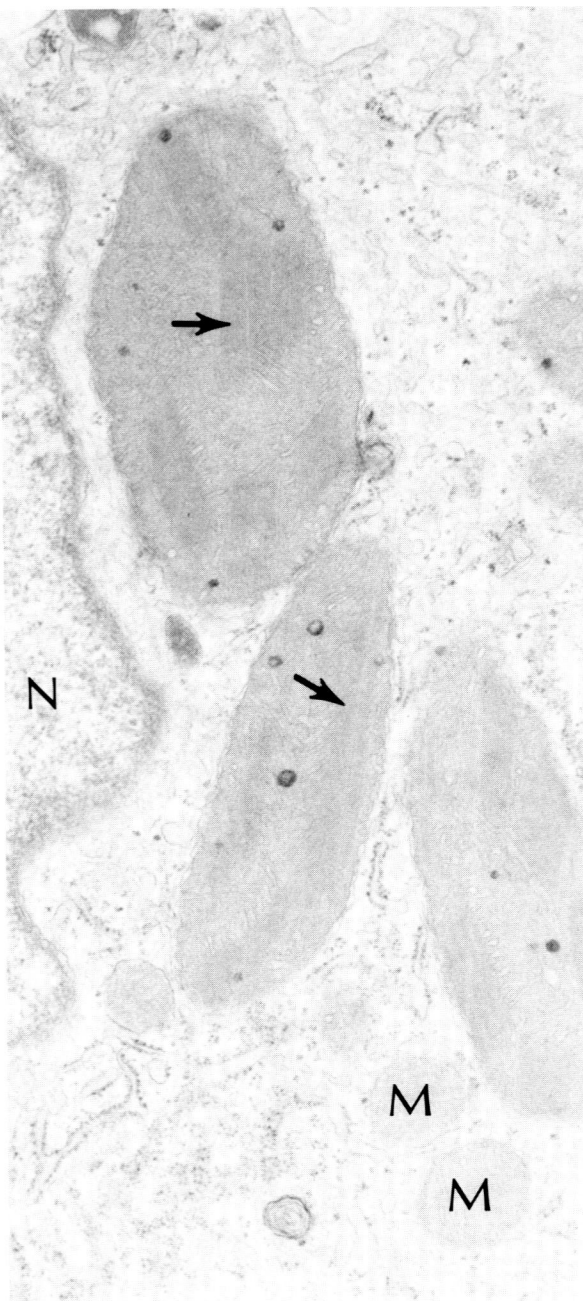

Figure 6–71. Megamitochondria are seen in this liver specimen from an alcoholic patient. They begin to aproach the size of the nucleus (N) and are dramatically enlarged when compared to several nearby normal-sized mitochondria (M). Unusual paracrystalline arrays (arrows) are also seen within the megamitochondria.

Table 6–32. *Examples of Diseases Associated with Megamitochondria*

Agents or Conditions	Disease	Tissue
Physical pressure	Obstructive jaundice	Liver
Nutritional imbalance	Starvation	Liver
	Riboflavin deficiency	Liver
Viral infections	Reye's syndrome	Liver
Drugs	Alcoholic hepatitis	Liver
Hormones	Hyperadrenalism	Adrenal
Neoplasia	Erythroleukemia	Bone marrow
	Myeloid leukemia	Bone marrow
	Oncocytoma	Salivary gland
	Pheochromocytoma	Adrenal

mia, erythroleukemia, Reye's syndrome, and extra-adrenal pheochromocytoma (Table 6–32 and Fig. 6–71).

A large group of distinctive *abnormal* mitochondrial *cristae* has been described (see Fig. 6–70).

Inclusions

Examples of mitochondrial *inclusions* are iron in sideroblastic anemia, glycogen in glycogen storage diseases, lipids, and protein crystals. Hepatic intramitochondrial crystalloid inclusions have been demonstrated in three previously unreported entities: anicteric hepatitis, type 1 lipoproteinemia, and exogenous obesity with latent diabetes mellitus.

Mitochondria with dense calcium salt granules may be seen in osteocytes, osteoblasts, and osteoclasts. *Calcium phosphate precipitates* are an early sign of mitochondrial injury.

Specific Agents of Injury

Genetic Agents

Congenital Mitochondrial Myopathies. In several of the many diseases that may have abnormal mitochondria, clinical features reflect primary mitochondrial functional alterations. The concept of *genetic mitochondrial myopathies* was introduced in 1959 by Luft, who described a rare skeletal-muscle disorder *(Luft's syndrome)* with enlarged mitochondria, excessive respiration, uncoupled oxidative phosphorylation, and nonthyroidal hypermetabolism.[307] Large collections of abnormal, oversized mitochondria with tightly packed cristae and crystalline inclusions were seen in muscle cells. Chloramphenicol, which may depress protein synthesis in abnormal mitochondria, has been beneficial in a patient with this syndrome.[308]

Other myopathies have been associated with mitochondrial alterations. The *cerebrohepatorenal-skeletal* syndrome is characterized by hypotonia and iron and lipid storage, and the disorder usually results in death within six months.

Mitochondria are distorted, peroxisomes are missing in renal tubules and hepatocytes, and glycogen stores are increased in the liver. Oxygen consumption of isolated brain and liver mitochondria, incubated with succinate, is decreased secondary to a defect in succinate dehydrogenase protein and coenzyme Q.[309]

These diseases represent a family of myopathies with multiple inherited metabolic defects and are manifested by symptoms associated with altered mitochondrial structure and function.[310] These disorders are sometimes diagnosed by specific histochemical (NADH) stains.

A number of encephalopathies are characterized by specific mitochondrial abnormalities (Table 6–33).

Table 6–33. *Mitochondrial Encephalomyopathies*

Disorder	Tissue Involvement
Menke's syndrome (inherited defect in copper absorption, cytochrome aa$_3$ deficiency)	Muscle neurons, liver
Leigh's disease (lactic acidemia, inhibition of TPP-ATP transferase)	Muscle
Zellweger's disease (peroxisomal defects, defect in succinate oxidation)	Astrocytes, hepatocytes, muscle
Disease described by Spiro et al. (loose coupling of oxidative phosphorylation, cytochrome b deficiency)	Muscle
Syndrome described by Tsairis et al. (lactic and pyruvic acidemia)	Muscle
Disease described by Shapira et al. (lactic and pyruvic acidemia, increased lactate to pyruvate ratio, defect in NADH oxidation)	Muscle

(Modified from Shapira, Y., Harel, S., and Russell, A.: Mitochondrial encephalomyopathies: a group of neuromuscular disorders with defects in oxidative metabolism. Isr. J. Med. Sci., *18*:162, 1977.)

Wilson's Disease. Sternlieb and Feldman[311] have described pleomorphic, vacuolated, electron-dense crystalline inclusions in the mitochondrial matrix in *Wilson's disease*. These researchers have found that the inner and outer membranes are redundant and form buds and whorls. The simultaneous occurrence of several such alterations in the same mitochondrion is believed to be pathognomonic of Wilson's disease. After three to five years of treatment with *D-penicillamine*, these alterations either became less prominent or disappeared in five out of seven patients.

Physical Agents

Hypoxia. The best-studied physical agent that damages mitochondria is *oxygen deficit*. In hypertrophied muscles, significant mitochondrial alterations have occurred either spontaneously or as a result of hypertension and oxygen deficiency.[312] Increase in mitochondrial size and number has been seen in cardiac hypertrophy associated with aortic stenosis, in patients undergoing cardiopulmonary bypass operations, and in chronic anemia and chronic hypertension.[313]

Structural mitochondrial changes associated with hypoxia are reflections, in part, of the ion and water shifts that occur among the various cellular compartments. These shifts result in profound functional changes in the mitochondrial membrane. This membrane behaves as an "osmometer," and mitochondrial swelling or contraction reflects membrane permeability to solutes. Such changes further alter ion transport and oxidative phosphorylation.

Hypoxia, with a lack of ATP, often changes the *"orthodox" standard* form of mitochondria to the *condensed form,* that is, the condensation of matrix protein and swelling of the outer membrane. This change is frequently followed by *high-amplitude swelling* and eventual rupture of the outer membrane. Fluffy deposits consisting of denatured protein, tubular forms, and calcification are end-stage mitochondrial changes. Mitochondria may be incorporated into telolysosomes as well as segregated into intracisternal channels of the ER. Both calcium and phosphorus have been demonstrated in these intramitochondrial dense deposits by x-ray microanalysis.[314,315]

Temperature. Freezing and thawing of cells is associated with structural mitochondrial alterations, a concomitant loss of oxidative capacity, and a reduction in cytochrome C oxidase activity.[316-318]

Radiation. The effect of *radiation* on mitochondrial function is different from that of the physical agents of injury previously discussed because the primary target of radiation is the *DNA,* and much of mitochondrial protein is coded for by nuclear DNA. It is known that small doses of radiation stimulate replication of DNA, division of cells, and protein synthesis. Larger doses of radiation inhibit or completely stop synthesis of DNA, RNA, and protein.[319]

Nutritional Factors

Diet affects mitochondrial structure and function. French and Todoroff noted that young male rats fed *ethanol* and *choline-deficient diets* developed *abnormal liver mitochondria,* with increased fragility, permeability, and enzyme activity.[320] If diets containing large amounts of fat are consumed, megamitochondria develop, as do intramitochondrial inclusions such as glycogen and lipid droplets.

Human fatty livers associated with alcoholism, diabetes, or obesity also contain abnormal hepatic mitochondria, including megamitochondria with paracrystalline arrays.[321]

Enlarged mitochondria have been seen with riboflavin deficiency (liver),[321] vitamin C deficiency, vitamin E deficiency, and in chronic renal disease.[322] Intramitochondrial calcification has been seen following magnesium deficiency.

Mitochondrial *iron overload* is characteristically seen in *sideroblastic anemia* associated with *pyridoxine* deficiency. Ultrastructurally, the sideroblasts have dense clumps of iron in the space between the cristae. The iron-laden mitochondria are distorted and swollen. Exposure to excessive iron levels produces peroxidation of mitochondrial membranes and mitochondrial disruption.[323]

Infectious Agents

Bacteria. These microorganisms cause mitochondrial abnormalities principally by the elaboration of toxins. Endotoxins release lysosomal phospholipase C, decrease pH, increase lactic acid, and hydrolize mitochondrial membrane lipids. Endotoxins may also uncouple oxidative phosphorylation and cause a reduction in respiratory activity that is accompanied by a complete block of ion transport. Escherichia coli endotoxin produces mitochondrial whorls, herniations, and bulges, whereas cholera exotoxin leads to large-amplitude swelling and disruption of the cristae.[305]

Viruses. *Hepatitis virus* has been associated with mitochondrial shrinkage and involution, whereas *herpesvirus* infection produces sequential swelling, first by expanding the membrane and later by swelling the matrix.[324]

Studies on other intramitochondrial viral structures indicate that these virions are similar to C-type viruses. They are synthesized in close association with the inner mitochondrial membrane, which contributes to the formation of a trilaminar viral envelope.[325]

Another interesting disease involving mitochondria is *Reye's syndrome,* a serious disease characterized by postviral encephalopathy and fatty changes in the viscera. The mortality rate is about 40%, and many of the clinical features are consistent with an abnormality of mitochondrial function. Severe morphologic abnormalities are seen in the mitochondria of the liver, brain, and skeletal muscles in such patients.[251]

Drugs, Chemicals, and Hormones

Damage to mitochondria by drugs and chemicals is classified in several general groups. There are those agents whose primary effect is to alter the inner mitochondrial membranes and to uncouple oxidative phosphorylation.[326] Another class of agents primarily interacts with mitochondrial ribonucleoproteins, and finally, some agents usually produce megamitochondria or act as ionophores (Table 6–34).

Table 6–34. *Alterations in Mitochondria Associated with Chemical Agents and Hormones*

Agent	Change
Dinitrophenol Azide Hashish Valinomycin Arsenic Cyanide Mersalyl N-ethyl-maleimide	Uncoupling of oxidative phosphorylation
Actinomycin D Cycloheximide Chloramphenicol Puromycin Ethidium bromide Doxorubicin (Adriamycin) Rifampicin	Inhibition of protein synthesis
Ionophores	Increase in mitochondrial permeability
Hormones	
Parathormone	Increase in calcium deposits
Calcitonin	Decrease in calcium deposits
Thyroxine	Increase in oxidative phosphorylation
Glucocorticoids	Defect in ability to generate ATP

Uncoupling of Oxidative Phosphorylation. When the uncouplers of oxidative phosphorylation were studied by Hanstein and Hatefi,[327] these researchers found that classic uncouplers bind to specific binding sites. All the agents listed in Table 6–34 are examples of *uncouplers* of oxidative phosphorylation, and many of them exhibit competitive binding for these sites. The lack of ATP production as the result of the action of these and other drugs results in morphologic alterations of the mitochondria, including swelling and rupture. *Valinomycin* causes a rapid potassium influx and an expanded mitochondrial matrix in liver cells.

Inhibition of Protein Synthesis. Several drugs have been associated with the *inhibition of protein synthesis*.[328] As a result of altered protein synthesis, ruptured membranes, longitudinal cristae, rings, intramatrical iron deposits, and lipid droplets are seen.[329] *Ethidium bromide* binds to the DNA (see the section of this chapter on the nucleus), and normal mitochondrial development is hampered. In addition to its action on general protein synthesis, *chloramphenicol* specifically inhibits the synthesis of the cytochromes.[330]

Ionophores. A class of agents known as *ionophores* (ionophoroproteins) or *ion-channel-forming complexes* renders the mitochondrial membrane more permeable to cations.[331]

Hormones. Mitochondrial function is altered by the hormonal environment. *Parathormone* and *calcitonin* affect *calcium* metabolism, and mitochondria are major sites of cellular calcium accumulation. The number of calcium granules is increased in osteoblasts in teeth.[332]

Abnormalities in inner mitochondrial membrane function have also been identified in hypothyroid states, characterized by decreased oxidative phosphorylation. It is postulated that a metabolic defect in unsaturated fatty acid metabolism may be partially responsible.[333] *Thyroxine* increases respiration and oxidative phosphorylation.

Glucocorticoids, when present in excess, cause a defect in the ability of mitochondria to generate ATP and to prevent accumulations of intramitochondrial Ca^{++}.[334]

Immune Agents

Primary Biliary Cirrhosis (PBC). This chronic, destructive, bile duct disorder of the liver is associated with anti-mitochondrial antibodies *(AMA)*. These antibodies are specific for this disease, although low titers of AMA have been seen in chronic hepatitis and other biliary diseases. Studies of the immune system in *PBC* have shown that immune complexes, histocompatibility antigens on bile duct epithelium, and T-cell and killer-cell function are all at work, whether in primary or secondary roles. The exact reason for the specificity of AMA for PBC, however, remains unexplained.[335]

Cellular Blastogenesis. Purified *mitochondrial membranes* obtained from a variety of diseased tissues have stimulated lymphocytes to undergo *blast transformation* in vitro. These membranes were obtained from patients with PBC, Hashimoto's thyroiditis, Addison's disease, pernicious anemia, and diabetes mellitus.

LYSOSOMES

Structure

Lysosomal bodies (Fig. 6–72), cytoplasmic membrane-bound organelles containing a variety of hydrolytic enzymes active at an acid pH, were discovered by DeDuve in 1955.[336] At present at least 40 hydrolases, virtually all glycoproteins, are known to reside in lysosomes (Table 6–35), and they function in the degradation of proteins, carbohydrates, lipids, and nucleic acids. Lysosomal hydrolases are synthesized on membrane-associated polysomes, gain access to ER cisternae, are transported to the Golgi region, and are concentrated and packaged into lysosomes in the GERL.

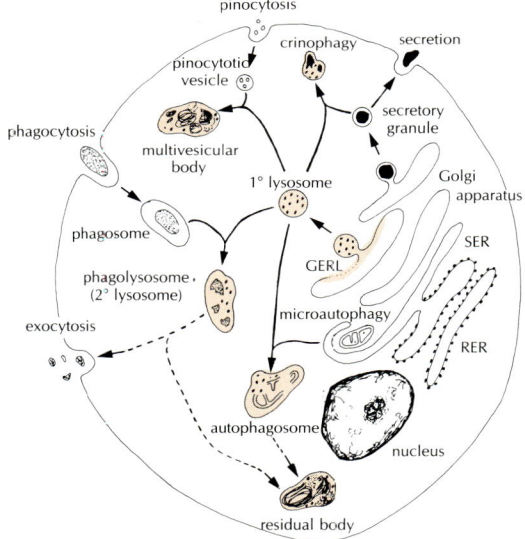

Figure 6–72. The genesis of the primary (1°) lysosome from GERL and the disposition of cellular products. Vesicles of "waste products" such as phagolysosomes and autophagosomes may ultimately come to rest near the nucleus as residual bodies. Organelle turnover by microautophagy and destruction of secretory granules by crinophagy are also shown.

Table 6–35. *Lysosomal Enzymes*

Protein Hydrolases
Cathepsins A, B, C, D, IV
Dipeptidyl aminopeptidase II
Dipeptidase

Exoglycosidases
α-Glucosidase
β-Glucosidase
β-Xylosidase
α-Galactosidase
β-Fucosidase
α-L-fucosidase
α-Mannosidase
β-Glucoromidase
α-L-Iuronidase
N-acetyl-β-hexosaminidase
N-acetyl-α-hexosaminidase
O-seryl-N-acetyl-α-galactosaminidase
Neurominidase (sialidase)

Endoglycosidases
Hyaluronidase
Lysozyme (muramidase)

Sulfatases
Arylsulfatase A
Arysulfatase B
Chondrosulfatase

Amidase
Aspartylglucosylamine
Amidohydrolase

Galactosidases
Galactocerebroside-β-galactosidase
Monosialoganglioside-β-galactosidase
Lactosylcoramide-β-galactosidase
Digalactosylglucosyl ceramide-α-galactosidase

Lipases
Acid lipase
Phosphatidate phosphatase
Phospholipase A_1 and A_2
Acid phosphatase
Sphingomyelinase
Ceramidase
Galactocerebrosidase
Glucocerebrosidase

Endonucleases: Nucleases and Nucleotidases
Acid deoxyribonuclease (deoxyribonuclease II)
Acid ribonuclease

Exonucleases
Acid exonuclease
Acid phosphodiesterase
Acid pyrophosphatase

Respiratory Burst Enzymes
Superoxide dismutase
Myeloperoxidase

Lysosomes are found in all cells, but are particularly prominent in neutrophils, eosinophils, and macrophages, both circulating monocytes and tissue histiocytes; in renal tubular cells, as hyaline droplets; in liver, as peribiliary dense bodies; in lymphoreticular cells containing hemo-

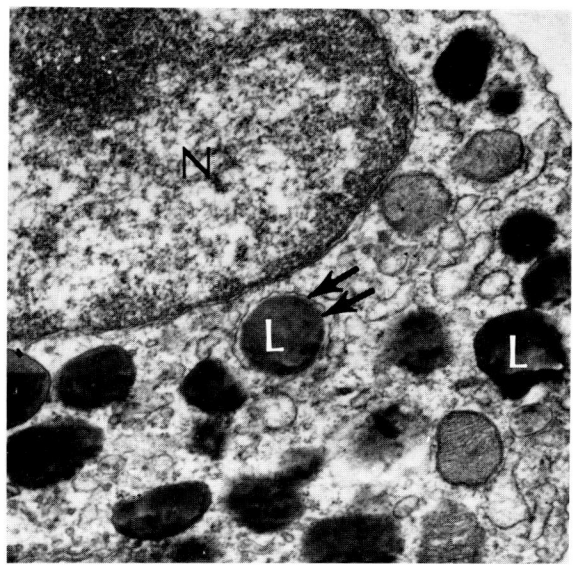

Figure 6–73. Lysosomes (L) frequently appear as electron-dense granules in the cytoplasm. Occasionally, the membrane lining these is prominent (arrows). The nucleus (N) is also present in this electron micrograph.

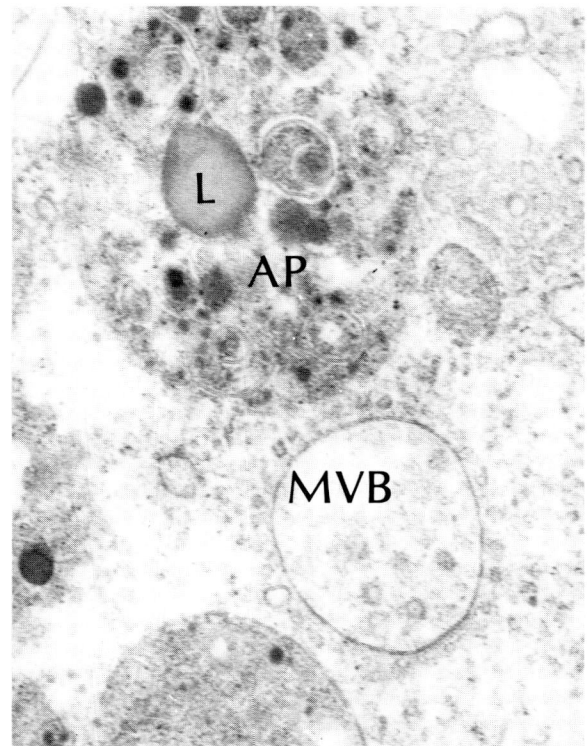

Figure 6–74. Autophagosomes (AP) contain primary lysosomes (L) as well as numerous membranous profiles. Multivesicular bodies (MVB) are membrane-bound structures containing small, membranous vesicles.

siderin; and in heart, adrenal, liver, or brain cells containing lipofuscin.

The classic, *primary*, pure *lysosome* is the neutrophilic granule of the polymorphonuclear leukocyte (PMN) (Fig. 6–73). These granules are of two types: *azurophilic* and *specific*. Azurophilic granules contain myeloperoxidase, elastase, cathepsin G, lysozyme, and several acid hydrolases, including acid phosphatase.[337] Specific granules contain lactoferrin and lysozyme.[338]

A tripartite division of neutrophilic granules into primary (azurophilic), secondary, and *tertiary types* has also been described; the last two types lack myeloperoxidase (Table 6–36).

Table 6–36.   *Enzymes of Lysosomal Granules of Neutrophils*

1° (azurophilic) granules
Myeloperoxidase
Elastase
Cathepsin G
Lysozyme
Acid hydrolases, including acid phosphatase
2° (specific) granule
Alkaline phosphatase
Lactoferrin
Lysozyme
3° granule
Acid hydrolases

Endocytosis, Lysosomes, Phagosomes, Phagolysosomes

Exogenous materials enter the cell by endocytosis and are incorporated into phagocytic vacuoles. The *phagosome* then merges with a *1° lysosomal* vesicle containing hydrolases that have not yet been active in intracellular digestion. Once merged, they form a *2° lysosome (phagolysosome)*.

Multivesicular Bodies

Pinocytosed exogenous or endogenous substances are sometimes transported to distinctive digestive multivesicular bodies (Fig. 6–74) characterized by internal vesicles. These bodies consist of a vacuole containing acid phosphatase-staining vesicles resting on a lucent or dense matrix. *Multivesicular bodies* are also seen in *type II pneumocytes* in the lung and are believed to be responsible for the release of surfactant to the alveolar luminal surface. The surfactant itself is stored in *lamellar bodies*.[339]

Residual Bodies (Telolysosomes)

Secondary lysosomes (phagolysosomes) are derived from phagosomes and 1° lysosomes or from *multivesicular bodies* that cannot degrade or extrude all undigested material. They persist as *residual bodies* or *telolysosomes*. The undigestible materials appear as membrane-bound, electron-opaque granules, membranous whorls, myelin figures, and amorphous aggregates.

Autophagosomes

The cell may digest bits of its own cytoplasm *(autophagy)* by forming *autophagic vacuoles,* which are also a form of 2° phagolysosome (Fig. 6–74). Autophagocytosis is the postulated mechanism for the degradation of subcellular organelles.[340] This event is not random, but is part of the normal cellular turnover mechanism of the cell. Autophagic vacuoles may contain fragments of membranes, mitochondria, ribosomes, and other organelles. Cell membranes in this process are removed from cell surfaces in vesicles. The fate of these vesicles may be a function of their net charge. Only those portions with a net negative charge fuse with the lysosomal system, whereas those with a positive charge fuse with the lysosomal system, with Golgi cisternae, or with condensing vacuoles.[159]

Although lysosomal membranes are single, those of autophagic vacuoles are often double, owing to the delimitation of sequestered cytoplasm by the ER. It has been suggested, however, that the double membrane originates from the Golgi apparatus; it may also be newly synthesized within the cytoplasm.[159] Autophagic turnover of organelles may eventually result in the formation of residual bodies (see Fig. 6–72). *"Crinophagy"* denotes the process whereby a 1° or 2° lysosome fuses with a secretory granule membrane (see Fig. 6–72).

Peroxisomes (Microbodies): Lysosome-like Structures

Structure

Peroxisomes, which appear to be ubiquitous organelles,[341,342] are particularly prominent in hepatocytes[343] and red blood cells.[344] They vary in size and shape, but are usually 0.5 to 1.0 μ in diameter (Fig. 6–75). These single, membrane-bound organelles may be in continuity with the ER, the Golgi apparatus, or the nuclear membrane.

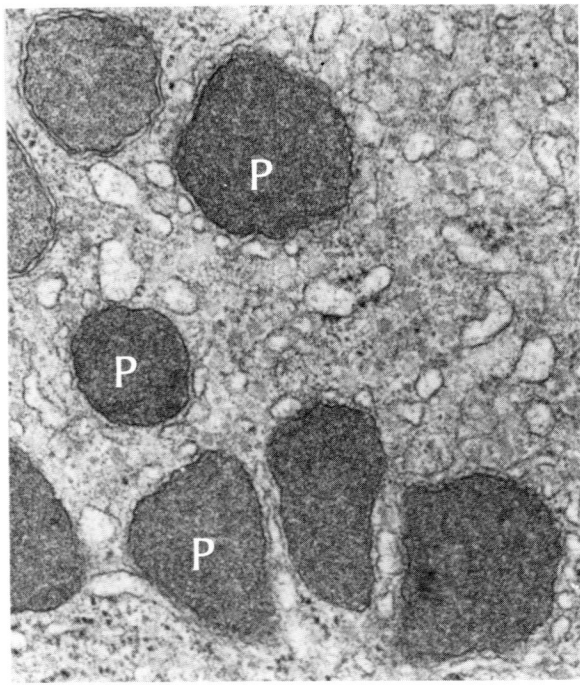

Figure 6–75. Hepatocyte containing numerous peroxisomes (P). (Courtesy of Dr. I. Sternlieb, Albert Einstein College of Medicine of Yeshiva University, New York.)

Enzymes

Some investigators believe that peroxisomes represent locally differentiated zones of the ER.[345] They contain six major enzymes: urate oxidase, d-amino oxidase, alpha-hydroxy acid oxidase, isocitrate dehydrogenase, enoyl-CoA-hydratase, and catalase. The first four enzymes are synthesized on the ER and enter the peroxisome as a unit (Table 6–37).

Catalase enters the organelle as four separate subunits and is assembled with iron into a complete enzyme when incorporated into the granule. It converts H_2O_2 to CO_2 and H_2O.

Table 6–37. *Enzymes of Peroxisomes*

urate oxidase
D-amino acid oxidase
alpha-hydroxy acid oxidase
L-amino acid oxidase
catalase
enoyl-CoA hydratase

Function

Peroxisomes are commonly found where lipid transport, storage, and secretion occur, and they are particularly prominent in cells during fetal and postnatal development or after hepatectomy.[346] Following their proliferation, peroxisomes are believed to be degraded in part by lysosomes in a manner similar to that seen in other organelles.[347] They may also be retracted into the SER, or they may simply dissolve without incorporation into other membrane systems.[347]

Because lipids are a respiratory fuel for the continuous work of the contracting myocardium, the close association between peroxisomes and the sarcoplasmic reticulum, which is the site of triglyceride synthesis in the heart, has been considered as evidence for the relationship between catalase and lipid metabolism.[342] Evidence of this relationship is further strengthened by the observation that peroxisomes proliferate when animals are given hypocholesterolemic agents.[348,349] Conversely, drugs that block the synthesis of catalase produce hyperlipidemia.[340]

Lysosomal Enzymes

The broad spectrum of lysosomal enzymes is indicated in Table 6–35 and is discussed in detail in the following sections. The actions of these enzymes in hydrolysis of macromolecules are shown in Table 6–38.

Table 6–38. *Hydrolysis of Macromolecules Relevant to Tissue Injury by Lysosomal Hydrolases*

Enzyme	Substrate
Collagenase	Collagen
Hyaluronidase	Protein polysaccharides, hyaluronate, chondroitin sulfate
Neutral protease	Protein polysaccharides, C1q, C3, C5
Cathepsin D	Protein polysaccharides, cartilage matrix
Cathepsins D, E	Basement membranes, histones, thyroglobulin
Elastase	Elastin, arterial walls
Deoxyribonuclease	Deoxyribonucleic acid
Ribonuclease	Ribonucleic acid
Histonase (pH 7.4)	Histones
Acid peptidases	Kinins, fibrin
Neutral acid proteases	γ-globulin
Urokinase	Plasminogen

Digestion of Peptides and Proteins

Endo- and *exopeptidases* may act synergistically to degrade sequentially proteins to peptides and amino acids. Among these are several *cathepsins*, including two exopeptidases, cathepsin A and C, and two endopeptidases, cathepsin B and D.

Cathepsin A is a carboxypeptidase that attacks polypeptide chains at the COOH terminal. *Cathepsin D* is a major acid endoproteinase in liver and other tissues that acts on hemoglobin, globin, and other proteins. Other peptidases include thyroid acetylphenylalanyl tyrosinase hydrolase (APAT hydrolase), which acts synergistically with cathepsin D to degrade thyroglobulin.

Cathepsin D is responsible for degradation of extracellular cartilage protein-polysaccharide matrix during autolysis. Lysosomal collagenolytic cathepsin and a neutral collagenase present in tissues may also degrade extracellular matrix collagen. *Neutral collagenase*, activated outside the cell, initiates the attack on insoluble collagen fibers and produces fragments that can be endocytosed by cells and further degraded by the collagenolytic lysosomal cathepsin. *Elastase*, an enzyme capable of degrading insoluble extracellular elastin to soluble fragments, has been identified in lysosomal granules of PMN and may play a role in the various processes leading to vascular basement membrane destruction, such as in the immune-mediated *Arthus phenomenon*.[350]

Digestion of Carbohydrates

Some *disaccharides,* such as maltose and lactose, are digested in vivo in lysosomes and form monosaccharide products that diffuse freely out of these organelles. Other disaccharides are not digested. Once in lysosomes, these disaccharides cannot freely escape through the lysosomal membranes, and their accumulation causes progressive swelling and vacuolization of the lysosomal system. Subsequently, they may be hydrolyzed into diffusible monosaccharides by an exogenous hydrolase that has been taken up by pinocytosis into the same lysosomes.

Liver lysosomes contain, among other enzymes, an *alpha-glucosidase* capable of hydrolysis of maltose and glycogen. This enzyme is deficient in type II glycogenosis *(Pompe's disease),* characterized by accumulations of glycogen in lysosomal vacuoles in a variety of tissues.[351]

Digestion of Mucopolysaccharides

A prototype of lysosomal hydrolysis of these complex substances is the degradation of the chondroitin sulfate-protein complex of cartilage or chondromucoprotein. *Proteolytic enzymes,* including cathepsin D, release peptide-bound chondroitin sulfate together with free peptides and amino acids; the action of *hyaluronidase,* on the other hand, releases oligosaccharide and leaves intact the protein core to which some oligosaccharide fragments are still attached.[352]

Digestion of Glycoproteins

The *lysosomal acid hydrolases* degrade covalent glycoproteins to individual monomeric units. Examples of these degradable membrane components include sialic acid (apparently always located at the free, nonreducing end of the carbohydrate chain, next to either a galactose or an N-acetyl galactosamine residue), fucose, and mannose residues. Lysosomal enzymes act both on the carbohydrate moieties and on the glycopeptide bonds that attach the carbohydrate to the protein portion of the glycoprotein.[353]

Digestion of Lipids

Lysosomal enzymes can extensively degrade neutral fats, phospholipids, and sphingolipids. Fatty acids are released from human chylomicrons by the action of acid *lipase,* an enzyme congenitally absent in *Wolman's disease,* in which triglycerides[353] accumulate in liver and other tissues. Lysosomes of liver and kidney contain enzymes capable of degrading ceramide galactoside and glucocerebroside *(galactocerebrosidase* and *glucocerebrosidase,* respectively). Four distinct galactosidases are active in degradation of glycolipids. Studies of *Tay-Sachs disease* indicate that at least two different forms of *N-acetyl β-hexosaminidase (A* and *B)* are involved in the hydrolytic degradation of the gangliosides and globoside.[353]

Digestion of Nucleic Acids and Nucleotides

The primary attack on nucleic acids at the carbon 5′ phosphate bond is due to *acid deoxyribonuclease* or *acid ribonuclease*, both present in hepatic lysosomes. These endonucleases release oligonucleotides, 10 to 12 nucleotide units long, which are in turn hydrolyzed by a lysosomal acid exonuclease of broad specificity that may be related to lysosomal acid phosphodiesterase or acid pyrophosphatase. Released are 3′ phosphomononucleotides that are split into phosphate and nucleosides by lysosomal acid phosphatases.[354]

Function

One of the principal functions of lysosomes is *cellular defense* because lysosomal enzymes allow digestion of foreign molecules and organisms. Proteins, complex carbohydrates, nucleic acids, neutral fats, phospholipids, and sphingolipids are all broken down to their respective end products in lysosomes.

Lysosomal enzyme systems also provide a basis for the study of normal cellular biodegradation machinery. Scores of abnormal *storage diseases*, in which congenital or acquired deficiencies of certain enzymes result in distinct biochemical and morphologic changes, provide excellent models for the study of disease.

Phagocytosis and Pinocytosis

Phagocytosis consists of a sequence of events commencing with the attachment of a particle to the plasma membrane and ending with its internalization. We have discussed it extensively in the chapter on inflammation. Pinocytosis follows a similar pattern.[355]

Turnover of Organelles

We have previously alluded to the function of lysosomes in the normal turnover of cell organelles. Organelles such as mitochondria, ER, and ribosomes may be enclosed and digested inside a vesicle into which hydrolytic enzymes have been introduced. The half-life of mitochondria is 7 to 13 days; that of cytoplasmic RNA is 5 days; and that of peroxisomes is 1 to 2 days. These half-lives represent combined effects of molecular replacement and degradation in autophagic vacuoles.[356] Those products that cannot be degraded are sequestered in residual bodies. *Lipofuscin, ceroid* and *hemofuscin* are all likely part of the same substances, that is, polymers of glycolipoproteins, in different stages of oxidation.[357]

Regeneration

The lysosomal system is altered in normal cells preparing for division. Hyaluronidase and cathepsin D are increased during G_1, and hyaluronidase, β-N-acetylglucosaminidase, acid phosphatase, and cathepsin D are lost before the S period begins. Lysosomes and lysosomal enzymes are also lost just prior to mitosis, but the enzyme levels return to normal after mitosis.[358]

Tissue Remodeling

Menstruation is one example of physiologic tissue destruction and remodeling that is the result of lysosomal hydrolase release.[359] Some postulate that the source of these hydrolases is the endometrial granulocyte. The surface epithelium of the *ovary* also undergoes remodeling following each *ovulation*. The surface epithelium in the preovulatory phase contains numerous lysosomes that become pinched off from the Golgi cisternae. Maximal numbers of lysosomes are present before ovulation, with a decrease in numbers just before follicle rupture. It is at this time that the *tunica albuginea* undergoes focal dissolution.[360]

In the remodeling of *bone* during the repair of fracture, in growth, and in certain disease states, lysosomal enzymes are released by *osteoclasts* and *osteoblasts*. The presence of collagenase in *lysosomes* of *fibroblasts* indicates an important role for these organelles in wound repair[361] (see Chap. 2).

Special Secretory Mechanisms

Although *insulin* and *catecholamines* are apparently synthesized and then directly secreted from the cell by the process of emiocytosis, *thyroxine* is initially stored in the acinar lumen as thyroglobulin. Upon stimulation of the thyroid follicular cell, the thyroglobulin is taken back into the cell from which it was synthesized. The pinocytic vesicle is then fused with a lysosome, and the globulin fraction is enzymatically removed, allowing the thyroxine (T_4) *(tetraiodotyrosine molecule)* to be released into the circulation.[362]

Specific Agents of Injury

Lysosomal activity is present in most states of cell injury. In certain diseases, pathogenesis is directly related to altered lysosomal function, structure, and enzyme content.

Genetic Factors (Storage Diseases)

The concept of lysosomal storage diseases proposed by Hers and Van Hoof[353] pertains to a genetic deficiency of specific hydrolytic enzymes in lysosomes (Table 6–39). In genetic lysosomal defects, the 2° lysosome *(phagolysosome)* becomes engorged with the material it would ordinarily degrade. Cell function may be compromised by the increased lysosomal size, but most investigators believe the

Table 6–39. *Alterations in Lysosomes Associated with Genetic Disease*

Disease	Enzyme Deficiency	Major Accumulating Metabolites
GLYCOGENOSIS		
Type 2 (Pompe's disease)	α-Glucosidase	Glycogen
SPHINGOLIPIDOSES:		
G$_{M1}$-Gangliosidosis	G$_{M1}$-ganglioside	G$_{M1}$-Ganglioside, galactose-containing oli-
Type 1 (infantile generalized)	β-galactosidase	gosaccharides
Type 2 (juvenile)		
G$_{M2}$-Gangliosidosis		
Tay-Sachs disease	Hexosaminidase A	G$_{M2}$-Ganglioside
Sandhoff-Jatzkewitz disease	Hexosaminidases A and B	G$_{M2}$-Ganglioside, globoside
Sulfatidoses		
Metachromatic leukodystrophy	Aryl sulfatase A	Sulfatide
Multiple sulfatase deficiency	Aryl sulfatase A, B, C steroid sulfatase, iduronate sulfatase, heparan N-sulfatase	Sulfatide, steroid sulfate, heparan sulfate, dermatan sulfate
Krabbe's disease	Galactocerebroside β-galactosidase	Galactocerebroside
Fabry's disease	α-Galactosidase	Ceramide trihexoside
Gaucher's disease		
Infantile form	Total β-glucosidase	Glucocerebroside
Adult form	Membrane-bound β-glucosidase	Glucocerebroside
Niemann-Pick disease	Sphingomyelinase	Sphingomyelin
Farber's disease	Ceramidase	Ceramide
MUCOPOLYSACCHARIDOSES:		
Hurler-Scheie syndrome	α-Iduronidase	Dermatan sulfate, heparan sulfate
Hunter's syndrome	Iduronate sulfatase	Dermatan sulfate, heparan sulfate
Sanfilippo's syndrome:		
Type A	Heparan N-sulfatase	Heparan sulfate
Type B	α-N-acetylglucosaminidase	Heparan sulfate
Morquio's syndrome	N-acetylhexosamine-6-sulfate sulfatase	Keratan sulfate, chondroitin-6-sulfate
Maroteaux-Lamy syndrome	Aryl sulfatase B	Dermatan sulfate
β-Glucuronidase deficiency	β-Glucuronidase	Dermatan sulfate, heparan sulfate
MUCOLIPIDOSES:		
I-cell disease and pseudo-Hurler polydystrophy	Cellular deficiency of many lysosomal enzymes; increased levels of same enzymes extracellularly	Mucopolysaccharide, glycolipid
Types 1 and 4	Unknown	Unknown
OTHER DISEASES OF COMPLEX CARBOHYDRATES:		
Fucosidosis	α-Fucosidase	Fucose-containing sphingolipids and glycoprotein fragments
Mannosidosis	α-Mannosidase	Mannose-containing oligosaccharides
Aspartylglycosaminuria	Aspartylglycosamine amide hydrolase	Aspartyl-2-deoxy-2-acetamidoglycosyl-amine
OTHER LYSOSOMAL STORAGE DISEASE:		
Wolman's disease	Acid lipase	Cholesterol esters, triglycerides
Acid phosphatase deficiency	Lysosomal acid phosphatase	Phosphate esters

(Modified from Kolodny, E.H.: Lysosomal storage diseases. N. Engl. J. Med., 294:1217, 1976.)

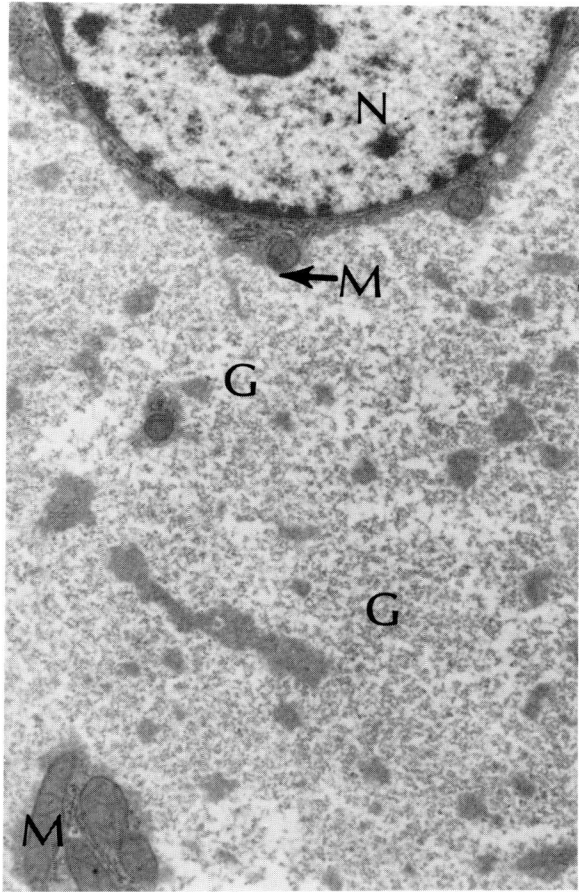

Figure 6–76. Hepatocyte from a patient with glycogen storage disease. There is a paucity of normal organelles, which have been compressed to the cell periphery by masses of glycogen (G). Several mitochondria (M) are also compressed against the nucleus (N).

metabolic defect, rather than the morphologic change, is the major problem.[363]

The increased lysosomal storage of various substrates and cell products is the result of a variety of lysosomal enzyme deficiencies and leads to many inborn errors of metabolism. These diseases include storage of glycogen (Fig. 6–76) (Pompe's disease),[353] ganglioside (Fig. 6–77) (Tay-Sachs disease), mucopolysaccharide (Fig. 6–78) (Hurler's disease),[364] glycolipid (Fabry's disease), and sphingomyelin (Niemann-Pick disease).[353,365]

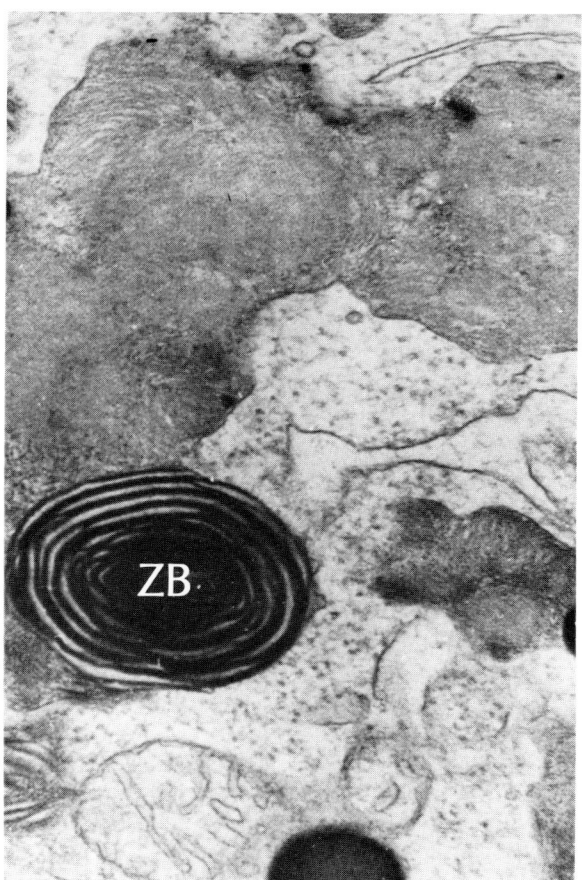

Figure 6–78. In Hurler's disease, there is an accumulation of mucopolysaccharide in neurons forming zebra bodies (ZB).

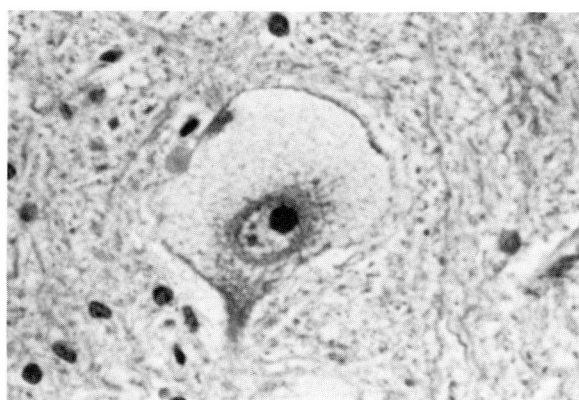

Figure 6–77. In Tay-Sachs disease, swelling of the neuron is secondary to the accumulation of lipid.

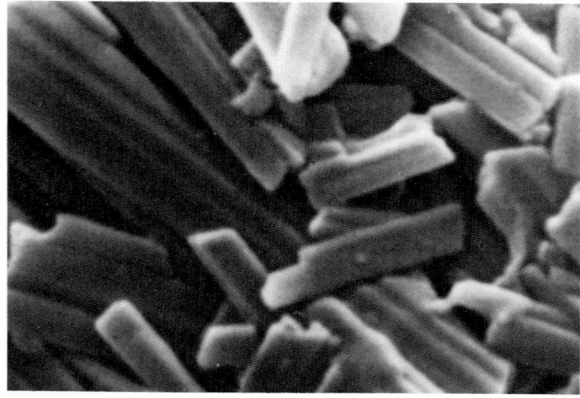

Figure 6–79. Scanning electron micrograph showing a urate crystal from the joint surface of a patient with gout. (Courtesy of Dr. K.P.H. Pritzker, Mount Sinai Hospital, Toronto, Canada.)

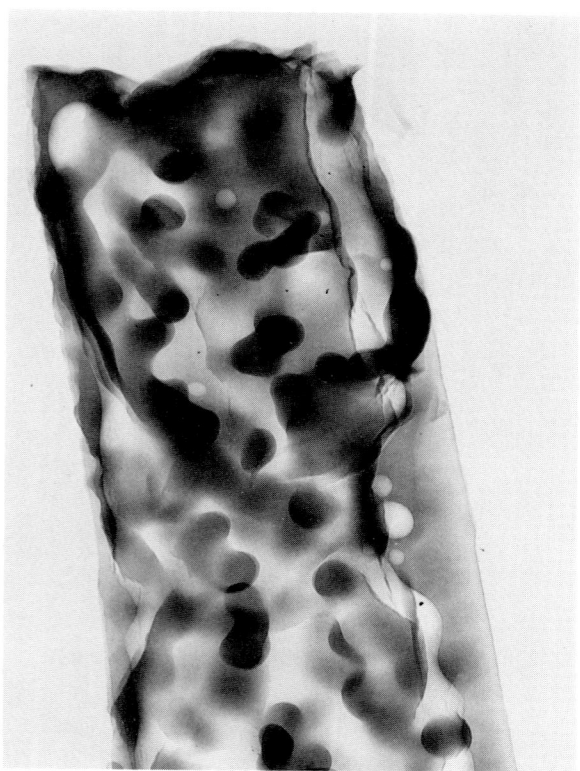

Figure 6–80. Scanning electron micrograph showing the internal structure of a urate crystal from the joint surface of a patient with gout. (Courtesy of Dr. K.P.H. Pritzker, Mount Sinai Hospital, Toronto, Canada.)

The stored substance may appear as electron-dense or lucent masses with multimembrane formations, that are lamellar, reticular, or zebra-like whorls. Lysosomal accumulations of LDL are seen in the autosomal dominant disorder, familial hypercholesterolemia, in which defective or limited LDL receptors on parenchymal cell membranes increase plasma cholesterol levels and engorge lymphoreticular cells.[42] Iron may be stored in lysosomes in one form of hemochromatosis, and copper is stored in Wilson's disease. Copper inhibits both acid phosphatase and β-glucuronidase activity of lysosomes.[351]

The definitive diagnosis of *gout* is made by the demonstration of needle-like monosodium urate crystals in lysosomes of tissues or in joint fluid. The disease results from *elevated uric acid* levels secondary to increased purine biosynthesis, decreased renal excretion of uric acid, or both. Crystals of monosodium urate rupture lysosomes and form hydrogen bonds with biomembranes. They present "donor phenolic" hydrogens at their surfaces that can interact with membrane phospholipids and rupture the lysosomal membrane in a manner which Weissmann and Rita have termed *"perforation from within"*[366] (Figs. 6–79 and 6–80).

Physical Agents

Autophagic vacuoles are *increased* following physical damage by a variety of injurious agents including *trauma, radiation* (UV and x-ray), and *hypoxia.* Degeneration of myocardial cells following hypoxia is associated with the release of lysosomal enzymes from the sarcoplasmic reticulum.[367] Exposure of macrophages to particulate matter stimulates a release of lysosomal enzymes including β-glucuronidase, a β-galactosidase, and cathepsin D.[368]

Nutritional Factors

Malnutrition is associated with an increased susceptibility to infections. This factor is important in tuberculosis. A defect in macrophage function in protein-deficient rabbits may account for their altered inflammatory responses.[369]

In *starvation,* in which sufficient metabolic precursors are lacking for normal organelle turnover, the *increase* in *autophagic vacuoles* is marked. Unusual lysosomes that contain lipid droplets have been termed *lipolysosomes* by Nehemiah and Novikoff.[370] These are found in livers of animals fed cholesterol-rich diets (Fig. 6–81) and differ from usual lipid droplets in cells in that they are membrane bound and contain lysosomal enzymes. These lysosomes are also found in hepatocytes of patients with minimal-to-severe fatty infiltration, as well as in some genetic diseases. An excess of vitamin A increases lysosomal membrane lability in vitro and in vivo, with the resultant release of hydrolytic enzymes.[371]

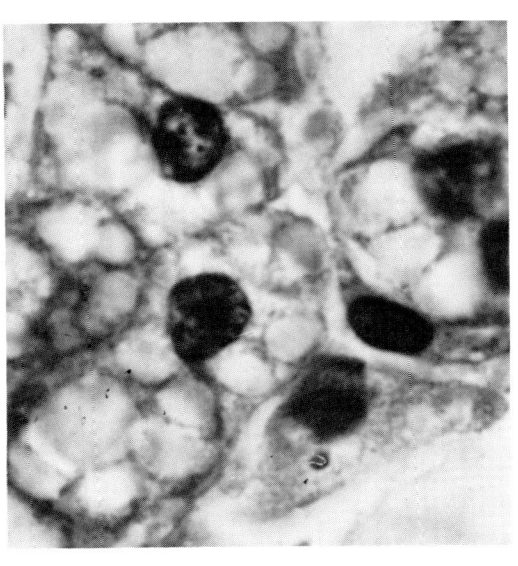

Figure 6–81. Hepatocytes with prominent lipid droplets.

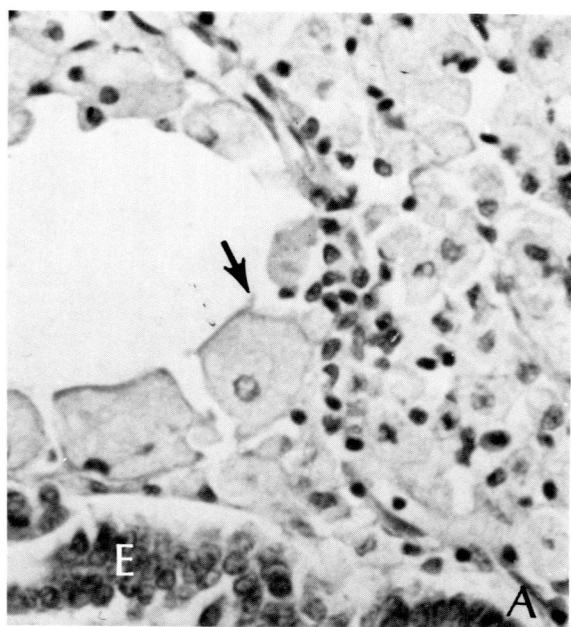

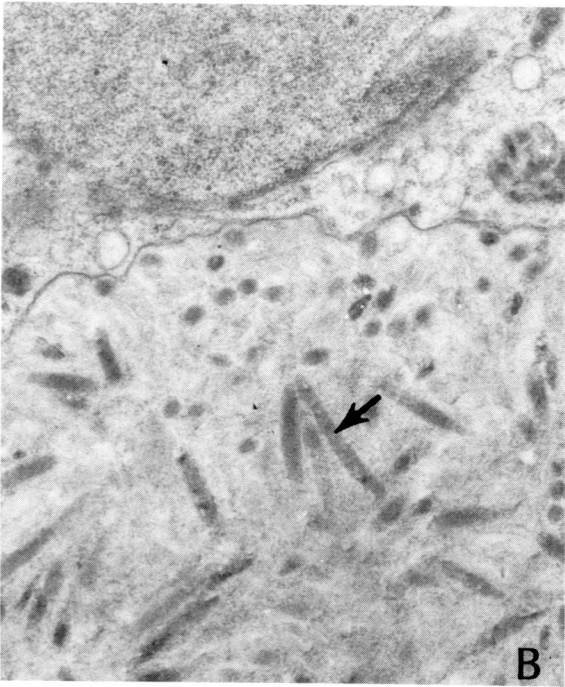

Figure 6–82. Whipple's disease. *A*, Light micrograph of small intestine showing foamy histiocytes (arrow) in the lamina propria between the epithelium (E) lining the glands. *B*, Bacilli (arrow) are present in the cytoplasm of these cells.

Infectious Agents

Phagocytes normally degrade both dead and live bacteria, fungi, and sometimes viruses. This process is accomplished by the transfer of lysosomal enzymes to phagosomes containing the organism. If unsuccessful, areas of *focal cytoplasmic degeneration* caused by bacterial exo- and endotoxins and viruses may result.[372]

Intracellular bacteria such as mycobacteria, for example, Mycobacterium tuberculosis, and M. leprae, stimulate an increase in autophagic vacuoles. Unlike other bacteria, the mycobacteria are resistant to lysosomal degradation even when dead. The ability of certain organisms to survive and to multiply within phagolysosomes is well known, notably M. leprae.[373] Bacilliform bodies have been found in jejunal villus cells in Whipple's disease (Fig. 6–82), and Leishmania donovani have been seen in macrophages in leishmaniasis.[373,374]

Malacoplakia[375] is discussed in the section of this chapter on *inclusions*, and *Chédiak-Higashi* disease and *chronic granulomatous disease of childhood*[376–378] are discussed in Chapter 2.

Drugs and Chemicals

Lysosomal Movement in Phagocytosis. Lysosomal degranulation in cells probably uses the microtubular system for transport to the cell membrane. Two drugs, *colchicine* and *vinblastine*,[258] solubilize microtubules and prevent or interfere with lysosomal degranulation. The administration of vinblastine or colchicine induces large numbers of autophagic vacuoles followed by transformation to residual bodies. *Cytochalasin B*, which interferes with microfilaments, impairs phagocytic uptake.[259] *Concanavilin A* inhibits phagocytosis, and secondarily, lysosomal movement.[259]

Autophagic Vacuoles. *Glucagon, chloroquine, Con A,* and *cAMP* increase the number of autophagic vacuoles in the liver. In addition, chloroquine alters the permeability of these organelles. It may be that this drug inhibits the release of lysosomal enzymes.[379] Autophagic vacuoles are also augmented in the kidney after *bacitracin* administration. *Vinblastine* may augment autophagocytosis because of the breakdown of microtubules. The importance of adequate ATP energy stores in autophagy is emphasized by the inhibited formation of autophagic vacuoles in animals when treated with *ethionine* and *cyanide*, blockers of electron transport.[380]

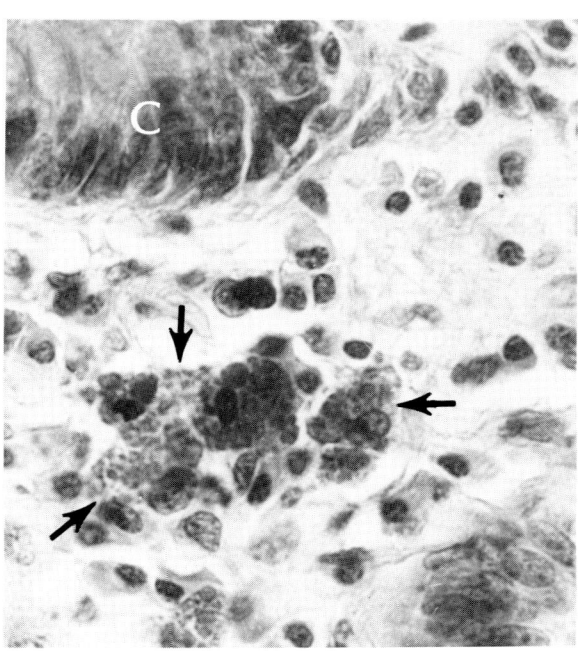

Figure 6–83. In melanosis coli, the histiocytes (arrows) in the lamina propria between the intestinal crypts (C) contain prominent collections of brownish pigment.

Residual Bodies. In *melanosis coli*, a condition associated with chronic constipation and the ingestion of the cathartic, *cascara*, residual bodies containing *lipofuscin* may be seen (Fig. 6–83). The lipofuscin may be produced from the oxidation of cyclic phenol compounds similar to melanin.

Other substances that have been given experimentally and sequestered in lysosomes include copper, gold, iron, lead, phosphorus, and mercury. Although lead and gold appear to enter lysosomes through autophagy of poisoned organelles such as mitochondria, the mechanism of mercury entry is unclear.[381]

Proliferation of Peroxisomes. Of particular interest are the actions of the hypolipidemic drugs, *clofibrate* and *nafenopin*. These agents induce the preferential expansion of the peroxisomal compartment of liver cells in much the same way as phenobarbital increases the SER. Not only do these drugs cause a *proliferation* of the *peroxisomes*, but characteristic tubular inclusions may form as well.[343]

Hormonal Injury

Labilization of lysosomal membranes with resulting leakage of acid hydrolases occurs in target cells exposed to *trophic hormones.* Lysosomes or multilysosomal aggregates may then be seen close to the nucleus. Eventually, lysosomal vesicles are seen in deep invaginations of the nuclear membrane. Electron micrographs have shown fusion of dense-body lysosomal and outer nuclear membranes, as well as striking nuclear inclusions whose membranes often stained for acid phosphatase. The cytoplasmic redistribution of lysosomes may be a response to cAMP generation following the interaction of a hormone with its receptor.[382]

Cortisone stabilizes lysosomal membranes by an unknown mechanism, but its significance in therapeutic dosages remains controversial. In vivo, corticosteroid therapy is also associated with the impaired ability of monocytes to kill staphylococci and Candida albicans,[383] and in vitro, corticosteroid administration impairs macrophage tumoricidal activity.

Immune Agents

Lysosomes have been implicated in the pathogenesis of rheumatoid arthritis. It is believed that gamma globulin and rheumatoid factor, a 19S IgM antibody to gamma globulin, are phagocytosed into macrophages; this process ruptures lysosomes, releases hydrolytic enzymes,[384] and causes severe synovial cell necrosis in acute attacks of arthritis. It is known that substances that labilize lysosomes, such as vitamin A, streptolysin, and filipin, also produce this acute phenomenon when injected into joints. Substances used to treat arthritis, for example, corticosteroids, gold, colchicine, and chloroquine, stabilize lysosomes, inhibit the release

Response of the Cell **499**

of hydrolytic enzymes, and thereby help to prevent acute attacks.[385]

Role of Lysosomes in Immune and Inflammatory Responses

Lysosomal cationic proteins from inflammatory cells function as mediators of tissue injury in acute and chronic inflammation.

Lysosomes, of major importance in the generation of immune responses, have been studied in all the principal cells of the *immune system.* They are key factors in the processing of particulate antigens by macrophages. Following endocytosis of antigens, the lysosomal enzymes degrade antigenic materials into active peptide subunits, which function as better *immunogens.*

Newly formed endocytic vacuoles with particulate antigens move from the plasma membrane to the Golgi apparatus, where they fuse with primary lysosomes to form secondary lysosomes. Hydrolysis of the antigenic material then begins. Some of this material may be sequestered in macrophage lysosomes for long periods of time.

Weissmann and Dukor have discussed lysosomal function in relation to the four major types of immune injury suggested by Coombs and Gel.[386]

Type I: Acute Hypersensitivity. Anaphylactic reactions are acute allergic reactions mediated by IgE. Vasoactive amines released from basophils and mast cell granules do not involve true lysosomes. Nevertheless, lysosomes are released with tissue destruction and remodeling, for example, in chronic asthma.

Type II: Hypersensitivity: Cytotoxic Reactions Mediated by Complement. When circulating antibodies have attached to the surface antigens of target cells, the lysosomes of target cells are disrupted, and lysosomal contents diffuse through the cytoplasm.

Type III: Hypersensitivity of Immune Complex Reactions. Circulating antigen-antibody complexes may be endocytosed, particularly by eosinophils. These complexes may become activated during lysosomal degradation with ensuing cell injury.

Type IV: Cellular Hypersensitivity. These reactions are mediated by activated T lymphocytes. Each time lymphokines are released from such cells, the lysosomal system becomes activated, as does the ER and the Golgi apparatus. Lysosomes are also involved in the early phases of blastogenesis.

Chemotactic Properties. *Chemotactic factors,* important in the recruitment of inflammatory cells, also affect lysosomal function. The complement-derived chemotactic factors *C3a, C5a,* and *C567* can induce lysosomal release from neutrophils.[387]

Prostaglandins *(PGF),* mediators of inflammatory reactions that increase vascular permeability, are found in inflammatory exudates secondary to their release during antigen-antibody reactions and have leukotactic properties.[388] It has been shown that *PGF$_2$ induces lability* of *lysosomal membranes* and incites release of lysosomal enzymes and a subsequent chain of inflammatory events. These effects can be inhibited by *aspirin*, a potent *inhibitor* of PGF synthesis.

INCLUSIONS

Intracellular inclusions are often detectable by standard microscopic techniques and are seen in all the organelles discussed previously. The exact characterization of the substances within such inclusions often requires specialized analysis, however. Immunohistochemical, ultrastructural, x-ray dispersive microanalysis, chemical ashing, or UV spectrophotometric techniques are used in this regard.

Inclusions result from accumulations of intracellular or extracellular materials. In many instances, they represent accumulations of material resulting from an enzyme deficiency or other metabolic disturbance. In other situations, altered membrane permeability, pinocytosis, or phagocytosis causes accumulations of substances that are partially metabolized and are later segregated within the cytoplasm or nucleus as an inclusion.

Inclusions seen by the light or electron microscope are often not distinctive enough to be characteristic of any specific disease. Normal cells often have temporary excessive accumulations of water, glycogen, lipid, minerals, pigments or proteinaceous crystals. These deposits are usually *reversible* and disappear once the normal intracellular milieu returns. Examples are shown in Table 6–40.

Table 6–40. *Examples of Types of Inclusions*

Water	Pigment deposition
Cloudy swelling	Hemosiderin
Hydropic degeneration	Melanin, neuromelanin
	Lipofuscin, ceroid
Nucleic acid inclusion	Homogentisic acid (ochronosis)
Uric acid deposits	
Nuclei with DNA-Ab complexes (LE cell)	Mineral and metal deposits
	Iron
Carbohydrates inclusion	Calcium
Glycogen	Cadmium
Muco- and glycoproteins	Zinc
	Mercury
Protein inclusions	Lead
Kidney tubule absorption granules	Copper
Councilman bodies	Aluminum
Mallory bodies	
	Infectious agents
Immunoglobulin and secretory products	Bacteria
Amyloid (e.g., light chains, insulin)	Viruses
Hormones	Fungi
Peptides	Parasites
	Chlamydiae, rickettsiae
Lipid inclusions	
Neutral fat	Crystals
Liposomes	Reinke
	Tyrosine

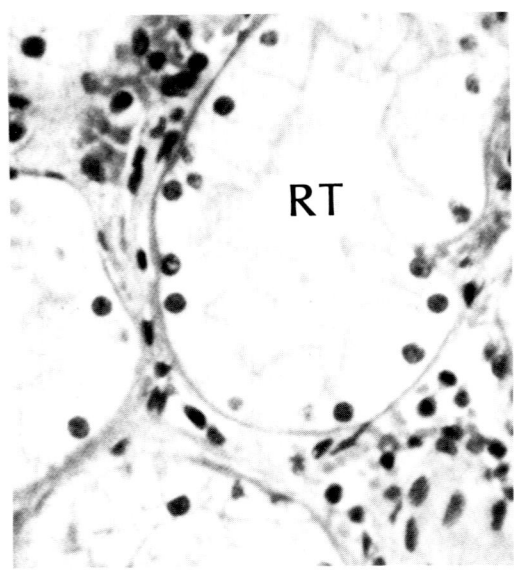

Figure 6–84. During swelling of the renal tubular (RT) epithelium, the cells become large, clear, and vacuolated.

Water Inclusions

The ionic composition of the intracellular fluid is different from that of the extracellular fluid. To maintain normal cellular osmolality, sodium is actively excluded from and potassium is retained in the cell by the *sodium-potassium pump*. If the normal cell membrane permeability is disturbed, or if oxidative respiration and ATP synthesis are impaired, then cellular osmolality increases, ion balance is disturbed, water enters, and swelling results.

By light microscopy, cellular imbibition of water is manifested by *cloudy swelling;* the swollen cytoplasm takes on the appearance of *ground glass* (Fig. 6–84). Initially, a marked increase of water and ions is present in the cisternae of the endoplasmic reticulum. Later, an increased mitochondrial outer membrane permeability results in a loss of ADP and respiratory cofactors such as NAD. Mitochondrial matrix condensation is followed by swelling and disappearance of the cristae. Swelling and rupture of many ER cisternae with larger inclusions of water is known as *hydropic degeneration.* The final result of excessive intracellular water accumulation is nuclear swelling, although the plasma membrane may rupture before this occurs.

Nucleic Acid Inclusions

Inclusions containing ribosomal nucleic acid can be seen in cytoplasmic autophagosomes in various disease states. Membrane-bound inclusions of DNA may be trapped in the cytoplasm following mitosis. In *gout, uric acid crystals,* resulting from purine degradation, are phagocytized by macrophages and may produce lysosomal hydrolysis. The crystals are first formed by precipitation of urate in the synovial fluid, followed by adherence of protein.[366] Phagocytosis of nucleoprotein nuclear fragments in systemic *lupus erythematosus* by PMN results in the characteristic *LE cells.*

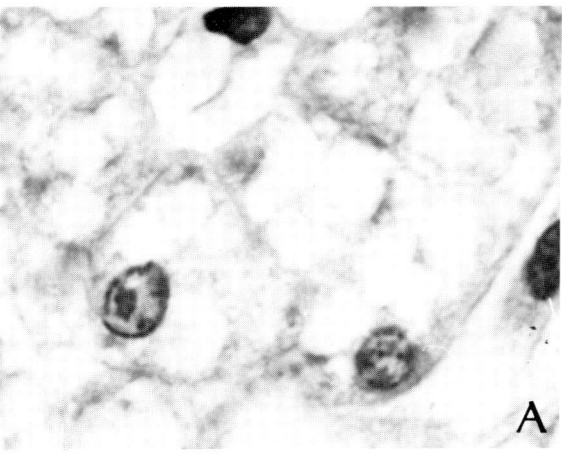

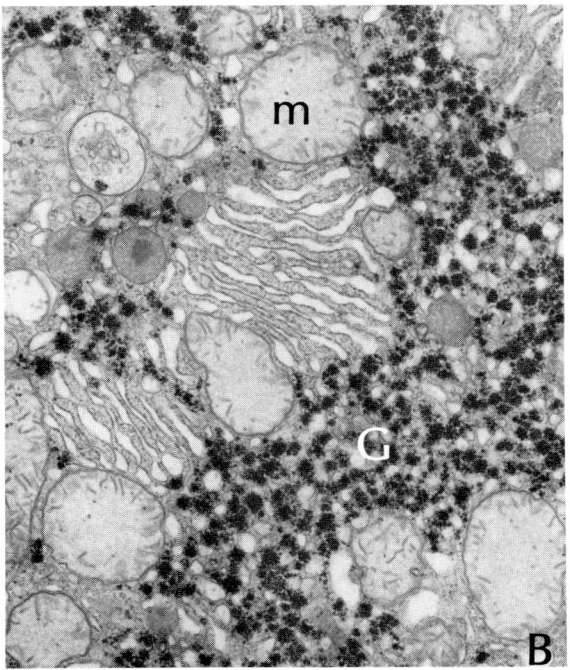

Figure 6–85. Glycogen in a hepatocyte. *A,* Light micrograph showing clear cytoplasm due to glycogen accumulation. *B,* Electron micrograph showing glycogen (G) dispersed between other cytoplasmic structures, including mitochondria (M).

Carbohydrate Inclusions

Structure of Glycogen

Glycogen is normally present in many cells, particularly liver and muscle (Fig. 6–85), and the amount correlates with the nutritional and physiologic state of the cells.[389] When glycogen is present in large amounts, the inclusion appears as a clear vacuole, but the presence of the carbohydrate aldehyde group can be confirmed by positive staining with the periodic acid-Schiff *(PAS)* reaction.

Glycogen may also be identified ultrastructurally as dense or occasionally lightly stained particles in routine electron-microscopic material. It usually consists of a *beta monomeric form,* approximately 150 to 300 Å in diameter and is sometimes confused with free cytoplasmic ribosomes. A rare, *polymeric form* of glycogen ranges in size from 600 to 1000 Å in diameter.[390]

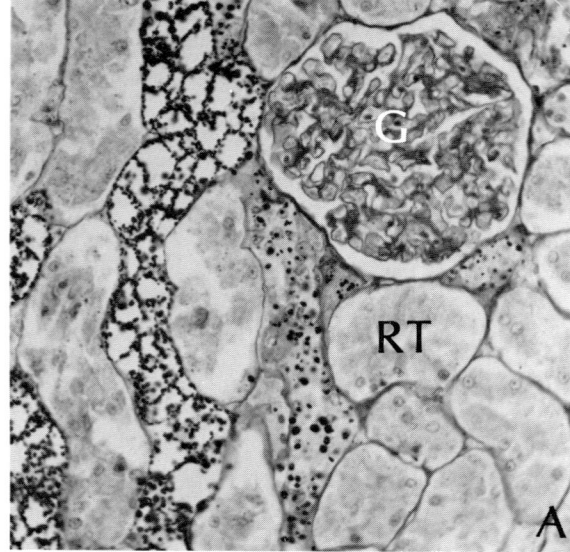

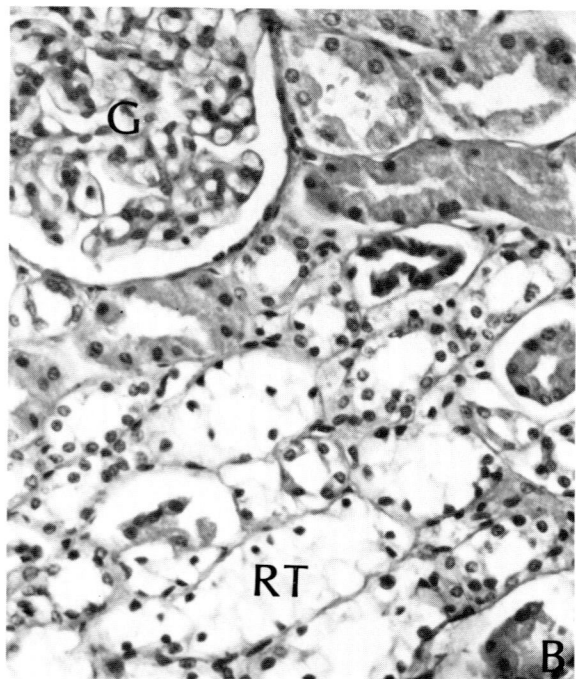

Figure 6–86. *A*, Normal kidney with glomerulus (G) and renal tubules (RT). *B*, This diabetic kidney has normal-appearing glomerulus (G) and clear renal tubular (RT) cells due to glycogen accumulation. This is known as the Armanni-Ebstein change.

Diabetes Mellitus

The amount of glycogen may be increased in genetic storage diseases and in certain metabolic states such as *diabetes mellitus.* Large collections of cytoplasmic glycogen in the renal collecting tubular epithelium produce the characteristic *Armanni-Ebstein change;* hepatic glycogen inclusions may also be present in the nucleus, as noted by Ehrlich in 1883[391] (Fig. 6–86).

Glycogen Storage Diseases

In glycogen storage diseases, glycogen may be prominent in myocardial cells, red blood cells, hepatocytes, and lymphoreticular cells. In *Pompe's disease,* with a deficiency of the lysosomal enzyme, *alpha-glucosidase,* the glycogen appears in the lysosomes of liver and myocardial cells.[351]

Neoplasms

Certain neoplastic cells contain large amounts of glycogen, especially in clear cell tumors of the kidney and the female genital tract.

Nuclear Glycogen Inclusions

Most of the inclusions previously discussed are associated with increased cytoplasmic glycogen, but glycogen may also be present in specific organelles. Nuclear glycogen inclusions occur in infectious hepatitis, diabetes, Graves' disease, lupus erythematosus, and a variety of tumors including Hodgkin's disease.

Mitochondrial Glycogen Inclusions

Glycogen inclusions are occasionally found between cristae in the matrix of mitochondria. Such mitochondrial inclusions are seen in *cardiomyopathy,* in *dystrophic axoplasm,*[392] in mouse liver cells deficient in riboflavin, and in human *adenocarcinomas* and *lymphomas.*

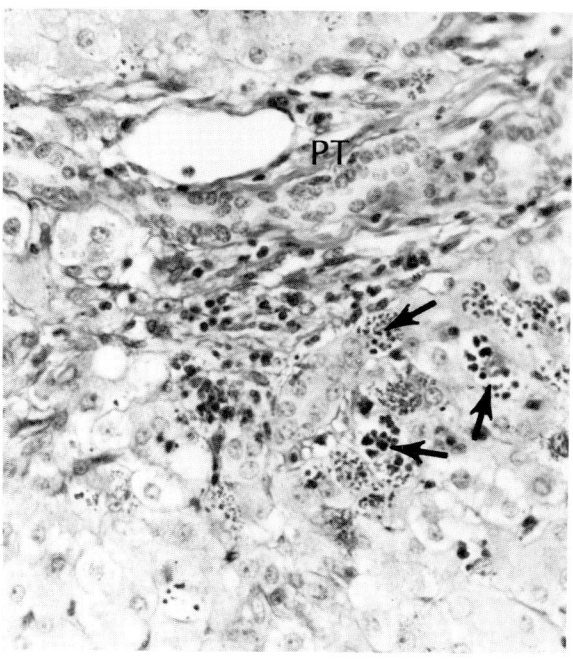

Figure 6–87. Liver biopsy specimen from a patient with alpha-1-antitrypsin deficiency. The portal tract (PT) is shown at top. This PAS stain with diastase digestion shows varied sized globules of alpha-1-antitrypsin (arrows) within the cytoplasm of periportal hepatocytes.

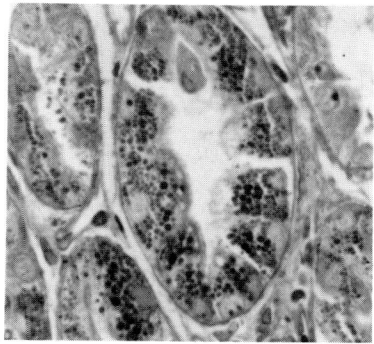

Figure 6–88. Protein accumulations in renal tubules appear as prominent dark cytoplasmic droplets.

Other Carbohydrate Inclusions

Carbohydrate inclusions may also be seen as a component of mucopolysaccharide genetic diseases, especially *Hurler's disease*. Inclusions of nonglycogen carbohydrate material may also occur in normal and abnormal livers and are believed by Popper and others to be related to both lipofuscin and bile pigment metabolism.[393] Ultrastructurally, these inclusions appear to arise from the sequestration and degradation of small parts of hepatocellular cytoplasm and are therefore partly autophagic in nature.

Some cellular PAS positive inclusions are not comprised purely of glycogen, but contain carbohydrate-protein complexes. These inclusions may be important indicators of an underlying disease, as in *alpha-1-antitrypsin deficiency*[394] (Fig. 6–87). These deposits in the ER are membrane bound, diastase resistant, PAS positive, sialic acid deficient, and immunologically characteristic of serum alpha-1-antitrypsin.

Protein Inclusions

Protein inclusions may represent degeneration of cellular components,[395] coagulation necrosis of the ER, autophagic vacuoles, or absorption of protein from outside the cell. Protein overloading of the glomerular filtrate in nephrosis can produce cytoplasmic proteinaceous deposits in tubular cells[396] (Fig. 6–88).

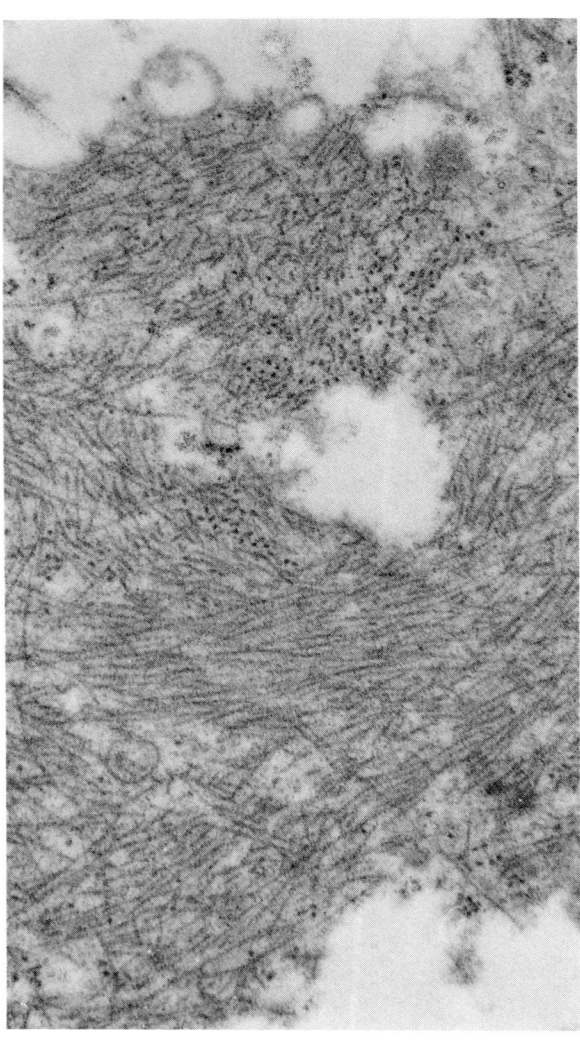

Figure 6–89. Portion of a Mallory body demonstrating its fibrillar nature. (Courtesy of Dr. S. French, Veterans Administration Hospital, Martinez, California.)

Mallory Bodies

Mallory bodies are eosinophilic proteinaceous bodies commonly seen in hepatocytes of patients with alcoholic hepatitis and several other conditions.[397] Ultrastructurally, they appear as fibrillar deposits without limiting membranes (Fig. 6–89). Synonyms include alcoholic hyalin or Mallory's hyalin.

Three distinct morphologic variants exist: (1) bundles of *filaments* in parallel arrays, (2) clusters of randomly oriented *fibrils*, and (3) granular or *amorphous arrays* containing only scattered remains of fibrils. The nature of these structures has been controversial since their original description.

Early histochemical studies showed that Mallory bodies contained unconjugated basic protein, ribonucleic acid, glycogen and other nonacidic carbohydrate components, as well as phospholipid. On the basis of these findings, it was concluded that Mallory bodies contained partially decomposed mitochondria, lysosomes, ribosomes, and endoplasmic reticulum. Evidence based on ultrastructural and immunologic studies, however, now indicates that these bodies may be partially derived from a misdirected synthesis, degeneration, or degradation of microtubules and microfilaments, which forms a particular type of intermediate filament related biochemically to prekeratin and tonofilaments.[398]

Although originally described in alcoholic hepatitis, Mallory bodies are also associated with long-standing cholestasis, nonalcoholic cirrhosis, Wilson's disease, Indian childhood cirrhosis,[399] and liver cell carcinomas.[400] Mallory bodies may be induced experimentally by griseofulvin therapy.[401]

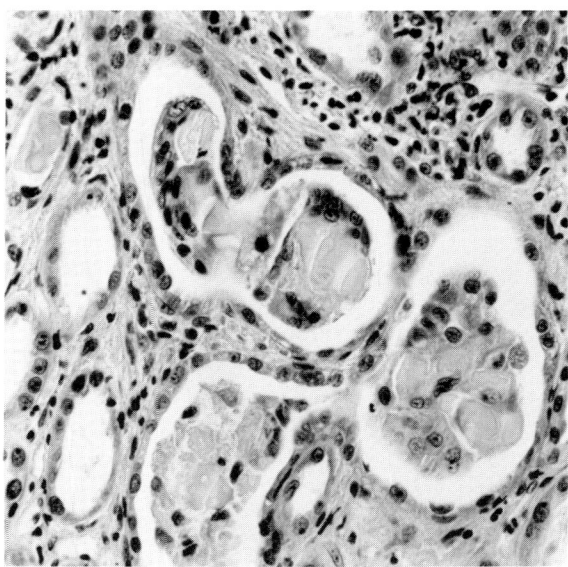

Figure 6–90. In multiple myeloma, immunoglobulin casts are seen in renal tubules.

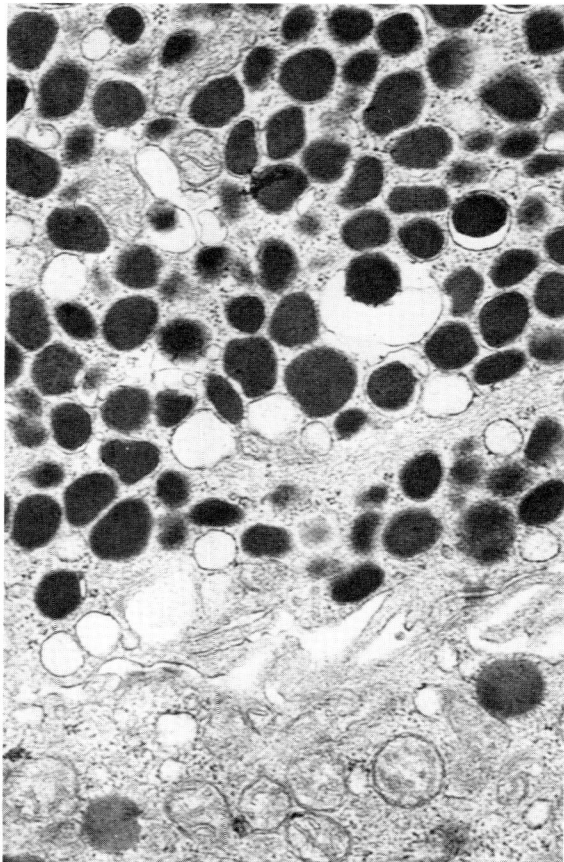

Figure 6–91. Portion of an argentaffin cell containing numerous electron-dense neurosecretory granules.

Immunoglobulins

Crystalline Bence Jones protein, the light chain polypeptide of an abnormal gamma globulin in multiple myeloma and other plasma cell dyscrasias, may form inclusions within renal tubular cells (Fig. 6–90). Protein inclusions are produced experimentally by injection of excessive amounts of kappa chains.[402]

Myeloma cells may contain deposits of *para-amyloid* in the cytosol or in membrane-bound vacuoles. This amyloid is composed of light chains of IgG or IgA linked to a glycoprotein matrix. These deposits give a negative reaction with the characteristic histochemical amyloid stains (crystal violet and Congo red), but display a moderate green birefringence in polarized light. In addition, these deposits display a greenish yellow fluorescence when stained with thioflavin.[403]

Other Protein Inclusions and Amyloid

A class of proteinaceous inclusions occurs in Hurlers' disease, a genetic disease with altered mucopolysaccharide synthesis, and in Marfan's syndrome, a genetic disease with altered elastin structure. Eosinophilic hyaline inclusions are seen in a variety of other disorders. These inclusions may also be induced by certain drugs, the most notable being spironolactone, the antihypertensive diuretic agent. These deposits, seen in the cytoplasm of the zona glomerulosa cells of the adrenal cortex, are believed by some to represent specific morphologic indices of excessive spironolactone therapy.[404]

Amyloid is generally believed to be a ubiquitous substance with several origins. In multiple myeloma, it represents light chains complexed to carbohydrate. The amyloid of diabetes represents crystalline insulin, whereas the amyloid of medullary carcinoma of the thyroid represents calcitonin. Another type of amyloid represents the AA protein. AA protein complex, perhaps prealbumin, is particularly associated with age.[405] All are discussed in Chapter 5.

Hormone Inclusions

Peptide, steroid, and *catecholamine* hormones are present in their respective cells of synthesis as membrane-bound inclusions (Fig. 6–91). In general, defective membrane transport and secretory or metabolic blocks may increase the accumulation of granular inclusions within swollen endocrine cells. Accumulation of hormones in target cells occurs because of deficiencies of hormone receptors on these cells.

Lipid Inclusions

Cytosol, ER, Golgi Apparatus

Lipid inclusions occur in normal fat cells. Fatty inclusions may be seen with or without a membrane and ultrastructurally appear either as electron-lucent or electron-dense areas. These inclusions are composed of large amounts of fatty acids, are osmiophilic in electron-micrographic preparations, and are positive with Sudan stains on light microscopy. Some normal cells contain *lamellar lipid inclusions* resembling *myelin figures,* for example, type II alveolar pneumocytes have surfactant-containing lamellar bodies.[406]

One of the earliest manifestations of injury to cells, particularly in heart, liver, kidney, and brain, is the appearance of cytoplasmic lipid inclusions. These inclusions are characteristic in alcoholic hepatitis, in which protein synthesis is abnormal and lipoprotein assembly is altered.[407] Lipid-laden macrophages and myointimal cells are prominent in atherosclerotic plaques.

In addition to lying free in the cytosol, lipid vacuoles may be seen within the ER or Golgi system. These vacuoles are termed *liposomes* and are not to be confused with artificial lipid sacs that are used for experiments on phagocytosis by cells in vitro.[408]

Mitochondrial Lipid

Lipid inclusions in *mitochondria* often lack a membrane and exist either as solitary or as multiple irregular forms. Mitochondria often appear near *lipid vacuoles,* and it has been suggested that these vacuoles represent an *energy source* for mitochondrial metabolism. Mitochondrial lipid inclusions may arise from cytoplasmic invaginations and disruption of the wall followed by rehealing of the mitochondrial membrane. These inclusions have been seen in degenerating giant mitochondria of the adrenal cortex following injection of *ethionine* in rats or after the ingestion of experimental carcinogens.[409]

Nuclear Lipid

Nuclear lipid inclusions may appear with or without membranes. Many are *pseudoinclusions* trapped after mitosis by resealing of the nuclear membrane; however, lipid transport through nuclear pores is also possible. Nuclear lipid inclusions are seen occasionally in normal liver, in synovial cells following hemorrhage into the joint, in diabetes mellitus, and in a variety of human and experimentally induced tumors.[410]

Pigment Inclusions

Hemosiderin and Hematin

The breakdown of hemoglobin in red blood cells during hemorrhage or hemolysis releases iron. *Hemorrhage* is commonly seen in cerebrovascular accidents, trauma, and ulcers, and as a complication of tuberculosis and carcinoma. *Hemolysis* occurs in a variety of conditions including hemolytic anemia, malaria, thrombosis, emboli, and thrombocytopenia. *Hemosiderin,* a breakdown product of hemoglobin, is a yellowish brown intra- or extracellular pigment that appears black *(hematin)* when oxidized. Ultrastructurally, hemosiderin has the characteristics of lysosomal dense bodies and contains aggregates of carbohydrates, proteins, lipid, and iron. Another breakdown product of hemoglobin is *bilirubin,* which may be incorporated into liver and other epithelial or mesenchymal cells. *Urobilinogen,* a later degradation product of bilirubin, may also be found intracellularly, particularly in kidney tubular epithelium or intestinal mucosal cells.

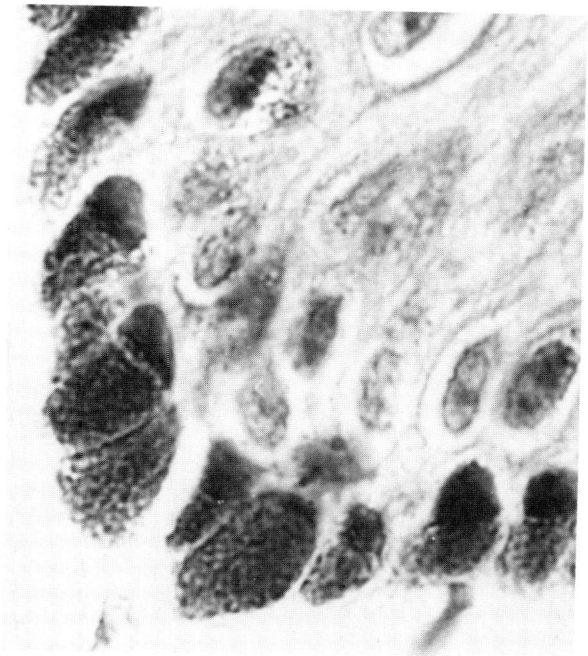

Melanin

A normal pigment found in melanosomes in melanocytes, particularly in retinal and skin epithelium, melanin is also accumulated in inclusions in cells in malignant melanoma, pheochromocytoma, and dermatopathic lymphadenitis[411] (Fig. 6–92). When macrophages acquire melanin, they are known as melanophages.

Lipofuscin (Ceroid)

One of the most prominent intracellular inclusion pigments is the pigment of aging, *lipofuscin;* this term is generally used synonymously with *ceroid* (Fig. 6–93). This pigment is present in all cells, but is particularly prominent in the myocardium, adrenal, liver, and neurons, and increases with age. Lipofuscin is believed to represent a complex of unsaturated fatty acids combined in a glycolipid proteinaceous matrix. It is often found in lysosomes[412] (see Chap. 5, "Morphologic Alterations").

Excessive lipofuscin accumulations are seen in the thyroid glands of patients with *mucoviscidosis* and appear to be age-related. The excessive accumulation, which may be related to chronic vitamin E deficiency, possibly results in auto-oxidation of lipids within acinar cells of the thyroid gland.[413] In *Gilbert's disease* (constitutional hyperbilirubinemia), intracellular lipofuscin-containing deposits are seen in greater numbers near the canalicular pole of liver cells. These deposits appear as coarsely granular heterogeneous aggregates of membrane-bound electron-dense material ranging in size from 1 to 3 μ.

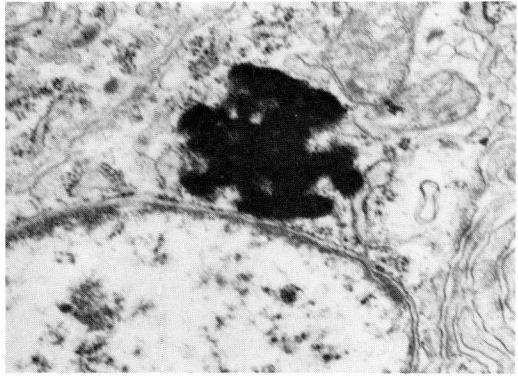

Figure 6–92. Melanocytes at the base of the epidermis are so full of melanin that they make the cells appear granular.

Figure 6–93. Ceroid in cells appears as irregular, electron-dense deposits in the cytoplasm.

Chédiak-Higashi disease is a rare disorder in which large, ceroid-filled lysosomal granules are seen in white blood cells.[414]

Alkaptonuria

A block in tyrosine metabolism in *alkaptonuria* results in the excretion of *homogentisic acid* and the tissue deposition of a characteristic black pigment in bone cells, a condition known as *ochronosis.*[415,416]

Other Pigments

Other pigmented lysosomal deposits may be seen in lymph nodes from patients with *sarcoidosis*[417] and from patients with a history of heavy *smoking.* In smokers, x-ray microanalysis of the lymph nodes has confirmed that the lysosomal deposits are composed of *aluminum silicate kaolinite,* presumably from inhaled tobacco smoke.[418]

Mineral and Metal Deposits

Inclusions containing copper, iron, calcium, mercury, lead, arsenic, cadmium, and zinc have all been seen in human cells. Of these, *carbon, iron,* and *calcium* are the most common. *Anthracosis,* with carbon deposits in macrophages of the lungs and thoracic lymph nodes, is seen in all urban dwellers and particularly in coal miners. It probably is of little physiologic or pathologic significance.

Iron

Iron deposits are commonly seen near sites of previous hemorrhage, in *hemosiderosis,* in *hemochromatosis,*[419] and in *hemolytic anemias.* Iron most commonly appears within *siderosomes,* that is, lysosomes containing iron. These are bounded by a single membrane and enclose aggregates of iron consisting of electron-dense particles 50 to 60 Å in diameter[420] (Fig. 6–94). Groups of siderosomes clumped

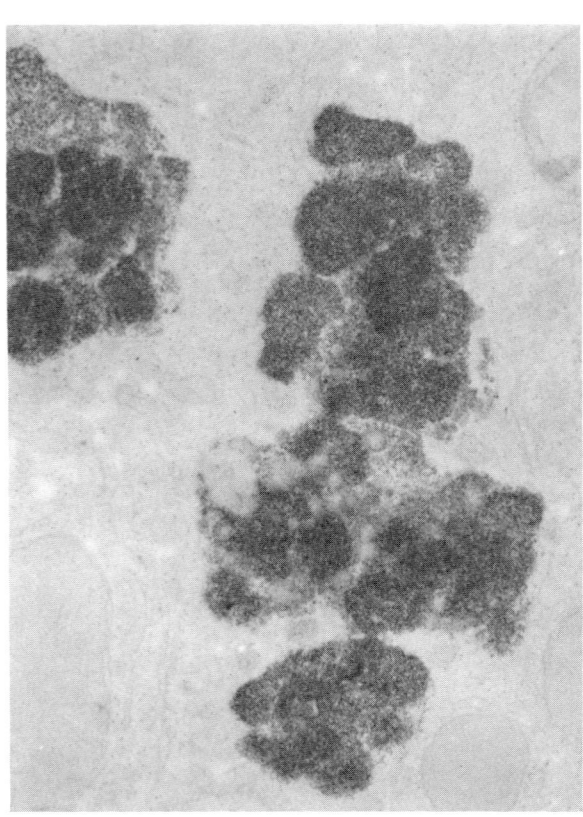

Figure 6–94. Hemosiderosis following transfusion therapy for anemia. Siderosomes are prominent in the hepatocytes. (Courtesy of Dr. I. Sternlieb, Albert Einstein College of Medicine, Yeshiva University, New York.)

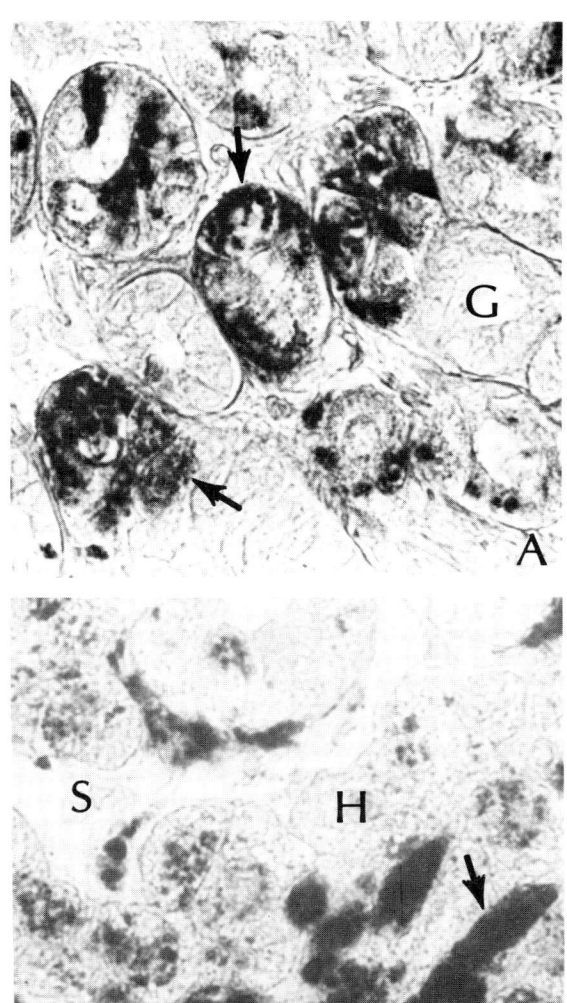

Figure 6-95. Hemochromatosis. *A*, Portions of gastric glands (G) contain iron (arrows). The iron stain makes pigment appear black in the photograph. *B*, This portion of liver with hepatocytes (H) near sinuscid (S) containing abundant iron (arrow).

together make iron visible by light microscopy when stained with the *Prussian blue* reaction. An increase in iron is seen in lymphoreticular cells following *blood transfusions*, in macrophages and synovial cells following *hemorrhage* into joints, and in intestinal cells following the absorption of blood from the intestine. It is also present in *Kupffer cells*, liver cells, and pancreatic acinar cells in hemochromatosis (Fig. 6-95).

Iron rarely appears in the nucleus, but occasionally it is seen there in sideroblastic anemia. It presumably enters through the nuclear pores. Similar deposits are also seen in mitochondria.

Calcium

Calcium plays an important role in secretion, transport, muscle contraction, nerve transmission, activation of hormones, and bone formation. Pathologically, calcium phosphate precipitates in tissue, particularly in mitochondria, are evidence of injury. Calcium binds occasionally to oxalates and appears as calcium oxalate crystals in tissues in the genetic condition known as *oxalosis*.[421]

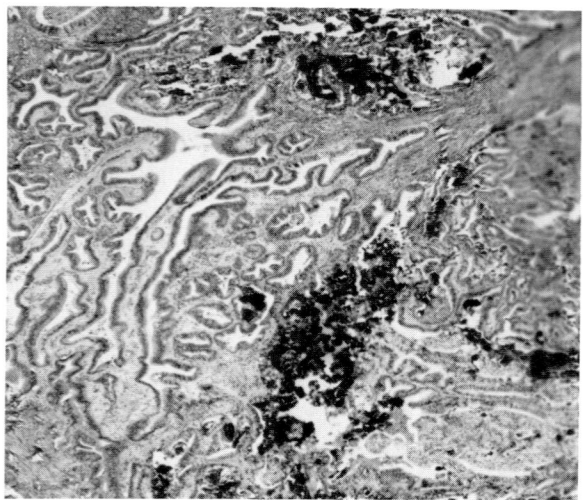

Figure 6–96. Section of bile duct carcinoma with abundant calcium deposits (appearing black in the micrograph).

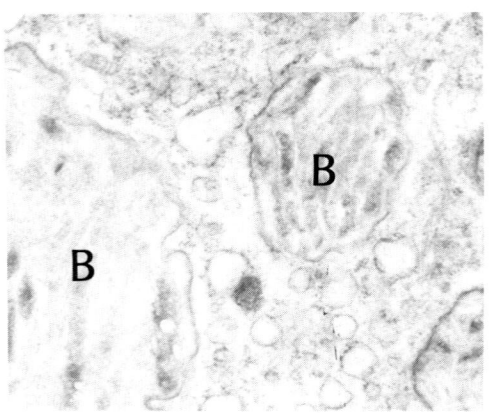

Figure 6–97. In Whipple's disease, the bacteria (B) are frequently segregated from the cytoplasm in membrane-bound vacuoles.

A peculiar form of degeneration, called *calcific degeneration,* is seen intra- and extracellularly in the pancreas, heart, and muscle following necrosis and release of fatty acids, as well as in atherosclerotic blood vessels. *Dystrophic* and *metastatic calcifications* are seen in many sites with a variety of diseases. Crystalline calcium deposits appear in *psammoma bodies.* Microcalcifications may be seen in breast and other carcinomas (Fig. 6–96).

Cadmimum, Zinc, Mercury, Lead, Arsenic, and Copper

That the ingestion of cadmium, zinc, and mercury leads to deposits in kidney tubule cells has been reported. *Lead poisoning* is associated with intracellular deposits in the oral mucosa and in bone. *Arsenic poisoning* is primarily associated with increased concentrations of the metal in bone, kidney, liver, skin, and hair. In *Wilson's disease,* copper is deposited in the cornea as *Kayser-Fleischer rings,* as well as in the liver and in basal ganglia.[353]

Infectious Agent Inclusions

Some infectious agents such as mycobacteria, parasites, fungi, and viruses live for long periods in inclusions in a symbiotic relationship with the host.

Bacteria

Mycobacteria may lie free in the cytosol or in membrane-bound inclusions in the cytoplasm of macrophages or epithelioid or giant cells. Other intracellular bacteria include *shigella,* found in inclusions of the colonic mucosa,[422] and *meningococcus,* found in white blood cells of the spinal fluid.

Whipple's disease causes significant intestinal malabsorption and is characteristically associated with the presence of intracellular rod-shaped bacilli within PAS-positive, glycoprotein-laden foamy macrophages in the small intestine and lymph nodes[423] (Fig. 6–97).

Fungi

Fungal inclusions are frequently found in the cytoplasm of cells of the gastrointestinal, genitourinary, and respiratory tracts. Both *filamentous* and *yeast* forms may be discerned, depending upon the type of fungus. Fungi may live for months in tissue culture in vitro, but often overwhelm host cells in vivo within a few days. They may live quietly for years on epithelial surfaces; however, fungi are opportunistic agents and invade mucosa when host resistance is decreased.[424]

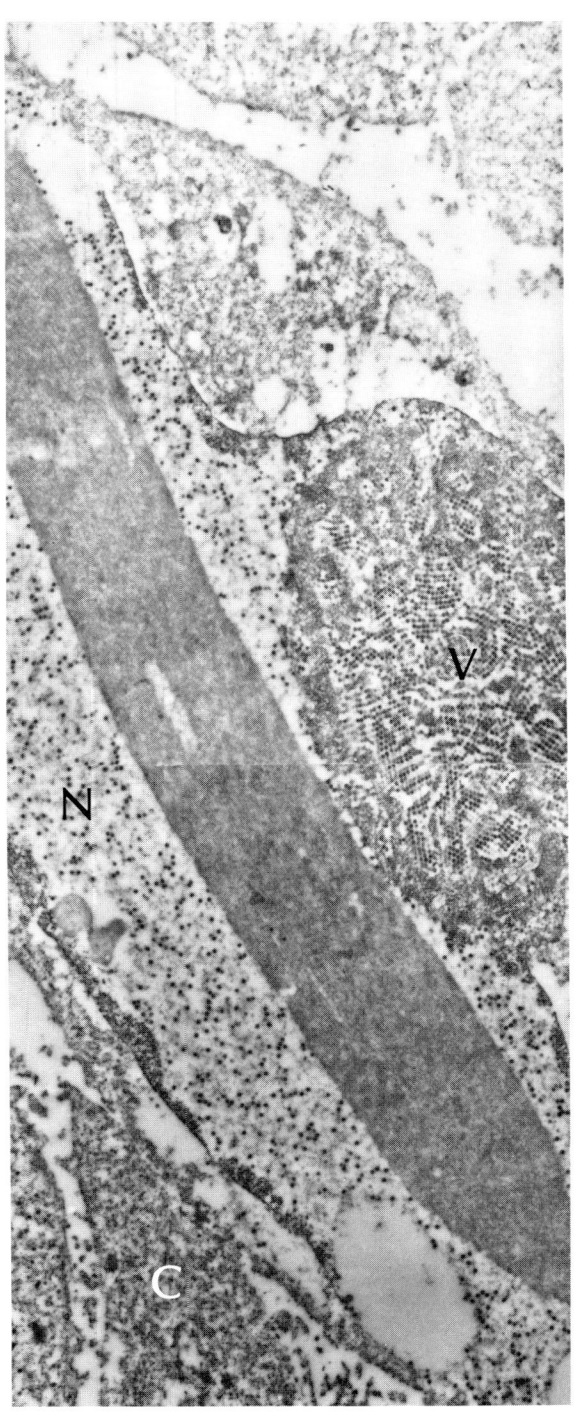

Figure 6–98. Accumulation of adenovirus particles (V) in the nucleus (N). No particles are present in the cytoplasm (C).

Parasites

Many parasites may also live for days, weeks, or months in lymphoreticular as well as mesenchymal cells. Toxoplasma organisms can be found in neutrophils,[425] and malarial parasites[426] complete part of their cycle in red blood cells. Endothelial cells are characteristically invaded by rickettsiae,[427] although these organisms may be found in the cells of a variety of other tissues. Chlamydia are found in intracellular cytoplasmic inclusions.[428]

Viruses

Viral inclusions may be seen in either the cytoplasm or the nucleus (Fig. 6–98). Histologically, characteristic nuclear *viral* inclusions are seen in herpesvirus[429] and cytomegalovirus infections. Measles and myxoviral inclusions may be seen within either the nucleus or the cytoplasm. Most viruses can be seen with the electron microscope during the absorption or penetration period, but they are generally not visible during the eclipse period, when DNA and RNA replication occurs. Virions become visible again during the assembly and release process.

Many viruses appear as *paracrystalline arrays*. Both adeno- and herpesviruses synthesize their DNA in the nucleus and may appear as nuclear clusters of the aggregated or crystalline deposits with a dense DNA core.[430] Measles (RNA) virus may also appear in the nucleus as a deposit of aggregated tubules, although replication takes place in the cytoplasm. Viruses may be seen in the cytosol,[431] ER, or nucleus, but are usually not found in mitochondria or in lysosomes.

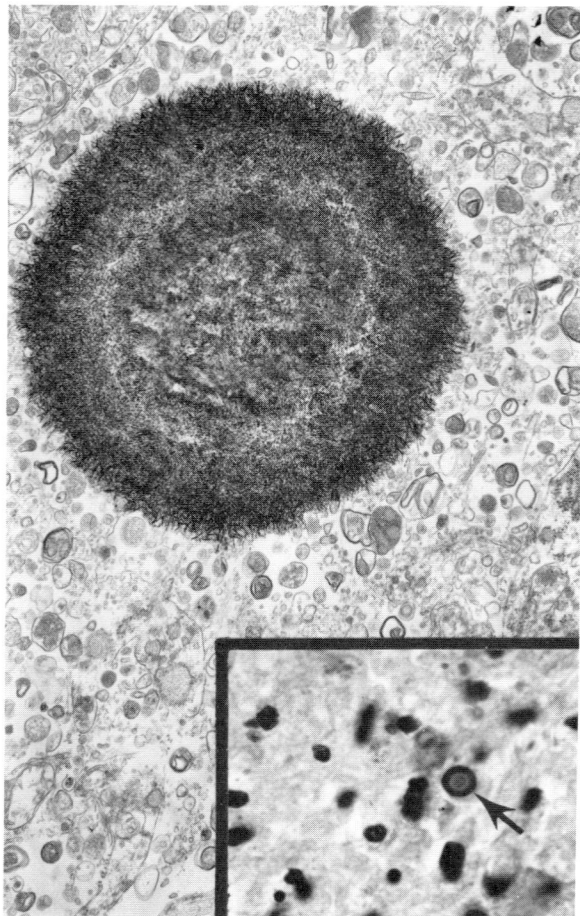

Figure 6–99. In malacoplakia, characteristic Michaelis-Gutmann bodies can be seen histologically (inset arrow) and ultrastructurally. (Courtesy of Dr. A. Ferenczy, McGill University, Montreal, Canada.)

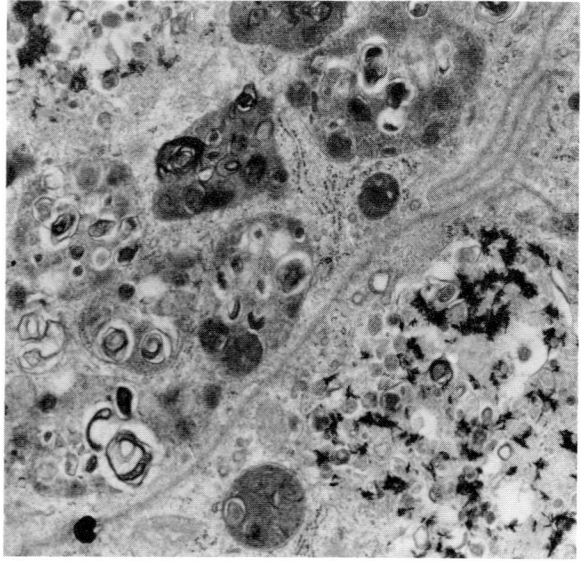

Figure 6–100. Portions of Hansemann cells with large numbers of lysosomes and telolysosomes. (Courtesy of Dr. E. Kuthy, University of Mediou, Szegel, Hungary.)

All the RNA viruses, with the exception of myxoviruses, are assembled in the cytoplasm and produce inclusions in this region. Even the small, nonenveloped RNA viruses, such as polio-,[432] and echoviruses, produce large inclusions in the cytoplasm. In both herpes, a DNA virus, and rubella, an RNA virus, nucleocapsids can be seen in the ER. Murine leukemia virus appears in the ER cisterna in Ehrlich ascites cells. Hepatitis B virus structural components may be seen ultrastructurally in liver cells, including core particles in nuclei and surface antigen within ER cisternae.[433]

Malacoplakia

A rare chronic inflammatory disease, *malacoplakia*,[375] is classically seen in the genitourinary tract.[434] This disorder is characterized by special phagosomal activity of the macrophage cells that give rise to the *Hansemann cells* and then to the *Michaelis-Gutmann body* (Figs. 6–99 and 6–100). The latter is formed by gradual calcification of the material in the phagolysosome.[435]

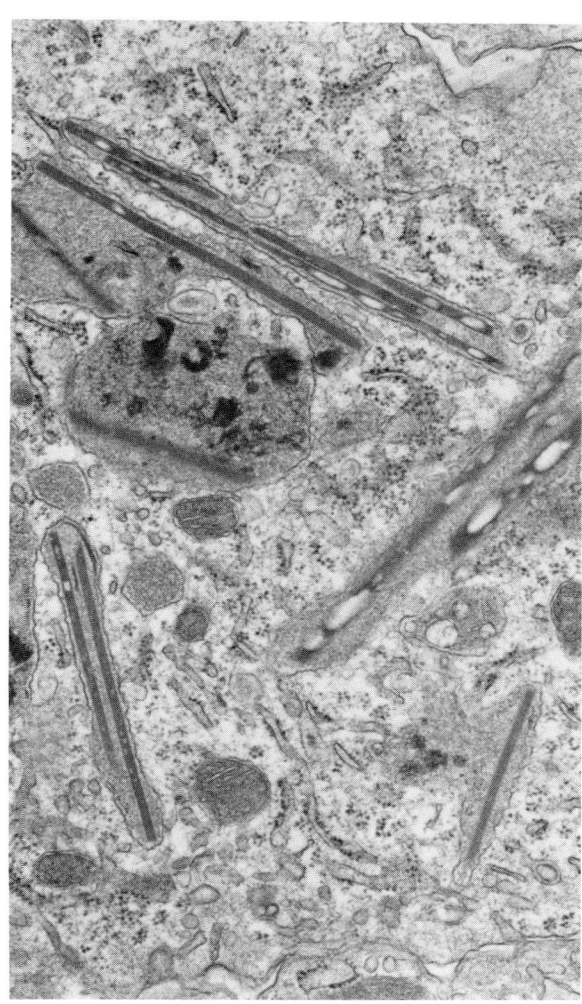

Figure 6–101. Alveolar macrophages with crystalline structures in the GERL of a beige mouse. (Courtesy of Dr. E. Essner, Wayne State University, Michigan.)

Two types of cytoplasmic inclusions are present in this disease: PAS-positive granules, corresponding to phagolysosomes, and Michaelis-Gutmann bodies, which develop later within the lysosomes. The cells that contain these structures are known as *Hansemann macrophages. Bacteria,* usually E. coli or klebsiella, are phagocytosed by malacoplakic macrophages and are incorporated into *phagolysosomes* in which they are incompletely digested.[436] The bacteria persist as dense amorphous aggregates, and the phospholipid membranes become encrusted with calcium phosphate crystals.[437]

Some postulate that the intralysosomal digestion processes are impaired by a defect in lysosomal acidification processes. Defective microtubular-mediated phagocytic function has also been implicated.[438] Ultrastructurally, tetrad-shaped particles resembling ferritin may be present; however, immunocytohistochemical reactions indicate that glycolipids are the main constituents of these particles.

Michaelis-Gutmann bodies have been noted in the gastrointestinal, genitourinary, respiratory, and lymphoreticular systems. Although some researchers suggest that these deposits are only remnants of phagocytosed E. coli, others believe that these bodies also contain erythrocyte membranes as well as degenerated cellular organelles.

Crystal Inclusions

One frequently sees large, amorphous intracellular crystalline or tubular deposits, presumably representing altered glycolipids, protein, or nuclear proteins (Fig. 6–101).

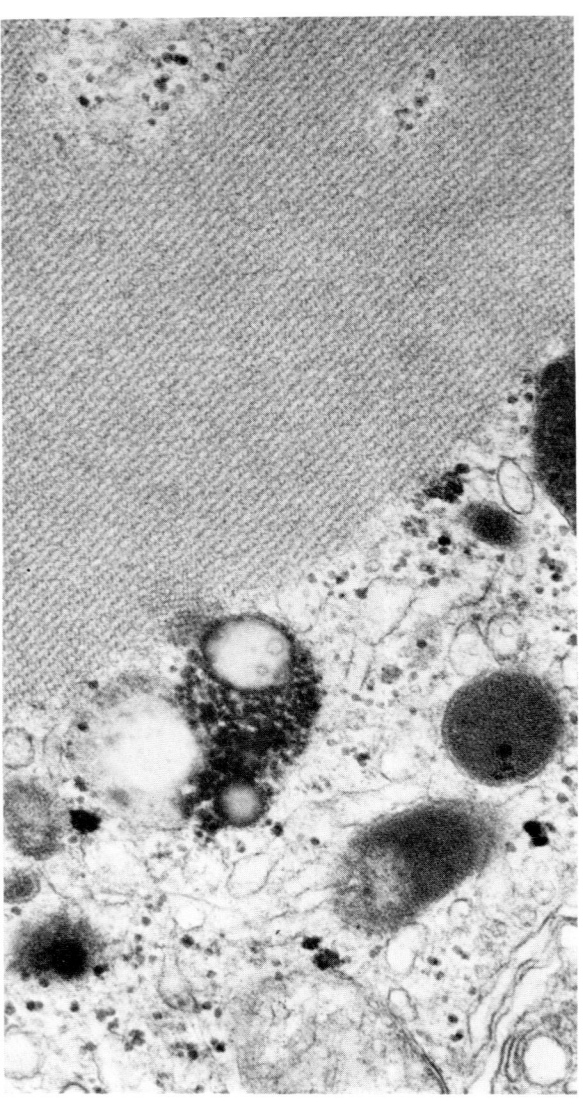

Figure 6–102. Interstitial cell with a Reinke crystal. A prominent latticework is present within the crystal. (Courtesy of Dr. A. Ferenczy, McGill University, Montreal, Canada.)

Reinke Crystals

Among the most interesting crystals are the *Reinke crystals,* which von Winiwarter calls *"rice-form bodies."*[438a] They are hexagonal units composed of filaments 50 Å thick (Fig. 6–102). Reinke crystals are not associated with the SER, so that they differ from crystals occurring in other steroid-producing cells. They are seen in interstitial cells of the testis or the ovarian hilus, or in tumors derived from them.[439]

A similar structure is the *crystal of Lubarsch,* a filament of 130 to 450 Å, which appears in the spermatogonia of the human testis.[440] Similar crystalline deposits have been seen in the lymphocytes of peripheral blood in Down's syndrome and in L cells treated with vinca alkaloid. These deposits may represent microtubular degeneration.

Tyrosine, Uric Acid, and Pyrophosphate Crystals

Tyrosine crystals have been identified in *salivary gland tumors* and in normal fibroid tissues.[441] *Uric acid* crystals are commonly deposited in *gout.*[442] In pseudogout the tissue is infiltrated with calcium pyrophosphate crystals. The products of *porphyrin* metabolism are deposited in the liver as needle-like inclusions in *porphyria cutanea tarda.*[443]

Lattice Crystalline Deposits

Lattice crystalline deposits of unknown constituents, appearing in spherical or cylindrical forms, have been noted in mitochondria both of the renal tubules and of the liver associated with obstructive jaundice, viral hepatitis, alcoholism, diabetes, and other diseases.[444]

It is not uncommon to find crystals arranged in lattice-like arrays either in the nucleus or the cytoplasm. In many instances, they represent viral particles. In other diseases, such as multiple sclerosis or systemic lupus erythematosus, such crystals may or may not represent degenerated viruses.

Crystals may be induced experimentally by the administration of *drugs,* such as *parachlorophenylalanine,* or by injection of *kappa light chains* of immunoglobulins.[445]

REFERENCES

1. Singer, S.J., and Nicolson, G.L.: The fluid mosaic model of the structure of cell membranes. Science, *175*:720, 1972.
2. Scott, R.E., and Furcht, L.T.: Membrane pathology of normal and malignant cells. A review. Hum. Pathol., *7*:519, 1976.
3. Cooper, R.A.: Abnormalities of cell membrane fluidity in the pathogenesis of disease. N. Engl. J. Med., *297*:371, 1977.
4. Jackson, R.L., and Gotto, A.M.: Phospholipids in biology and medicine. N. Engl. J. Med., *290*:24, 1974.
5. Chiu, T-C., and Babitch, J.A.: Protein asymmetry in chick synaptosomal plasma membrane. J. Biol. Chem., *252*:3862, 1977.
6. Fowler, V., and Branton, D.: Lateral mobility of human erythrocyte integral membrane proteins. Nature, *268*:23, 1977.

7. Marchesi, V.T.: Recent membrane research and its implications for clinical medicine. Annu. Rev. Med., 29:593, 1978.
8. Da Silva, P.P., and Nicolson, G.L.: Freeze-etch localization of concanavalin A receptors to the membrane intercalated particles of human erythrocyte ghost membranes. Biochim. Biophys. Acta, 363:311, 1974.
9. Prives, J., and Shinitzky, J.: Increased membrane fluidity precedes fusion of muscle cells. Nature, 268:761, 1977.
10. Inbar, M., et al.: Fluidity difference of membrane lipids in human normal and leukemic lymphocytes as controlled by serum components. Cancer Res., 37:3037, 1977.
11. Miller, J.B., and Koshland, D.E., Jr.: Membrane fluidity and chemotaxis: effects of temperature and membrane lipid composition on the swimming behavior of Salmonella typhimurium and Escherichia coli. J. Mol. Biol., 111:183, 1977.
12. Frye, L.D., and Edidin, M.: The rapid intermixing of cell surface antigens after formation of mouse human heterokaryons. J. Cell Sci., 7:319, 1970.
13. Pontecorvo, G., Croce, C., and Sisskin, E.: Cell fusion. Adv. Pathobiol., 6:258, 1977.
14. Okada, Y., et al.: Specific movement of cell membranes fused with HVJ (Sendai virus). Proc. Natl. Acad. Sci. USA, 71:2043, 1974.
15. Herman, B.A., and Fernandez, S.M.: Changes in membrane dynamics associated with myogenic cell fusion. J. Cell. Physiol., 94:253, 1978.
16. Linthicum, D.S., et al.: Endocytosis and exocytosis of phytohemagglutinin (PHA) cell surface receptors of human lymphocytes during blast transformation. Exp. Cell Res., 110:237, 1977.
17. Marchesi, V.T.: Topical review. Spectrin: present status of a putative cyto-skeletal protein of the red cell membrane. J. Membr. Biol., 51:101, 1979.
18. Jacob, H.S.: Tightening red cell membranes. N. Engl. J. Med., 294:1234, 1974.
19. Bennett, V., and Stenbuck, P.J.: The membrane attachment protein for spectrin is associated with band 3 in human erythrocyte membranes. Nature, 280:468, 1979.
20. Nicolson, G.L., and Painter, R.G.: Ionic sites of human erythrocyte membranes. Antispectrin-induced transmembrane aggregation of the binding sites for positively charged colloidal particles. J. Cell Biol., 59:395, 1973.
21. Mircevova, L.: The role of Mg^{++}-ATPase (actinomysin-like protein) in maintaining the biconcave shape of erythrocytes. Blut, 35:323, 1977.
22. Tannenbaum, J., Tannenbaum, S.W., and Godman, G.C.: The binding sites of cytochalasin D. I. Evidence that they may be peripheral membrane proteins. J. Cell. Physiol., 91:225, 1977.
23. Tannenbaum, J. Tannenbaum, S.W., and Godman, G.C.: The binding sites of cytochalasin D. II. Their relationship to hexose transport and to cytochalasin B. J. Cell. Physiol., 91:239, 1977.
24. Franke, W.W., et al.: Paracrystalline arrays of membrane-to-membrane cross bridges associated with the inner surface of plasma membrane. J. Cell Biol., 77:232, 1978.
25. Spicer, S.S., and Schulte, B.A.: Identification of cell surface constituents. Lab. Invest., 47:2, 1982.
26. Ito, S.: Form and function of the glycocalyx on free cell surfaces. Philos. Trans. R. Soc. Lond. [Biol.], 268:55, 1974.
27. Hosey, M.M., and Tao, M.: Protein kinases of rabbit and human erythrocyte membranes. Solubilization and characterization. Biochim. Biophys. Acta, 482:348, 1976.
28. Hosey, M.M., and Tao, M.: Phosphorylation of rabbit and human erythrocyte membranes by soluble adenosine 3':5'-monophosphate-dependent and -independent protein kinases. J. Biol. Chem., 252:102, 1977.
29. Snyder, S.H.: Receptors, neurotransmitters and drug responses. N. Engl. J. Med., 300:465, 1979.
30. Bennett, J.: Drug receptors and their effectors. Nature, 285:192, 1980.
31. Pietras, R.J., and Szego, C.M.: Specific binding sites for oestrogen at the outer surfaces of isolated endometrial cells. Nature, 265:69, 1977.
32. Kahn, C.R.: Membrane receptors for hormones and neurotransmitters. J. Cell Biol., 70:261, 1976.

33. Kolata, G.B.: Cyclic GMP: cellular regulatory agent? Science, *182*:149, 1973.
34. Valdimarsson, H., Agnarsdottir, G., and Lachmann, P.J.: Measles virus receptor on human T lymphocytes. Nature, *225*:554, 1975.
35. Miller, L.H., et al.: Erythrocyte receptors for *(Plasmodium knowlesi)* malaria: Duffy blood group determinants. Science, *189*:561, 1975.
36. Hart, D.A.: Evidence for the non-protein nature of the receptor for the enterotoxin of *Vibrio cholerae* on murine lymphoid cells. Infect. Immun. *11*:742, 1975.
37. Sharon, N.: Lectins as mitogen. *In* Mitogens in Immunobiology. Edited by J.J. Oppenheim and D.L. Rosentereich. New York, Academic Press, 1976.
38. Snyder, S.M.: Opiate receptors in the brain. N. Engl. J. Med., *296*:266, 1977.
39. Loh, H.H., et al.: Possible involvement of cerebroside sulfate in opiate receptor binding. Fed. Proc., *37*:147, 1978.
40. Simon, E.J., and Miller, J.M.: *In vitro* studies on opiate receptors and their ligands. Fed. Proc., *37*:141, 1978.
41. Akera, T.: Membrane adenosinetriphosphatase: a digitalis receptor? Science, *198*:569, 1977.
42. Anderson, R.G.W., Goldstein, J.S., and Brown, M.S.: A mutation that impairs the ability of lipoprotein receptors to localize in coated pits on the cell surface of human fibroblasts. Nature, *270*:695, 1977.
43. Greaves, M.F.: Membrane receptor-adenylate cyclase relationships. Nature, *265*:681, 1977.
44. Haga, T., et al.: Adenylate cyclase permanently uncoupled from hormone receptors in a novel variant of A49 mouse lymphoma cells. Proc. Natl. Acad. Sci. USA, *74*:2016, 1977.
45. Korenbrot, J.I.: Ion transport in membranes: incorporation of biological ion-translocating proteins in model membrane systems. Annu. Rev. Physiol., *39*:19, 1977.
46. Carlsen, S.A., Till, J.E., and Ling, V.: Modulation of membrane drug permeability of Chinese hamster ovary cells. Biochim. Biophys. Acta, *455*:900, 1976.
47. McNamee, M.G., and McConnell, H.M.: Transmembrane potentials and phospholipid flip-flop in excitable membrane vesicles. Biochemistry, *12*:2951, 1973.
48. Kovacs, L., Rios, E., and Schneider, M.F.: Calcium transients and intramembrane charge movement in skeletal muscle fibres. Nature, *279*:391, 1979.
49. Farquhar, M.G., and Palade, G.E.: Junctional complexes in various epithelia. J. Cell Biol., *17*:375, 1963.
50. Friend, D.S., and Gilula, N.B.: Variations in tight and gap junction in mammalian tissues. J. Cell Biol., *53*:758, 1972.
51. Copeland, D.D., Bell, S.W., and Shelburne, J.D.: Hemidesmosome-like intercellular specializations in human meningiomas. Cancer, *41*:2248, 1978.
52. Pannese, E., et al.: Intercellular junctions and other membrane specializations in developing spinal ganglia: a freeze-fracture study. J. Ultrastruct. Res., *60*:169, 1977.
53. Kelley, B.O.: Development of the aging cell surface: a freeze-fracture analysis of gap junctions between human embryo fibroblasts aging in culture. A brief note. Mech. Aging Dev., *5*:339, 1976.
54. Dallai, G.: Septate and continuous junctions associated in the same epithelium. J. Submicrosc. Cytol., *8*:163, 1976.
55. Fukushima, M.: Intercellular junctions in the human developing preovulatory follicle and corpus luteum. Int. J. Fertil., *22*:206, 1977.
56. Korneliussen, H.: Tubules invaginating from the sarcolemma in the subneural region of muscle fibers. Cell Tissue Res., *181*:73, 1977.
57. Mokri, B., and Engel, A.G.: Duchenne dystrophy: electron microscopic findings pointing to a basic or early abnormality in the plasma membrane of the muscle fiber. Neurology, *25*:1111, 1975.
58. Palek, J.: Red cell membrane injury in sickle cell anaemia. Br. J. Haematol., *35*:1, 1977.
59. Markesbery, W.R., and Butterfield, D.A.: Scanning electron microscopy studies of erythrocytes in Huntington's disease. Biochem. Biophys. Res. Commun., *78*:560, 1977.
60. Pickard, N.A., et al.: Systemic membrane defect in the proximal muscular dystrophies. N. Engl. J. Med., *299*:841, 1978.
61. Brown, M.S., and Goldstein, J.L.: Familial hypercholesterolemia: a genetic defect in the low density lipoprotein receptor. N. Engl. J. Med., *294*:1386, 1976.

62. Orci, L., et al.: Occurrence of low density lipoprotein receptors within large pits on the surface of human fibroblasts as demonstrated by freeze-etching. Exp. Cell Res., *113*:1, 1978.

63. Goldstein, J.L., Anderson, R.G.W., and Brown, M.S.: Coated pits, coated vesicles, and receptor-mediated endocytosis. A review article. Nature, *279*:679, 1979.

64. Segal, S.: Disorders of renal amino acid transport. N. Engl. J. Med., *294*:1044, 1976.

65. El-Mofty, S.K., et al.: Early, reversible plasma membrane injury in galactosamine induced liver cell death. Am. J. Pathol., *79*:579, 1975.

66. Dingle, J.T.: Studies on the mode of action of excess of vitamin A. 3. Release of a bound protease by the action of vitamin A. Biochem. J., *79*:509, 1961.

67. Farrow, S.P., and Lawrence, J.C.: Thermal injury and the sodium, potassium and water exchanges of skin. Br. J. Exp. Pathol., *58*:327, 1977.

68. Hansen, H.J.M., Karle, H., and Stender, S.: The effect *in vitro* of ionizing irradiation and small rises in temperature on the uptake and release of labelled lipids by the human erythrocyte membrane. Biochim. Biophys. Acta, *528*:230, 1978.

69. Metz, J., et al.: Morphological alterations and functional changes of interhepatocellular junctions induced by bile duct ligation. Cell Tissue Res., *182*:299, 1977.

70. Ashraf, M., and Halverson, C.A.: Structural changes in the freeze-fractured sarcolemma of ischemic myocardium. Am. J. Pathol., *88*:583, 1977.

71. Seeman, P., Cheng, D., and Iles, G.H.: Structure of membrane holes in osmotic and saponin hemolysis. J. Cell Biol., *56*:519, 1973.

72. Okada, Y., et al.: Modification of cell membranes with viral envelopes during fusion of cells with HVJ (Sendai virus). Exp. Cell Res., *93*:368, 1975.

73. Morgan, C., et al.: The application of ferritin-conjugated antibody to electron microscopic studies of influenza virus in infected cells. II. The interior of the cell. J. Exp. Med., *114*:833, 1961.

74. Norkin, L.C.: Cell killing by simian virus 40: impairment of membrane formation and function. J. Virol., *21*:872, 1977.

75. Deisseroth, A.: Isolation of hybrid cells that exhibit markers of erythroid differentiation. N. Engl. J. Med., *294*:148, 1976.

76. Grant, C.K., et al.: Lysis of feline lymphoma cells by complement-dependent antibodies in feline leukemia virus contact cats. Correlation of lysis and antibodies to feline oncornavirus-associated cell membrane antigen. J.N.C.I., *60*:161, 1978.

77. Nakazawa, A., and Suzuki, N.: Induction of colicin E1 synthesis in recombination-defective mutants in both the RecBC and RecF pathways. J. Bacteriol., *131*:1011, 1977.

78. Calabrese, V.P.: The effect of small quantities of phospholipase C on ionic and protein permeabilities of red cell membranes. Physiol. Chem. Phys., *8*:285, 1976.

79. Wadstrom, T., and Jeljaszewicz, J.: Bacterial Toxins and Cell Membranes. London, Academic Press, 1978.

80. Singer, S.J.: Structure of membranes. Adv. Pathobiol., *1*:5, 1975.

81. Appleton, J.C., and Kemp, R.B.: Effects of cytochalasins on the initial aggregation *in vitro* of embryonic chick cells. J. Cell Sci., *14*:187, 1974.

82. Stagno, P.A., and Low, F.N.: Effects of cytochalasin B on the fine structure of organized endodermal cells of the early chick embryo. Am. J. Anat., *151*:159, 1978.

83. Smuckler, E.A., Koplitz, M., and Striker, G.E.: Cellular adenosine triphosphate levels in liver and kidney during CCl₄ intoxication. Lab. Invest., *19*:218, 1968.

84. Repke, K.: Influence of cardioactive principles on pump ATP-ases. *In* Proceedings of the First International Pharmacological Meeting. Vo. 3. New Aspects of Cardiac Glycosides. Edited by W. Wilbrandt and P. Lindgren. Oxford, Pergamon Press, 1963.

85. Carlsen, S.A., Till, J.E., and Ling, V.: Modulation of drug permeability in Chinese hamster ovary cells. Possible role for phosphorylation of surface glycoproteins. Biochim. Biophys. Acta, *467*:238, 1977.

86. Marchand, A., et al.: Studies on the mechanism of lithium action: preliminary report. Commun. Psychopharmacol. Comm., *1*:139, 1975.

87. Scott, R.E., and Maercklein, P.B.: Plasma membrane vesiculation: correlation between macrophage spreading and the shedding of cell surface vesicles. Lab. Invest., *37*:430, 1977.

88. Hammer, C.H., Nicholson, A., and Mayer, M.M.: On the mechanism of cytolysis by complement: evidence on insertion of C5b and C7 subunits of the C5b,6,7 complex into phospholipid bilayers of erythrocyte membranes. Proc. Natl. Acad. Sci. USA, *72*:5076, 1975.

89. Muller-Eberhard, H.J.: Chemistry and function of the complement system. Hosp. Pract., *12*:33, 1977.

90. Law, S.K., and Levine, R.P.: Interaction between the third complement protein and cell surface macromolecules. Proc. Natl. Acad. Sci. USA, *74*:2701, 1977.

91. Hu, C.H., Michel, B., and Schiltz, J.R.: Epidermal acantholysis induced *in vitro* by pemphigus autoantibody: an ultrastructural study. Am. J. Pathol., *90*:345, 1978.

92. Nordheim, A., et al.: Antibodies to left-handed Z-DNA bind to interband regions of *Drosophila* polytene chromosomes. Nature, *294*:417, 1981.

93. Gurley, L.R., et al.: Heterochromatin and histone phosphorylation. Exp. Cell Res., *111*:373, 1978.

94. Weisbrod, S.: Active chromatin. Nature, *297*:289, 1982.

95. Poon, N.H., and Seligy, V.L.: Comparative bright field microscopy of isolated nucleosomes, ribosomes and histone aggregates. Exp. Cell Res., *113*:95, 1978.

96. Axel, R.: Transcription and chromatin subunit structure. Adv. Pathobiol., *3*:27, 1976.

97. Musich, P.R., Brown, L., and Maio, J.: Subunit structure of chromatin and the organization of eukaryotic highly repetitive DNA: nucleosomal proteins associated with a highly repetitive mammalian DNA. Proc. Natl. Acad. Sci. USA, *74*:3297, 1977.

98. Philip, M., et al.: Nucleosome core histone complex isolated gently and rapidly in 2 M NaCl is octameric. Proc. Natl. Acad. Sci. USA, *10*:5178, 1979.

99. Weintraub, H.: Assembly of an active chromatin structure during replication. Nucleic Acids Res., *7*:781, 1979.

100. Ris, H.: Chromosome structure. Adv. Pathobiol., *3*:5, 1976.

101. Latt, S.A.: Localization of sister chromatid exchanges in human chromosomes. Science, *185*:74, 1974.

102. Lewin, R.: Repeated DNA still in search of a function. Science, *217*:621, 1982.

103. Kuo, M.R., Meinke, W., and Saunders, G.F.: Localization of cytoplasmic-membrane-associated DNA in human chromosomes. Proc. Natl. Acad. Sci. USA, *72*:5004, 1975.

104. Huberman, J.A., and Riggs, A.D.: On the mechanism of DNA replication in mammalian chromosomes. J. Mol. Biol., *32*:327, 1968.

105. Carter, M., and Ross, P.M.: Cutaneous DNA damage and repair. *In* Biochemistry and Physiology of the Skin. Edited by L.A. Goldsmith. New York, Oxford University Press, 1982.

106. Ruddle, F.H.: A new era in mammalian gene mapping: somatic cell genetics and recombinant DNA methodologies. Nature, *294*:115, 1981.

107. Borek, E.: Possible role of nucleic acid methylases in the induction of cancer. Cancer Res., *31*:641, 1971.

108. Miller, O.J., et al.: Chromosome identification. Nobel Symposium 23. New York, Academic Press, 1973.

109. Gilbert, W.: DNA sequencing and gene structure. Science, *214*:1305, 1981.

110. Kabat, E.A., Wu, T.T., and Bilofsky, H.: Evidence supporting somatic assembly of the DNA segments (minigenes), coding for the framework, and complementarity-determining segments of immunoglobulin variable regions. J. Exp. Med., *149*:1299, 1979.

111. Schimke, R.T.: Gene amplification and drug resistance. Experiments on the development of drug resistance in cultured mammalian cells serve as a laboratory model of the mechanism whereby duplicate genes are created in the course of evolution. Sci. Am., *243*:60, 1980.

112. Maniatis, T., et al.: The isolation of structural genes from libraries of eukaryotic DNA. Cell, *15*:687, 1978.

113. Goessens, G.: The nucleolar fibrillar centres in various cell types *in vivo* or *in vitro*. Cell Tissue Res., *173*:315, 1976.

114. Rao, M.S., Rothblum, L.I., and Busch, H.: Presence of elongation factor 1 in nuclei and nucleoli of rat liver. Cell Biol. Int. Rep., *2*:25, 1978.

115. Ghosh, S.: The nucleolar structure. Int. Rev. Cytol., *44*:1, 1976.
116. Ghosh, S., Paweletz, N., and Ghosh, I.: Cytological identification and characterization of the nuclear matrix. Exp. Cell Res., *111*:363, 1978.
117. Monk, M.: Biochemical studies on mammalian X chromosome activity. *In* Development in Mammals. Vol. 3. Edited by M.H. Johnson. New York, North Holland Publishing, 1978.
118. Virtanen, I., and Wartiovaara, J.: Lectin receptor sites on rat liver cell nuclear membranes. J. Cell Sci., *22*:335, 1976.
119. Kirschner, R.H., Rusli, M., and Martin, T.E.: Characterization of the nuclear envelope, pore complexes, and dense lamina of mouse liver nuclei by high resolution scanning electron microscopy. J. Cell Biol., *72*:118, 1977.
120. Abelson, H.T., and Smith, G.H.: Nuclear pores: the pore-annulus relationship in thin section. J. Ultrastruct. Res., *30*:558, 1970.
121. Pickett-Heaps, J.D., Tippet, D.H., and Porter, K.R.: Rethinking mitosis. Cell, *29*:729, 1982.
122. Hastings, P.J., Quah, S-K., and Von Borstel, R.C.: Spontaneous mutation by mutagenic repair of spontaneous lesions in DNA. Nature, *264*:719, 1976.
123. Lehmann, A.R., and Stevens, S.: The production and repair of double strand breaks in cells from normal humans and from patients with ataxia telangiectasia. Biochim. Biophys. Acta, *474*:49, 1977.
124. Lambert, B., and Ringborg, U.: Review article: DNA repair and human disease. Acta Med. Scand., *200*:433, 1976.
125. Darzynkiewicz, A., et al.: Different sensitivity of DNA *in situ* in interphase and metaphase chromatin to heat denaturation. J. Cell Biol., *73*:128, 1977.
126. Roth, D., and London, M.: Acridine probe study into synergistic DNA-denaturing action of heat and ultraviolet light in squamous cells. J. Invest. Dermatol., *69*:368, 1977.
127. Tan, J.C., Huang, C.C., and Fiel, R.J.: Effects of radiation and porphyrin on mitosis and chromosomes in human hematopoietic cell lines. J. Med., *7*:169, 1976.
128. Day, R.S.: Xeroderma pigmentosum variants have decreased repair of ultraviolet-damaged DNA. Nature, *253*:748, 1975.
129. Chan, G.L., and Little, J.B.: Induction of oncogenic transformation *in vitro* by ultraviolet light. Nature, *264*:442, 1976.
130. Cohen, S.S.: On biochemical variability and innovation. Science, *139*:1017, 1963.
131. Kato, H., and Sandberg, A.A.: Chromosome pulverization in human binucleate cells following colcemid treatment. J. Cell Biol., *34*:35, 1967.
132. Rebhun, L.I.: Cyclic nucleotides, calcium, and cell division. Int. Rev. Cytol., *49*:1, 1977.
133. Freed, J.J., and Schatz, S.A.: Chromosome aberrations in cultured cells deprived of single essential amino acids. Exp. Cell Res., *55*:359, 1969.
134. Kaplan, J.C., Zamansky, G.B., and Black, P.H.: Parallel induction of sister chromatid exchanges and infectious virus from SV40-transformed cells by alkylating agents. Nature, *271*:662, 1978.
135. Nichols, W.W.: Virus-induced chromosome abnormalities. Annu. Rev. Microbiol., *24*:479, 1970.
136. Wolinsky, S., et al.: Ultrastructure of mumps virus replication in newborn hamster central nervous system. Lab. Invest., *31*:403, 1974.
137. Stenram, U.: Autoradiographic, biochemical, and ultrastructural studies into the effect of actinomycin, 5-fluorouracil, and adenosine on nucleolar and cellular structure and function. Natl. Cancer Inst. Monogr., *23*:379, 1966.
138. Kähkönen, M., et al.: Mutagenicity of Bacillus thuringiensis exotoxin III. Sister chromatid exchange in rats *in vivo*. Hereditas, *91*:1, 1979.
139. Nagatsum, M., Richart, R.M., and Lambert, A.: Effects of bleomycin on the cell cycle of Ehrlich ascites carcinoma. Cancer Res., *32*:1966, 1972.
140. Iverson, O.H., et al.: Effects of bleomycin on the epidermal content of growth-regulatory substances (chalones). Cell Tissue Kinet., *10*:71, 1977.
141. Von Hoff, D.D., Slavik, M., and Muggie, F.M.: 5-Azacytidine: a new anticancer drug with effectiveness in acute myelogenous leukemia. Ann. Intern. Med., *85*:237, 1976.
142. Moreno Diaz de la Espina, S., and Risueno, M.C.: Observations of a certain arrangement in the nucleolar chromatin after continuous ethidium bromide treatment. Experientia, *33*:1033, 1977.

143. Fritzler, M.J., and Tan, E.M.: Antibodies to histones in drug-induced and idiopathic lupus erythematosus. J. Clin. Invest., 62:560, 1978.

144. Godman, G.: The effect of colchicine on striated muscle in tissue culture. Exp. Cell Res., 8:488, 1955.

145. Brasch, K., and Sinclair, G.D.: The organization, composition and matrix of hepatocyte nuclei exposed to x-amanitin. Virchows Arch. [Cell Pathol.,], 27:193, 1978.

146. O'Malley, B.W., et al.: Effects of steroid hormone receptors on gene transcription. Adv. Pathobiol., 6:79, 1977.

147. Ferenczy, A., and Richart, R.M.: Female Reproductive System: Dynamics of Scan and Transmission Electron Microscopy. New York, John Wiley & Sons, 1974.

148. Alspaugh, M.A., and Miller, J.J.: Study of specificities of antinuclear antibodies in juvenile rheumatoid arthritis. J. Pediatr., 90:391, 1977.

149. Nakamura, R.M., and Tan, E.M.: Recent progress in the study of autoantibodies to nuclear antigens. Hum. Pathol., 9:85, 1978.

150. Tatal, N., et al.: Biological significance of IgM and IgG antibodies to DNA and RNA in autoimmune disease. Am. J. Clin. Pathol., 68:643, 1977.

151. Gerber, M.A., Sarno, E., and Vernace, S.J.: Immune complexes in hepatocyte nuclei of HB Ag-positive chronic hepatitis. N. Engl. J. Med., 294:922, 1976.

152. Novikoff, A.B.: The endoplasmic reticulum: a cytochemist's view (a review). Proc. Natl. Acad. Sci. USA, 73:2781, 1976.

153. Lake, J.A.: The ribosome. Sci. Am., 245:84, 1981.

154. Frank, J., Verschoor, A., and Boublik, M.: Computer averaging of electron micrographs of 40S ribosomal subunits. Science, 214:1353, 1981.

155. Warner, J.R., Knof, P.M., and Rich, A.: A multiple ribosomal structure in protein synthesis. Proc. Natl. Acad. Sci. USA, 49:122, 1963.

156. Kreibich, G., and Sabatini, D.D.: Microsomal membranes and the translational apparatus of eukaryotic cells. Fed. Proc., 32:2133, 1973.

157. Unwin, P.N.T.: Three-dimensional model of membrane-bound ribosomes obtained by electron microscopy. Nature, 269:118, 1977.

158. Chedid, A., and Nair, V.: Diurnal rhythm in endoplasmic reticulum of rat liver: electron microscopy study. Science, 175:176, 1972.

159. Waley, W.G.: The Golgi Apparatus. Vol. 2. Cell Biology Monographs. New York, Springer-Verlag, 1975.

160. Godman, G., and Lane, N.: On the site of sulfation in the chondrocyte. J. Cell Biol., 21:353, 1964.

161. Dallner, G., Siekevitz, P., and Palade, G.E.: Biogenesis of endoplasmic reticulum membranes. I. Structural and chemical differentiation in developing rat hepatocyte. II. Synthesis of constitutive microsomal enzymes in developing rat hepatocyte. J. Cell Biol., 30:73, 97, 1966.

162. Eagon, P.K., and Heath, E.C.: Glycoprotein biosynthesis in myeloma cells. J. Biol. Chem., 252:2372, 1977.

163. Shimotohno, K., et al.: Importance of 5'-terminal blocking structure to stabilize mRNA in eukaryotic protein synthesis. Proc. Natl. Acad. Sci. USA, 74:2734, 1977.

164. Tate. W.P., and Caskey, C.T.: The mechanism of peptide chain termination. Mol. Cell. Biochem., 5:115, 1974.

165. Jackson, R.C., and Blobel, G.: Post-translational cleavage of presecretory proteins with an extract of rough microsomes from dog pancreas containing signal peptidase activity. Proc. Natl. Acad. Sci. USA, 74:5598, 1977.

166. Campbell, P.N., and Blobel, G.: The role of organelles in the chemical modification of the primary translation products of secretory proteins. FEBS Lett., 72:215, 1976.

167. Caskey, C.T., and Konecki, D.S.: Release factor binding to ribosome requires an intact 16S rRNA 3' terminus. J. Biol. Chem., 252:4435, 1977.

168. Sabatini, D.D., et al.: Mechanisms for the incorporation of proteins in membranes and organelles. J. Cell Biol., 92:1, 1982.

169. Jamieson, J.D., and Palade, G.E.: Production of secretory proteins in animal cells. In International Congress on Cell Biology Symposium. Edited by B.R. Brinkley and K.R. Porter. New York, Rockefeller University Press, 1977.

170. Morse, J.O.: Alpha₁-antitrypsin deficiency. N. Engl. J. Med., 299:1045 & 1099, 1978.

171. Clawson, C.C., Repine, J.E., and White, J.G.: The Chediak-Higashi

syndrome. Quantitation of a deficiency in maximal bactericidal capacity. Am. J. Pathol., *94*:539, 1979.

172. Bernelli-Zazzero, A., et al.: Further studies on ribosomal damage in liver ischemia. Exp. Mol. Pathol., *17*:121, 1972.

173. Tappel, A.L.: Lipid peroxidation damage to cell components. Fed. Proc., *32*:1870, 1973.

174. Hamberg, H., et al.: Cytoplasmic effects of x-irradiation on cultured cells in nondividing stage. I. Establishment of an experimental model. Acta Pathol. Microbiol. Scand. [A], *84*:201, 1976.

175. Hamberg, H., et al.: Cytoplasmic effects of x-irradiation on cultured cells. 2. Alterations in lysosomes, plasma membrane, Golgi apparatus, and related structures. Acta Pathol. Microbiol. Scand. [A], *85*:625, 1977.

176. Sidranksy, H.: Regulatory effect of amino acids on polyribosomes and protein synthesis of liver. Prog. Liver Dis., *4*:31, 1973.

177. Ramsey, J.C., and Steele, W.J.: Effect of starvation on the distribution of free and membrane-bound ribosomes in rat liver and on the content of phospholipid and glycogen in purified ribosomes. Biochim. Biophys. Acta, *447*:312, 1976.

178. Scott, E.B.: Histopathology of amino acid deficiencies. IX. The ultrastructure of the Leydig cells of rats receiving lysine-deficient or hypocaloric diets. Arch. Pathol., *90*:294, 1970.

179. Estes, L., and Lombardi, B.: Effect of choline deficiency on the Golgi apparatus of rat hepatocytes. Lab. Invest., *21*:374, 1969.

180. Bollesman, R.A., et al.: Ribosomal proteins in normal simian cells infected with SV40, adenovirus 5, and vesicular stomatitis virus. Intervirology, *9*:8, 1978.

181. Bouquet, P., and Pappenheimer, A.M., Jr.: Interaction of diphtheria toxin with mammalian cell membranes. J. Biol. Chem., *251*:5770, 1976.

182. Daskal, I., et al.: The effects of cycloheximide on the ultrastructure of rat liver cells. Exp. Cell Res., *93*:395, 1975.

183. Gonzalez-Cadavid, N.F., and Quijada, F.H.: Inhibition of translation in liver polyribosomes by a new substituted thiopseudourea with antitumour action. Biochem. J., *138*:129, 1974.

184. Tsurugi, K., and Ogata, K.: Preferential degradation of newly synthesized ribosomal proteins in rat liver treated with a low dose of actinomycin D. Biochem. Biophys. Res. Commun., *75*:525, 1977.

185. Van Venrooij, W.J., Eenbergen, J., and Janssen, A.P.M.: Effect of anisomycin on the cellular level of native ribosomal subunits. Biochemistry, *16*:2343, 1977.

186. Aterman, K., and Yüce, G.: Hepatoprotective substances: a partial assessment. *In* Pathogenesis and Mechanisms of Liver Cell Necrosis. Edited by D. Keppler. Baltimore, University Park Press, 1975.

187. Jones, A.L., and Fawcett, D.W.: Hypertrophy of the agranular endoplasmic reticulum in hamster liver induced by phenobarbital (with a review on the functions of this organelle in liver). J. Histochem. Cytochem., *14*:215, 1966.

188. Hutterer, F., et al.: Hepatocellular adaptation and injury: structural and biochemical changes following dieldrin and methyl butter yellow. Lab. Invest., *20*:455, 1969.

189. Gutteridge, J.M.C.: The effect of calcium on phospholipid peroxidation. Biochem. Biophys. Res. Commun., *74*:529, 1977.

190. Pavazzola, M.: Golgi complex induced by X537A in chief cells of rat parathyroid gland. Lab Invest., *35*:425, 1976.

191. Sturgess, J.M., et al.: The Golgi complex. II. The effects of aminonucleoside on ultrastructure and glycoprotein biosynthesis. Lab. Invest., *31*:6, 1974.

192. Nicod, I., Girard, J.P., and Cruchaud, A.: Membrane associated immunoglobulins of human lymphocytes in immunologic disorders. Clin. Exp. Immunol., *15*:365, 1973.

193. Porter, K.R.: Statement. *In* Research Frontiers in Aging and Cancer: International Symposium for the 1980's. Natl. Cancer Inst. Monogr., *60*, 1980.

194. Longley, W.: A new crystalline form of tropomyosin. J. Mol. Biol., *115*:381, 1977.

195. Yagi, N., et al.: Return of myosin heads to thick filaments after muscle contraction. Science, *197*:685, 1977.

196. Katz, A.M.: Congestive heart failure: role of altered myocardial cellular control. N. Engl. J. Med., *293*:1184, 1975.

197. Bray, D.: Membrane movements and microfilaments. Nature, *273*:265, 1978.

198. Marx, J.L.: Actin and myosin: role in nonmuscle cells. Science, *189*:34, 1975.
199. Squire, J.M.: Structure and force generation in muscle. Nature, *281*:99, 1979.
200. Buckley, I.K., and Raju, T.R.: Form and distribution of actin and myosin in non-muscle cells: A study using cultured chick embryo fibroblasts. J. Microsc., *107*:129, 1976.
201. Fawcett, D.W.: The Cell. Its Organelles and Inclusions. Philadelphia, W.B. Saunders, 1966.
202. Taylor, D.L., et al.: The contractile basis of amoeboid movement. I. The chemical control of motility in isolated cytoplasm. J. Cell Biol., *59*:378, 1973.
203. Lazarides, E.: Intermediate filaments as mechanical integrators of cellular space. Nature, *283*:249, 1980.
204. Gordon, W.E., Bushnell, A., and Burridge, K.: Characterization of the intermediate (10nm) filaments of cultured cells using an autoimmune rabbit antiserum. Cell, *13*:249, 1978.
205. Paulson, J.C., and McClure, W.O.: Microtubules and axoplasmic transport: inhibition of transport by podophyllotoxin: an interaction with microtubule protein. J. Cell Biol., *67*:461, 1975.
206. Erickson, H.P.: The structure and assembly of microtubules. Ann. NY Acad. Sci., *253*:60, 1975.
207. Bryan, J.: Biochemical properties of microtubules. Fed. Proc., *33*:152, 1974.
208. Tucker, J.B.: Shape and pattern specification during microtubule bundle assembly. Nature, *266*:22, 1977.
209. Wilson, L.: Pharmacological and biochemical properties of microtubule proteins. Fed. Proc., *33*:151, 1974.
210. Herzog, W., and Weber, K.: *In vitro* assembly of pure tubulin into microtubules in the absence of microtubule-associated proteins and glycerol. Proc. Natl. Acad. Sci. USA, *74*:1860, 1977.
211. Alicea, H.A., and Renaud, F.L.: Actin-tubulin homology revisited. Nature, *257*:601, 1975.
212. Albertini, D.F., and Anderson, E.: Microtubule and microfilament rearrangements during capping of concanavalin A receptors on cultured ovarian granulosa cells. J. Cell Biol., *73*:111, 1977.
213. Bhisey, A.N., and Freed, J.J.: Remnant motility of macrophages treated with cytochalasin B in the presence of colchicine. Exp. Cell Res., *95*:376, 1975.
214. Hirsimaki, Y., Arstila, A.U., and Trump, B.F.: Autophagocytosis: *in vitro* induction by microtubule poisons. Exp. Cell Res., *92*:11, 1975.
215. Skosey, J.L., et al.: Effect of cytochalasin B on response of human polymorphonuclear leukocytes to zymosan. J. Cell Biol., *57*:237, 1973.
216. Kowal, C.D.: Phagocytosis and microtubules. N. Engl. J. Med., *290*:1202, 1974.
217. Malaisse, W.J.: Insulin secretion: multifactorial regulation for a single process of release. Diabetologia, *9*:167, 1973.
218. Dales, S., Hsu, K.C., and Nogayama, A.: Fine structure and immunological labeling of the achromatic mitotic apparatus after disruption of cell membranes. J. Cell Biol., *59*:643, 1973.
219. Bajer, A.: Interaction of microtubules and the mechanisms of chromosomal movement (zipper hypothesis). 2. Dynamic architecture of the spindle. *In* Mechanisms and Control of Cell Division. Edited by T.L. Rost and E.M. Gifford. Stroudsburg, PA, Dower, Hutchinson and Ross, 1977.
220. Nicklas, R.B.: Mitosis. Adv. Cell Biol., *2*:225, 1971.
221. Roth, L.E., Wilson, H.J., and Chakraborty, J.: Anaphase structure in mitotic cells typified by spindle elongation. J. Ultrastruct. Res., *14*:460, 1966.
222. Cashon, J., et al.: Movement generated by interactions between the dense material at the ends of microtubules and non-actin-containing microfilaments in Sticholonche zanclea. J. Cell Biol., *72*:314, 1977.
223. Anderson, R.G.W.: The three-dimensional structure of the basal body from the Rhesus monkey oviduct. J. Cell Biol., *54*:246, 1972.
224. Miki-Noumura, T.: Studies on the de novo formation of centrioles: aster formation in the activated eggs of sea urchin. J. Cell Sci., *24*:203, 1977.
225. Dirksen, E.F.: Centriole morphogenesis in developing ciliated epithelium in the mouse oviduct. J. Cell Biol., *51*:286, 1971.

226. Anderson, R.G.: Isolation of ciliated or unciliated basal bodies from the rabbit oviduct. J. Cell Biol., 60:393, 1974.

227. Stearns, M.E., Connolly, J.A., and Brown, D.L.: Cytoplasmic microtubule organizing centers isolated from Polytomella agilis. Science, 191:188, 1976.

228. Fawcett, D.W., and Porter, K.R.: A study of the fine structure of ciliated epithelia. J. Morphol., 94:221, 1954.

229. Sale, W.S., and Satir, P.: Direction of active sliding of microtubules in tetrahymena cilia. Proc. Natl. Acad. Sci. USA, 74:2045, 1977.

230. Warner, F.D., and Satir, P.: The structural basis of ciliary bend formation. J. Cell Biol., 63:35, 1974.

231. Headington, J.T., McNamara, J.O., and Brownell, A.K.: Centronuclear myopathy: histochemistry and electron microscopy. Arch. Pathol., 99:16, 1975.

232. Lenard, H.G., Goebel, H.H., and Weigel, W.: Smooth muscle involvement in congenital myotonic dystrophy. Neuropaediatrie, 8:42, 1977.

233. Stracher, A., McGowan, E.B., and Shafiq, S.A.: Muscular dystrophy: inhibition of degeneration in vivo with protease inhibitors. Science, 200:50, 1978.

234. Hartman, K.S., and Standish, S.M.: Muscle regeneration in the dystrophic Syrian hamster tongue. Arch. Pathol., 98:126, 1974.

235. Ionescu, V., Radu, H., and Nicolescu, P.: Identification of Duchenne muscular dystrophy carriers. Electron microscopical investigation of skeletal muscle. Arch. Pathol., 99:436, 1975.

236. Eliasson, R., et al.: The immotile-cilia syndrome: a congenital ciliary abnormality as an etiologic factor in chronic airway infections and male sterility. N. Engl. J. Med., 297:1, 1977.

237. Afzelius, B.A.: Human syndrome caused by immotile cilia. Science, 193:317, 1976.

238. Golan, D.T., and Kursbaum, A.: Anti-heart autoantibodies in ischaemic heart disease patients. Clin. Exp. Immunol., 26:86, 1976.

239. Shiverick, K.T., Hamrell, B.B., and Alpert, N.R.: Structural and functional properties of myosin associated with the compensatory cardiac hypertrophy in the rabbit. J. Mol. Cell. Cardiol., 8:837, 1976.

240. Skosey, J.L., et al: Biochemical correlates of cardiac hypertrophy: V. Labeling of collagen, myosin, and nuclear DNA during experimental myocardial hypertrophy in the rat. Circ. Res., 31:145, 1972.

241. Anversa, P., Loud, A.V., and Vitali-Mazza, L.: Morphometry and autoradiography of early hypertrophic changes in the ventricular myocardium of adult rat: an electron microscopic study. Lab. Invest., 35:475, 1976.

242. Laks, M.M., et al.: Presence of widened and multiple intercalated discs in the hypertrophied canine heart. Circ. Res., 27:391, 1970.

243. Henry, W.L., et al.: Asymmetric septal hypertrophy. Ann. Intern. Med., 81:650, 1974.

244. Yang, V.V., Stearner, S.P., and Tyler, S.A.: Radiation-induced changes in the fine structure of the heart: comparison of fission neutrons and ^{60}Co gamma rays in the mouse. Radiat. Res., 67:344, 1976.

245. Rieder, C.L., and Bajer, A.S.: Effect of elevated temperatures on spindle microtubules and chromosome movements in cultured newt lung cells. Cytobios, 18:201, 1977.

246. Warner, E.D., Dahl, C., and Ewy, G.A.: Myocardial injury from transthoracic defibrillator countershock. Arch. Pathol., 99:55, 1975.

247. Fleet, J.F., Ferans, V.J., and Ruth, G.R.: Ultrastructural alterations in nutritional cardiomyopathy of selenium-vitamin E deficient swine. Lab. Invest., 37:188, 1977.

248. Vedder, E.B.: The pathology of beriberi. JAMA, 110:893, 1938.

249. Ebina, T., Staake, M., and Ishida, N.: Involvement of microtubules in cytopathic effects of animal viruses: Early proteins of adenovirus and herpesvirus inhibit formation of microtubular paracrystals in HeLa-23 cells. J. Gen. Virol., 38:535, 1978.

250. Damsky, C.H., et al.: Is there a role for actin in virus budding? J. Cell Biol., 75:593, 1977.

251. Iancu, T.C., Mason, W.H., and Neustein, H.B.: Ultrastructural abnormalities of liver cells in Reye's syndrome. Hum. Pathol., 8:421, 1977.

252. Marsh, J.C.: The effects of cancer chemotherapeutic agents on normal hematopoietic precursor cells. A review. Cancer Res., 36:1853, 1976.

253. Dousa, T.P., and Hie, Y.S.F.: Microtubule assembly in renal medullary slides: effects of vasopressin, vinblastine, and lithium. J. Lab. Clin. Med., *92*:252, 1978.
254. Gemmell, R.T., and Stacy, B.D.: Effects of colchicine on the ovine corpus luteum: role of microtubules in the secretion of progesterone. J. Reprod. Fert., *49*:115, 1977.
255. Wilson, L., and Bryan, J.: Biochemical and pharmacological properties of microtubules. *In* Advances in Cell and Molecular Biology. Vol. 3. Edited by E.J. DuPraw. New York, Academic Press, 1974.
256. Wen-Jen Wang, R., Rubhun, L.I., and Jupchan, S.M.: Antimitotic and antitubulin activity of the tumor inhibitor steganacin. Cancer Res., *37*:3071, 1977.
257. Rasmussen, S.A., and Davis, R.P.: Effect of microtubular antagonists on lymphocyte mitogenesis. Nature, *269*:249, 1977.
258. Andrews, P.M.: The effect of vinblastine-induced microtubule loss on kidney podocyte morphology. Am. J. Anat., *150*:53, 1977.
259. Goldman, I.D., et al.: The effect of microtubular inhibitors on transport of a-amino-isobutyric acid: inhibition of uphill transport without changes in transmembrane gradients of Na^+, K^+, or H^+. Biochim. Biophys. Acta, *467*:185, 1977.
260. Rathke, P.C., et al.: Rod-like elements from actin-containing microfilament bundles observed in cultured cells after treatment with cytochalasin A (CA). Exp. Cell Res., *105*:253, 1977.
261. Coster, H.G.L., and Zimmermann, U.: The mechanism of electrical breakdown in the membranes of *Valonia utricularis*. J. Membr. Biol., *22*:73, 1975.
262. Godman, G.C., et al.: Action of cytochalasin D on cells of established lines. III. Zeiosis and movements at the cell surface J. Cell Biol., *64*:677, 1975.
263. Price, H.M., et al.: New evidence for excessive accumulation of Z-band material in nemaline myopathy. Proc. Natl. Acad. Sci. USA, *54*:1398, 1965.
264. Yamaguchi, M., Robson, R.M., and Stromer, M.H.: Actin filaments form the backbone of nemaline myopathy rods. Nature, *271*:265, 1978.
265. Itabashi, H.H., and Kokman, E.: Chloroquine neuromyopathy. Arch. Pathol., *93*:209, 1972.
266. Jaenke, R.S.: An anthracycline antibiotic-induced cardiomyopathy in rabbits. Lab. Invest., *30*:292, 1974.
267. Poisner, A.M., and Bernstein, J.: A possible role of microtubules in catecholamine release from the adrenal medulla: effect of colchicine, vinca alkaloids and deuterium oxide. J. Pharmacol. Exp. Ther., *177*:102, 1971.
268. Petersen, P.: Alcoholic hyalin, microfilaments and microtubules in alcoholic hepatitis. Acta Pathol. Microbiol. Scand. [A.], *85*:384, 1977.
269. Tinberg, H.M., et al.: Mallory bodies. Isolation of hepatocellular hyalin and electrophoretic resolution of polypeptide components. Lab. Invest., *39*:483, 1978.
270. Sim, J.S., et al.: Mallory bodies compared with microfilament hyperplasia. Arch. Pathol. Lab. Med., *101*:401, 1977.
271. Fredericsson, B.: Proliferation of rabbit oviduct epithelium after estrogenic stimulation, with reference to the relationship between ciliated and secretory cells. Acta Morphol. Neerl. Scand., *2*:193, 1959.
272. Ichikawa, Y., Maeda, M., and Horiuchi, M.: Induction of differentiated functions which are reversibly suppressed by cytochalasin B. Exp. Cell Res., *90*:20, 1975.
273. Rydgren, L.: The role of cytoplasmic microtubules in polymorphonuclear leukocyte chemotaxis. Exp. Cell Res., *99*:207, 1976.
274. Skosey, J.L., et al.: Effect of cytochalasin B on response of human polymorphonuclear leukocytes to zymosan. J. Cell Biol., *57*:237, 1973.
275. Wills, E.J., et al.: Cytochalasin B fails to inhibit pinocytosis by macrophages. Nature [New Biol.], *240*:58, 1972.
276. Boxer, LA.: Correction of leukocyte function in Chediak-Higashi syndrome by ascorbate. N. Engl. J. Med., *295*:1041, 1976.
277. Gabbiani, G., et al.: Granulation tissue as a contractile organ. J. Exp. Med., *135*:719, 1972.
278. Chaponnier, C., Kohler, L., and Gabbiani, G.: Fixation of human anti-actin autoantibodies on skeletal muscle fibres. Clin. Exp. Immunol., *27*:278, 1977.

279. Husby, G., Pierce, P.E., and Williams, R.C., Jr.: Smooth muscle antibody in heroin addicts. Ann. Intern. Med., 83:801, 1975.
280. Nordal, H.J., and Vandvik, B.: Evidence of a local synthesis of smooth-muscle antibodies in the central nervous system in isolated cases of multiple sclerosis and chronic lymphocytic meningoencephalitis. Scand. J. Immunol., 6:327, 1977.
281. Kessel, R.G.: Annulate lamellae. J. Ultrastruct. Res. [Suppl.], 10:1, 1968.
282. Maul, G.G.: The presence of intranuclear annulate lamellae shortly after mitosis in human melanoma cells in vitro. J. Ultrastruct. Res., 31:375, 1970.
283. Krishan, A., Hsu, D., and Hutchins, P.S.: Hypertrophy of granular endoplasmic reticulum and annulate lamellae in Earle's L cells exposed to vinblastine sulfate. J. Cell Biol., 39:211, 1968.
284. Ghadially, F.N., and Parry, E.W.: Intranuclear annulate lamellae in Ehrlich ascites tumour cells. Virchows Arch. [Cell Pathol.], 15:131, 1974.
285. Schwartz, R.M., and Dayhoff, M.O.: Origins of prokaryotes, eukaryotes, mitochondria, and chloroplasts: a perspective is derived from protein and nucleic acid sequence data. Science, 199:395, 1978.
286. Myklebust, R., Dalen, H., and Saetersdal, T.S.: A comparative study in the transmission electron microscope and scanning electron microscope of intracellular structures in sheep heart muscle cells. J. Microsc., 105:57, 1975.
287. Friede, R.L., and Ho, K-C.: The relation of axonal transport of mitochondria with microtubules and other axoplasmic organelles. J. Physiol., 265:507, 1977.
288. Koukl, J.F., Vorbeck, M.L., and Martin, A.P.: Mitochondrial three-dimensional form in ascites tumor cells during changes in respiration. J. Ultrastruct. Res., 61:158, 1977.
289. Dewey, W.C., and Fuhr, M.A.: Quantification of mitochondria during the cell cycle of Chinese hamster cells. Exp. Cell Res., 99:23, 1976.
290. Clayton, D.A.: Replication of animal mitochondrial DNA. Cell, 28:693, 1982.
291. Albring, M., Griffith, J., and Attardi, G.: Association of a protein structure of probable membrane derivation with HeLa cell mitochondrial DNA near its origin of replication. Proc. Natl. Acad. Sci. USA, 74:1348, 1977.
292. Bogenhagen, D., and Clayton, D.A.: Mouse L cell mitochondrial DNA molecules are selected randomly for replication throughout the cell cycle. Cell, 11:719, 1977.
293. Schatz, G., and Mason, T.L.: The biosynthesis of mitochondrial proteins. Annu. Rev. Biochem., 43:51, 1974.
294. Davenport, L.W., Taylor, R.H., and Dubin, D.T.: Comparison of human and hamster mitochondrial transfer RNA. Physical properties and methylation status. Biochim. Biophys. Acta, 447:285, 1976.
295. Sacchi, A., et al.: Mitochondrial and cytoplasmic ribosomes from mammalian tissues: further characterization of ribosomal subunits and validity of buoyant-density methods for determination of the chemical composition and partial specific volume of ribonucleoprotein particles. Biochem. J., 168:245, 1977.
296. Schatz, G.: How mitochondria import proteins from the cytoplasm. FEBS Lett., 103:203, 1979.
297. Weber, N.E.: Ultrastructural studies of beef heart mitochondria. J. Cell Biol., 55:457, 1972.
298. Tzagoloff, A.: Genetic and translational capabilities of the mitochondrion. Bioscience, 27:18, 1977.
299. Poyton, R.O., and Kavanagh, J.: Regulation of mitochondrial protein synthesis by cytoplasmic proteins. Proc. Natl. Acad. Sci. USA, 73:3947, 1976.
300. Scarpa, A., et al.: On the problem of the release of mitochondrial calcium by cyclic AMP. J. Membr. Biol., 29:205, 1976.
301. Mitchell, P.: Keilin's respiratory chain concept and its chemiosmotic consequences. Science, 206:1148, 1979.
302. Berger, E.R.: Two morphologically different mitochondrial populations in the rat hepatocyte as determined by quantitative three-dimensional electron microscopy. J. Ultrastruct. Res., 45:303, 1973.
303. Acosta, D., and Wenzel, D.G.: A permeability test for the study of mitochondrial injury in in vitro cultured heart muscle and endothelioid cells. Histochem. J., 7:45, 1975.

304. King, M.E., and King, D.W.: Respiratory enzyme activity and mitochondrial morphology of L-cells under prolonged oxygen deprivation. Lab. Invest., 25:374, 1971.
305. Douglas, S.D., Zuckerman, S.H., and Ooka, M.P.: Effects of cholera exotoxin on the mitochondrial morphology of lymphoid cells and mononuclear phagocytes. Lab. Invest., 35:607, 1976.
306. Thureson-Klein, A.: Giant mitochondria in Schwann cells of bovine splenic nerve. Tissue Cell, 4:519, 1972.
307. DiMauro, S., et al.: Luft's disease. Further biochemical and ultrastructural studies of skeletal muscle in the second case. J. Neurol. Sci., 27:217, 1976.
308. Haydar, N.B., et al.: Severe hypermetabolism with primary abnormality of skeletal muscle mitochondria. Functional and therapeutic effects of chloramphenicol treatment. Ann. Intern. Med., 74:548, 1971.
309. Goldfischer, S., et al.: Peroxisomal and mitochondrial defects in the cerebro-hepato-renal syndrome. Science, 182:62, 1973.
310. Dodson, R.F., et al.: Mitochondrial abnormalities in progressive ophthalmoplegia.. Cytobios, 15:57, 1976.
311. Sternlieb, I., and Feldman, G.: Effects of anticopper therapy on hepatocellular mitochondria in patients with Wilson's disease. An ultrastructural and stereological study. Gastroenterol., 71:457, 1976.
312. Wollenberger, A., Kleitke, B., and Raabe, G.: Some metabolic characteristics of mitochondria from chronically overloaded, hypertrophied hearts. Exp. Mol. Pathol., 2:251, 1963.
313. Datta, B.N., and Silver, M.D.: Cardiomegaly in chronic anemia in rats. An experimental study including ultrastructural, histometric, and stereologic observations. Lab. Invest., 32:503, 1975.
314. Ashraf, M., and Bloor, C.M.: X-ray microanalysis of mitochondrial deposits in ischemic myocardium. Virchows Arch. [Cell Pathol.], 22:287, 1976.
315. Somlyo, A.P., et al.: Electron microscopy and electron probe analyis of mitochondrial cation accumulation in smooth muscle. J. Cell Biol., 61:723, 1974.
316. Araki, T.: Freezing injury in mitochondrial membranes. I. Susceptible components in the oxidation systems of frozen and thawed rabbit liver mitochondria. Cryobiology, 14:144, 1977.
317. Araki, T.: Freezing injury in mitochondrial membranes. II. Degradation of phospholipid in rabbit liver mitochondria during freezing and storage at low temperatures. Cryobiology, 14:151, 1977.
318. Araki, T.: Inactivation of mitochondrial 2-oxoglutarate dehydrogenase complex as a result of phospholipid degradation induced by freeze thawing. Biochim. Biophys. Acta, 496:532, 1977.
319. Aitar, A.S., and Alexander, K.C.: Radiation-induced alterations in mitochondrial protein synthesis in rat liver. Radiat. Res., 73:510, 1978.
320. French, S.W., and Todoroff, T.: Hepatic mitochondrial fragility and permeability. Effect of ethanol and choline deficiency. Arch. Pathol., 89:329, 1970.
321. Tandler, B., Erlandson, R.A., and Wynder, E.L.: Riboflavin and mouse hepatic cell structure and function: I. Ultrastructural alterations in simple deficiency. Am. J. Pathol., 52:69, 1962.
322. Suzuki, T., et al.: Giant mitochondria in the epithelial cells of the proximal convoluted tubules of diseased human kidneys. Lab. Invest., 33:578, 1975.
323. Cartwright, G.E., and Deiss, A.: Sideroblasts, siderocytes, and sideroblastic anemia. N. Engl. J. Med., 292:185, 1975.
324. Trump, B.F., and Jones, R.T. (Eds.): Diagnostic Electron Microscopy. Vol. 1. New York, John Wiley & Sons, 1978.
325. Lunger, P.D., and Clark, H.F.: An ultrastructural study and model of membrane-intramitochondrial virus relationships. Intervirology, 7:240, 1976.
326. Hanstein, W.G., and Hatefi, Y.: Characterization and localization of mitochondrial uncoupler binding sites with an uncoupler capable of photoaffinity labeling. J. Biol. Chem., 249:1356, 1974.
327. Hanstein, W.G., and Hatefi, Y.: Trinitrophenol: a membrane-impermeable uncoupler of oxidative phosphorylation. Proc. Natl. Acad. Sci. USA, 71:288, 1974.
328. Jaenke, R.S., and Fajardo, L.F. (Eds.): Adriamycin-induced myocardial lesions. Am. J. Surg. Pathol., 1:55, 1977.
329. Albring, M., Radsak, K., and Thoenes, W.: Giant mitochondria. II. Induction of matrix enriched megamitochondria in mouse liver pa-

renchymal cells by ethidium bromide. Virchows Arch. [Cell Pathol.], *14*:373, 1973.

330. Skinnider, L.F., and Ghadially, F.N.: Chloramphenicol-induced mitochondrial and ultrastructural changes in hemopoietic cells. Arch. Pathol. Lab. Med., *100*:601, 1976.

331. Blondin, G.A.: Isolation, properties, and structural features of divalent cation ionophores derived from beef heart mitochondria. Ann. NY Acad. Sci., *264*:98, 1975.

332. Sayegh, F.S., and Abousy, A.: Mitochondrial granule distribution in tooth germ cells. Anat. Rec., *189*:451, 1977.

333. Ida Chen, Y-D., and Hoch, F.L.: Mitochondrial inner membrane in hypothyroidism. Arch Biochem. Biophys., *172*:741, 1976.

334. Fujioka, T., Kai, O., and Yasuda, M.: Unusual mitochondrial ultrastructure in the pig adrenal cortex. Cell Tissue Res., *187*:129, 1978.

335. Ben-Yoseph, Y., Shapira, E., and Doniach, D.: Further purification of the mitochondrial inner membrane autoantigen reacting with primary biliary cirrhosis sera. Immunology, *26*:311, 1974.

336. deDuve, C., and Wattiaux, R.: Functions of lysosomes. Annu. Rev. Physiol., *28*:435, 1966.

337. Spitznagel, J.K., et al.: Character of azurophil and specific granules purified from human polymorphonuclear leukocytes. Lab. Invest., *30*:774, 1974.

338. Leffell, M.S., and Spitznagel, J.K.: Association of lactoferrin with lysozyme in granules of human polymorphonuclear leukocytes. Infect. Immun., *6*:761, 1972.

339. Hallman, M., Miyai, K., and Wagner, R.M.: Isolated lamellar bodies from rat lung. Lab. Invest., *35*:79, 1976.

340. Arstila, A.U., Nuuja, I.J.M., and Trump, B.F.: Studies on cellular autophagocytosis. Exp. Cell Res., *87*:249, 1974.

341. Veenhuis, M., van Dijken, J.P., Pilon, S.A., and Harder, W.: Development of crystalline peroxisomes in methanol-grown cells of the yeast Hansenula polymorpha and its relation to environmental conditions. Arch. Microbiol., *117*:153, 1978.

342. Herzog, V., and Sariush Fahimi, H.: Microbodies (peroxisomes) containing catalase in myocardium: morphological and biochemical evidence. Science, *185*:271, 1974.

343. Hruban, Z., et al.: Structure of hepatic microbodies in rats treated with acetylsalicylic acid, clofibrate, and dimethrin. Lab. Invest., *30*:64, 1974.

344. Breton-Gorium, J., and Guichard, J.: Fine structural and cytochemical identification of microperoxisomes in developing human erythrocytic cells. Am. J. Pathol., *79*:523, 1975.

345. Moody, D.E., and Reddy, J.K.: Morphometric analysis of the ultrastructural changes in rat liver induced by the peroxisome proliferator SaH 42–348. J. Cell Biol., *71*:768, 1976.

346. Staubli, W., et al.: The proliferative response of hepatic peroxisomes of neonatal rats to treatment with SU-13 r37 (nafenopin). J. Cell Biol., *74*:665, 1977.

347. Glaumann, H., et al.: Lysosomal degradation of cell organelles. II. Ultrastructural analysis of uptake and digestion of intravenously injected microsomes and ribosomes by Kupffer cells. Lab. Invest., *33*:252, 1975.

348. Moody, D.E., and Reddy, J.K.: The hepatic effects of hypolipidemic drugs (clofibrate, nafenopin, tibric acid, and Wy-14, 643) on hepatic peroxisomes and peroxisome-associated enzymes. Am. J. Pathol., *90*:435, 1978.

349. Hruban, Z., et al.: Effects of some hypocholesterolemic agents on hepatic ultrastructure and microbody enzymes. Lab. Invest., *30*:474, 1974.

350. Sandberg, L.B., Soskel, N.T., and Leslie, J.G.: Elastin structure, biosynthesis, and relation to disease states. N. Engl. J. Med., *304*:566, 1981.

351. Resibois, A., et al.: Lysosomes and storage diseases. Int. Rev. Exp. Pathol., *9*:93, 1970.

352. Kint, J.A., et al.: Mucopolysaccharidosis: secondarily induced abnormal distribution of lysosomal isoenzymes. Science, *181*:352, 1973.

353. Hers, H., and Van Hoof, R. (Eds.): Lysosomes and Storage Diseases. New York, Academic Press, 1973.

354. Hundgen, M.: Potential and limitations of enzyme cytochemistry: studies of the intracellular digestive apparatus of cells in tissue culture. Int. Rev. Cytol., *48*:281, 1977.

355. Sbarra, A.J., et al.: Biochemical, functional, and structural aspects of phagocytosis. Int. Rev. Exp. Pathol., *16*:249, 1976.

356. Glaumann, H., et al.: Lysosomal degradation of cell organelles. I. Ultrastructural analysis of uptake and digestion of intravenously injected mitochondria by Kupffer cells. Lab. Invest., *33*:239, 1975.

357. Brody, H.: The nervous system and aging. Adv. Pathobiol., *7*:200, 1980.

358. Papadimitriou, J.M., and Wee, S.H.: Selective release of lysosomal enzymes from cell populations containing multinucleate giant cells. J. Pathol., *120*:193, 1976.

359. Baron, D.A., and Esterly, J.R.: Histochemical demonstration of lysosomal hydrolase activity in endometrial mononuclear cells. II. Abnormal endometrium. Am. J. Obstet. Gynecol., *123*:797, 1975.

360. Cajander, S., and Bjersing, L.: Further studies of the surface epithelium covering preovulatory rabbit follicles with special reference to lysosomal alterations. Cell Tissue Res., *169*:129, 1976.

361. Grillo, H.C., and Gross, J.: Collagenolytic activity during mammalian wound repair. Dev. Biol., *15*:300, 1967.

362. Van Herle, A.J., Vassart, G., and Dumont, J.E.: Control of thyroglobulin synthesis and secretion. N. Engl. J. Med., *301*:239, 307, 1979.

363. Kolodny, E.H.: Lysosomal storage diseases. N. Engl. J. Med., *294*:1217, 1976.

364. Kint, J.A., et al.: Mucopolysaccharidosis: secondarily induced abnormal distribution of lysosomal isoenzymes. Science, *181*:352, 1973.

365. Schneck, L., Amsterdam, D., and Volk, B.W.: Antenatal diagnosis and therapeutic trends in sphingolipidoses. JAMA, *228*:615, 1974.

366. Weissmann, G., and Rita, G.A.: Molecular basis of gouty inflammation interaction of monosodium urate crystals with lysosomes and liposomes. Nature [New Biol.], *240*:167, 1972.

367. Hoffstein, S., et al.: Cytochemical localization of lysosomal enzyme activity in normal and ischemic dog myocardium. Am. J. Pathol., *79*:193, 1975.

368. Welscher, H.D., and Cruchaud, A.: The influence of various particles and 3', 5' cyclic adenosine monophosphate on release of lysosomal enzymes by mouse macrophages. J. Reticuloendothel. Soc., *20*:405, 1976.

369. Bhuyan, U.N., and Ramalingaswami, V.: Systemic macrophage mobilization and granulomatous response to BCG in the protein-deficient rabbit. Am. J. Pathol., *76*:313, 1974.

370. Nehemiah, J.I., and Novikoff, A.B.: Unusual lysosomes in hamster hepatocytes. Exp. Mol. Pathol., *21*:398, 1974.

371. Dingle, J.T., and Lucy, J.A.: Vitamin A, carotenoids and cell function. Biol. Rev., *40*:422, 1965.

372. Levy, E., and Reubner, B.H.: Endotoxin effect. Am. J. Pathol., *52*:485, 1968.

373. Job, C.K.: Lysosomal activity of macrophages in leprosy. Arch. Pathol., *90*:547, 1970.

374. Chang, K., and Dwyer, D.M.: Multiplication of a human parasite (Leishmania donovani) in phagolysosomes of hamster macrophages *in vitro*. Science, *193*:678, 1976.

375. Lou, T.Y., and Teplitz, C.: Malakoplakia: Pathogenesis and ultrastructural morphogenesis. Hum. Pathol., *5*:191, 1974.

376. Curnutte, J.T., Whitten, D.M., and Babior, B.M.: Defective superoxide production by granulocytes from patients with chronic granulomatous disease. N. Engl. J. Med., *290*:593, 1974.

377. Curnutte, J.T., Kipnes, R.S., and Babior, B.M.: Defect in pyridine nucleotide dependent superoxide production by a particulate fraction from the granulocytes of patients with chronic granulomatous disease. N. Engl. J. Med., *293*:628, 1975.

378. Gold, S.B., et al.: Abnormal kinetics of degranulation in chronic granulomatous disease. N. Engl. J. Med., *291*:332, 1974.

379. Abraham, R., and Ringwood, N.: Effects of lysosomotropic agents on the hepatic uptake and storage of degraded carrageenan: disparity in response of hepatocytes and Kupffer cells. Exp. Mol. Pathol., *26*:13, 1977.

380. Orfei, E., et al.: Effect of iron loading on the hepatic injury induced by ethionine. Am. J. Pathol., *52*;547, 1968.

381. Fowler, B.A., et al.: Mercury uptake by renal lysosomes of rats ingesting methyl hydroxide. Ultrastructural observations and energy dispersive x-ray analysis. Arch. Pathol., *98*:297, 1974.

382. Shelburne, J.D., Arstila, A.U., and Trump, B.F.: Studies on cellular autophagocytosis cyclic AMP- and dibutyryl cyclic AMP-stimulated autophagy in rat liver. Am. J. Pathol., 72:521, 1973.

383. Rinehart, J.J., et al.: Effects of corticosteroid therapy on human monocyte function. N. Engl. J. Med., 292:236, 1975.

384. Ignarro, L.J.: Release of neutral protease and B-glucuronidase from human neutrophils in the presence of cartilage treated with various immunologic reactants. J. Immunol., 113:298, 301, 1974.

385. Kelley, W.N.: Current therapy of gout and hyperuricemia. Hosp. Pract. 11:69, 1976.

386. Weissmann, G., and Dukor, P.: The role of lysosomes in immune responses. Adv. Immunol., 12:283, 1970.

387. Becker, E.L., et al.: The ability of chemotactic factors to induce lysosomal enzyme release. II. The mechanism of release. J. Immunol., 112:2055, 1974.

388. Zurier, R.B.: Prostaglandins. In Mediators of Inflammation. Edited by G. Weissmann. New York, Plenum Press, 1974, pg. 163.

389. Revel, J.P., Napolitano, L., and Fawcett, D.W.: Identification of glycogen in electron micrographs of thin tissue sections. J. Biophys. Biochem. Cytol., 8:575, 1960.

390. Biava, C., Grossman, A., and West, M.: Ultrastructural observations on renal glycogen in normal and pathologic human kidneys. Lab. Invest., 15:330, 1966.

391. Ehrlich, P.: Ueber das Vorkommen Von Glykogen im diabetischen und in normalen Organismus. Arch. Klin. Med., 6:33, 1883.

392. Lampert, P.W.: A comparative electron microscopic study of reactive, degenerating, regenerating and dystrophic axons. J. Neuropathol. Exp. Neurol., 26:345, 1967.

393. Popper, H.: Mechanism of cholestasis. In Liver and Bile. Edited by L. Bianchi, W. Gerok, and K. Sickinger. Lancaster, England, MTP Press, 1977.

394. Eriksson, S., and Larsson, C.: Purification and partial characterization of PAS-positive inclusion bodies from the liver in alpha$_1$-antitrypsin deficiency. N. Engl. J. Med., 292:176, 1975.

395. Klion, F.M., and Schaffner, F.: The ultrastructure of acidophilic "Councilman-like" bodies in the liver. Am. J. Pathol., 48:755, 1966.

396. De Duve, C., and Wattiaux, R.: Functions of lysosomes. Annu. Rev. Physiol., 28:435, 1966.

397. Ma, M.H.: Ultrastructural pathologic findings of the human hepatocyte. Arch. Pathol., 94:554, 1972.

398. Phillips, M.J.: Mallory bodies and the liver. Lab Invest., 47:311, 1982.

399. Popper, H., et al.: Cytoplasmic copper and its toxic effects: studies in Indian childhood cirrhosis. Lancet, 1:1205, 1979.

400. Keeley, A.F., Iseri, O.A., and Gottlieb, L.S.: Ultrastructure of hyaline cytoplasmic inclusions in a human hepatoma: relationship to Mallory's alcoholic hyalin. Gastroenterology, 62:280, 1972.

401. Franke, W.W., et al.: Ultrastructural, biochemical, and immunologic characterization of Mallory bodies in livers of griseofulvin-treated mice. Fimbriated rods of filaments containing prekeratin-like polypeptides. Lab. Invest., 40:207, 1979.

402. Clyne, D.H., et al.: Renal effects of intraperitoneal kappa chain injection. Lab Invest., 31:131, 1974.

403. Waldrop, F.S., et al.: Fluorescence microscopy of amyloid. Arch. Pathol., 95:37, 1973.

404. Fisher, E.R., and Horwat, B.: Experimental production of so-called spironolactone bodies. Arch. Pathol., 91:471, 1971.

405. Glenner, G.G.: Amyloid deposits and amyloidosis. The B-fibrilloses. N. Engl. J. Med., 302:1283, 1980.

406. Schultz, H.: The Submicroscopic Anatomy and Pathology of the Lung. Berlin, Springer, 1959.

407. Hoyumpa, A.M., et al.: Fatty liver: biochemical and clinical considerations. Am. J. Dig. Dis., 20:1142, 1975.

408. Marx, J.L.: Liposomes: research applications grow. Science, 199:1056, 1978.

409. Ghadially, F.N.: Ultrastructural Pathology of the Cell: A Text and Atlas of Physiological and Pathological Alterations in Cell Fine Structure. London, Butterworths, 1975.

410. Schulz, H., and Hahnel, E.: Die Ultrastruktur des Glykogens in Lochkernen der menschlichen Leberepithelzellen bei Diabetes Mellitus. Virchows Arch. [Cell Pathol.], 3:282, 1969.

411. Bagnara, J.T., et al.: Common origin of pigment cells. Science, *203*:410, 1979.
412. Pearse, A.G.E.: Histochemistry: Theoretical and Applied. 3rd Ed. Edinburgh, Churchill Livingstone, 1972.
413. Barden, H.: Interference filter brain microfluorometry of neuromelanin and lipofuscin in human. J. Neuropathol., *39*:598, 1980.
414. Oliver, C., et al.: Age-related accumulation of ceroid-like pigment in mice with Chediak-Higashi syndrome. Am. J. Pathol., *84*:225, 1976.
415. Kutty, M.K., et al.: Ochronitic arthropathy: a comparative study of light microscopic and ultrastructural features. Arch. Pathol., *96*:100, 1973.
416. Kutty, M.K., et al.: Ochronitic arthropathy: an electron microscopical study with a view on pathogenesis. Arch. Pathol., *98*:5557, 1974.
417. Belcher, R.W., Czarnetzki, B.M., and Campbell, P.G.: Ultrastructure of inclusions in peripheral blood mononuclear cells in sarcoidosis. Am. J. Pathol., *78*:461, 1975.
418. Brody, A.R., and Craighead, J.E.: Cytoplasmic inclusions in pulmonary macrophages of cigarette smokers. Lab. Invest., *32*:125, 1975.
419. Cartwright, G.E., et al.: Hereditary hemochromatosis: phenotypic expression of the disease. N. Engl. J. Med., *301*:175, 1979.
420. Erickson, J.L.E.: Transport and digestion of hemoglobin in the proximal tubules. II. Electron microscopy. Lab. Invest., *14*:16, 1965.
421. Arbus, G.S., and Sniderman, S.: Oxalosis with peripheral gangrene. Arch. Pathol., *97*:107, 1974.
422. Takeuchi, A., Formal, S.B., and Sprinz, H.: Experimental acute colitis in the Rhesus monkey following peroral infection with Shigella flexneri. Am. J. Pathol., *52*:503, 1968.
423. Mansbach, C.M. II, et al.: Lymph-node bacilliform bodies resembling those of Whipple's disease in a patient without intestinal involvement. Ann. Intern. Med., *89*:64, 1978.
424. Drutz, D.J.: Urban coccidioidomycosis and histoplasmosis. N. Engl. J. Med., *301*:381, 1979.
425. Godfrey, O.G.: Identification of economically important parasites. Nature, *273*:600, 1978.
426. Aikawa, M., Miller, L.H., and Rabbege, J.: Caveola-vesicle complexes in the plasmalemma of erythrocytes infected by *Plasmodium vivax* and *P. cynomolgi*. Unique structure related to Schuffner's dots. Am. J. Pathol., *79*:285, 1975.
427. Walker, D.H., and Cain, B.G.: The rickettsial plaque. Evidence for direct cytopathic effect of *Rickettsia rickettsii*. Lab. Invest., *43*:388, 1980.
428. Schatu, J.: Chlamydial infections. N. Engl. J. Med., *298*:540, 1978.
429. Baringer, J.R., and Swoveland, P.: Persistent herpes simplex virus infection in rabbit trigeminal ganglia. Lab. Invest., *30*:230, 1974.
430. Morgan, C., et al.: A correlative study by electron and light microscopy of the development of type 5 adenovirus. I. Electron microscopy. J. Exp. Med., *112*:373, 1960.
431. Morgan, C., et al.: The application of ferritin-conjugated antibody to electron microscopic studies of influenza virus in infected cells. II. The interior of the cells. J. Exp. Med., *114*:833, 1961.
432. Horne, R.W., and Nagington, J.: Electron microscope studies of the development and structure of poliomyelitis virus. J. Mol. Biol., *1*:333, 1959.
433. Nowoslawski, A., et al.: Tissue localization of Australia antigen immune complexes in acute and chronic hepatitis and liver cirrhosis. Am. J. Pathol., *68*:31, 1972.
434. Ranchod, M., and Kahn, L.B.: Malacoplakia of the gastrointestinal tract. Arch. Pathol., *94*:90, 1972.
435. Abdou, N.I., et al.: Malakoplakia: evidence for monocyte lysosomal abnormality correctable by cholinergic agonist *in vitro* and *in vivo*. N. Engl. J. Med., *297*:1413, 1977.
436. Lewin, K.J., et al.: Malacoplakia: An electron-microscopic study: demonstration of bacilliform organisms in malacoplakic macrophages. Gastroenterology, *66*:28, 1974.
437. Thorning, D., and Vracko, R.: Malakoplakia: defect in digestion of phagocytized material due to impaired vacuolar acidification? Arch. Pathol., *99*:456, 1975.
438. Editorial: Malfunctioning microtubules. Lancet, *1*:697, 1978.
438a. von Winiwarter, H.: Contribution à l'étude de l'ovaire humain. (I.

Appareil nerveux et phéochrome. II. Tissu musculaire. III. Cordons médullaires et corticaux). Arch. Biol. (Paris), *25*:683, 1910.

439. Merkow, L.P., et al.: Ultrastructure of an interstitial (hilar) cell tumor of the ovary. Obstet. Gynecol., *37*:845, 1971.

440. Sohval, A.R., et al.: Ultrastructure of crystalloids in spermatogonia and Sertoli cells of normal human testis. J. Ultrastruct. Res., *34*:83, 1971.

441. Nochomoritz, L.E., and Kahn, L.B.: Tyrosine crystals in pleomorphic adenoma of the salivary gland. Arch. Pathol., *97*:141, 1974.

442. Pritzker, K.P.H., et al.: The ultrastructure of urate crystals in gout. J. Rheumatol., *5*:7, 1978.

443. Biempica, L., et al.: Hepatic porphyrias. Cytochemical and ultrastructural studies of liver in acute intermittent porphyria and porphyria cutanea tarda. Arch. Pathol., *98*:336, 1974.

444. Roy, S., and Wolman, L.: Electron microscopic observations on the virus particles in *Herpes simplex* encephalitis. J. Clin. Pathol., *22*:51, 1969.

445. Koss, M.N., Pirani, C.L., and Osserman, E.F.: Experimental Bence-Jones case nephropathy. Lab. Invest., *34*:579, 1976.

Appendix

A GUIDE TO A LECTURE SCHEDULE

We have used the style and approach of this book to formulate a series of over 20 lectures delivered in a first-year general pathology course at the College of Physicians & Surgeons of Columbia University and feel that a similar experience might be afforded students in other university, graduate, and undergraduate programs. The 5 major text chapters can be divided into 20 or more lectures. The suggested lecture order is indicated in the following table of contents, in parentheses after section headings. Lecture 1 may be supplemented with material from Chapter 6 in the form of additional lectures, which are also noted in this table of contents.

TABLE OF CONTENTS

Index

Cell adhesion, 310–311, 395
Cell agglutination, 310
Cell cycle, 11, 71
  mitosis in, 11, 71, 414, 426, 461
  S phase in, 129, 330, 331
Cell death, 16–17, 348
Cell differentiation, 2, 3
Cell division, 71
Cell fusion, 112
Cell hybridization, 112
Cell injury, 15–16, 391
Cell loss, 355
Cell transport, 5. See also *Plasma membrane*
Cellulitis, 79
Central nervous system (CNS), 3, 198, 296
  in aging, 372–373
Centriole(s), 417, 454, 461
Centromere(s), 414
Cerebral cortex, 356, 372
Cerebral hemorrhage, 347
Cerebrohepatorenal syndrome, 480–481
Ceroid, 128, 358, 509. See also *Lipofuscin*
Cervix, carcinoma of, 175, 203, 274, 279, 290, 293, 320, 327, 329, 376
  intraepithelial neoplasia of, 323
Chalone(s), 55, 70
Chediak-Higashi syndrome, 89, 282, 448, 470, 510
Chemical agents of injury, 5, 193–214.
  See also specific agents
Chemical-induced antigen(s), 29, 317
Chemiosmotic theory of oxidative phosphorylation, 478
Chemotactic factor, 225, 500
  of anaphylaxis, 33
Chemotaxis, 33, 54, 57, 59–60, 353, 470
Chemotherapeutic agent(s), 98, 204. See also specific agents
Childhood, 346
Chlamydia, 162, 184, 513
Chloramphenicol, 200, 451, 480, 484
Chloride, 141, 143
Chloroform, 201
Chloroquine, 468, 498, 499
Cholecystokinin, 138
Cholelithiasis, 125, 371
Cholera, 400
Cholestasis, 506
Cholesterol, 6
  deficiency of, 449, 482
Cholinergic cell(s), 356
Chondroma, 274
Chondrosarcoma, 274
Choriocarcinoma, 314, 330
Christmas disease, 93
Christmas-tree configuration of RNA, 421
Chromatid, 357, 414
Chromatin, 297, 307, 414, 416, 426
  ischemia and, 141
  margination of, 13
Chromium, 131, 295
Chromomeric band, 416
Chromonema, 416
Chromosome(s), 3, 13–14, 307, 414
  aneuploid, 13, 306
  banding of, 112, 416
  banding patterns of, 357, 416
  eukaryotic, 417
  hyperdiploid, 14, 366

hyperplasia of, 13
karyotypes of, 307
mutations of, 427
octaploid, 371
polyploid, 371
tetraploid, 371
Chromosome abnormality(ies), 427, 431.
  See also *Deoxyribonucleic acid (DNA); Genetic disease(s)*
  additions as, 427
  breaks as, 149, 304, 427, 431, 432
  bridges as, 427
  damage in, 13
  deletions as, 307, 427
  dicentric chromosomes as, 430, 431
  exchanges as, 427, 431
  gaps as, 149, 431
  nondisjunctions as, 13, 115
  rings as, 427, 431
  translocations as, 13, 115, 307, 308, 427
Chylomicron(s), 127, 207
Cigarette smoking, 150, 196, 274, 298, 366, 510
Cilia, 454, 463
Cirrhosis, 78, 127, 190, 347, 370, 384, 506. See also *Alcohol toxicity; Hepatitis*
  inactive, 180
  Indian childhood, 506
  macronodular, 180
  primary biliary, 228, 235, 485
Citrovorum rescue, 331, 433
Clofibrate, 499
Clones, forbidden, 353
Clostridia, 97
Clotting factor(s), 65. See also *Coagulation*
Cloudy swelling, 8, 446, 450, 502
Coagulase, 167
Coagulation, 63–68, 353. See also specific disorders
  clot formation in, 68
  clotting factors in, 65
  diseases of, 91–93
  disseminated intravascular, 97, 144, 167
  drugs and, 98–99
  embolus and, 65
  extrinsic pathway of, 67
  fibrin and, 64, 65
  fibrinogen and, 65–67, 218
  fibrinolysis and, 65, 167
  fibrinopeptides and, 65
  Hageman factor in, 58, 68, 91
  hemostasis and, 63–68
  intrinsic pathway of, 67
  platelets in, 67–68
  prothrombin and, 130
  thrombosis and, 64, 68
Coagulative necrosis, 17
Coal tar, 198
Coated pit(s), 401, 407
Coated vesicle(s), 440
Cobalt, 10, 131
Cocci. See *Bacteria*
Coccidioidomycosis, 81, 176
Codon, 421
Coenzyme(s), 478
Colcemid, 466
Colchicine, 13, 99, 204, 411, 433, 459, 466, 467, 498, 499
Cold injury, 145

Colicin(s), 410
Collagen, 2, 16, 74–78, 128, 354, 357, 365, 371, 377, 379, 380, 450
  collagenase and, 78, 167, 490
  cross linking and, 78, 380, 382
  deficiencies of, 78, 93
  degradation of, 78
  isotypes of, 77, 209
  production of, 76
Collagen vascular disease(s), 434. See also specific diseases
Colon, absorption and, 370
  amyloid in, 370
  angiodysplasia of, 370
  carcinoma of, 274, 277, 284, 289, 293, 308, 329, 347, 384
  bulk and, 370
  constipation and, 370, 382
  diarrhea and, 370, 410
  diverticula of, 370
  hemorrhoids and, 364, 370
  polyp of, 284, 359, 370
  prolapse of, 362, 370
  rectocele and, 370
  secretion of, 370
Complement, 3, 20, 26–27, 32–35, 54, 57, 60, 218, 238, 413, 435, 500
  alternate pathway of, 32
  biologic activities of, 33
  classic pathway of, 33–35
  components of, 33
  genetic control of synthesis of, 33
  osmotic lysis of, 34–35, 413
  properdin and, 32
Complement receptors. See *Lymphocyte(s), markers of*
Conconavalin A, 47, 204, 310, 459, 467, 498
Condensing vacuole(s), 435, 439, 440
Condyloma(s), 293
Congenic mice, 350, 353
Congenital malformation(s). See *Genetic disease(s)*
Congenital neutropenia, 56
Congestive heart failure, 160
Connective tissue, fascia as, 359, 362. See also *Collagen*
  in aging, 356
  ligaments as, 359, 362
  tendons as, 359, 362
Constipation, 370, 382
Contraceptive(s), 302
Copper, 131, 380, 496, 510, 512
Corynebacterium diphtheriae, 168–170, 400, 451
  effect of on ribosomes, 168–169, 451
  lysogenization of, 168–169
  morphology of, 169–170
  pseudomembrane in, 168
  toxin of, 168–169, 400, 451
Coronary artery disease. See *Myocardial infarct*
Corpora amylacea, 362
Corticosteroid(s), 128, 301, 507
  cortisone as, 203, 330, 384, 453, 499
  glucocorticoids as, 374, 485
  in aging, 357, 374
  in inflammation and repair, 99–100
Councilman-like body(ies), 188, 450
Coxsackie virus, 176, 184, 432
Creatine phosphokinase (CPK), 409
Creutzfeldt-Jakob disease, 383

type II, 407
Liposarcoma, 276
Liposome(s), 508
Liquefaction necrosis, 17
Lithium, 412, 467
Liver, 3, 12, 17, 36, 194, 199, 285
  acute yellow atrophy of, 189
  adenoma of, 203, 301, 302
  albumin-globulin ratio in, 371
  alcohol and. See *Cirrhosis; Hepatitis*
  amyloid in, 371
  balloon cells in, 188
  carcinoma of, 203, 279, 285, 290, 293,
    296–297, 300, 307, 314, 506
  cells of, 72
  cirrhosis of. See *Cirrhosis*
  hypertension and, 370
  in aging, 361, 371
  in hemochromatosis, 132
  necrosis of, 189
  peliosis hepatis in, 203
  viral hepatitis in. See *Hepatitis, viral*
Locus ceruleus, 356
Longevity, 353
Low-density lipoprotein(s) (LDL), 71,
    154–155, 401, 407, 496
Lucké virus, 125, 290
Luft's syndrome, 480
Lung, 12
  aging changes in, 366
  alveolar ducts of, 365
  bronchioles of, 359, 366
  carcinoma of, 274, 277, 279, 285, 289,
    298, 314, 347, 366, 384
  cells of, 72
  fibrosis of, 16, 78, 198
  pneumonia in, 72, 383
  residual volume of, 366
  type II pneumocytes of, 487, 508
  vital capacity of, 366
Lupus erythematosus, systemic. See
  Systemic lupus erythematosus
Luteinizing hormone, 400
Lymph node(s), 17, 37, 204, 285
  atrophy of, 364
  fibrosis of, 364
  metastasis in, 327
Lymphatic(s), 2, 3, 17, 56, 325
Lymphocyte(s), 39–45, 59, 60, 137, 165,
    276, 327, 356, 412
  B, 20, 37–39, 48–50, 52–53, 80, 214,
    217, 412
  cortisone and, 39
  cytotoxic, 21
  deficiencies of, 84–87
  distribution of, 39
  identification of, 41
  markers of, 41–45
    B cell antigens as, 44
    complement receptors as, 43, 46
    Epstein-Barr virus receptors as, 43,
      292
    erythrocyte rosettes as, 44–46
    esterase as, 46
    Fc receptors as, 43, 46
    Ia antigens as, 23, 25, 39, 46
    surface immunoglobulin as, 43, 46
  memory cells of, 49, 224
  mitogens of, 47
  natural killer (NK) cells of, 46, 225,
    302, 327

null cells of, 42, 136, 218, 225, 302,
    412
  recirculation of, 41
  sensitized, 328
  T, 20, 37, 48, 63, 80–82, 136, 214,
    217, 224–225, 353, 360, 378, 412
    helper, 21, 40, 48, 224, 225
    suppressor, 21, 40, 225, 356, 378
    cytotoxic, 21, 23, 26, 136, 214, 218,
      225, 302, 327
Lymphocytic meningoencephalitis, 471
Lymphocytosis, 56
Lymphogranuloma venereum, 184
Lymphokine(s), 40, 63, 82, 328, 435,
    450. See also specific factors
Lymphoma(s), 133, 275, 276, 277, 282,
    287, 289–291, 304–305, 504. See
    also *Burkitt's lymphoma; Hodgkin's
    disease*
Lymphoreticular cell(s), 3
Lymphotoxin(s), 40, 82, 435
Lysosome(s), 7–8, 312, 357, 384, 408,
    440, 470, 485–501
  agents of injury to, 493
  autophagosome as, 7–8, 16, 357, 379,
    440, 488
  enzymes of, 8, 62–63, 194–195, 220
  lipolysosomes as, 497
  multivesicular body as, 487–488
  peroxisome(s) and, 488, 499
  phagolysosome as, 63, 487
  phagosome as, 63, 459, 487
  primary, 62, 487
  residual body (telolysosome), 128, 440,
    488, 499
  secondary, 487, 488
    autophagic vacuoles as, 7, 8, 488
  siderosomes as, 510
  storage diseases of, 111, 347, 492
  tertiary, 487
Lysozyme, 314, 487
Lysyl oxidase, 380

M line, 456
Macroglobulinemia, 8, 357, 361
Macrophage(s), 17, 20, 42, 48, 60,
    136–137, 165, 217, 327. See also
    Phagocytosis
  in aging, 357
  cytotoxic, 302
  Kupffer cells and, 286, 511
  in antigen processing, 48
  in antibody synthesis, 48–49
  in repair, 74, 78, 82
  neoplasm of, 276
Macrophage arming factor (MAF), 46,
    225
Macrophage cytotoxic factor, 225
Macrophage inhibition factor (MIF), 40,
    136, 214, 224
Macula adherens (desmosome), 405, 413,
    469
Magnesium, 10, 143, 156
Major histocompatibility complex, 48,
    304, 353
  H-2, 23
  HLA, 24–26
  Ia genes in, 23
  immune response in, 26
Malabsorption, 125, 133–135, 139, 384
Malacoplakia, 514

Malaria, 178–181, 292, 400, 513
  clinical features of, 181
  membrane alterations in, 180
  multiplication in, 180–181
  plasmodial life cycle in, 179
  red blood cells and, 180, 509
Malate, 478
Mallory body(ies), 208, 469, 506. See also
  Hepatitis
Mannose, 440
Marantic endocarditis, 365
Marfan's syndrome, 93, 507
Marek's disease virus, 175, 290
Mason Pfizer monkey virus, 288
Mast cell(s), 20, 38, 217, 500
Measles virus, 98, 140, 172, 176, 409,
    432, 466, 513
Mechanical injury(ies), 143, 150
Megamitochondria, 16, 211, 312, 479,
    482–483, 508. See also
    Mitochondria
Melanin, 14, 509
Melanin-stimulating hormone, 314
Melanocyte(s), 379
Melanoma(s), 321, 509
Melanosis coli, 499
Meningioma(s), 307
Meningococcus, 512
Menopause, 351, 376
Menstruation, 492
Mental disease, 347
Mercaptoethylamine (MEA) 2-
    hydrochloride, 382
Mercury, 198, 412, 510, 512
Meromyosin, 456
Mesothelioma(s), 197, 274, 279
Metabolic alkalosis, 144
Metabolism, 7, 9–10, 194–195
Metal(s), 131–132
  deficiency of, 95, 131–132. See also
    specific metal
Metaphase, 71, 461
Metaplasia, 16, 69, 275, 355, 358, 366,
    376
  squamous, 366, 372
Metazoa, 162, 182. See also specific
    agents
Methotrexate, 330, 331, 433
Methylcholanthrene, 196, 294, 300, 318
Michaelis-Gutmann body(ies), 514
Microbody(ies), 488, 499
Microcalcification(s), 512
Microfilament(s), 6, 16, 211, 357, 379,
    411, 454, 456
Micronucleus(i), 433
Microsomal fraction, 439
Microtubule(s), 16, 210–211, 391, 411,
    454, 458, 498
Microvillus(i), 141, 310, 395, 404, 412,
    457
Middle age, 347
Migration inhibition factor, 63
Minigene(s), 53, 421
Mintz experiment(s), 4
Mitochondria, 7, 9–10, 156, 157, 391,
    472
  agents of injury to, 480
  calcium in, 143, 211
  configurations of, 9, 482
  contraction of, 9, 478
  cristae in, 357, 473, 474
  crystals in, 312